ESSENTIALS OF
PEDIATRICS

<u>Test - Wed-</u> Growth + Development — 3 years
Disease conditions

<u>Fri</u> - Celiac, Cystic Fibrosis, Cerebral Palsy

<u>Mon</u> - Convulsions, Burns 4 + 5 year old

<u>Wed</u> - Chest (lungs heart) Croup , Bronchitis
Pneumonia

<u>Fri</u> - Kidney Disorders - Heart Conditions

~~Mon~~ - Rheumatic Heart Disease, Diabetic
<u>Fri</u> Blood Dyscrasias , Reumatic Fever,
Impetigo — Orthopedic + Neuralogical, Tu.

<u>Fri</u> - Test — 4 + 5 , 6 - 9 + above

Last Week - Communicable diseases

2nd test

Play room - <u>Tues</u>

Essentials of
PEDIATRICS

PHILIP C. JEANS, A.B., M.D.
Late Professor of Pediatrics,
State University of Iowa, Iowa City

F. HOWELL WRIGHT, B.S., M.D.
Professor of Pediatrics, University of Chicago

FLORENCE G. BLAKE, R.N., M.A.
Associate Professor of Nursing Education
(Nursing Care of Children),
University of Chicago

SIXTH EDITION

115 Illustrations, Including 7 Color Plates

J. B. LIPPINCOTT COMPANY
Philadelphia · Montreal

Preface to the Sixth Edition

The introductory chapter of this revision describes the widening scope of pediatric nursing. Like other branches of medicine, pediatrics is advancing along several fronts. One of these is the scientific study of disease which is continually producing new insights into the normal and the abnormal physiology of the body and is responsible for the exciting and dramatic improvements in methods of diagnosis, treatment and prevention. It is natural for the nurse to turn toward these new technics with curiosity and a desire to understand. But their highly technical nature often prevents an elementary text from offering more than general explanations. Further pursuit of details through the suggested reading must be left to the initiative of the individual reader.

More germane to the nurse's function are the efforts which are being made to understand children and parents as persons. To an increasing degree, doctors generally and pediatricians in particular are concerning themselves with the emotional aspects of disease, with psychological rehabilitation and with the task of improving intrapersonal and interpersonal adjustments in our complex modern society. By the nature of her occupation the nurse is on the firing line. She is continually dealing with children and parents and necessarily becomes a participant in the cultivation of personalities. Through her understanding and behavior she has countless opportunities to influence individual growth and to further satisfying family living. To do this well she must be versed in the expected changes of personality growth and the effects which parental attitudes toward health and disease may bear upon it. Throughout the text an effort has been made to analyze this role which the nurse inevitably plays in the lives of her patients.

The material of the book has been reorganized with the hope of improving the logic of its presentation and facilitating organization of curricula. Unit I confines itself to the expected growth and development of children, including the requirements for optimal nutrition. Unit II considers the kinds, the incidence and the severity of diseases among children and the measures which can be used to forestall them. Unit III treats the rudiments of nursing care, with attention to the interpersonal relationships of the nurse, as well as the physical care which she must render. The last two units offer more detailed consideration of disease and special problems related to the nursing care of the sick infant and child. Unit IV attempts to group together all of the aspects of infant nursing, while Unit V contains diseases which are more characteristic of the older child. The separation is patently artificial, since many of the disorders do not observe strict age limitations. A chapter on malformations has been placed in the section on infant nursing because many of the abnormalities are recognized early in life; and even though treatment may be delayed, the nurse needs some idea of what is in prospect for the malformed infant and his parents.

Again we wish to express our appreciation to the many persons at the University of Iowa and the University of Chicago who have helped in this and in previous revisions of the text. Thanks are also due to the interested readers who have been good enough to suggest improvements. We regret that it is impossible to incorporate all of the desired changes and still maintain a book of manageable size.

F. HOWELL WRIGHT
FLORENCE G. BLAKE

Preface to the First Edition

In preparing this textbook care has been taken to include all of the subject matter suggested in the curriculum for schools of nursing prepared by the National League of Nursing Education. Though the book contains the essentials of the technics which are peculiarly concerned with pediatric nursing and emphasizes the care of the child in health and in illness, more emphasis than perhaps is customary has been given to discussion of phases other than the technics of nursing. Many of the subjects are discussed in considerable detail, considering the space limitations of a small textbook. This is done with a realization that nurses usually are eager to extend their knowledge beyond that which is expected of them. A nurse should not be called upon to diagnose the nature of an illness and prescribe for a patient, yet a knowledge of these fields is an aid in understanding the reasons for those things which she is required to do. Better and more intelligent work results when the reasons for the task are understood.

The basic content of this book has been used as mimeographed text material in several training schools for some years and has thus been submitted to the searching criticism of classroom requirements. This plan provided a thorough checking up and has afforded a means of incorporating into the finished text all the valuable suggestions which have come through such a tryout. The text is illustrated by many cuts, each one of which has been carefully selected for its teaching value.

Chapters III and IV were contributed by Winifred Rand, R.N., Specialist in Parental Education, Merrill-Palmer School. The point of view presented by these chapters on child guidance and nursing care supplements in a useful manner that of the physician as represented by the remainder of the book. Knowledge of proper methods of managing children is fully as important to the nurse as knowledge of the physical aspects of the child in health and disease. When these fields of knowledge are combined, a more complete understanding of the child is attained.

P. C. J.

Contents

CHAPTER ONE

Introduction to Pediatric Nursing

THE DEVELOPMENT OF PEDIATRICS AND PEDIATRIC NURSING

A chapter introducing the subject of pediatric nursing might well begin with "once upon a time," for once upon a time there was no specialty of pediatrics and no pediatric nursing as we understand the term today.

Up until 1860, medical attention was centered on disease and the saving of life. Disease was taught as disease without reference to child or to man. The patient as a person was of comparatively little significance to the physician. This fact is reflected today in our tendency to speak of the patient as a "case." This did not mean that the physicians of that era had no understanding of their patients as persons. Many of the physicians of earlier days were intuitively psychologists; they had deep insight into personality and its relationship to disease. But this type of learning came through living; it was not taught in medical schools or learned from textbooks.

Preventing death was the physician's primary concern. It was also one of the major concerns of society. A comparative study of the medical problems of that era with those that exist today sheds light on the reason why medical and public interest was focused on the

curative aspect of medicine. Childbirth in hospitals was feared and dreaded because so many of the mothers who were delivered there died of childbed fever. The incidence of death and sickness among babies and young children was far greater than it is today. Because the causes of disease were obscure, preventive measures were relatively ineffective. Lay people looked upon disease as a visitation from evil spirits or as a punishment. Superstitions in relation to disease were rife. Even today superstitions and fears concerning disease, hospitalization, pregnancy and delivery have not been wholly eradicated from the minds of many lay people.

The word *pediatrics* is derived from the Greek word *pais, paidos,* meaning child; according to dictionary definition the word means "the medical treatment of children." Pediatrics as a specialty came into being in 1860. Dr. Abraham Jacobi established the first children's clinic in New York and gave special lectures on the diseases of children. The first department of pediatrics was established at the Harvard Medical School in 1888 with Dr. Thomas Morgan Rotch as its first professor. Dr. Jacobi and Dr. Rotch were among the first men to

1

teach that the diseases of children differed somewhat from the diseases of adults and so were deserving of special consideration.

At the time Dr. Rotch was appointed as head of the Pediatric Department of the Harvard Medical School, there were few schools of nursing in the United States and none in hospitals for children. The first school of nursing in the United States was established in 1872 in the first hospital which was built for the care of women and children—The New England Hospital. In 1889 The Children's Hospital in Boston opened the first school of nursing in a hospital for children only. Several hospitals for women and children continue to have schools of nursing, but Boston Children's Hospital is the only children's hospital which continues to maintain a basic school.

It is difficult to say when pediatric nursing came to be considered a specialty, for it arose gradually as the profession recognized children's need for care adapted to their individual requirements. Today pediatric nursing is recognized as an essential requirement for graduation from all schools of nursing, and graduate education is necessary for those nurses who wish to specialize in the field.

Thirty years ago the goals of pediatric nursing were very different from what they are today. In 1927 pediatric nursing instruction had for its goal the teaching of disease, its symptoms, etiology, treatment and the procedures and the hospital routines which were necessary to save lives and to restore children to physical health. The care of sick children in hospitals revolved about food, fluids, treatments, medicine and physical protection. Hospitalized children were rigidly isolated from each other and from their parents. If parents visited in wards, they were garbed in gowns that restricted the use of their hands and arms. Infectious diseases were rampant. There were no antibiotics and few

specific medicines or preventive measures. The majority of the children were kept in their beds. "Absolute bed rest" was a frequently written order for both medical and surgical patients and when necessary it was enforced with restraint jackets. The child's need for play and social experiences was rarely considered because the nurse's energy was being consumed in saving the lives of desperately ill children. Few play materials were available, and parents were rarely permitted to bring toys from home. The emotional impact of illness and hospitalization on the child and his parents was not a major subject of concern. The reason for this is conjectural. Perhaps the sight of the newly admitted young child was so painful to see that hospital personnel were forced to adopt a casual veneer of unconcern in order to protect themselves against emotional strain. For many the lack of such a professional armor would have made it impossible to pursue their life-saving ministrations. Perhaps part of the attitude arose from frustration at lack of time and preparation for dealing with the psychological needs which arose in response to maternal deprivation. The acquisition of this detached professional attitude toward sick children gradually desensitized the novice until she became emotionally blind to the feelings of the children in the ward. Perhaps in a similar fashion hospital personnel were frustrated by their inability to deal with the anxiety of parents who at that time had a real fear of hospitals as places in which sick people usually died. The considerations of limited time and energy thus made it necessary for the hospital staff to isolate itself as much as possible from parents with whom it was ill-prepared to deal.

Many medical and health service advances have been made during the past 30 years. Some of them have resulted from the stimulus of The White House Conferences which began in 1909 and have been held at 10-year intervals ever since. These conferences are called by the President of the United States. Representatives from Federal Agencies, from national and voluntary organizations and from state and local areas come together to study children and their needs and to make recommendations designed to improve services to children and their families. The 1950 White House Conference on children and youth had for its theme, "A Healthy Personality for Every Child." Other important contributory factors in the advancement of medicine have come about through the leadership of individuals in the Children's Bureau, in the Federal Department of Labor (now the Department of Health, Education and Welfare), in the official and the nonofficial public health agencies and in the medical centers of this country. As a result of their leadership, the causes of many diseases have been discovered. Some of them are preventable; others are treated more easily and rapidly than before. Education of the public has reduced the incidence of gastro-intestinal, nutritional and some of the infectious diseases. Antibiotics and public health measures have brought infections under better control, so that prolonged isolation and hospitalization are required less often. More children are being treated in outpatient departments and cared for in homes. This change has increased the public health nurse's responsibilities. It has also freed many hospital beds for the study, the treatment and the rehabilitation of children with chronic disease, physical handicaps and congenital malformations.

Research into the cause and the correction of cardiac and other malformations, in the study and the treatment of children with emotional and psychosomatic disturbances and in the use of hormone therapy for such chronic illnesses as leukemia and rheumatic heart disease have changed the child clientele in pediatric wards and created new problems for the nurse of today. More

diagnostic tests and studies and major corrective and plastic surgery are being done. The nursing care of such children not only requires a high degree of technical skill but also demands supportive nursing measures which help them adjust in a healthy fashion to hospitalization and to the changes produced by corrective surgery. In pediatric wards there are many ambulatory patients and children with long-term illnesses. The care of these children requires the concerted effort of many professional people, both in pediatric wards and in community agencies which provide continuity of medical, nursing and social services to children and to their families. During the past 30 years the health team has expanded to include the social worker, the physiotherapist, the nutritionist, the occupational therapist, the speech therapist, the public health educator, the mental hygienist, the psychologist, the schoolteacher and auxiliary personnel. The health team has been expanded because the family's needs and goals are complex and cannot be met without the help of specialists in these allied professions.

Parents are more enlightened and sophisticated than they were 30 years ago. Public health education and the widespread circulation of progress reports concerning advances in medicine and the research findings pertaining to human development have made society "health conscious" and avidly interested in obtaining the best for their children and for themselves. The rapidity with which our society is changing is making parents acutely aware of their children's need for learning experiences which will prepare them to adjust to the social changes which are inevitable in a democracy.

As physical health problems have been reduced, more energy of persons in the fields of pediatrics, obstetrics and the allied professions has been directed toward the study of growth and development during the cycle from conception to the end of the child-rearing age. Research which has increased knowledge of growth and development particularly emphasizes the child's need for an intimate, warm and continuous relationship with his mother or with a permanent mother substitute. It has pointed out that the child needs nurture which helps him to master the steps of the socialization process leading toward maturity. It has also demonstrated his urgent need for protection from experiences which are beyond his capacity to master. Experiences which cannot be handled without residual feelings of fear, anger or revenge are commonly defined as psychic traumas or traumatic experiences. Research has pointed out how illness, deviations from normality and hospitalization affect children's and parents' feelings and their capacity for adjustment. Today professional people both here and abroad are studying sick and handicapped children and their parents to discover methods of helping them deal with the realities that they must face.

In a similar way the psychology and the needs of women during the reproductive cycle have come under scrutiny, and an understanding of the personality changes and of the emotional needs of women during the child-bearing age has evolved. In many medical centers health teams are focusing interest upon the unmet needs of expectant parents and parents of young children who are trying to adjust to this mightily important job of child-rearing.

Studies such as the above reflect a growing concern for the patient as a person rather than a case. Pediatric nurses are discovering that a child is a person with a mind and feelings which are closely knit together and are reacting on each other constantly. They are also perceiving the child as a part of a family which is of vital importance to him as a person. They are seeing the importance of keeping intact the bond that exists between child and parents.

Illness is now being viewed as an episode in the child's life during which his past experiences must be considered and his future needs safeguarded.

In their field, maternity nurses are not only viewing the expectant and postparturient mother as a person with a unique personality and needs but also as a key person in the family—a person who has profound influence upon the mental health of each member of her family. The interest of maternity nurses is being directed toward finding supportive measures which will help young couples make healthy adjustments to the developmental tasks which are a natural part of the maternity cycle. Parenthood, like any other career, requires preparation.

Through recognition of the young child's needs for continuity of warm maternal care during illness as well as in periods of health, nurses began to face their responsibilities toward parents. A few years ago parents were kept from pediatric wards because hospital personnel were fearful of cross-infections and were unprepared to deal with the behavior of anxiety-ridden parents. Gradually, however, nurses are becoming more ready to learn to be helpful to parents. They are approaching the problem slowly and thoughtfully, as all new problems should be faced. Pediatric nurses are finding that liberal visiting hours are of therapeutic value for the child. They are also discovering that a mother's anxiety lessens as her own needs are considered and she is given opportunity to be of help to her hospitalized child. In addition, nurses are finding that liberal visiting hours provide unique occasions to promote the health of the whole family. Opportunities for family-centered guidance are available that were rarely existent during a short, infrequent visiting hour. In maternity hospitals nurses are discovering that mothers profit immeasurably from experiences that keep them in close touch with their new baby and give them opportunities to become competent in understanding and caring for him. Helping the new family to become comfortably established with each other has become the challenge of family-centered maternity care.

The challenge of work with mothers motivated pediatric nurses to seek increased understanding of parents. Many pediatric nurses have obtained such help from maternity nurses, social workers and specialists in the field of dynamic psychiatry and mental hygiene. They studied the psychology of the reproductive cycle which evolved from study of women during pregnancy and the earliest periods of motherhood. They sought clinical experience in maternity hospitals and homes. As a result of these experiences they became aware of the biologically determined crises that often arise during pregnancy and their effect on the woman and her entire family. They also became aware of the problems that new parents encounter as they adapt to the responsibilities inherent in the parental role. They observed the expectant mother's need for a continuous relationship which would help her to understand herself, to become prepared for labor, to support her during it and to assist her in acquiring pleasure and confidence in her capacity to fulfill the mother role. In addition, these pediatric nurses felt anew the emotional investment that parents have in their children. From these experiences they developed a deeper understanding of the emotional impact on parents of the child's illness or deviation from normality.

Such experiences prepare pediatric nurses to work with parents more successfully than before. They acquire increased capacity to feel with parents (empathize) and thus to identify their needs. They have become more facile in dealing with parents who need help when illness, prematurity or a congenital anomaly necessitates an extended period of hospitalization of the child.

Pediatric nurses have also extended their skills to mothers of normal children seen in well-baby clinics and in homes.

In the same way that the pediatric nurse has learned from experiences with families during the maternity cycle, so the maternity nurse has studied in the pediatric field in order to deepen her appreciation of the developmental process and the problems of the reproductive cycle and to gain increased mastery of the mothering skills. The experiences which brought pediatric and maternity nurses together have motivated those in the two fields to view their responsibilities anew. They have come to see that *families need the help of specialists from all areas of nursing and from others of the helping professions.* These two fields are merging to encompass a field currently called Maternal and Child Health Nursing. Family-centered care has become the concern of nurses in both fields. They are working to protect the family's physical health and to promote the development of warm family relationships which safeguard the mental health of each member of the family. Mental hygienists view the maternity cycle and the periods immediately following it as periods of great importance in the prevention of juvenile delinquency and other emotional disturbances. They believe that important preventive work can be done then—preventive work that can foster the development of the parents and prepare them to nurture their child in ways which are satisfying to and productive for all members of the family.

Progress in pediatrics and obstetrics and in the allied professions has broadened the scope of medicine and nursing and changed their goals. Today professional workers are focusing their interest on the preventive aspects of their specialty and on the restoration of sick and handicapped individuals to a state of optimal physical and mental health. They are not losing interest in reducing the maternal and child death and sickness rates by any means. Research is going ahead in these areas, but the emphasis is on the study of causes and the methods of removing the obstacles that thwart the individual's attainment of optimal health. Unit II presents the characteristics of disease in childhood and its effects upon the individual child. It also presents the scope of pediatrics, its problems, goals and methods of carrying the protection derived from medical and psychological research to parents and to the children themselves.

To do preventive work the nurse needs a different kind of preparation than she had 30 years ago. The nursing profession grew out of society's need for the care of the sick. Hospitals were full of critically ill, bedridden people who needed much physical care. The nurse's education was concerned with knowledge and training essential to nurse the sick and to save lives. Most of the nurse's education came from teachers who were responsible for the care of physically ill children and adults. The nurse gained her experience in institutions established for sick people; she had no experience in homes, clinics or schools. It is little wonder that the nurse's education was lacking in the experience and the training which would help her to become "health conscious," to gain insight into the common human needs of the individual and the family, and to acquire the knowledge, the attitudes and the skills which are necessary to promote mental and physical health.

Through the course of the last 30 years many changes in pediatric nursing courses have occurred as the result of the research which has been cited. Early in this century our knowledge of child growth and development was limited. We did not understand the dynamics of the growth process and of behavior as well as we do today. As nurses became aware of research findings, curriculum changes were made. At first the content of pediatric nursing courses was expanded to help nurses gain understanding of the growth process and to plan play and social experiences for hospitalized children. Soon nursery schools were used for the purpose of broadening the student's knowledge of the nature and the needs of the normal child. As nurses' awareness of children's and parents' feelings increased, curriculum changes were required to assist the student in expanding her capacity to help children feel understood and to adjust to illnesses, to handicaps and to the frightening and painful experiences of hospitalization. Throughout this book *the words "healthy adjustment" and "mastery" will be used to indicate a mode of adjustment which ensures to the child a continuation of warm relationships with others, respect for himself and maximum opportunities for further emotional development. The words, "unhealthy adjustment," will be used to indicate a mode of adjustment which produces residual feelings of hopelessness, anger, anxiety or revenge.*

Today further curriculum changes are being made because faculties recognize society's need for nurses who are prepared to meet the challenge of family-centered preventive care. Some faculties are concentrating on the enrichment of the basic educational foundation upon which supportive nursing in all areas depends. Some faculties are emphasizing the development of their individual courses in pediatric and maternity nursing. Others are combining maternity and pediatric nursing experiences and broadening and weaving together the content of these two fields into an integrated whole. The central objective of these newly developed courses is to help the student of nursing to gain a broad concept of the scope of Maternal and Child Health Nursing. These newly developed courses provide education and clinical experience which expand the student's capacity to understand the biophysiologic and psychological aspects of growth and development from conception to maturity and through the marriage, the child-bearing and the child-rearing stages of development. The student's experience is not confined to work with patients in hospitals as it was 30 years ago. Students are placed in community agencies which provide preventive health services to expectant parents and to parents and children in homes, clinics and schools. Instructors are becoming aware that the student nurse's feelings toward patients and their families, toward her co-workers and toward the knowledge she is gleaning from study are important in the learning process. As a result they are focusing more attention upon methods of supervision which are designed to help the students meet their needs for professional and personal growth.

To supplement the education which has been outlined briefly above, the student of nursing must have knowledge from the biologic, physical and nursing sciences which provides her with special information about disease, physiology and practical means of relieving the physical discomfort of patients. *Perfecting the nurse's curative and physically comforting skills is as important today as it was a century ago.* To the student's theoretical knowledge must be added clinical experience with patients in pediatric and maternity wards in order that she may learn to function successfully as the nurse member of the health team which provides comprehensive care: (1) to the family during the maternity cycle and (2) to the child during periods of illness, rehabilitation or convalescence.

UNDERSTANDING GROWTH AND DEVELOPMENT

Nurses in the field of Maternal and Child Health are concerned with the care of individuals in all periods of growth. They work with the helpless, primitive and rapidly growing infant. They work with the preschool child who is struggling to acquire the ability to control his asocial impulses, to socialize with children and adults outside his family and to master his environment. They care for the school-age child who has developed wider intellectual and social interests and acquired a desire to gain increased inner controls. The active preadolescents who are making strides in adaptation to the realities of society's demands and expectations are also individuals who turn to nurses for help.

Today adolescents are placed in many pediatric wards because the word *child* now includes them. Up until recent years the generally accepted meaning of the word *child* included only infants and children to the beginning of puberty. Pediatricians dismissed their patients at adolescence. The upper age limit in children's wards used to be 12 to 13 years. This left the adolescent at that important threshold, the period of transition from childhood to maturity, without the special help he required. Today pediatricians are aware of the adolescent's need for a continuing relationship until maturity is reached and until separation from home makes a change in medical care inevitable. Pediatricians, along with school and pediatric nurses, are trying to meet the challenge of helping teen-agers discover their place in a world that is continually changing at a very rapid rate. Not only are many pediatric wards accommodating adolescents today but also some children's hospitals are providing special wards for their care.

The pediatric nurse also deals with adults who are in vitally important stages of development. Development does not cease at adolescence; it continues as long as there is life in the individual. The young adult has growing to do during the marriage and the child-bearing stages of development. He, too, has new learning experiences to master. Marriage, pregnancy and the arrival of children produce changes in the adult's life. Taking on a new role often creates conflict and stress; it always presents problems and responsibilities that the individual never has faced before. The manner in which young adults adjust to these periods of growth not only affects personal development but also influences that of the spouse and of the children which result from this union.

Knowledge pertaining to growth and the developmental process is presented in Unit I. It is the first unit of this book because one of the greatest concerns of the pediatrician and the nurse working in the field of Maternal and Child Health is the protection of the family's potentialities for maximum physical, social, mental, emotional and spiritual development. Because the nurse needs more knowledge on this subject than one textbook and a short clinical experience can provide, supplementary reading and educational experiences are being suggested. The nurse can glean broader concepts of the health goal toward which she is working from reading and observation and participation in well-baby clinics, in nursery, primary and secondary schools, in organized recreational programs for children, on playgrounds and in homes.

COMPREHENSIVE CARE THAT SUPPORTS GROWTH AND DEVELOPMENT

Nursing entails support which fosters the growth and the development of the individual. To provide the physical support that the growing individual requires during periods of illness and convalescence or during periods when he is in the throes of meeting new problems and responsibilities, the nurse needs knowledge which is derived from the biologic and physical sciences. Units IV and V are presented to expand the student's capacity to understand the child's health problem and to provide symptomatic nursing care.

To provide the emotional support that the growing individual requires the nurse needs additional knowledge, attitudes, training and skills which are derived chiefly from dynamic psychiatry, preventive medicine and the social sciences. She needs knowledge of the individual's background of family and cultural experiences and the manner in which they affect his response to illness, treatment and rehabilitation or toward pregnancy and child-rearing if the individual is a prospective or actual parent. She needs healthy attitudes and awareness of herself and others. She also needs special skills to study the individual, to identify his psychological needs, to interpret them and to help him find ways to get the satisfactions he requires for successful adaptation to the reality of the problems he faces.

Emotional support becomes paramount when illness strikes; it also becomes essential when the individual is facing major changes in himself or in those closest to himself or in his life situation. Illness, treatment and hospitalization produce anxiety in the child and his parents. Anxiety is an intrinsic part of other life situations which produce major changes in a person's life. Growth produces biologic and psychological change. Mastery of one learning experience changes the individual and prepares and motivates him to tackle the next step in the developmental process. Some phases of growth and development produce minor changes; others produce major changes which require the help of persons outside the family— the doctor, the nurse and others of the health team. All children do not come to the hospital equally well-prepared to adapt to the experience. Growth-producing past experiences build inner resources which prepare the individual to meet life situations which would produce a crisis in an ill-prepared person. Not all women come to the child-bearing and child-rearing stages of development equally well fitted to meet the changes and the responsibilities inherent in them. In contrast with the poorly prepared woman, the well-prepared one needs minimal support to adjust to her changing role. The poorly prepared woman and child need infinitely more support, and the kind must be based on the health team's study of the individual.

Emotional support helps the individual adapt to the reality he is facing in the healthiest possible way for himself and for society. This kind of support strengthens the individual's ego. The ego is a portion of the personality which is very difficult to define. It develops as the nervous system grows and is stimulated. Its development is further influenced as the child has the pleasurable feelings which are derived from mutually satisfying relationships with his mother and others who are important to him personally. The ego functions to preserve the individual's sense of reality; it perceives the demands and the expectations of his society; it determines the manner in which he will respond to inner drives and environmental standards and expectations. It also functions to maintain the emotional equilibrium or balance the child or adult requires for growth or for recuperation from disease. The individual's ego determines how he will adjust to the reality of his current life-situation. It is the person's ego which determines the kind of emotional support that he requires. The newborn has no ego resources. Emotional support for him must contain elements different from those required by the school-age child. The ego is that part of the personality which matures in a healthy way when the child is nurtured by persons who understand growth and the developmental process; who perceive his physical and psychological readiness to learn to adjust himself to society's expectations; who see things from his point of view; who supply the physical and ego support which helps him to complete each stage of development. Throughout the book the words *ego resources* and *inner strengths* will be used synonymously to indicate the personality characteristics which must be acquired to achieve emotional equilibrium (personal happiness and security) and socially acceptable adjustment. This subject will be developed more fully in Chapter 4.

The capacity to establish and maintain an ego-supporting relationship with the individual and his family is one of the most fundamental ingredients of comprehensive Maternal and Child Health Nursing. Providing clinical experiences and supervision which strengthen the student's competence to study the individual's ego-strengths and limitations and to maintain a constructive relationship which helps him to meet his needs are of utmost importance in the education of professional nurses and those who assist them in meeting their goals in the care of patients. Chapters 7 and 8 are presented to stimulate the student's interest in gaining awareness of herself and others and to help her to adapt her knowledge of the developmental process and the dynamics of behavior to the care of patients and to the support of their families.

Comprehensive care which promotes the growth and the development of the individual requires the concerted effort of all members of the health team who are providing services to the individual and his family. The capacity to understand and respect the contribution of each member of the team and to work in a way which helps the troubled person to profit from their special skills are two important attributes of the professional nurse.

The ability to detect the child's or the parent's need for help from others of the health team is another quality which enhances the nurse's service to humanity. "Case-finding" or recognition that a problem exists is one of the first essentials in the prevention of juvenile delinquency and other forms of mental ill-health. The nurse's education should make her aware of the danger signs which indicate deviation from normality, either in physical development or in the behavior of children or parents—

danger signs which may forecast unhealthy life adjustment for children unless appropriate care is obtained. It is vitally important that the nurse be able to provide psychological first-aid and to help the disturbed person to realize his need for expert help. The effects may be far-reaching not only for the individual but also for his entire family and even for society.

BIBLIOGRAPHY

Bowlby, John: Child Care and the Growth of Love, London, Penguin Books, 1953.

Caplan, Gerald: Psychological aspects of maternity care, Am. J. Pub. Health 47:25, 1957.

Chaloner, Len: British experiments in the care of sick children, Children 3:91, 1956.

Church, Gertrude M.: Understanding each other to achieve a common goal, Am. J. Nursing 56:201, 1956.

Deutsch, Helene: The Psychology of Women, vol. 2, New York, Grune, 1945.

Hohle, Bertha M.: We admit parents, too, Am. J. Nursing 57:865, 1957.

Kirkwood, Samuel: Complete maternity care, Am. J. Pub. Health 46:1547, 1956.

Kreuter, Frances Reiter: What is good nursing care? Nursing Outlook 5:302, 1957.

Lesser, Marion S., and Keane, Vera R.: Nurse-Patient Relationship in a Hospital Maternity Service, St. Louis, Mosby, 1956.

Liberal visiting policies for children in hospitals, J. Pediat. 46:710, 1955.

Robertson, James: Some responses of young children to the loss of maternal care, Nursing Times 49:382, 1953.

Thompson, Morton: The Cry and the Covenant, New York, Signet Books, 1949.

U. S. Dept. Health, Education and Welfare: Four Decades of Action for Children; A Short History of the Children's Bureau, Washington, D. C., 1956.

———: Your Children's Bureau; Its Current Program (pamphlet), Washington, D. C., 1956.

The Healthy Child

In contrast with adult medicine, pediatrics deals with individuals who are in a dynamic, rapidly changing period of life. Whereas the adult possesses a body which will alter relatively little during the remainder of his life, the child must accommodate to more than a 3-fold increase in length and an approximate 20-fold increase in weight between birth and adolescence. Simultaneously, his muscular and intellectual skills and his emotional controls progress from the rudimentary state of the newborn to the complex, highly integrated level of modern civilized man. The term "growth and development" is used to encompass the changes which take place during this dramatic transition. Strictly speaking, growth implies an increase in size, while development denotes an improvement in functional capacity. For example, the child's brain increases very little in size (growth) after the age of 6, but the operations it can perform (development) continue to advance for years afterward. Since it is often difficult to make a clear distinction between growth and development, it has become common practice to use the terms jointly or even interchangeably.

The rapid changes which a child undergoes in response to the growth impulse complicate the task of evaluating his health and progress. Any standard against which he is measured must take due account of his age. In addition, some allowance must be made for individual variation in rates of growth and development. Thus in assessing the growth of a 1-year-old boy it is not expected that his weight will exactly match the 22 pounds which is average for his age. But if his weight falls outside the range of 19½ to 25½ pounds, the figure begins to assume significance when it is understood that four fifths of year-old males fall within these boundaries. In the same way the evaluation of developmental progress must be made in terms of a normal range rather than a precise average. An infant who fails to sit alone until 8 months should not be considered as abnormally slow merely because the average age of this achievement is 7 months. But if the child still is not sitting by 12 months the delay exceeds the normal range, and a reason must be sought. Ranges are more cumbersome than averages, but without them individuality may be maligned unjustly.

The growth and the development of a child is a complex process which, for purposes of description, is usually dissected into several components such as

11

its physical, physiologic, motor, intellectual, emotional and social aspects. The separation of these facets of growth is admittedly artificial, for they merge into and depend upon each other. Thus motor development (walking, for example) depends upon normal growth of bone and muscle (physical), supplied by adequate food and energy (physiologic), and guided by the developing nervous system (intellectual). In extreme circumstances it may be impeded by maternal neglect (emotional) or by the cultural mores of a society which overprotects its infants (social).

Within a given child growth does not necessarily proceed at the same pace along each of these channels. A child who is growing slowly in the physical aspects of height and weight often outstrips his peers in motor achievement and social adaptation. Or an intellectually precocious schoolboy may lag behind in his athletic skills and social adjustment. Proper understanding of the child thus depends upon an evaluation of the several phases of his growth and the manner in which they interrelate.

In this unit the first chapter sketches the physical and physiologic changes which can be anticipated. In general these aspects of growth are readily measured and can be referred to standards of normal with some exactness. The second chapter deals with the food requirements necessary to provide building materials for the growing body and to supply energy for its operation. The final chapter treats those phenomena which depend upon the development of the central nervous system—the motor skills, the intellectual powers and the emotional sensitivity to the environment which constitute the unique biologic heritage setting the human infant apart from all other animals.

CHAPTER TWO

Physical and Physiologic Aspects of Growth

THE GENERAL PATTERN OF GROWTH

FETAL GROWTH

Hidden from direct observation and relatively inaccessible to study, the fetus receives scant attention in considerations of growth and development. Yet these early stages are the most remarkable and in some ways the most crucial period of human growth. The new individual starts as a microscopic cell (the fertilized ovum) which in some incredible manner contains the impulse to direct it through a series of carefully controlled subdivisions which mimic the evolutionary history of man and result after 9 months in the emergence of an infant endowed not only with the universal structure of his race but with many of the individual traits of his parents.

When compared with the postnatal growth which we are able to observe, fetal growth takes place at an extraordinarily rapid rate. The adult weighs about 20 times what he did at birth; but the newborn infant weighs about 6 billion times what he did at conception. Within this period he has changed structurally from a single-celled organism to a complex of organ systems which can support life outside his mother's body. During the first 8 weeks of the period of gestation growth proceeds at its most frantic pace, and rearrangements are made which bring most of the organ systems close to their final forms. It is during this critical period of organ formation that errors in the sequence of developmental changes are particularly apt to result in malformation or even death of the fetus. Careful prenatal care is designed to maintain an optimum environment for the fetus by shielding the health of his mother.

POSTNATAL GROWTH

At birth the rate of increase in body size has begun to slow down, yet growth during the first year will far outstrip any that occurs in later life. The average increases of 50 per cent in length and 200 per cent in weight never will be approached subsequently. These annual percentage increases in size taper off rapidly and after a temporary rise during adolescence fall to zero, indicating

13

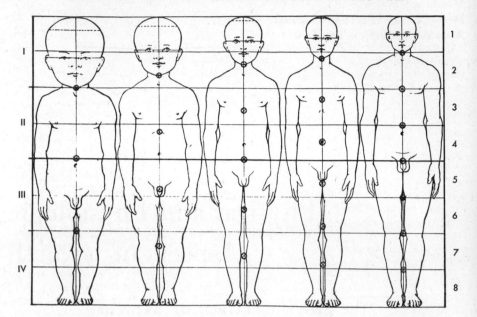

FIG. 1. Outlines of the body at different ages reduced to the same size to show the changing proportions between head size, trunk length and extremity length. (After Stratz, Der Körper des Kinder, E. Enke, Berlin, p. 64)

that growth is complete. The calculation of percentages of increase is too cumbersome for general use. Instead, the changes which take place are usually described in terms of the number of pounds or inches added to the body per month or per year. Even with this less-exact method the over-all view of childhood growth presents a similar picture. The number of inches added during the first year is more than double the increase in height which occurs during the second year, and this in turn exceeds any increment of later years. From 3 years to puberty annual increases in height remain between 2 and 3 inches, then they spurt up slightly but rapidly dwindle as growth trails off. Changes in weight parallel the changes in height in a rough fashion but are more subject to deviation from average values.

The growth pattern of girls is slightly but significantly different from that of boys. During infancy and the early school years girls are on the average a little shorter and a little lighter than boys of the same age. Because they enter puberty with its attendant spurt in growth about 2 years before boys do, girls often overtake boys of a similar age during the early part of the second decade of life. However, this advantage is temporary, for by the middle teens most girls are slowing down in growth rate to a final stature which will be less than that of the adult male. The pubertal growth spurt of boys begins later but lasts longer and then carries them to a final height which is generally above that reached by the girls.

Sex is only one of a number of influences which determine the ultimate size to which a child will grow. The final result appears to depend upon a balance among the hormones of the pituitary, thyroid, adrenal cortex and gonads which determines the number of years over which growth will continue and the rate at which it proceeds. Behind the hormonal control lie the influences of race, individual heredity, chronic illness, nutrition and perhaps climate. It is not always easy to decide the relative importance of these different factors in determining the growth pattern of an individual child.

The over-all progress of growth is not necessarily a steady one. Children may grow in short-term spurts and lags. Frequently, the period between 18 months and 3 years of age is characterized by slow or irregular growth activity. Acute illness, emotional disturbances, inadequate intake of food or vitamins and decrease in exposure to sunlight with the change of seasons are commonly associated with temporary slowing of the rate of growth.

DIFFERENTIAL GROWTH

The infant is not a miniature man, for the relative sizes of various parts of his body does not correspond to that of the adult (Fig. 1). The upper portion of his body is further advanced than the lower regions. His head is large and represents about one fourth of his total length. It will grow fairly rapidly for a year and then slow down, permitting the more rapid growth of trunk and legs to produce a body in which the head is reduced to one eighth of the total length. The circumference of the trunk is slightly less than that of the head at birth, but growth of the thoracic organs pushes it ahead of the cranial circumference within the first few months of life; and by the time a heavy deposition of muscle has been added at puberty, the chest is half again as large around as the head. In a similar way the lower extremities grow faster than the upper. The particularly marked growth of the legs during childhood drops the center of the body from a point which is about an inch above the umbilicus at birth down to the symphysis of the pubes at maturity. These are but a few of the many indices which can be measured by the student of body morphology in describing the effect of growth on body contour. The changes which take place in localized portions of the body will be considered later on in this chapter.

MEASURING GROWTH

Height and weight are the usual measurements of growth. For many years attempts have been made to compile tables of growth which could serve as guides in evaluating the progress of children. Such tables have a definite field of usefulness, but it is important to remember that they can represent only averages and may not adequately account for factors such as race, nutrition, previous illness or socio-economic condition. Whenever feasible a child should be measured against standards derived from the study of a large group of children living in comparable circumstances. Common sense tells us that it will be futile to measure Peruvian Indian children living in poverty at an altitude of 12,000 feet against the growth standards of well-to-do youngsters in Stockholm. But it is easy to overlook lesser degrees of discrepancy between the child and the presumed normal standards.

GROWTH CHARTS

In the United States the growth tables compiled by the Children's Bureau in 1918 from weights and measurements of preschool children all over the country served as a tremendous impetus to public interest in the health of the young. Subsequently, a number of studies have been made which show a progressing increase in the rate of growth of American children decade by decade, which is presumably related to an improvement in standards of nutrition. Most widely used today are the Iowa growth charts prepared by Jackson, the Harvard charts by Stuart, and the Wetzel grid. Each of these tables presents the data in a somewhat different fashion.

Iowa Growth Charts

The use of growth charts may be illustrated by considering the Iowa standards reproduced in Figures 2 through 7. Separate growth curves are given for each sex covering the first year of life, the pre-school years and the school years, including adolescence. Height and weight for age are included on the same sheet so that a ready comparison of progress in the two aspects of growth can be made.

The curves show a mean value at the different age levels represented by the middle line of the three lines shown. The

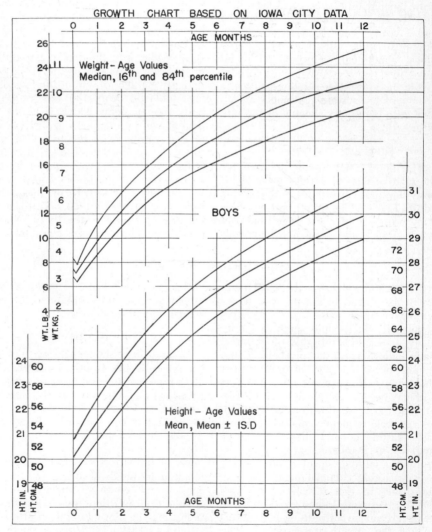

Fig. 2. Average measurements of boys from 0 to 12 months of age.

other two lines represent one standard deviation° on each side of the mean. Heights and weights falling within the ranges shown are considered to be normal, provided that certain criteria are met. Growth may be considered normal

° A standard deviation is the amount of variation above or below the mean which will include ⅓ of all the observations made. Thus, between the lines which represent plus 1 S.D. and minus 1 S.D. will be found exactly ⅔ of the observations from which the graphs were drawn. At a given age, the heights or the weights of ⅙ of normal children will be above the top line; ⅓ will fall between the top and the middle lines; ⅓ will fall between the middle and the lower lines; and ⅙ will fall below the bottom line.

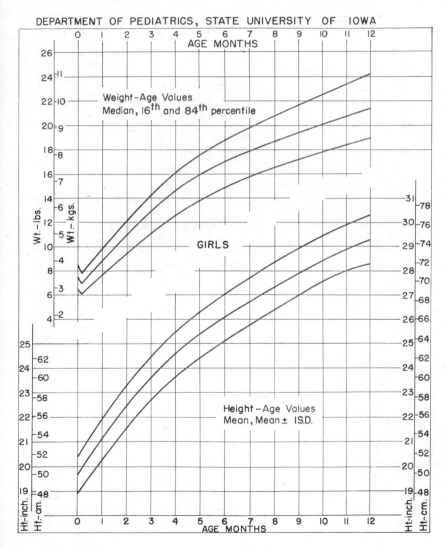

FIG. 3. Average measurements of girls from 0 to 12 months of age.

if it parallels the general course of the curves, even though the height or the weight may be above or below the median curve. Change in position in relation to the curve may represent abnormality of growth, especially if relative decrease is found from one observation to another. From these curves it is apparent that the norm consists of a range of values. A tendency exists to discontinue the use of "average" in relation to growth and to consider growth only in terms of the normal range. A general picture of the expected growth in height and weight is useful as a guide, although it must be remembered that the word

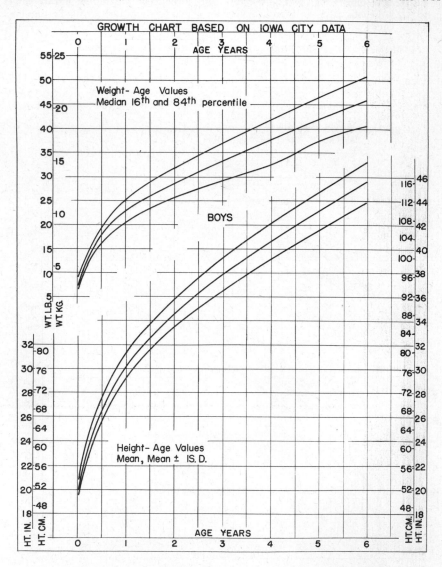

FIG. 4. Average measurements of boys from 0 to 6 years of age.

approximate may represent a wide range.

Body build is reflected in the relationship between height and weight. The child with a slender skeleton and small muscles will likely fall at a lower level on the weight-age portion of the graph than he does on the height-age portion. Conversely, if his bones are broad and covered by large muscles or a heavy layer of fat, he will occupy a higher position on the weight graph than he does on the height standard. Orientation should be made from height, since growth in length is less fluctuant and offers a more consistent picture through the years. The degree to which weight

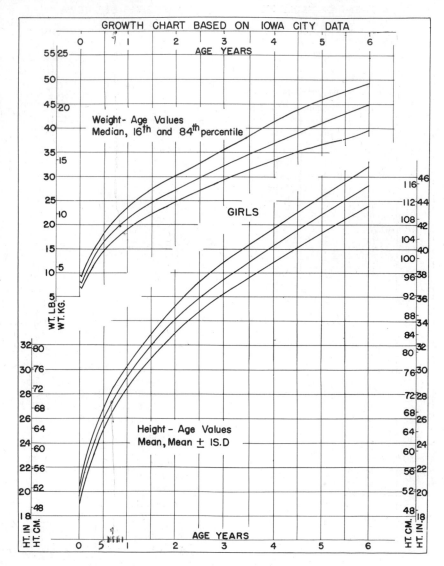

FIG. 5. Average measurements of girls from 0 to 6 years of age.

can be expected to deviate because of body build is difficult to say. Usually if it is more than 10 per cent below or 20 per cent above the corresponding point on the height graph, suboptimal health should be suspected.

Measurement of the length of infants is often omitted because it is relatively difficult and inexact. However, proper interpretation of weight changes during the early months should depend upon knowledge of the infant's length. In contrast with the older child, infants rather commonly shift their positions on the

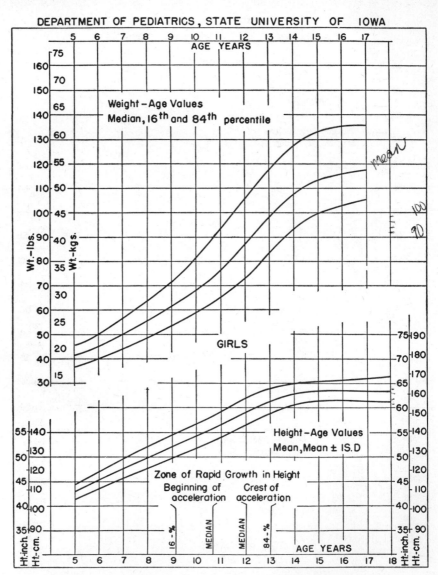

FIG. 6. Average measurements of girls from 5 to 18 years of age.

height graphs between birth and the end of the second year. The direction and the speed of this change should be taken into account when evaluating the weight progress with which interested parties are more commonly preoccupied.

By the end of the second year most infants reveal a steady pattern of height increase which remains characteristic until adolescence. Persistent decrease of the rate of growth may be an early warning of unrecognized illness or abnormality.

Changes in weight are more quixotic.

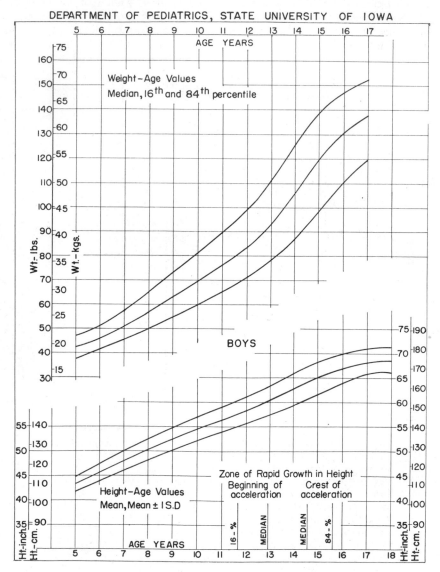

FIG. 7 Average measurements of boys from 5 to 18 years of age.

Many factors such as illness, poor diet, too little or too much physical activity, overeating and insufficient rest may be responsible for brief or more protracted alterations in the weight curve. Decline in a previously satisfactory rate of weight gain is an earlier harbinger of disease than a change in the rate of growth in length. It is obvious that such changes in the rates of increase in height or weight cannot be observed unless re-peated measurements of the child are made and preserved for later reference.

Harvard Growth Curves

The curves compiled by Stuart and his associates are very similar to those of the Iowa group and can be used in the same fashion. The main difference in their construction is that instead of indi-cating the mean and one standard devia-tion on either side of it, the data is ar-

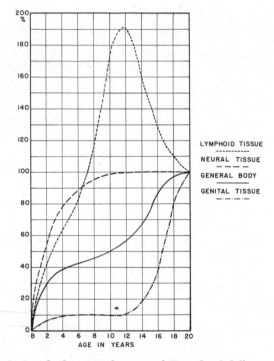

FIG. 8. Graph showing the rate of growth of different body tissues from birth to adult size at 20 years. Genital tissue which includes the internal and the external reproductive organs grows very little during the prepubertal years and then sud-denly enlarges to reach its final size. Neural tissue which is the brain, the spinal cord and their coverings, grows rapidly to-ward final size which it reaches at about the time of puberty. Lymphoid tissue, which includes the lymph nodes, the thymus, adenoids and the tonsils, not only increases very rapidly in the early years but surpasses its ultimate size and then regresses during puberty. (Adapted from Harris, J. A., *et al.*, The Meas-urement of Man, Minneapolis, University of Minnesota Press, 1930)

ranged in percentiles. The line of the 50th percentile corresponds to the mean. One quarter of all children at a given age fall below the 25th percentile line, and another quarter of the group fall above the 75th percentile line. Additional lines indicate the positions of the 3rd, 10th, 90th and 97th percentiles. The graphs include a similar chart of head circumferences.

The Wetzel Grid

Based upon the conviction that normal growth follows a predictable pattern which varies primarily with body build, Wetzel has constructed a graph on which the relation between height and weight is plotted. This index of body build places the child in one of 9 channels ranging from obesity to poor nutrition. Healthy children fall into and progress along the middle channels. The speed of a child's progress along his channels depends upon the rate of maturation and can be correlated with other aspects of growth. Although the grid provides a graphic view of consistent individual growth, the complex theory upon which it is based has limited its wide acceptance.

Use of Growth Curves

Plotting heights and weights against appropriate standards is an efficient and graphic method for the preliminary assessment of growth of individual children or of groups such as school populations. But the partial nature of this evaluation requires emphasis lest the child's position on a height-weight graph assume unwarranted importance. Some of the allowances which must be made for individual variation have been indicated above. Mensuration must be supplemented by an evaluation of food intake, of motor, mental and emotional progress, and by a search for the effects of disease or abnormalities. Thus proper evaluation of the child's total health requires a careful history, physical examination and appropriate laboratory tests.

DEVELOPMENT OF THE ORGAN SYSTEMS

For the more detailed study of physical growth and development, the body is conveniently subdivided into a collection of organ systems each of which has a particular role to play. The sizes and the functional abilities of these several aspects of body physiology change at different rates as they prepare for the assumption of their duties as part of the final mature individual (Fig. 8). For example, changes in the bones parallel the changes in height; but the brain moves quickly toward its ultimate size. The reproductive organs remain rudimentary in size and function until the final spurt of adolescence; but the digestive organs maintain a constant relationship to total body size with only minor changes in functional ability. Only a general view of these changes can be attempted here. Further details may be sought in the sections devoted to disease of the various organ systems.

Osseous System

Bone Growth

Growth in length is dependent entirely on bone growth, and bone growth is largely dependent on the mineral supply which the body is given and can use. During growth, bones change in composition, number and size. The skeleton as a whole increases in size about 20 times from birth to maturity. Bones consist of an organic matrix, cartilage, fibrous tissue, mineral salts, fat and water. The fat is largely in the marrow cavities.

At birth, the amount of mineral matter in the bones (chiefly a complex calcium phosphate carbonate) is relatively small, and the amount of water large (75%) in

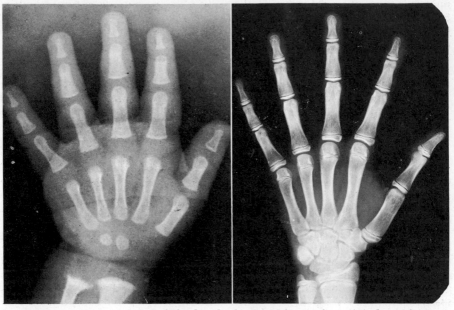

Fig. 9. Roentgenogram of the hand: (*Left*) Of an infant. (*Right*) Of an adolescent. Note the appearance of additional bony centers in the wrist and at the ends of the bones of the forearm and the hand. Bone age can be calculated from the number of such centers which are present.

comparison with adult bone. As growth progresses, the amount of mineral increases, and the water decreases. At 1 year, the skeleton is about 60 per cent water, at which level it remains for the next 2 years. After this time, the mineral gradually increases, and the water decreases until the adult level of 40 per cent mineral and 10 to 25 per cent water is reached at about 12 years. As the amount of mineral increases and ossification takes place, the pliant bones of infancy, easily subject to changes due to muscle pull and pressure, become the rigid bones needed to protect the organs of the child and to give the adult his sturdy framework.

Since growth in length is so largely dependent on the mineral supply, and since that in turn is so dependent on the food we eat, it is to be expected that those with an inadequate or poor food supply, through either poverty or igno-

rance, will not reach their optimum growth in stature, and certain studies have borne out this supposition. It has been noted that when the mineral intake is decreased only moderately, growth continues at the normal rate, but the bones have a low mineral and high water content. With a still lower intake of mineral, bone growth is slower, and with greater deprivation it is stopped.

In the cartilaginous and membranous structures destined to become bone, mineralization starts at one or more points and gradually spreads throughout the bone. Approximately 800 of these ossification centers exist, more than half of them appearing after birth. During growth, the epiphyses or ends of the long bones grow from their own ossification centers independently of the bone shaft. It is chiefly by the growth in the length of the bone shaft that growth in body length occurs. This growth takes place at the end of the shaft, between the shaft and the ununited epiphysis. Growth ceases when shaft and epiphysis unite. Union of the epiphyses with the neighboring bones begins in the innominate bone at about 12½ years in girls and 14 years in boys. It ends in the upper end of the humerus at from 19 to 20 years with good nutrition, but often later with poor nutrition. Closure of the epiphyses is largely under the influence of the sex hormones.

Roentgenograms have become an important implement in studying skeletal development. By their use we can study bone growth and so are able to talk of *bone age* as well as chronologic or mental age. For example, a 5-year-old child whose height and weight indicate him to be within the average range expected for that age might prove by x-ray examination to have a bone age of a much younger child if ossification had not taken place in some of the cartilaginous and fibrous tissue to the extent that would be expected. Roentgenograms of the hand and the wrist (Fig. 9) which have been found to give a reliable picture of the skeletal development of the young child show no carpal bones at birth and no epiphyses. Succeeding roentgenograms will trace the appearance and the development of these bones and epiphyses. The rate of appearance of epiphyses from which bone age is calculated depends in large measure upon the activity of the thyroid gland.

Bones of the Skull

The upper part of the skull is made up of 7 "membranous" bones still separate and ununited at birth. The boundary lines between them are known as sutures, and the point of juncture of 3 or more bones is a fontanel. Six fontanels exist at birth, but only 2 of them are normally palpable in a full-term baby—the anterior and the posterior. The posterior fontanel closes at approximately 2 months. The average time for closure of the anterior fontanel is usually stated as 18 months. However, in many robust, well-developed babies, it may be closed at 1 year or even earlier. The most common cause of delayed closure is rickets. Closure is delayed also in mongolism and cretinism. The sutures become ossified at from 6 to 9 months of age, though still capable of expansive growth. Premature closure of some of the sutures leads to growth of the skull in other directions, with consequent deformity. Separation of the sutures occurs with hydrocephalus.

The cranium enlarges in response to the growth of the brain for which it provides a closely fitting protective armor. Both the brain and the cranium are relatively far advanced at birth, continue to grow rapidly for the first 2 years and then slow down, since they have reached about 90 per cent of their final size by the age of 4 or 5 years. The functional changes which take place in the cranial contents, i.e., the main portion of the nervous system, are considered in Chapter 4.

At birth the facial portion of the skull is dwarfed by the overhanging cranium which is 8 or 9 times as large. The universal "cuteness" of babies is due in large measure to the smallness and the lack of differentiation of features. Facial growth proceeds downward and outward, at first slowly, later steadily continuing after cranial enlargement has practically ceased, until with puberty there is a rapid transformation into the final, grosser physiognomy of the adult. During this process the small edentulous jaw undergoes the greatest relative enlargement as it grows forward and downward to accommodate first the baby teeth and then the permanent set. The upper jaw enlarges also but at a somewhat slower rate. The retroussé nose, the flat cheekbones and the shallow orbits of the infant are slowly altered as the face grows to almost half the size of the cranium.

Teeth

Although newborn infants rarely display erupted teeth, the formation of both the first and the second set is well advanced within the substance of the jaw and can be demonstrated by x-ray examination. The enamel (outer) and the dentin (inner) portions of the crowns of the first teeth begin to form as early as the fourth month of fetal life. The permanent teeth, which do not appear until 6 years of age, begin to develop just before birth. Thus, since tooth formation is part of fetal development, the mother's

PERMANENT TEETH

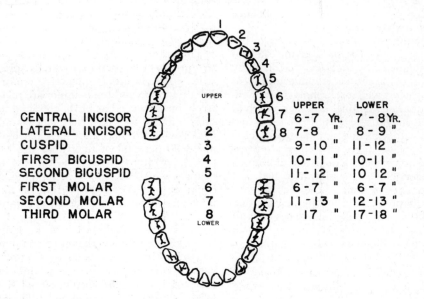

		UPPER	LOWER
CENTRAL INCISOR	1	6-7 YR.	7 - 8 YR.
LATERAL INCISOR	2	7-8 "	8 - 9 "
CUSPID	3	9-10 "	11-12 "
FIRST BICUSPID	4	10-11 "	10-11 "
SECOND BICUSPID	5	11-12 "	10 12 "
FIRST MOLAR	6	6-7 "	6 - 7 "
SECOND MOLAR	7	11-13 "	12-13 "
THIRD MOLAR	8	17 "	17-18 "

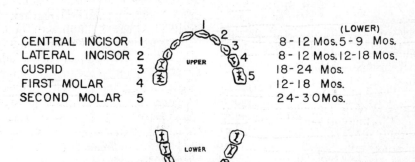

		(LOWER)	
CENTRAL INCISOR	1	8 - 12 Mos.	5 - 9 Mos.
LATERAL INCISOR	2	8 - 12 Mos.	12-18 Mos.
CUSPID	3	18-24 Mos.	
FIRST MOLAR	4	12-18 Mos.	
SECOND MOLAR	5	24-30 Mos.	

FIG. 10. Showing time of eruption of the teeth.

health, diet and nutrition play a considerable role in the character of the first dentition. In a similar way the early health and diet of the infant influences the soundness of his permanent teeth.

The time at which teeth erupt is subject to the same variation as other aspects of growth and development. The usual times of appearance of both the 20 deciduous, or first, set of teeth and the 32 permanent, or second, set are presented in Figure 10. In a rough way tooth development parallels the maturation of the bony structure and is under the same hormonal control. Because tooth eruption is so easily observed it is often a source of concern about the speed of maturation. Wide individual differences occur in otherwise normal infants. Sometimes the first tooth will erupt as early as 3 months; in others it may not appear until 14 months. However, delay in eruption which is associated with other signs of immaturity has greater significance.

The usual sequence of eruption of the deciduous teeth is tabulated below:

2 lower central incisors	
2 upper central incisors	6-12 months
2 upper lateral incisors	
2 lower lateral incisors	
4 anterior molars	12-15 months
4 canines	
4 posterior molars	15-30 months

By subtracting 6 from the age in months, the approximate number of teeth expected at each age up to 18 months is obtained. Excessive drooling which usually appears several weeks before the teeth is due to maturation of the salivary glands which are relatively inactive at birth. Drooling is due to the infant's inability to swallow saliva automatically. It has no particular relation to impending eruption of teeth. In most infants no symptoms of illness accompany teething. Occasionally irritability, slight fever or mild diarrhea may be associated. Since an infant is always in a potential teething period, symptoms of illness are too readily ascribed to this normal process, and the treatment of significant disease may be delayed by such an assumption.

The teeth of the first set are shed as those of the second set which are to replace them push against their roots. Thus the age at which deciduous teeth are lost corresponds closely to the time of eruption of the underlying permanent teeth. The permanent teeth are 32 in number and begin to erupt at about 6 years. The process is not completed until the 3rd molars or wisdom teeth erupt between 17 and 23 years of age. The following is an approximate schedule for the eruption of the permanent teeth:

4 first molars		
("6-year" molars)	5 to	7 years
4 central incisors	6½ to	8 years
4 lateral incisors	7 to	9 years
4 first bicuspids	9 to	11 years
4 second bicuspids	10 to	12 years
4 cuspids ("canines")	11 to	14 years
4 second molars	11½ to	13 years
4 third molars	14 to	23 years
		or more

The 4 first teeth of the permanent teeth to appear, the so-called "6-year" molars, do not replace any of the first set but come in behind the deciduous posterior molars and are exceedingly important teeth. Too often they are neglected because they are thought to be some of the first set of teeth, and caries in them remains untreated. Seventy-five per cent or more of school children are said to have caries of the first molars. It is around these teeth that the whole denture develops, and their loss affects the relation of all the teeth to the skull and modifies the shape of the face. The jaw from which these teeth have been lost prematurely remains much shorter than it would be normally, and the teeth do not meet effectively for mastication. Premature loss of the first teeth, often due to neglected caries, is a common cause of poor alignment of the second set. The child with carious or lost first teeth will not and cannot chew food well, thereby suffering a disadvantage in regard to both nutrition and jaw development.

SKIN AND HAIR

As part of the picture of physical growth we should note the changing picture in regard to skin and hair. At birth, the skin of the Caucasian is dark or bluish red, changing to a light pink in 2 weeks. "Rosy cheeks," a part of the traditional picture of healthy childhood, are not always present in the older child, since they seem to have a relationship to other factors as well as health, such as general coloring and racial inheritance. The newborn's color may be modified by jaundice, a not uncommon occurrence in the first week. A certain amount of desquamation is normally present during the first month, the amount and the depth varying widely with different babies. The sweat glands are inactive at birth. Their function gradually increases, and many babies are able to perspire freely after 1 month. "Goose flesh" is not an accomplishment of the very young baby.

Newborn babies present various pictures so far as hair is concerned, from the bald-headed baby to the one with hair that is relatively abundant and long. The hair at birth is very soft and usually dark. Loss of the first hair may occur soon, either because it falls out or because it is rubbed off by friction against the bed. The new hair, which will come in slowly, is of a firmer texture than the first and usually lighter. The very fair hair of early childhood tends to darken as the child grows older, although it may stay very fair throughout the growing years and for some years after maturity is reached.

At birth, fine downy hairs (lanugo) are often thickly distributed over the body, especially on the back and the legs. These disappear largely by the end of the first week. Occasionally, excessive hair is found, particularly on arms and legs in early childhood, but usually there is no noticeable hair on a child's body until puberty is reached.

The condition of the hair in childhood often gives us a clue to the child's nutrition. The child who is in good nutritional condition reflects it in glossy, strong hair. Dull, lifeless-looking hair is often part of the picture of poor nutrition.

HEART AND LUNGS

The thorax undergoes significant changes in both contour and movement between birth and adolescence. The newborn chest is short, thick in the anteroposterior dimension, and because of the horizontal direction of the ribs, it seems to remain in a position of full inspiration. These contours actually do limit the degree of change which the young infant can make in the volume of the underlying lungs. In order to maintain an adequate exchange of oxygen he must breathe more rapidly than the older individual and depend upon the activity of his diaphragm to augment pulmonary ventilation. Thus the small baby's chest moves through a very narrow range while his abdomen rises and falls in a wide arc. The stresses of exercise, excitement or fever markedly disturb the rate and the rhythm of the small infant's breathing. Even under ideal conditions of rest wide fluctuations in rate may occur. During growth the chest elongates, and the ribs adopt a downward slant, which permits a wider respiratory excursion. By the age of 5 or 6 years the adult configuration is present, and the respiratory rate has fallen accordingly.

The changes which take place in the heart at or shortly after birth are described in Chapter 18. Adaptation to extra-uterine circulation is usually complete within a day or two. The infant's heart is larger than the adult's relative to his total weight. While his body as a whole increases about 20 times during maturation, his heart enlarges only about 13 times. The more rapid metabolism of the infant is mainly responsible for the acceleration of heart rate which is normally observed. The volume of blood in his body is a little greater (slightly more than 10% of his body weight) than it will be in later life. Blood pressure is low in infancy, increases gradually during childhood and often undergoes a rise at adolescence which carries it temporarily above the adult range. These changes as well as changes in pulse and respiration rates are outlined in Table 1. Blood flow to the distal parts of the body is often sluggish in the small infant so that his feet in particular become cold and even blue in the absence of illness or chilling. This parsimonious distribution of blood to the legs is accounted for by their relative uselessness. Most of the infant's blood is being shunted around to more important organs in the head, the thorax and the abdomen.

DIGESTIVE SYSTEM

The abdomen of the infant and the young child often appears to be proportionally large. The weak abdominal muscles which cannot compress the loops of intestine when they distend with gas do not acquire sufficient strength to prevent his "pot-bellied" look until the infant has been walking erect for several years. In addition, his liver, which also must be housed in the abdominal cavity, is about twice as heavy relative to total body size as it will be at maturity. In spite of its size the liver is not as efficient in carrying out functions such as bilirubin excretion, the fabrication of plasma proteins and some of the steps in the metabolism of fat and carbohydrate as it will be later. The digestive tube itself is essentially a miniature copy of its adult counterpart. The minor differences in anatomy and physiology which have been described have only occasional clinical significance.

URINARY SYSTEM

Before birth the task of ridding the body of waste products is assumed by the mother through the placental circulation. The kidneys develop late but rapidly during the fetal period. At birth their size, like that of the heart and the liver, is nearly twice that of the adult when related to total body weight; but they are not as efficient in controlling the excretion of water and chemicals from the body until most of the first year of postnatal life has elapsed. Since the infant body contains a relatively large percentage of water which it turns over at a rapid rate it is not surprising that the immature kidneys fall short of the proper regulation of water and chemicals during the stress of disease. This accounts for the relative frequency of dehydration and acidosis among sick infants.

Rapid turnover of water within his body also results in a large daily excretion of urine in the infant and the small child. Since his bladder capacity is roughly proportional to his size, it is

TABLE 1. PULSE, RESPIRATION AND BLOOD PRESSURE RANGES
OF NORMAL CHILDREN AT VARIOUS AGES

| | RATE PER MINUTE | | MILLIMETERS OF MERCURY | |
Age	Respiration	Pulse	Systolic B.P.	Diastolic B.P.
First Month	30-80	120-150	....	....
First Year	20-40	100-140	....	....
Second Year	20-35	90-120	....	....
2-6 Years	20-30	90-110	60-110	40-75
6-10 Years	18-25	85-100	75-120	40-75
11-16 Years	16-23	75- 90	85-130	45-85

(Blood pressure data adapted from Downing, E. M.: Am. J. Dis. Child. 73:293, 1947)

necessary for him to urinate at shorter intervals than the older child or adult.

REPRODUCTIVE SYSTEM

During the conversion from functionally sexually immature child to fully developed adult, pronounced changes occur in body size and in social and emotional development. The latter will be considered in Chapter 4. The infant at birth possesses a full complement of the reproductive organs which mark him definitely as male or female. These organs, the primary sex characteristics, are small in size and remain functionally dormant until the second decade of life. Then, under the stimulus of hormones secreted by the pituitary gland, profound changes take place which convert the child from an individual who is relatively sexless in appearance to one who displays the distinctive appearance (the secondary sex characteristics) of his sex and is able functionally to play his part in reproduction.

The pubertal changes which occur in girls affect all tissues of the body. In girls, such changes may begin as early as the 10th year. Under the influence of estrogens produced by the developing ovaries, the bony pelvis enlarges and broadens, and the hips become rounded. First the nipples and then the breasts begin to bud. Later the nipples become pigmented. Hair appears in the pubic region and later in the axilla. The vagina enlarges, and its secretions become more profuse and acid in reaction. While these external changes are taking place, the ovaries and the uterus are enlarging and are beginning to acquire the periodicity of function which eventually produces menstruation. The first menstrual period is termed the menarche and is the official onset of puberty. In the United States it occurs most commonly between 11 and 15 years but occasionally is seen earlier or later. Irregularities in the appearance and the duration of the periods is not uncommon during the first 2 years. At some point during this time interval the girl acquires the ability to reproduce. The estrogenic substances not only influence the skeleton by stimulating growth in height but they also limit this growth by fostering closure of the epiphyseal lines. Consequently, while the girl initiates her spurt in growth earlier than the boy, she is likely to approach her ultimate height early in her teens, whereas the boy may continue to grow into his twenties.

The pubertal changes which occur in boys are equally marked. They begin about 2 years later than in girls. Under the influence of androgenic substances produced in the testes, the penis and the testes begin to enlarge. Hair appears in the pubic region, then on the face and in the axilla. Changes take place in the larynx which make the voice more resonant and lower in pitch. For a time the control over pitch may be uncertain, so that sudden breaks occur during speech. The skeleton is not only influenced to grow in length but also tends to become broader and more sturdy, and there is a dramatic increase in the mass of muscles. There is no externally apparent sign which signalizes the ability to reproduce. Production of spermatozoa probably begins at 13 to 15 years of age but cannot be determined readily.

LYMPHATIC TISSUE

Lymphatic tissue plays an important role in resistance to disease. It is the seat of origin of the predominant white blood cell of infancy (the lymphocyte). The lymph nodes act as filters through which infectious agents must pass on their way from the outside of the body toward general dissemination by the blood stream. Recently it has been recognized that antibodies are produced in lymphatic tissues. At birth the elements of this tissue are well developed but not particularly conspicuous. During infancy and childhood, perhaps in part due to normal maturation and in part due to repeated exposure to new infectious agents, the various lymphatic centers enlarge. Those which are observed easily are the tonsils, adenoids and the palpable subcutaneous lymph nodes in the neck, the axilla and the groin. For a time enlargement is cumulative. The immediate response to an acute infection subsides incompletely, leaving the lymph node or the tonsil a bit larger than it was. Later in childhood infections make less impression, and there is actually a regression in size of the lymphatic structures. In recent years there is a growing tendency to leave large adenoids and tonsils alone, waiting for spontaneous atrophy to take place rather than subjecting the child to a surgical operation.

The thymus and the spleen are also part of the lymphatic apparatus. These masses are comparatively large at birth and tend to diminish in relative size. Formerly, the dramatic shadows cast in the chest roentgenogram by a large thymus gland were regarded as dangerous to the child's safety, foreshadowing possible obstruction of the trachea. From careful study of the development of the normal thymus it has now been concluded that such shadows are harmless and that they melt away rapidly during the first 2 years of life.

SITUATIONS FOR FURTHER STUDY

1. Observe a normal newborn baby and a 5-year-old child during an hour of wakefulness and describe their muscular and intellectual skills and emotional controls. Contrast the body proportions and the behavior of these 2 individuals. What changes have come about as the result of growth? What changes have come about as a result of development? What factors influenced the growth changes? The developmental changes? What did you learn from this observational study which has professional significance to you?

2. What factors must a nurse take into account when she evaluates a child's health and progress?

3. Why are ranges in growth measurements more meaningful than averages?

4. In what period of fetal life is growth must crucial? What makes it a crucial period? How can prenatal care during that period influence growth of the fetus? Why is prenatal care during that period so often neglected? Would health education during adolescence be one way of ensuring better health for the pregnant woman and her unborn child? How would it?

5. How does the rate of growth during the first year of life compare with that which occurs during fetal life?

6. How does knowledge of rapid growth during the first year of life influence your feelings toward babies?

7. Growth occurs in spurts and lags. What effect might this knowledge have on a mother's feelings toward and care of her child?

8. Describe the use of growth curves.

9. In what ways might a nurse use knowledge of bone growth?

10. What do you consider to be the most important facts concerning dentition?

11. What purpose does knowledge of infant kidney function serve on behalf of the nurse?

BIBLIOGRAPHY

Jackson, R. L., and Kelly, H. G.: Growth charts for use in pediatric practice, J. Pediat. 27:215, 1945.

Stuart, H. C., and Stevenson, S. S.: Physical growth and development in Nelson's Textbook of Pediatrics, ed. 6, Philadelphia, Saunders, 1954.

Washburn, A. H.: The appraisal of

healthy growth and development from birth to adolescence *in* Brenneman's Practice of Pediatrics, vol. 1, Hagerstown, Md., Prior, 1957.

Watson, E. H., and Lowrey, G. H.: Growth and Development of Children, ed. 2, Chicago, Year Book Pub., 1954.

Wetzel, N. C.: Assessing physical condition of children, J. Pediat. **22**:82, 208, 329, 1943.

CHAPTER THREE

Nutritional Requirements and Diet

The human body requires a continuing supply of oxygen, water and food to support its vital functions.

Oxygen is the most critical of these imports, for the body has no reserve on which to draw. During health the supply is monitored by reflex control of respiration which operates automatically no matter what the state of consciousness. If the intake is interrupted for more than a few minutes, the oxidative chemical reactions which drive the body machinery come to a halt, and life ebbs rapidly. Hence disease or accident which threatens the oxygen supply is an immediate medical emergency.

Deprivation of fluid can be tolerated for a few days while the body draws upon its reserves. But the continuance of water loss from the skin and the lungs and through the urine and the stools eventually concentrates the body fluids and seriously impedes its vital chemical reactions. The instinct of thirst assures an adequate water intake when the accessible supply is unlimited and when losses from the body are not excessive.

During complete starvation the body may survive for 2 or 3 weeks or even longer by consuming its normal nutrient reserves and its own tissues. In health and with a plentiful supply, the instinct of hunger forces a sufficient quantitative intake of food and to some degree guides the selection of types of food. Unlike oxygen and water, which are simple chemical substances and subserve straightforward functions within the body, food is a broad category enclosing a very wide variety of substances needed by the body as fuel to provide energy, and as building blocks to repair old tissues and to fabricate the new ones required by growth.

The science of nutrition is concerned with determining the amounts of the various food components—protein, carbohydrate, fat, vitamins and minerals—which are required not merely to support life but also to provide the best opportunity for growth and the maintenance of health. For many of the dietary constituents *minimum* levels of intake have been determined with some accu-

33

racy. It is usually more difficult to fix *optimum* levels; consequently, authorities are not always in agreement when recommending goals in dietary construction. To supplement knowledge of requirements, the nutritionist must be skilled in making foods attractive and acceptable. Science can put a complete diet on the plate, but it often requires art to convey it to the stomach.

WATER

Approximately 70 per cent of the body weight is water. It is the basic constituent of the cells in which the important chemical reactions take place, of the interstitial fluid which lies between the cells, of the transport fluids such as blood, lymph and spinal fluid, and of the various excretions from the body—sweat, urine, bile and intestinal juices. Under usual conditions of climate and physical activity a grownup gets along with about a quart of fluid per day. But a small infant, only one twentieth of the adult's weight, will need one third as much. The reason lies in the greater speed of the infant's metabolism. Consequently, his fluid requirements parallel his heat production or oxygen consumption which are considered below.

The older child can be expected to cover his modest water needs (30 to 50 ml. per Kg. per day) by satisfying his thirst. He obtains fluid not only from the liquid components of his diet but also from the significant water content of many foods which we commonly regard as "solid." Technics for assuring an adequate fluid intake during illness are considered in Chapter 9.

In infancy the rate of water turnover within the body is much more rapid; from 100 to 150 ml. per Kg. of weight must be ingested each day in order to keep pace with normal fluid losses. Both the natural and the artificial sources of food for the infant are very dilute liquids so that his water needs are usually satisfied if he is being fed properly. But since the infant is unable to go after water when he becomes thirsty, closer supervision of his intake is essential. An uncertain breast milk supply, hot weather, fever, or losses in the stool or by vomiting can lead to dehydration much more rapidly than in the adult or even in the older child. In practice it is usually sufficient to offer water once or twice a day during health and to permit the infant's thirst to decide whether or not he is in arrears.

ENERGY

Like any machine the body must have a source of energy in order to perform its work. Food serves two purposes: (1) it provides fuel which is burned in the body, consuming oxygen in the process and liberating energy and heat, and (2) it provides chemical substances needed in the construction of new tissues. Both purposes must be considered in determining requirements or in planning or evaluating diets. In practice it is simplest to begin by considering the total amount of fuel or energy needed per day. Then the proportion of different types of fuel (protein, carbohydrate and fat) within the total amount is determined. Finally, a check is made to be sure that the necessary vitamins and minerals are included.

The energy content of foods is rated in calories, i.e., the amount of heat they will produce when burned in the body. A large calorie (the unit employed in metabolic work) is defined as the amount of heat necessary to raise 1 liter of water by $1°$ C. By experimental methods it can be shown that carbohydrates and proteins when burned in the body yield on the average about 4 calories per gram; whereas fat provides about 9 calories per gram.

The speed at which the body uses energy is called the metabolic rate. It can be determined directly by measuring the amount of heat given off from the body. If 1,500 calories are given off per day, an equivalent amount of fuel will have to be ingested as food in order to provide this amount of energy. In clinical practice it is less cumbersome to measure the amount of oxygen used in the combustion, a figure which necessarily parallels exactly the rate of heat production. This can be done by determining the amount of oxygen extracted from the air which goes into and out of the lungs during a standard period of time. Metabolic measurements of this kind are made under standardized conditions called the *basal state*. Ideally, this is a state of minimum body work in which the subject should be in good health, rested, relaxed, not digesting food and performing no unnecessary muscular work. Such conditions are obviously difficult to obtain when working with infants or small children, but a number of patient investigators have been able to determine fairly accurately the basal requirements of children and even of premature infants.

Basal energy requirements are proportionately high during the early months of life (55 to 60 calories per Kg. of body weight per day) and taper off gradually to approximately half this level at maturity. In addition to this fuel which is required for the minimum housekeeping activities of the body, energy is needed for muscular contraction, for growth, for the work of digesting food (specific dynamic activity) and to cover an inevitable loss in the stools. Individual infants and children vary considerably both in the speed at which they grow and in the amount of physical activity they perform. Consequently, it is difficult to make precise predictions of the total amount of fuel that a given child will require. Few infants will remain satisfied and grow on less than 80 calories/Kg./day; most of them require from 100 to 120; and a few rapid growers or physically live wires may burn up 150 or even more. Similar individual variations must be allowed for older children. Psychological factors and cultural eating habits play an increasing role in total food consumption as the child grows older. A rough method of predicting the minimum number of total calories required by children between infancy and adolescence is to allow 1,000 calories plus 100 additional for each year of age.

FOODS

PROTEIN

Protein is an essential part of all living cells. As the cells function, protein is used up and needs to be replaced. Additional supplies are demanded by growth. Protein or proteinlike substances serve important specialized functions such as plasma proteins, hemoglobin, antibodies, enzymes and hormones. Unlike plants, which can manufacture proteins from simple substances which they absorb from the air and the soil, animals are unable to build proteins anew and must consume them preformed in their food. During digestion the complex proteins are broken down into their basic units, the amino acids, which are then absorbed and rearranged into new protein substances specifically designed to suit the needs of the human tissues. They are indispensable. Neither men nor animals can live for any considerable portion of time without them. In their absence, growth ceases, the muscles become feeble, resistance to infection is low, and anemia develops.

Composition

Proteins are alike in that they are all made up of amino acids in various combinations. At least 22 amino acids are known to be constituents of proteins. The possible combinations of amino acids to form proteins are almost infinite, each combination having its own special characteristics as a protein. Ten of these amino acids are essential in the diet, in that the body must have them and cannot construct them. Others are useful to the body, though they are not essential. Proteins are said to be complete when they contain all the essential amino acids. Many proteins are incomplete. In order to be useful in meeting the protein need, they must be supplemented by other proteins which contain the remainder of the essential amino acids. Most animal proteins are complete, e.g., those of milk and meat. Relatively few vegetable proteins supply all the essential amino acids adequately when taken alone.

One of the constituents of protein is nitrogen. It occurs in all proteins in approximately the same proportion. The amount in the diet in materials other than protein is quantitatively unimportant. Consequently, the determination of the amount of nitrogen in foods constitutes an easy method of estimating the amount of protein. From the amount of nitrogen excreted in the urine may be estimated the amount of protein which has been split in the body to its physiologic end-products. After growth has ceased, the amount of nitrogen (protein) ingested and the amount excreted should be equal, a condition known as nitrogen equilibrium. If the amount excreted is greater than the amount ingested, body protein is being burned. If ingestion exceeds excretion, protein is being stored. During growth, protein is being added to the body constantly and the amount of nitrogen ingested is in excess of that excreted. A growing child requires more protein in proportion to size than one who has stopped growing.

Protein Requirement of the Infant

Estimates of the protein requirement of the infant have been based largely on the amounts of protein received when infants are breast-fed and thriving. In these circumstances the amount of protein ingested is from 2 to 2.5 Gm. daily for each Kg. of body weight. When human milk is unavailable, cow's milk is the customary substitute. It is a widely accepted concept that cow's-milk protein is biologically inferior to human-milk protein because of the difference in relative proportions of essential amino acids. On the basis that it may be inferior by approximately 20 per cent, the protein requirement when cow's milk is fed is from 2.5 to 3 Gm. for each Kg. When cow's milk is fed to infants in customary quantities, the protein intake is at least 3.5 Gm. for each Kg., sometimes as much as 4.5 Gm. The excess over the theoretical requirement is well utilized and produces increased growth. Infants tolerate well any amount of protein that it is possible to give them as undiluted milk provided that some means has been used to adapt it to their digestion. Sometimes, when babies are allergic to cow's milk, vegetable preparations, such as soybean "milk," are used in substitution. Soybean protein is complete, but a much larger quantity must be fed in order that all essential amino acids be present in sufficient amount. The amount of soybean protein fed is commonly 50 per cent more than that of cow's milk.

Protein Requirement of the Child

The total amount of protein required by the child increases with the age, but the amount for each unit of body weight gradually decreases. The requirement is met amply by 3 Gm. daily for each Kg. at from 1 to 3 years of age, 2.75 Gm. at from 4 to 6 years, 2.5 Gm. at from 7 to 9 years, 2 Gm. at from 10 to 14 years, 1.5 Gm. at from 16 to 20 years, 1 Gm. for adults. These values have been computed on the basis of a mixed diet in which some of the protein is not of high biologic value. Of the foods supplying a good type of protein in abundance, the more important are milk, eggs, meat, cheese and the legumes. The animal proteins are to be emphasized particularly, and special emphasis is to be placed on milk. A quart of milk supplies most of the protein requirement of the young child and half the requirement at 12 years. Without milk, a satisfactory protein intake for the child is not possible when only customary diets are considered. Protein deficiency among children is much more common than is generally recognized. Insufficient protein leads to impairment of growth, often in ways undetectable by physical examination. For example, the amount of muscle in the body, as determined by creatinine excretion, is commonly less than that which may be considered as normal and is easily attainable by ingestion of the stated protein allowances.

FAT

Fats consist of a chemical combination of glycerin and fatty acids. They differ from each other by reason of the differences in the fatty acids. Certain fatty acids (linoleic and arachidonic) have been found to be essential for some animals on which experiments were made. It is possible that they may be important also for the human, but the necessity for them has not been proved. In fact, young children have been maintained in an excellent state of nutrition for long periods with negligible amounts of fat in the diet. Aside from the possibility that certain fat components may be essential, fat does not appear to be a necessary constituent of the diet, and so no fat requirement exists. The chief nutritional function of fat in the diet is to supply energy, and in this respect it can be replaced completely by carbohydrate. However, certain fats are highly desirable in the diet because they contain fat-soluble vitamins which are essential, though these vitamins may be supplied by special preparations if necessary. Fats are desirable also because they furnish considerably more energy for each unit of weight than protein or carbohydrate, thus conserving the functions of digestion and absorption and distributing the burden of energy production among a greater number of body functions. Also, fats contribute materially to the palatability of the diet, and without them insufficient total food is likely to be ingested if the amount is left to choice.

CARBOHYDRATE

The chief function of carbohydrate is to supply energy. It is an essential constituent of the body. Carbohydrate becomes available through the breakdown of protein and, to some extent, of fat. While it is theoretically possible to derive sufficient carbohydrate from these sources, it is much more practical to consider that a carbohydrate requirement exists. A certain amount of energy must be derived from sources other than fat in order to spare fat combustion. The capacity of the body to burn fat completely is limited. When the energy requirements demand that an excessive amount of fat be consumed, ketone bodies are formed which in excessive amount may create acidosis. Incomplete combustion of fat may be avoided if at least one fifth as much carbohydrate is burned simultaneously. In the usual diet, the amount of carbohydrate taken in is far in excess of this minimum, and it is seldom necessary to worry about the carbohydrate requirement. When carbohydrate is consumed, as it frequently is, in amounts which exceed immediate energy needs, it is stored in the body as fat.

MINERALS

Numerous minerals are essential for life and growth. Most of them are present in customary diets in ample amount. Only those likely to be deficient will be discussed.

In the case of the infant, all the essential minerals are supplied by either human or cow's milk with the exception of iron and possibly copper. Normally, at birth the liver contains a small store of iron and copper. The store of iron is increased considerably in the first 2 months by the breakdown of hemoglobin in the change from the high level of hemoglobin at birth to the lower level normal for infancy. During good health, this store is not exhausted for several months. In order to maintain the store, the addition of iron to the diet is necessary at 2 or 3 months of age. Although it is not essential that the store be fully maintained, the addition of iron is desirable before the store is exhausted. Iron-containing foods should be given not later than 4 months of age. Special attention to copper seems to be unnecessary.

Infants born prematurely are handicapped in numerous ways, among others by small stores of iron and calcium. The percentage of hemoglobin is the same as for babies born at term, and the total amount of blood is proportionate to body size, but the size is small, and the infant is expected to grow rapidly to overcome his size handicap. Thus proportionately larger amounts of iron are required and they are needed earlier than for the baby born at term. A somewhat similar situation exists in regard to calcium. Almost all the calcium of the body is present as a part of bone structure. Most of the prenatal calcification of bone occurs in the last 3 months of fetal life, and about one half of it occurs in the last 4 weeks.

In order that prematurely born babies may maintain normal bone structure, it is necessary that special consideration be given to the calcium content of the food.

For the child over 2 years of age, the minerals requiring discussion are chiefly calcium and iodine. Deficiency of iron is not common. Iron is supplied by meat, liver, eggs and green vegetables. Iodine is present in sufficient amounts in foods grown and produced in regions where iodine exists in the soil and the water. Sea foods are excellent natural sources of iodine. Iodine is lacking in the soil of a large area round the Great Lakes and in the Pacific Northwest. Since iodine is an essential, the small amounts necessary should be supplied to those living in iodine-deficient regions. The most convenient method of obtaining satisfactory, though minimum, amounts is the use of iodized salt. Iodine is discussed further under Simple Goiter.

Sufficient calcium is obtained by children who receive at least 1½ pints of milk up to adolescence and a quart during the rapid growth period of adolescence. Milk, including milk products, is the one good food source of calcium. A quart of milk supplies from 4 to 6 times as much calcium as all the remainder of the day's diet. Calcium deficiency of some degree is extremely common because for one reason or another many children do not receive their quota of milk. These same children are very likely also to be receiving insufficient protein and certain other nutritional essentials. Deficiency of calcium is one of the factors responsible for tooth decay. It also causes osteoporosis, a condition of undermineralization of bone which is independent of rickets.

VITAMINS

Vitamin is a term applied to certain organic substances which are essential in minute amounts and cannot be synthesized in the body. A few of the vitamins have a somewhat similar function, but most of them are entirely unrelated, and their inclusion in a single group is a result of historic development. One vitamin cannot replace another. Each must be supplied in the required amount in order to ensure good growth and health. As a part of the historic development of our knowledge, the vitamins have been divided into fat-soluble and water-soluble groups. The fat-soluble group includes vitamins A, D and K; the water-soluble group includes the vitamins of the B complex and vitamin C. The designation of the vitamins by letter resulted from the recognition of the existence of the materials by identification of their functions before their chemical structures became known. Most of them have been identified chemically and have been synthesized. Gradually, the chemical names are replacing the letter designations. When vitamins were known only in terms of their function, they were measured quantitatively in terms of biologic units. Now that most of these materials have been identified chemically, units are being replaced gradually by weight. The present mixture of letters and chemical names and of units and milligrams represents a stage in the development of knowledge.

VITAMIN A

Vitamin A is a term usually applied to both vitamin A itself and certain carotenoid pigments which are converted to vitamin A in the liver. Vitamin A is colorless; carotene or provitamin A is yellow. Most of the vitamin A of the usual diet is present as carotene. Its chief sources are the leafy and the yellow vegetables. Vitamin A is present along with carotene in milk and products prepared from milk fat and in egg yolk. Liver is an excellent source, the fish-liver oils being the richest natural source. Vitamin A is utilized more efficiently than is carotene. Neither material is affected to an important degree by the usual processes of cooking. Vitamin A

is stored in the body, chiefly in the liver, and a goodly store is to be considered as normal.

The functions of vitamin A, as of other vitamins, have been studied first with animals by depriving them of it. It is not known whether all the findings of experiments apply to the human, as, for example, defective ovulation in the mature animal and the occurrence of certain congenital malformations (cleft lip and palate) in the offspring when the mother has been maintained in a state of partial deficiency. Vitamin A is essential for growth, for the formation of normal teeth and bones, for ability to adapt quickly to vision in a dim light from that in a bright light, and for the maintenance of a normal state of epithelial structures.

The vitamin-A requirement varies with the size or the weight of the body. The requirement of the young infant is met easily by the content of either human or cow's milk when these are average. The customary additions to the milk diet as the infant becomes older increase the intake to maintain it at a level fully adequate. In fact, at all ages any reasonably good diet supplies adequate vitamin A without resort to special preparations of this material. Important deficiency of intake occurs only with diets which depart markedly from a satisfactory pattern. Even with a good intake of vitamin A, deficiency may arise from poor utilization. Utilization becomes markedly impaired by illness, particularly acute infection. The allowance of vitamin A recommended has been placed at 2,500 units at from 4 to 6 years, 3,500 units at from 7 to 9 years, 4,500 units at from 10 to 12 years, and 5,000 units at all periods after 13 years, except in the case of women during pregnancy and lactation and of boys from 16 to 20 years of age, when it is larger.

VITAMIN D

Vitamin D can be produced in the

body by the action of ultraviolet light upon cholesterol in the skin. In this way primitive children can manufacture enough to meet their needs if they have a daily exposure to the midday sun lasting about 15 minutes. The civilized child can obtain the same effect on a beach in summer or from a shorter exposure to a mercury vapor lamp indoors in the winter. However, civilized living in temperate climates is likely to interfere with the natural formation of vitamin D in adequate amounts. The ultraviolet rays which have waves less than 320 millimicrons in length, are filtered out by ordinary window glass and by atmospheric conditions such as clouds, smog and the oblique passage of light from the sun through the earth's atmosphere. Adequate exposure of the child's skin is further hampered by clothing and by the fact that he spends much time indoors, particularly during the cold seasons. Consequently, it is unwise to rely upon the automatic production of vitamin D in the skin, and adequate amounts must be supplied with the diet.

Vitamin D is present in ordinary foods in unimportant quantities only. It occurs in small amounts in milk, butter and egg yolk. Liver is a good source, the liver oils of fish being the richest natural source. Vitamin D is prepared artificially by irradiation of cholesterol, an animal product, or ergosterol, a vegetable product. Activated ergosterol, when purified to contain only vitamin D, is known as calciferol. Inconclusive evidence indicates that activated cholesterol and naturally occurring vitamin D may be somewhat superior to activated ergosterol in effectiveness for humans, but the difference, if any, is small. Vitamin D is relatively stable and resists destruction in the various processes of cooking food. Vitamin D may be stored to some extent, chiefly in the liver.

The function of vitamin D is to improve and regulate the utilization of calcium and phosphorus of the diet. Vitamin-D deficiency is known to lead to rickets and tetany in the infant and to osteomalacia in the adult. It leads also to subnormal mineralization of teeth and bones in the growing child, even though rickets may not be clinically evident.

Except for children who are consistently exposed to the sun, vitamin D should be offered regularly as part of the diet. The speed of growth and consequently of bone formation determines to a considerable degree how much vitamin D is required. For this reason the infant's small body must have between 400 and 800 units per day, the same amount required by the much larger body of the adolescent or the adult. Premature infants who grow at the most rapid rate of all require from 800 to 1,200 units per day. Originally, vitamin D was given as cod-liver oil in a dose of 1 or 2 teaspoonfuls per day. The large volume and the objectionable smell have been overcome by preparing concentrates of other fish-liver oils with approximately 100 times the vitamin D content of cod-liver oil. These and synthetic preparations of vitamin D have largely replaced the old-fashioned vehicle. Vitamin D can also be added to milk in amounts which almost completely satisfy the child's daily requirement. In the United States most large dairies so fortify the fresh milk they produce, and nearly all brands of evaporated milk contain 400 units in each reconstituted quart. When practically all the available milk is fortified, rickets disappears. A common practice in infant feeding is to make assurance doubly sure by giving fortified milk and a vitamin D supplement in addition. Although overdosage of vitamin D may interfere with appetite and result in abnormalities of the calcium metabolism of the body, these toxic symptoms generally appear only when intakes of 5 to 10 times the minimum daily requirements are maintained consistently for several weeks.

Vitamin E

Vitamin E (tocopherol) deficiency in animal experimentation leads to sterility in both sexes, and when females have received only minimum amounts their young have muscular dysfunction similar to muscular dystrophy of the human. It is believed that vitamin E may be necessary for muscle development. Satisfactory evidence of deficiency in the human has not been presented. Vitamin E has a distribution so wide that any mixed diet contains an abundance. It is present in foods of animal origin—less abundant in those tissues rich in vitamin A, more abundant in muscle. It is present in green vegetables and vegetable oils, and it is particularly abundant in wheat germ oil. It is relatively stable, though it may be destroyed under conditions which produce rancidity.

Vitamin K

Vitamin K as found naturally in food is a fat-soluble material, chemically a naphthoquinone which has been given the name *menadione*. Other and synthetic derivatives of naphthoquinone have vitamin-K activity, and some are water-soluble. Vitamin K is found in many foods and also is synthesized in the intestinal tract by fecal bacteria. Deficiencies occur in the newborn infant before abundant implantation of bacteria in the intestine and at any age when absorption is impaired by absence of bile. Vitamin K is necessary for the formation of prothrombin, a material essential for blood coagulation. Deficiency leads to a tendency to bleed, a condition discussed under Hemorrhagic Disease of the Newborn.

Vitamin B Complex

Vitamin B complex includes thiamine (B$_1$), riboflavin (B$_2$ or G), niacin (nicotinic acid) and many other components. These substances are found in the same foods, though the proportion of each to the others varies in different foods. Deficiency of only one B vitamin is rare, but often one may be more deficient than others. Thiamine, riboflavin and niacin, and probably other members of the complex, are components of enzymes necessary for cell respiration.

Thiamine

Thiamine deficiency, when severe, causes beriberi. Deficiency of lesser degree may cause certain varieties of neuritis and neurosis (see Beriberi). Thiamine is necessary for normal appetite and gastro-intestinal function and for successful lactation. Impairment of growth may result from poor appetite. Thiamine has been synthesized on a commercial scale and is available abundantly in crystalline form. In nature it is found in important amounts in whole-grain cereals, peanuts, yeast and lean meat, especially pork and liver. It is found in smaller amounts in many foods, including milk, eggs, vegetables and fruits. It has been added in small amounts to enriched flour and bread. Despite its fairly wide distribution, it is the B component most likely to be deficient in the average diet. It is easily destroyed by heat, the usual cooking processes resulting in an average loss of 25 per cent or more. It is water-soluble and often is discarded with the water of cooking. Thiamine is necessary for the combustion of carbohydrate, and the requirement is proportional to the nonfat calories of the diet. Recommended allowances vary from 0.4 mg. in the first year to 1.5 mg. at 15 years for average diets, or 0.05 mg. for each 100 calories of the diet.

Riboflavin

Riboflavin deficiency in the human, when severe and chronic, produces characteristic changes in the eyes and about the mouth. The eye changes show first in the conjunctiva about the cornea, where small blood vessels become enlarged and visible. These changes are associated with photophobia, lacrimation, burning sensation and dimness of vision known as twilight blindness. Subsequently, interstitial keratitis may develop. In the mouth, the tongue becomes inflamed, and inflammatory fissures and maceration appear in the skin and the mucous membrane at the corners of the mouth (cheilitis). More severe effects have been observed in experiments on animals. Riboflavin is necessary for growth, and probably also for successful lactation. Riboflavin is a yellow pigment, stable to the heat of cooking but destroyed by exposure to light. The best source in the daily diet is milk. The customary milk formula supplies the requirement of the infant, and a quart of milk supplies most, if not all, of the requirement of the child. Riboflavin is present in important amounts also in liver, egg yolk, meat, whole-grain cereals and green vegetables, but the requirement is not likely to be met from these sources without the inclusion of milk in the diet. The appropriate allowance for riboflavin is approximately 50 per cent greater than that for thiamine, namely 0.6 mg. in the first year, increasing to 2.0 mg. at 15 years.

Niacin (Nicotinic Acid)

Niacin deficiency causes pellagra. This vitamin exists commercially both as the acid and as its amide. No common food is a rich source of this material, but liver, lean meat, eggs, whole-grain cereals, enriched bread, wheat germ and yeast have it in important amounts. The amount in milk is small, both human and cow's, approximately 1 mg. to the liter. However, it is well established that the dietary requirement for niacin decreases when milk is contained in the diet, presumably because of bacterial synthesis in the intestine. The appropriate allowance of niacin is 10 times that of thiamine in all age groups. The material is stable to usual food handling.

Other B-Complex Factors

Other B-complex factors exist which are known to be essential for experimental animals and presumably are important in human nutrition. Folic acid under ordinary circumstances is produced in the intestine by the bacteria that dwell therein. After heavy antibiotic therapy this source of supply may be cut off because the bacteria are destroyed. Folic acid normally requires an adequate amount of vitamin C to convert it into folinic acid (citrovorum factor) which in turn is essential in the formation of nucleic acids. Disturbance of this complicated chain of chemical events may result in megaloblastic anemia because of inadequate formation of red blood cell protein. Pyridoxine (B_6) is also essential in human metabolism but can be lacking from the average diet only under very special circumstances. A few instances of convulsions in infants have been traced to its destruction during the preparation of commercial canned milk formulas. The remaining members of the B-complex are choline, biotin, inositol and pantothenic acid. Their essentiality in human nutrition has not been proved. The incompleteness of our knowledge about the details of vitamin requirements emphasizes the wisdom of depending upon a mixed diet for nutritional essentials rather than on special preparations of the known vitamins.

ASCORBIC ACID (VITAMIN C)

Ascorbic-acid deficiency causes scurvy. Vitamin C probably is necessary for all living cells. It is found most abundantly in actively growing cells. The effects of deficiency are most apparent in bones, teeth and small blood vessels. Capillary hemorrhages are characteristic of severe deficiency, the hemorrhages presumably being caused by defective growth of connective tissue supporting structure about the capillaries and loss of cement substance between the cells of capillary walls. ~~Ascorbic acid is essential for growth of connective tissue and consequently for normal wound healing~~. Ascorbic acid is destroyed easily by oxidation in neutral or alkaline media, less easily in an acid medium. Destruction is hastened by heat, and cooking often destroys a high proportion. In view of these facts, the importance of fresh foods in the diet becomes apparent. Ascorbic acid is present in many fruits and vegetables. The citrus fruits are relatively rich sources. The juice of ripe oranges may be considered to contain an average of 50 mg. of ascorbic acid to 100 cc. Canned frozen orange juice retains nearly all of this vitamin C activity but should be used soon after thawing and diluting. Tomato juice, fresh or canned, is a good source of vitamin C, although it has a content smaller and more variable than orange juice. The vitamin C content varies with the soil and the region in which the tomatoes are grown. It varies with the amount of sunshine during the ripening stage. Some tomato juices contain approximately 25 mg. of ascorbic acid to 100 cc., while other samples contain only half as much. When the poorer varieties are used, the volume required to meet the needs of an infant are excessive. Fresh cow's milk contains approximately 20 mg. to the quart, pasteurized milk about one third less. Reconstituted dried milk contains 12 mg., and reconstituted evaporated milk 6 mg. to the quart. The amount in human milk depends on the diet of the mother. With a good intake of vitamin C the milk may contain as much as 75 mg. to the quart. However, average human milk contains much less, possibly from 40 to 50 mg. to the quart. The requirement of the young infant may be considered to be 20 mg. daily. Such an amount cannot be received by the artificially fed baby without supplementing the milk formula. At birth the amount of ascorbic acid in the blood is proportionately greater than that in the mother's blood. The amount decreases rapidly, and by the 10th day in artificially fed babies it reaches a level that would lead to scurvy if allowed to persist. Thus vitamin C supplements should be given to artificially fed babies soon after birth. The recommended allowance for ascorbic acid increases with size or age from about 30 mg. in the first year to 80 mg. at 15 years.

MULTIPLE-VITAMIN PREPARATIONS

A great many preparations are marketed for the purpose of ensuring protection against deficiency of any of the known vitamins. For infants such preparations are prepared as drops that may be squirted into the mouth or admixed with formula; for older children they take the form of capsules or palatable liquids to be given by spoon. The virtue of the daily administration of such preparations has been grossly overstated by the advertising campaigns of the manufacturers, and it is undoubtedly true that many children take quantities that are superfluous, particularly when they are receiving adequate well-mixed diets. If carried to extremes the lavish use of some of the vitamins may result in toxic reactions. It is doubtful if any but economic harm results from the practice of giving 2 or 3 times the calculated daily requirement.

SELECTION OF THE DIET

The rate of growth of the child is determined to a considerable extent by the kind and the amount of food he is given. Defects in the diet may cause malnutrition and sometimes serious illness; they may lead to lowered resistance to infection and to intellectual inertia. A lack of knowledge even of general dietary principles and the mistaken belief that whatever satisfies hunger is suitable food often are reasons why mothers permit children to make

TABLE 2. A DIET OF COMMON FOODS SUITABLE FOR A 12-YEAR-OLD CHILD, WITH TABULATION OF ITS CONTENT OF CERTAIN ESSENTIAL NUTRIENTS

	WEIGHT (GM.)	CALORIES	PROTEIN (GM.)	FAT (GM.)	CHO (GM.)
Milk (fortified), 1 qt.	976	666	34.2	38.1	48.0
Egg[1]	54	77	6.1	5.1	0.3
Meat,[1] 1 serving	65	130	15.9	7.3	0
Fruit,[2] 2 servings	200	157	1.4	0.6	36.6
Nonstarchy vegetables,[3] 2 servings	185	66	4.8	0.4	10.8
Starchy vegetables or substitutes,[4] 2 servings	200	205	6.6	0.8	43.0
Enriched bread, 5 slices	125	338	11.0	4.0	64.8
Cereal (breakfast),[5] 1 serving	20	76	2.1	0.5	15.9
Starchy dessert,[6] 1 serving	120	261	4.4	9.9	38.5
Butter, 3 tblsp.	42	300	.3	33.9	.3
Cheese	10	43	2.8	3.5	. . .
Peanut butter, 1 tbsp.	16	92	4.2	7.6	3.4
Sugar*	30	120	0	0	30.0
Cooking fat, 1 tbsp.	15	135	0	15.0	. . .
Total		2,666	93.8		
Recommended allowance 12-year-old		2,500	70.0		

Average figures for the given food classes were determined as listed above. All figures are in grams.

Vitamin values for the foods *as served* have been used whenever available.

[1] *Meat:* Pork 75, bacon 20, ham 75, beef 75, hamburger 75, wieners 50, chicken 60, liver 25, salmon 25, fresh fish 25. Total considered as 8 servings and averaged.

[2] *Fruit:* Average of orange 100, grapefruit 100, apple (fresh) 130, apples (canned) 100, pear (fresh) 150, pears (canned) 100, peach (fresh) 100, peaches (canned) 100, plum 50, dried prunes 50, cherries (pitted) 100, strawberries (fresh) 100, pineapple (canned) 100, apricots (canned) 100, apricots (dried) 25, banana 100, watermelon 250, cantaloupe 150, grapes 100, raspberries 75, raisins 60, rhubarb 100. Total, 22 servings.

[3] *Nonstarchy vegetable:* Average of tomato 400, lettuce 50, celery 30, cabbage 150, carrots 150, beets 100, peas 200, string beans 100, spinach 50, turnips 50, squash (yellow) 50, onion 50. Total, 15 servings.

SAMPLE MENUS

Breakfast

Fruit
Cereal with milk
1 or 2 eggs
Milk, 8 oz.
Toast, crackers or zwieback
with butter

Dinner

Beef, chicken, fish, liver or other meat
Mashed potato with butter
⅔ cup vegetable
Fresh vegetable or fruit
1 slice of bread with butter
Simple pudding
Milk, 8 oz.

their own food selection. Thus, a most important factor in physical development is left to chance. Even when opportunities for food selection by the child are minimal, it often happens that the food habits of the family do not permit the ingestion of a complete and adequate diet. That the average diet of the people of this country is incomplete in several essentials has been pointed out many times by various observers. Much nutritional education still is

TABLE 2. A DIET OF COMMON FOODS SUITABLE FOR A 12-YEAR-OLD CHILD, WITH TABULATION OF ITS CONTENT OF CERTAIN ESSENTIAL NUTRIENTS—(*Continued*)

CA (MG.)	FE (MG.)	VITAMIN A (I. U.)	THIA- MINE (MG.)	RIBO- FLAVIN (MG.)	NIACIN (MG.)	ASCORBIC ACID (MG.)	VITAMIN D (I. U.)
1,150	0.7	1,550	0.35	1.68	1.1	12.0	400
26	1.3	550	0.05	0.14	Tr	0	25
9	2.0	880	0.385	0.245	3.3	1.2	. . .
40	1.4	1,420	0.116	0.120	0.8	30.0	. . .
54	1.6	5,080	0.150	0.124	1.0	34.0	. . .
24	2.0	200	0.220	0.106	2.4	16.0	. . .
75	2.0	0	0.24	0.15	2.2	0	. . .
37	1.8	45	0.052	0.045	0.7	0	. . .
56	0.7	320	0.100	0.125	0.5	0.6	. . .
9	0.0	1,380	Tr	Tr	Tr	0	. . .
93	0.1	170	0.010	0.060	0	0	. . .
12	0.3	. . .	0.02	0.02	2.6	0	. . .
0	0	0	0	0	0	0	. . .
0	0	0	0	0	0	0	. . .
1,585	13.9	13,595	1.693	2.815	14.6†	93.8	425
1,200	12.0	4,500	1.2	1.8	12.0	75.0	400

⁴ *Starchy vegetable or substitute:* Average of potato 100, lima beans 35, corn 150, noodles 50, macaroni (cooked) 100, white rice 50, navy beans, 35. Total, 15 servings.

⁵ *Cereal, dry weight:* Average of oatmeal 20, farina 20, cornflakes 20, cream of wheat 20, Wheaties 20, shredded wheat 25, puffed rice 10. Total, 7 servings.

⁶ *Starchy desserts:* Ice cream and 2 plain cookies, rice pudding with raisins, bread pudding, chocolate cornstarch pudding, brown betty, chocolate cake, fruit pie. Total, 7 servings, ⅔ cup each.

* Includes sugar of jam, etc.

† The full allowance of niacin is not necessary when sufficient milk is included in the diet, because tryptophan of milk can substitute for niacin.

SAMPLE MENUS

Supper
Egg or fish or liver or cottage cheese
Baked potato or legumes
⅔ cup vegetable
1 slice of bread with butter
Fruit
Milk, 8 oz.

Bedtime
Glass of milk

needed. Yet, over the years diets of children have improved with increase and spread of knowledge of nutrition and with improved economic status. When diets of children are deficient, they are likely to be low in calcium, protein, ascorbic acid and vitamin A more often than in other nutrients. Older children tend to have poorer diets than younger, and girls poorer diets than boys even in the same family. Adolescent girls are particularly prone to inadequate intakes. Distressed by rapid changes in their body contours they easily fall prey to advertising blandishments and fads for slenderizing and may seriously deplete their diets of nutritional essentials. Adolescent boys, on the other hand, usually develop voracious appetites which they make no effort to restrain.

From a knowledge of the requirements of individual nutrients and their concentrations in particular foods it is possible to construct completely adequate diets for children at any age. In the case of the small infant this is a relatively easy task (Chap. 12) because milk alone contains most of what he requires. For the older child a wider variety of foods is necessary, and the construction of an exact diet is more complicated. The accompanying Table 2 illustrates how the foods of a complete diet contribute toward the quota of each essential nutrient. The sample menu shows how the daily intake can be distributed among the various meals.

Such detailed analysis of food intakes is used in planning ideal meals for hospitals, schools and institutions of various sorts and for the regulation of food consumption by diabetic and obese children. Few homes plan meals with such attention to scientific detail, but intelligent concern for the child's nutrition demands that mothers and their medical advisors take an interest in the relative value of common foods and evaluate weekly intakes. Often the goal of an ideal food intake is unattainable due to peripheral factors such as economic status, religious and cultural eating habits, fads, developmental changes in the child and psychological interplay between child and mother. Some of these difficulties will be considered in relation to the individual foods below; others are treated in more detail in Chapters 4 and 8.

MILK

Milk is a very important food for growing children at any age. The large contribution which milk makes to the total of each nutrient can be seen by comparing the top and the bottom lines of the table analyzing the diet of a 12-year-old. This amounts to about one fourth of the total calories; half of the protein; and practically all of the calcium, vitamin A, vitamin D and riboflavin. With this much of a start it is easy to fill out the other essentials from relatively small amounts of other foods. But if no milk is being consumed, an optimum diet is more difficult to achieve. In the United States and some other countries with a well-developed dairy industry milk is in plentiful supply at relatively low cost. But many populous areas of the world get along without it because of scarcity or tradition.

Lusty milk consumption is not always a blessing. Taken as the sole item of diet it can appease hunger but does not provide completely adequate nutrition. Serious anemia is a common outcome when a small child becomes overly fond of milk and satisfies his appetite with 1 or 2 quarts per day. Ordinarily from 1½ to 2 pints is considered a proper daily intake, but in some children stricter control must be exercised if a cosmopolitan appetite is to be cultivated.

MEAT AND FISH

Animal protein is generally superior to vegetable protein because it provides a more complete selection of the essential amino acids. Meat and fish are the chief source in addition to that obtained from milk. They also add considerably to the intake of iron and of the B-complex vitamins. They are a relatively expensive item of the diet, which is frequently scrimped by the underprivileged. A significant number of small children dislike meat because of its texture and because of the necessity for chewing. Modern trends which introduce meat early during infant feeding attempt to cultivate a taste which will be sufficiently strong to override the latter objection to chewing. Meat for small children should be well cooked and finely subdivided. The popularity of hamburgers and hot dogs in the United States may be a persistence of earlier attitudes toward chewing.

EGGS

Eggs are a concentrated source of high value animal protein which also contribute significant amounts of iron and vitamins to the diet. Like meat, they are relatively expensive and tend to drop out of the diet under poor economic circumstances. Some children object to the taste of eggs prepared in the usual ways, but many of these will accept a raw egg beaten up in a glass of milk or prepared in the form of a custard. A few children are unable to tolerate eggs at all because of specific allergic reactions to them. Of course, such idiosyncracies must be honored in the preparation of meals.

FRUITS AND VEGETABLES

Most of the vitamin C in the diet is derived from fruits, fruit juices and vegetables. These substances also supply carbohydrate calories in proportion to their content of natural sugars and starches. Their relatively indigestible cellulose residue forms most of the bulk of the diet. Nutritionists generally favor the inclusion of fresh fruits and vegetables twice a day in the food intake, but a growing fraction of American children find them unpalatable. Undoubtedly, some of this indifference is acquired from parents who themselves eat little or no garden truck. It is difficult to state how important is the omission of fruits and vegetables when the missing vitamins are made up from other food sources or from supplements.

BREAD AND CEREALS

The importance of cereal grains and starchy vegetables depends upon the total food supply. Children who are well fed require bread and cereal mainly as a source of thiamine and calories. Both of these may be satisfied from other foods. In many parts of the world where food is scarce, the cereal grains provide the major if not the sole item of diet. Their modest content of vegetable protein and vitamins and high energy value are sufficient for sustenance but do not provide an optimal intake of nutrients. Thus, for some children, items such as bread, rice and potatoes serve chiefly as fillers or as the medium of gratifying excessive appetites and making them fat. But elsewhere in the world the same foods may represent the stark necessity for survival.

CULTIVATION OF APPETITE

The art of inducing children to consume complete diets is a highly individualized process which must be tailored to suit special circumstances. Its roots lie in the early feeding experiences of the infant which are considered in Chapter 4. When the process of food-taking is habitually surrounded by a happy environment devoid of psychological battles, appetites generally flourish and need no special persuasion during health. It is easy to identify technics which undermine wholesome attitudes toward food so that the "don'ts" usually outnumber the "dos" when guidance is presented to mothers. Unraveling of feeding problems requires a study of the child in his total family environment. Only a few general principles will be mentioned here.

Appetites are too often deflated by chronic persuasion. The technics which range from forced feeding and severe disciplinary measures through polite nagging to bribery cannot be expected to increase the child's enjoyment of food. Instead, they pervert the meaning of food from a desirable means of satisfying hunger to a bone of contention or a psychological weapon between the feeder and the fed. To be effective, persuasive measures must be subtle, seductive and indirect. The imaginative use of color, seasoning and arrangement into special forms will achieve more than verbal debate over the value of foods and the dire consequences of their omission. The sociability of eating with others usually fosters better food intake, particularly when the group is one which enjoys its meal. However, some children are too easily excited or diverted by groups and do better when fed quietly by themselves. Occasionally, children refuse food in order to draw attention to themselves within a group which is preoccupied in tackling its meal.

Often aversion to food can be avoided if care is taken to present only quantities which are likely to be consumed. A child with limited appetite is often defeated at once by the size of the portions on his plate. By underestimating what he wants, an attitude of "I can't possibly eat all that" is converted to "Is that all I get?" and he is likely to have the satisfaction of cleaning his plate and perhaps asking for a second helping. Within reason, specific likes and dislikes should be honored. Particularly with young children, fixations on certain foods are only temporary and will change if indulged.

Catering to individual whims does not mean that all attempts to regulate the quality of food should be abandoned. If left entirely to themselves, some children will select a poor diet from a narrow range of foods. Then control must be exercised over the amounts of favored foods permitted and perhaps over the sequence in which foods are presented. Thus a child with a small appetite can easily satisfy his hunger by downing a glass of milk at the beginning of the meal, but if the milk is withheld he may appease his hunger with less favored foods and then find room for the milk after all.

Evaluation of home diets is not always easy. Care must be taken to obtain objective records of the food consumed. Summary statements that the child "eats enough" or "doesn't eat a thing" must be confirmed by a recital of exactly what and how much he takes. Often parents' notions of what is required are sketchy or incorrect, and memories tend to fix upon particularly good or bad feeding episodes. Therefore, serious dietary evaluation must be based upon actual records of food intake.

SITUATIONS FOR FURTHER STUDY

1. Why is an infant's need for water intake greater than the older child's?

2. What is the infant's daily water requirement? His daily basal energy requirement?

3. Why is protein so essential in the child's diet? What is the infant's protein requirement? What is the child's protein requirement?

4. Why should fats be included in the child's diet?

5. Why must iron-containing foods be introduced into the infant's diet before 4 months of age?

6. How do a premature infant's mineral requirements differ from those of the full-term infant? What is the cause of the difference in need?

7. Why is vitamin A essential in the child's diet? What is the function of vitamin D in the infant's diet? of vitamin K? of vitamin B? of vitamin C?

8. How do early feeding experiences affect appetite?

9. A disturbed mother-child relationship is often reflected in an infant's feeding habits. If you made a home call in a public health district and you discovered an infant of 7 months of age who refused to take solid foods, how would you approach the problem?

10. Visit a nursery school and observe the noon-meal period. How was the food served? What was the response of the children to the type of food service that was used? What did the teacher

do and say during the meal period? How did her behavior affect the children's response to the meal period and to food? Do you think that the kind of food service used in the nursery school would be practical for hospital use? What would be the advantages for the children and for student nurses? What prevents hospital personnel from instituting this type of food service?

BIBLIOGRAPHY

Martin, Ethel A.: Roberts' Nutrition Work with Children, Chicago, Univ. Chicago Press, 1954.

Wagner, Muriel Ginsberg: Appetites and attitudes, a viewpoint on feeding the young child, J. Am. Dietit. A. 30:329, 1954.

Nutrition and Healthy Growth (pamphlet), Washington, D. C., U. S. Dept. Health, Education and Welfare, 1955.

CHAPTER FOUR

The Nature and Nurture
of Personality

The changes taking place in body form and physical function during the years of growth have been traced in Chapter 2. The present chapter is concerned with the maturation of the central nervous system and the associated organs of special sense. From the function of this organ system several interrelated kinds of development emerge—sometimes in concert, sometimes in opposition. The instinctive reactions, the motor and the mental skills, and the emotional responses and their controls are all dependent upon the nervous system and are facets of a larger process which we call personality. Clear separation of these different processes is frequently impossible, for they are inextricably tangled. Similarly artificial is the necessity of describing development by age periods, for each merges into and overlaps with its antecedent and following eras.

The process of personality formation starts with an infant endowed with certain universal traits and drives which guide his neuromuscular development and behavior along lines which are necessary to his survival and to the perpetuation of the race. Throughout this chapter the term "instinctual drive" will be used to designate inherent biologic urges or needs which are characteristically directed toward one of two major goals: (1) obtaining that which produces feelings of pleasure (ultimately this will include the desire to give pleasure as well as to receive it) and (2) striking out against frustration. An infant does not have to learn to be hungry or to be aggressive when hunger makes him uncomfortable. An urge for pleasure and an urge to aggress when frustrated are biologically determined instincts. When a baby's biologic needs are satisfied by a giving mother, he feels loved. This state of fulfillment expands into a desire to be loved and

50

eventually to give love. When his needs are unfulfilled, he expresses his aggressive drive as primitively as he expresses his drive for love. *The drive for love and the urge to respond aggressively to frustration are often opposed to one another during childhood. When they are, the child is in conflict and is anxious. Anxiety is a painful warning signal; it alerts the individual to the impending danger of being overwhelmed by inner feelings or outer circumstances that he cannot master. If the individual's ego cannot cope with the anxiety and he gets no support from others which helps him to master it, he becomes traumatized.*

These built-in universal drives, largely genetically determined, comprise the personality nature of the infant (or the id of the personality). The instinctual drives vary in quality and intensity so that even at birth each child has his own peculiar individuality. Immediately after birth the infant begins to interact with his surrounding environment. The response of the persons about the child (chiefly the mother or her substitute at first) in appeasing, assuaging, encouraging and in helping him redirect, modify or control these innate instinctual drives is the aspect of personality formation implied by the term nurture.

Emotional maturation takes place as the child grows physically and gets the support he needs to make a healthy adjustment to the myriad of learning experiences which are necessary for personally satisfying and socially approved adjustment in our society. Adjustment to many learning experiences is easy for the child. Learning to walk is an example of an easy task. The baby works to learn but he does not have to give up any pleasure to accomplish this feat. Adjustment to learning experiences which involve sacrifice of the pleasure which direct expression of instincts provides is infinitely more difficult. Weaning and learning excretory control are

examples of the more difficult lessons in learning. When the child's mother introduces the weaning experience, he has to modify his sucking instinct. During the weaning period, observation will show that he sucks on objects other than a nipple until he discovers other activities which are more satisfying. During major learning experiences he has conflict between his two basic drives; he wants instinct satisfaction and the approval of his mother. Simultaneously, frustration makes him feel aggressive; he has the urge to strike out at the situation which brings pain. His id says, "Keep the bottle. Sucking is one of my greatest pleasures. I'm going to knock the cup from my mother's hand because it keeps me from having what my nature craves." The mother must act as the child's ego until it becomes strong enough to function independently of his mother. She must supply nurturing which helps him find ways to gratify or modify his two major drives in such a way that they cease to be opposed to one another. She must nurture him in a way which prevents him from forcing his need for love or his aggression out of his conscious mind. The mother's behavior in these major learning experiences must say: "Learning to adjust to society's expectations in regard to eating is a difficult experience. I accept your feelings about it. I will help you learn to enjoy it. I will not make you give it up all at once. You can learn gradually. I will give you something you will enjoy even more than sucking. You can suck on your toys whenever you need to and my pride in your accomplishment will give you the pleasure that feeling grown up produces." Support of this kind helps the child to solve his conflict between his two major drives. The comfortably adjusted adult has solved this conflict. His two major drives have become directed toward a common goal which is socially approved and personally satisfying. The aggression which was produced from frustration has become directed toward a goal which is personally satisfying and socially constructive. Because it meets the needs of society, he gets the approval and the recognition that his nature requires.

The timing of the socialization experiences and the quality of the support are important factors in personality development. *For growth, the timing must be based upon the child's readiness to* cope with the experience. The support must be based upon his individual needs for mastery. Support that makes mastery possible grows out of knowledge of the developmental process, out of understanding the complexity of each task from the child's point of view and out of wholesome attitudes toward the child and the learning process.

While opinions differ concerning the exact extent to which the ultimate personality depends upon its nature, there is little doubt that the quality of the

nurture has a very considerable influence upon the final outcome. Thus the optimal guidance of the child during the formative years requires an appreciation of his basic nature and a long-range view of efforts to modify it.

Particularly during the early months and years, the mother is almost the sole source of nurture. Mothering is highlighted in this chapter to show the important role that the mother plays in helping her child to modify the expression of his instinctual drives in the process of becoming a socially mature and happy individual. It is also highlighted to help the nurse gain insight into the emotional support that the child needs from her when circumstances require that he be separated from his mother. Furthermore, mothering is emphasized to increase the nurse's awareness of her important role in supporting the mother-child relationship both in health and during periods of illness.

THE PRENATAL PERIOD

The capacity for parenthood does not come automatically with the birth of a child; it evolves out of the complex of each parent's experience with his own family and acquaintances throughout the growth process and up to the time he assumes the parental role himself. The prenatal period is the time during which expectant parents are making their final preparations for parenthood. In our culture better preparation of individuals for parenthood could be achieved if all children were protected from physical disease; if they were provided with family interpersonal relationship experiences which fostered healthy personality development; and if they were understood by the professional workers who guide them during the maternity cycle and in the child-rearing years.

Although attitudes and feelings toward pregnancy and parenthood are formed largely from past experiences

within their own families, expectant parents can profit from ego support by professional workers. With interest in people, knowledge of the dynamic psychology of the reproductive cycle and skill in providing a helping relationship, the nurse can aid expectant parents in adjusting to the changes of pregnancy and to their parental roles.

Ego support helps expectant parents to adjust comfortably and healthily to pregnancy and to become prepared for their roles in nurturing the child from conception through the years of growth to the maturation which prepares him in turn to assume the reproductive role. *The expectant mother needs to learn about her health requirements during the reproductive cycle, to understand the changes in her body and in her emotional life and to cope constructively with the conflicting feelings and anxieties which arise. She needs to become prepared for labor and for the period which follows delivery and to acquire confidence that she will be able to play the mother role. She needs freedom from anxiety so she can store energy in preparation for dispensing it to her child.* Her ability to give is conditioned by her own reception of love during childhood and the recent pregnancy.

The expectant father needs help, too. *He should feel that he is a part of the experience.* He has an important role to play during the pregnancy, his wife's labor and in the period when she is adapting to new responsibilities entailed in the mother role. Pregnancy changes the life of the expectant father. *Anxieties stimulated by the pregnancy need to be allayed in order to preserve his health.* He needs energy to supply the love and the comfort which his wife needs. Her motherliness will be enhanced by the support, the security and the understanding that she received from her husband not only in the period when she is establishing her relationship with their child but also in the years to come. Through this increased reception of love she not only benefits their child but also matures and repays her husband's devotion with a more satisfying relationship with him.

A healthy woman who is making progress in her adjustment to pregnancy presumably is best supplied to give the fetus what it needs to grow from a minute cell into an individual who is prepared for life physically apart from his mother's body. *To cope with the adaptation required by extra-uterine life and to reach his full growth potentials, the fetus needs essential nutrients.* He probably profits from a peaceful, mutually interdependent emotional relationship with a mother who is becoming prepared to receive him with unconditional acceptance and motherliness.

Support during the maternity cycle has far-reaching effects for the whole family. In addition to those effects cited above, it also motivates parents to seek the help of professional workers in the guidance of their children. When a family's needs have been met during the maternity cycle, they become aware of the values of health supervision and seek help in using the resources of their community.

The prenatal period is important to the development of the fetus' personality because of the events taking place during this period of his parents' life. Pregnancy changes the lives of his parents and creates opportunities for further emotional development. When the expectant mother has the support of her husband and both expectant parents have the help of professional workers, healthy adjustment to change is better ensured. In the final analysis the most important factor in molding the personality of the fetus is the effect that maturation has on his parents who are preparing the emotional climate in which eventually he will live.

THE INFANT
(Birth to 1 Year)

Sometimes birth is called a traumatic experience because it abruptly separates the infant from his source of security (the mother's body) and forces him to participate immediately in his own adaptation to extra-uterine life. In the uterus the fetus experiences a close mutual interdependency with its mother and presumably is free of frustration, pain and fear. It is secure because it is protected from exposure to cold, from inappropriate stimuli and from psychologically traumatic experiences which would come if it were born before term. After 9 months of growth and intra-uterine existence which ideally and automatically fulfilled all his growth requirements, he is expelled into the outer world. No longer is he in a warm, dark place completely surrounded by water.

No longer is he physically supported in the gentlest fashion and rocked with his mother's movements. He comes into a world of bright light as well as darkness, a world of new noises and many new experiences.

Although the full-term baby must be ready to meet the frustrations of physical separation from his mother, he reacts to the birth experience with displeasure; his behavior manifests anger and fear. His cry serves a physiologic function; it forces air into his lungs and initiates the breathing process. His cry also expresses his feelings and reveals his need for supportive care which helps him adapt with ease and comfort. As one mother put it: "He sounds as if he didn't like this world. He acts as if he would like to go back where he came from."

EQUIPMENT FOR ADAPTATION AND LEARNING

Thrust into his new environment, the infant must begin to adapt himself to it immediately. He must oxygenate his own tissues, signal his needs for food, suck, swallow, digest and excrete. He must also signal his distress which arises when needs other than hunger remain unmet. He must communicate his discomfort from inappropriate temperatures, painful internal or external stimuli, an uncomfortable position, physiologic insufficiency or from loneliness which comes with separation from the mother's body.

The normal newborn is also equipped with organs of perception; he can receive sensory stimuli and respond emotionally to the people in the world about him. He feels their actions and reacts with feelings and attitudes toward them and toward himself. In other words he has the capacity for personality growth from the rudiments of personality with which he is born. Life in the outer world does not start at zero in personality as it does not start at the zero mark physically.

Rapid growth of the brain in utero prepares the normal newborn to adapt in the above ways and lays the groundwork for future physical and personality growth. The newborn's brain at birth is one of the farthest advanced in size of any of the organs of his body. The body increases approximately 20 times in size from birth to maturity, the brain slightly less than 4 times. This growth of the brain occurs in the first 7 or 8 years of life. By the fifth month of fetal life the individual has the 12 million or more nerve cells with their nerve fibers which make up the vast nervous system which will control every function of his total complex biophysiologic make-up. He is equipped with the network which will control every move which his body will make, be it under voluntary or involuntary control. He is equipped with the neurons which make it possible for him to communicate with others by means of language, to remember, to think, to learn, to imagine and to reason. Acquisition of these motor and mental skills will strengthen his ego resources and make it possible for him to adjust to increasingly more difficult situations.

INDIVIDUAL DIFFERENCES

No two newborns are alike; their constitutional make-up (physical heritage) differs in quality. Their instinctual drives and the energy which generates from them (the id) differ in intensity, rhythm, mode of expression and the way in which they can be satisfied. The first responses which the newborn makes to the frustration of birth and to the countless impressions that immediately come rushing in upon him show individual differences in biologic and psychological make-up. Each infant responds in his own way to internal and external stimuli —to hunger and pain and to the need for sleep, love and stimulation. He is not a personality if one thinks of the word as associated with awareness of self. But he is an individual with his own characteristic way of growing and behaving.

The infant's physical and personality growth and development will depend upon his constitutional make-up and the environmental factors which impinge upon him during the formative periods of his life. It will be a progression which follows a general pattern but it will have its own unique characteristics. Both heredity and environment will have a share in making the infant what he is and what he is to be. His personality growth will depend upon the culture into which he is born. It will depend upon his relationship with his parents, brothers and sisters, or siblings as they are often called, and with his playmates or peers, teachers and others who become important to him emotionally. If illness occurs during the formative periods of his life, his potentialities for personality growth will be influenced by the kind of experiences he encounters with nurses and others of the helping professions.

Each child in a family not only has a different constitutional make-up but also has a different environment. Each individual's place in the family in itself influences his environment. In addition, countless other factors make each child's environment different from that which is experienced by his siblings.

PLEASURE SUPPORTS PERSONALITY GROWTH

Without harm to himself the newborn cannot stand more frustration than that which he received at birth. Observation shows the newborn's complete dependency upon others for the satisfaction of his needs. He can scream to signal his need for food, but if it does not come, he can do nothing more to get it. Observation also shows the newborn's utter incapacity to wait for satisfaction. When he is hungry and food does not come, he quickly becomes disorganized. He screams, throws his arms and legs about, turns red in the face. Then he withdraws from exhaustion and goes to sleep. He acts that way because his nature makes him do so. His instinctual drives are potent, pleasure-seeking and inconsiderate. He has no inner strength which helps him to tolerate frustration or modify his wants; his brain is undeveloped; he cannot understand why his mother does not feed him; he cannot entertain himself while his mother finishes preparing dinner; he cannot say to himself: "Stop crying. You should be ashamed of yourself for wanting food so soon." He can only feel. He feels helpless and fearful of the unknown. These feelings must be mastered during the earliest years of his life if he is to reach his full potential.

Repeated satisfaction of needs lessens the infant's feelings of helplessness and increases his feelings of security in his new world. Separation from his mother's uterus was accompanied by physiologic changes which made him unstable physically and emotionally. *He needs consistent experiences which are mutually enjoyed by both him and his mother to become stabilized physiologically and to acquire feelings of trust, security and confidence in his own power to get what he needs when he needs it.* When the infant has acquired these feelings he has mastered his first and most important step in the socialization process. Throughout the remainder of this book these steps will be referred to as *developmental tasks*.

Because food combined with physical and emotional closeness to the mother is the infant's most urgent psychological need, hunger and feeding will be used to illustrate the mechanism which produces feelings of confidence and security in his own powers. When a baby's need for food and love is met consistently and promptly he eventually associates the hunger contractions which signal his need with the arrival of the food which satisfies his hunger. When he makes this connection between his need and the coming of food, he has acquired some degree of mastery over his feelings of helplessness and fear.

The consistent experience of being fed and loved when he is hungry makes him feel that his mother loves him and can be trusted to do his bidding. Little wonder Mother comes to be the source of his security and he comes to feel that he is master of all he surveys. This is the way he should feel. He *needs* to feel he is the king-pin during the first years of his life because it produces increased mastery of his feelings of helplessness and gives him the power to cope with the developmental tasks which are to come. It is true that he will have to discover the reality of his own power. He will need help to discover this little by little as he gains ego strength to face the reality of the limitations that every child possesses. Apportioning this discovery to the child's capacity to adjust to it is an important nurturing task.

Self-regulatory schedules which consistently recognize individual differences in need for food and love promote ego growth. They prevent the anxiety which conflict between the infant's two basic drives produces. Therefore, they conserve vital energy for growth. The intimate relationship which child and mother enjoy during periods of care help the infant to differentiate himself from his mother. It helps him to discover that his mother is the outside world and his self or ego is the inside. At birth he cannot differentiate himself from the external world—he is one with mother. But after months of loving care the external world begins to take form. He discovers his mother before he discovers himself, but it is through his intimate relationship with her that his ego begins to grow.

Consistent mutually enjoyed experiences with his mother promote ego growth in another way. They promote the development of feelings of security, self-confidence and trust—feelings that make it possible for the infant to begin to adapt to reality by withstanding small doses of frustration. Observation shows that his signals of need become less frantic after a period of experiencing consistent fulfillment; he grows increasingly more able to wait a longer time for gratification. He can wait because he feels *sure* that he will get what he needs. In the last quarter of the first year he can wait longer for food because the sight of his mother has been repeatedly associated with pleasure. If he can see her while she prepares his food, he gets something which gives him strength to tolerate his frustration. This capacity to tolerate frustration manifests the beginning growth of the ego. When he can wait, it shows his ego is beginning to develop powers to modify his instinctual drives so they can be in harmony with his mother's demands.

Supportive care which helps the infant master his first developmental task prepares him for growth in subsequent periods of life. The child learns to control or modify his instinctual drives through his relationship with his mother and eventually through interpersonal relationships with his father and others. If he has received bountifully from his mother during the first years of his life, he grows attached to her and becomes dependent upon her full acceptance for his security. Because of the need for security in the affections of his mother, he gradually learns to tolerate reality frustrations. Learning to tolerate reality frustrations has purpose for the child; it wins him the approval and the support of the mother upon which he is dependent. If his mother is sensitive to his need for readiness to tolerate frustration, he will be willing to forfeit the pleasure that comes from free expression of his drives to suck, bite, hit and soil, for the security of his mother's continuing approval and love. Giving up pleasures involves some conflict and hostility because the child's desires for instinctual satisfaction are often at variance with his mother's social mores. The ego's first task is to adapt to the mother's demands (reality) in a way which gives his instincts some measure of gratification. With cognizance of the child's need for readiness to learn to control or modify his instinctual drives, conflict can be minimized. With understanding guidance which supports his immature ego, he can learn to handle his hostile feelings constructively.

The child identifies with or imitates the behavior of those he admires, trusts and needs for security. When he is loved, he becomes motivated to be more grown-up, to acquire mastery of his instinctual urges and to gain gratification through his own accomplishments. He observes his parents' standards and forms a conscious picture of the way he must act to be constantly secure in his parents' affections and escape their punishment. In psychological terms this conscious formulation of the idealized self one strives to be is called the *ego-ideal.* Trust in his parents spreads to trust in other people. Understanding from his parents makes him anticipate and seek it from others. As he experiences meaningful relationships with others besides his parents, his ego-ideal will change. When he is an adult it will embody the ideals of all the people he has admired, had confidence in and trusted. This points out the reason why trust and confidence in others is such a basic ingredient of the personality. Trust in his parents and understanding from those who guide him support the growth impulse and give it the opportunities it needs to guide the child toward its goal —maturity.

Repeated frustrations traumatize the infant; they prevent him from mastering his first developmental task and color his response to later learning experiences. Feelings of trust and confidence provide the foundation upon which his personality must become structured or built. The infant who is consistently left to cry it out and is deprived of comfort and gentle handling cannot feel kindly toward others. Long before he recognizes his mother as a person, he will have hostile feelings toward the person he needs most to trust. His relationship with his mother will be disturbed because he never has felt truly loved. Since she has failed to meet his needs as they arose, he will acquire little motivation to please her. Thus, much of the normal interchange of pleasure between mother and baby is missing. But, most important of all, he will have unfulfilled desires, insecurity and hostility within him. Because he never has been unconditionally accepted, craving for that which he never had will remain a driving force within the deepest layers of his personality. How he will cope with these feelings depends upon his physical heritage and the guidance he receives during the years which are to come.

STIMULATION

Age-Adequate Stimulation

The special organs of sense through which the outer world is to reach the infant are present at birth but as yet not completely developed functionally. As his sense organs present him with impressions of the world about him, the infant gradually learns to associate certain emotional feelings with these experiences. Thus he begins to react very early to his mother's touch. If this touch usually brings comfort to him, his response is eventually one of pleasure to the touch itself. At a later age he will react with similar pleasure even to the sight of his mother who is about to touch him. By such a process of association, the infant gradually accumulates a group of emotional reactions to the sensory experiences that he feels.

Stimulation that is adjusted to the child's capacity to utilize it for growth is ego-supporting. During the first 3 months of life stimulation should be limited to satisfaction of the infant's biologic needs. He is ready to be held and loved during his feeding; he is ready to be cuddled when he shows signs of being afraid or lonely; he is ready to be fondled at bath time. If he receives too much stimulation at other times it may be fatiguing and painful. If it is excessive, he will show his feelings about it. He will either scream and become active or respond by withdrawing. Both hyperactivity and withdrawal show his rejection of the experience. His behavior says: "Leave me alone. I have had all I can take now. A little bit is pleasurable. Beyond that point it becomes painful. If you continue to give me what I am unready for, I will have to shut it out. I need it, but it must come gradually as I am able to assimilate it." Observation of the child's reaction to stimulation will guide the adult in adjusting the amount to his capacity to tolerate it. Too little results in apathy and a turning in upon the self for pleasure. The unstimulated baby develops mannerisms to get the pleasure he should be getting from another person. He may roll his head, rock his body or twist his hands in a bizarre fashion. The child signals his need for stimulation. He also signals the point at which it has ceased to bring pleasure and constructive activity.

Sensory Equipment

Sense of Touch. Although the extent to which there is sensory perception before birth is not known, the sense of touch seems to be the most highly developed at birth. It is certainly the most extensive of all senses, for the total body is the organ of the sense of touch. The child's sense of touch, to which pain and the feeling of temperature are related, comes to him from every part of his body. Some areas of his body are more sensitive than others. At birth he is less sensitive to some stimuli than he will be later. A touch on the lips causes the reflex of sucking in the newborn, and a light touch on the nose will cause the eyes to close.

Sensitivity to pain and temperature is present in early infancy. Sensitivity to physical pain exists at birth but it is less acute than it is in the older child. The newly born infant tolerates physical pain fairly well if he can suck on a nipple or a sugar-tit and be fondled during the procedure. The temperature sense is developed early. An unfavorable reaction to bath water which is too hot or too cold is often observed. If the temperature of the bath water is uncomfortable, a fear of the bath may arise which will be difficult to overcome. Bath water of 95° to 100° F. is comfortable for the baby. Lowering the baby into the water gradually and gently helps him adjust to the experience of being bathed.

The child's first impressions of life in this world come to him through the sense of touch. He feels the touch of hands at the moment of his birth. He feels the crib in which he lies and the touch of his mother's hands and body before he is aware of the world beyond his touch. Later, sight and sound will bring experiences of the world beyond. After 3 months the sense of touch is well developed over the body, and for many years the child will seek to understand his world through this sense. The mouth and the lips are sensitive tactile areas. The infant needs the stimulation that comes from toys. He will do much investigating by putting things into his mouth. From these experiences he will get pleasure and learn their properties. He will discover which things are edible and which are not; he will learn the difference between softness and hardness, warmth and cold. Mouthing is the natural avenue of investigation. Through the use of his mouth he takes in food and love from the person who feeds him. He is also stimulated to investigate and to learn.

As is true of all the senses, the sense of touch acquires meaning for the child through the variety of experiences it transmits. He will learn about the people in his world through his sense of touch long before he is aware of them as persons. The infant who is lifted and held lovingly and gently responds positively to people. His mother's hands will come to mean comfort to him. In fact, his mother's touch will contribute much to his eventual concept of his mother as a person who gives care and loves him, one whom he will love in return.

Sense of Sight. The extremely delicate organs of sight equipped with their 12 delicate muscles seem from a functional point of view to be the slowest of all the sense organs in development. Fine muscle control must be acquired before the baby is said to "see." The eyes must learn to move together. For some months and occasionally for much longer, the eyes may move independently, especially when an infant is trying to focus on a near object. This natural characteristic often makes mothers fearful. They think that their babies are cross-eyed because they do not know that it takes time for fine muscle coordination to develop.

Development of the eyes shows patterned progression. At birth, the baby's eyes move about without fixing themselves on a given object. There is a vague reaction to a moving light, and by the time the baby is about a month old he will fix his eyes on a bright object dangled above him and will follow it for a brief moment. As he grows and has the practice and the stimulation that he needs, he increases the arc of following. When he masters the ability to sit up, his horizons will broaden, thereby increasing his opportunity to see more of the things within his environment. By 3 to 4 months of age he is able to fix and follow well. At this time he enjoys and profits from new sight experiences.

Between 4 and 6 months of age the baby begins to recognize the person who constantly cares for him and objects such as his bottle which have become important to him. He has learned through many experiences to follow with his eyes. His mother begins to emerge from the as-yet-unknown world about him into something seen and recognized. If she has come to mean comfort and pleasure, he focuses on her, follows and responds to her smiles, words and gestures. He knows her only in part, but he is building those associations which eventually will mean a person called Mother. As his vision improves and he recognizes that she is the giver of comfort, he becomes more discriminating and prefers her to others who are less important to him personally.

Because the eye does not reach its full development until the child is 7 or 8 years of age, protection from eye strain is essential. The preschool child's play equipment should be large because his visual powers are incomplete and also because he has not developed the fine muscle co-ordination essential for delicate manipulation. For example, beads that the small child will enjoy stringing should be large and have large holes. Pictures should be large and simple in design to prevent strain and discomfort.

Sense of Hearing. Soon after birth babies respond to sounds. The deafness existent at birth is caused in part by absence of air in the eustachian tubes and in part by the persistence of embryonic tissue within the middle ear. However, fairly soon after birth response to sound becomes observable. A response which denotes pleasurable feelings is elicited from kindly spoken words or song; a response which denotes displeasure comes from sharp, harsh or sudden sounds. Association between a sound and its meaning may come as early as the second or the third month if it is a sound which has occurred frequently and has been associated with the same meaningful experience.

The recognized sound of his mother's voice will come to be associated with the meaning that she has come to have for the infant. If she has provided attention and comfort, the sound of her voice will bring a pleasurable response; he will smile and respond with his entire body. But if she has punished natural behavior (crying when he has urgent needs which are clamoring for satisfaction), the infant's response will be totally different. He may scream or withdraw because he has associated pain with what he hears. Thus sounds do their share in building up the concept of Mother.

Sense of Smell. The sense of smell seems to be present in young babies and grows more acute during preschool years. Young babies show more reaction to extremely strong odors. By 3 years of age, the preschool child shows definite preferences and dislikes for odors. If one observes the behavior of a group of preschool children, one will discover that there are marked variations in sensitivity to different odors.

Sense of Taste. Taste and smell are closely associated in infancy. The year-old baby, for example, who has learned to sniff in response to the stimulus of something fragrant held before him will open his mouth as if he expected to taste the fragrant flower. He does this because he has not yet learned complete discrimination between smell and taste. Doubtless, too, his interest in investigating by mouth plays a part in this reaction.

The sense of both taste and smell develops somewhat slowly in the first months of life. Although rejection of bitter and acceptance of sweet have been noted in very small infants, on the whole there seems to be an attitude of indifference toward taste in infancy. This fact has a bearing on the development of positive attitudes toward different kinds of food.

First rejections of solids, such as cereals and vegetables, in the diet seem to be more closely related to their consistency—a function of touch rather than of taste. Other factors, too, may impede the acceptance of solid food. The muscle activity which is required to get solid food from a spoon is more laborious for the infant than the sucking movements which are instinctively present at birth. In addition, the solid food is obtained more slowly than milk from the breast or the nipple, a fact which doubtlessly tends to frustrate him in his early attempts to eat this new variety of food. He spits because he has not yet learned to accept slowly flowing food and to manipulate his tongue muscles to get it into the back of his throat from whence it can be swallowed. It is not the taste to which he is reacting; it is the new experience with which he has had insufficient time to become familiar.

In the last quarter of the first year, changes in feeding behavior arise which worry some mothers when they discover that less food is being eaten at 9 to 10 months than was consumed at 4 to 5 months of age. In this period, the infant becomes more discriminating and he expresses his feelings about food more vigorously. Those he likes he eats greedily; those he dislikes he pushes away. This change in behavior is due partly to a slowing of the rate of somatic growth. It is also due partly to a myriad of social factors. At this stage, the infant is experimenting with locomotion and is consumed with interest in inspecting everything within reach. Often he is too busy or too easily distracted to gorge himself as he did a few months before. A developing interest in self-feeding is another factor in reducing intake. Between 7 and 10 months many babies cease to accept foods which their mothers offer to them. Even though they can hold their bottles by themselves, they have not developed sufficient motor skill to make self-feeding with a spoon possible. The mother's best solution is to provide bits of solid foods which can be grasped, or to allow her baby to dip his fingers into the food and carry some of it to his mouth. More often than not, more of the food lands in his hair, on his face, clothes and the floor. This display of independence is trying for a time but it usually increases his appetite and stimulates his interest in food.

The above characteristics show the infant's need to become accustomed to a variety of foods and consistencies before the 6th month of life. Prior to that time he will eat almost anything that is offered if new foods are introduced gradually and his need to learn is respected. Rapid growth stimulates appetite, and few things distract his goal for food if the mother-child relationship is mutually satisfying. However, the situation is different when introduction of a variety of foods is delayed past the 6th month. In these instances resistance to change is frequently observed.

Throughout the first year of life the infant's feeding experiences are of prime importance in personality development. The importance of prompt satisfaction of hunger and a need for closeness to the mother during the earliest months of life was cited above. When solid foods are introduced, understanding the infant's need to learn is essential to sustain the mother-child relationship. A well-prepared mother accepts her infant's reaction and finds ways to help him enjoy the experience; she remains poised throughout the learning period. She neither forces food nor gives up her responsibility in teaching. She also rewards her infant's efforts to withstand frustration with expressions of pride in his accomplishments. She gives of herself, which increases the infant's capacity to adjust himself to the frustration that he feels when a new feeding technic is introduced. Through consistent experiences of this kind he learns to enjoy new foods and new ways of feeding.

At the 8th or the 9th month when changes in eating behavior arise, under-standing will be necessary again to sustain the mother-child relationship. When feeding time continues to be a mutually enjoyed experience the mother-child relationship becomes strengthened. In the feeding experience all the infant's senses are utilized. He feels, hears his mother's voice, sees her facial expression and gestures and gets a taste of the outer world in the form of food.

Rest

The infant's schedule of care should be planned in accordance with his individual needs. The newborn sleeps most of the time. He needs all of his energy to make the physiologic adaptations that are necessary for extrauterine life. *He requires periods of undisturbed rest to gain the energy that he needs for growth of his body and adaptive capacities.* His behavior provides the clues which are necessary to plan his schedule of care. During the earliest months of life, his need for food and rest will vary from day to day. Gradually, however, his patterns of need will become more regular. He will establish a schedule of his own—sleeping when he is tired, and eating and playing when he requires food and stimulation. With growth his needs will change. When his needs change, he will establish new patterns of behavior which require respect.

It is important to provide environmental conditions which encourage restful sleep. Temperature and ventilation of the infant's room are often the subjects of parents' questions. Only one factor is important. The child should not become chilled or overheated. The infant's heat-regulating mechanism is imperfectly developed, and he cannot adjust to sudden changes in temperature as can an adult. In the daytime the infant's environment should range from 70° F. to 75° F., and he should have on enough clothing so that he does not need to be wrapped in a blanket when he is awake. His arms and legs should be free to move about so that he may have the pleasure of using them. At night or during the nap this temperature may be from 10° to 15° lower for the little baby and from 15° to 20° lower for the older child. The child needs a well-ventilated room which is warm enough for relaxed sleep. It is important to remember that one is ventilating a room that is inhabited by a person who cannot get up and close the window when he feels cold. Screens and window boards which can be bought or home-devised are helpful in protecting the baby from drafts. The amount of covering needed over a child at night is difficult to gauge. A baby's extremities should be warm, but he should not have so much covering that he perspires or is restless. When an infant is difficult to keep covered at night a sleeping bag which gives him the use of his hands and permits freedom of movement will bring comfort to both the baby and his mother.

Because there are individual differences in sleep needs, it is essential to follow the child's cues in providing care. The child should have enough rest for health and happiness. He should be free of signs of undue fatigue; he should be refreshed after sleep; his color should be good; his eyes bright; and he should be composed and productive. If he has no undesirable symptoms like irritability, loss of appetite, hyperactivity or apathy, he probably is getting sufficient sleep to meet his daily requirements.

As the infant grows older, he requires help in accepting his need for rest. Until 5 years of age, most children do not get enough sleep without a daily nap or two. With growth of sensory perception and motor skills, the infant becomes increasingly more stimulated by himself and by the persons and the things within his environment. He has difficulty in relaxing because he is carried away by his new-found powers and the joy of activity and exploration.

Guarding against overfatigue is an important responsibility of the adult. When beginning signs of fatigue are noted, the adult must help the child kindly but firmly to accept his need for rest. This is done by reducing the stimuli that impinge upon him, by preparing him for rest with quiet activity and by providing support that gives pleasure and helps him to relax.

MOTOR CONTROL

Motor Responses of the Newborn

The earliest responses which the infant makes to the sensory stimuli that impinge upon him in such countless numbers after birth are motor responses. The seemingly helpless infant can do a number of things. Many of his actions such as sucking, winking and pupillary movements are reflex. All of these reflexes continue throughout life. Other reflexes appear after birth, and some of them disappear.

The newborn infant's movements are random and un-co-ordinated. He wiggles, stretches, spreads his fingers and brings them together. His arms and legs move together, for he does not have the control necessary to inhibit the action of any extremity. When lying on his stomach, he can hold his head up for a moment, but for 3 or 4 months he must be held in such a way that support is given to his head and back. He has neither the skill nor the strength to hold his head or spine erect.

Relationship of Motor Development

Motor development does not progress independently of growth in other areas; it is an interrelated process. The child is growing physically, spiritually, mentally, socially and emotionally; maturation is taking place; he is getting ready in various ways to sit, crawl, walk, climb, run and master objects in his environment. The infant must grow bigger and stronger before he is ready to learn to control his body. His mind must learn to co-ordinate his movements into the complicated pattern of sitting, crawling, walking, and using his body. Also, he must be motivated to learn to use his body functionally.

People and his relationship to them are important factors in learning to master his body and environment. They must keep him physically fit and provide the encouragement and the support that he needs to learn to use his body. *The infant needs permission to grow more capable of independent activity; he needs play equipment and protection while he is discovering the use of his body and the properties of the things within his environment.* Unless his need for new experiences is understood and encouraged, he not only will have insufficient exercise but also he will feel thwarted and resentful toward those who inhibit his drive for self-mastery.

To appraise a child's progress in motor development, the interrelatedness of growth and the differences between individuals need to be considered. Standards of development must be flexible and used cautiously because there are wide variations in rate of growth and in the ages at which children develop given skills. The sequence in which developmental milestones are reached is more definitely fixed than are the chronologic ages at which they are reached. Individual differences exist; heredity and environment are both influencing factors.

Aldrich and Norval studied the neuromuscular development of 215 normal infants from birth to the early part of the second year and recorded the time of onset of various accomplishments. The infants were from all strata of society in Rochester, Minn. However, it is recognized that the population of Rochester is made up of more professional people than is usual in many other cities of its size. Each mother was informed about the usual sequence of neuromuscular development. Each was also advised to encourage her baby to use each new skill as it appeared. The investigators tested the infants at monthly intervals and instructed the mothers to observe the onset of achievement which would be elicited less easily in the clinic. The following steps in neuromuscular growth were chosen for study:

1. Smile—the baby begins to smile in response to an adult or to his voice.

2. Vocal—the infant utters such sounds as "ah," "eh" and "uh" spontaneously or on stimulation.

3. Head control—when the infant is lifted by his hands from the supine to the sitting position, the head does not lag but is supported by the anterior muscles of the neck.

4. Hand control—when a toy is dangled in the mid-line above his chest, the infant is able to close in on the toy with one or both hands and to grasp it.

5. Roll—the baby makes a complete roll from back to abdomen.

6. Sit—the baby sits alone for several moments.

7. Crawl—the baby is able to move across the room or the pen toward some distant object; this may be accomplished by rolling over and over, pushing himself along on his stomach or back, or by any individual modification of progression.

8. Prehension—this is the bringing together of the thumb and the index finger to pick up a small object. This can be tested with a bright-colored button.

9. Pull up—the infant pulls himself to a sitting position.

10. Walk with support—the infant walks by holding onto his playpen, a piece of furniture, or an adult.

11. Stand alone—without any support, the infant stands for several moments.

12. Walk alone—the infant takes several steps alone.*

Figure 11 is the developmental graph that Aldrich and Norval prepared. It is useful in following the neuromuscular growth of infants and in appraising their maturity.

Sequence

The variety of un-co-ordinated movements of the newborn gradually organize themselves and form patterns which result in the motor skills essential in our daily living. The newborn's movements *seem* to be without purpose, although within the first month one sees his hand make contact with his mouth, especially when he is hungry. It seems as though

* Aldrich, C. Anderson, and Norval, Mildred A.: A developmental graph for the first year of life, J. Pediat. 29:304, 1946.

he had some dim perception of the fact that hunger is assuaged by the putting of something into his mouth. His first movements are probably in response to internal tensions. Through the activity he obtains relief from tension (pleasure) and a pattern of behavior which serves his need.

Finger-sucking has purpose; it is a natural way for a baby to obtain pleasure. Sufficient sucking at the breast or on the bottle combined with closeness to the mother helps to prevent prolonged thumb-sucking. However, some babies seem to have an intense need for sucking which cannot be satisfied during the feeding experience. They use their fingers or objects to obtain the satisfaction that they crave.

Freedom to satisfy his sucking needs during the earliest months of the infant's life is supportive; it exercises the muscles

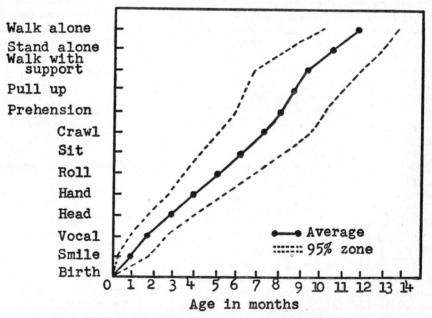

Fig. 11. A developmental graph for the first year, showing the average age for the beginning of the achievements selected and the zone in which 95 per cent of the infants' developmental graphs fell (Aldrich and Norval: J. Pediat. 29:304)

of his jaw and gives him the oral satisfaction he needs to relinquish eventually the pleasure for more grown-up modes of behavior. Finger-sucking continues until the infant discovers new ways of obtaining relief from tension. When his sucking and other emotional needs are satisfied and he is given opportunities to use his hands in play and in learning new skills, he discovers substitute activities which are more satisfying. Under these conditions, relinquishing finger-sucking comes about through a natural sequence of events.

Many people become concerned about thumb-sucking because they fear permanent deformity of the child's jaw. Studies have shown that thumb-sucking may be a cause of malocclusion in the deciduous teeth, but that this malformation tends to correct itself if the habit is broken before 5 years of age. However, persistence in the habit beyond that age tends to make the malformation permanent.

Prolonged thumb-sucking is a symptom of insecurity; it is a symptom which says that the child's life and living are not as emotionally satisfying as he needs them to be. Finding the cause of his discomfort and eliminating it is the only effective method of cure. This is true in all realms of therapy—psychological as well as physical.

By 3 to 6 months of age nervous system development increases the infant's powers of control. During the first months of extra-uterine life the infant learns to hold his head up for a longer time, and by 3 months of age usually he can hold it fairly steadily, although he still needs support for it. When lying on his stomach, he begins to lift his chest as well as his head. During this same time, he has been learning to control the tiny eye muscles and look *at* things. When lying on his stomach, his hands are brought into view without active volition, and he plays with them. As yet he probably does not know that they are

his, but he is beginning to exercise some control of them. He also finds them interesting playthings. In this period he attempts more control of his body, usually achieving first the ability to roll from back to side or side to back. Then will come the ability, at approximately 6 months, to roll completely over, a fact of significance to those caring for babies. When a baby is approaching the stage at which he will be able to roll over it is no longer safe to leave him lying on a bed, a bathinette or a davenport. In fact, a baby never should be left without the protection of cribsides or a railing because new skills are acquired rapidly when physical readiness is attained.

Growth of the nervous system and exercise prepares the infant for more complex achievements. The infant experiments and exercises constantly during the waking hours. He waves his arms and legs and moves his body in every way he can. Little by little the motor skills which will be necessary for the complex skill of walking are acquired. The 4-month-old baby cannot sit up but he is getting ready for that accomplishment. By 5 or 6 months of age he moves his legs and arms with good co-ordination and strength and springs up and down when held in his mother's lap. Within the next month or 2 he will acquire the power to sit alone. At first he will lean forward to hold himself up, and even then it will be evident that his sitting position is an unsteady one. In approximately another 4 weeks, he will have mastered the skill of sitting up straight.

During the early months of growing, the baby gets ready for the creeping, crawling, or hitching stage of locomotion. Most children creep, crawl or hitch before they walk, but occasionally one observes a child who walks at an early age and does not creep at all. He gets ready to crawl or hitch by pushing himself upward and downward, by kicking and stretching with increasing vigor and by making swimming movements with his arms and legs when he is in the bathtub. Through these experiences he gets pleasure and acquires the motor skills which make it possible for him to move about on all fours.

In the last quarter of the first year the infant will pull himself up on his feet. He has enjoyed stretching his legs out straight; he has felt their increased power. He has been held upright and has been allowed to press his feet against the bed or someone's lap and to make stepping motions against it. The inevitable next step in the orderly progression is to pull himself to his feet by taking hold of the side of his crib or playpen.

Learning to stand upright and walk is a triumphant feat of accomplishment. At this moment the child begins a new way of life; he is a different person because he has increased feelings of confidence and self-respect. He has mastered a feat in bodily control; he feels accomplished! One can detect his new feelings about himself in his behavior. He beams, chuckles and looks self-satisfied. From now on he will look at the world from a new angle and meet more of his own needs.

Experimentation soon produces the ability to sit down from a standing position and to walk. When a baby first gets onto his feet, he often does not know how to sit down and may stand until he tumbles in a heap. However, with practice and his mother's help he becomes agile and self-sufficient. Soon he begins to take a few steps when holding someone's hand. Then comes the day when he takes a few steps alone, and then more and more until he is off on his own adventuring about his home and yard. In learning to walk he has mastered the skill which will take him out into the world. At first he is awkward. He stands with a wide stance and wobbles as he walks, but with experience he gains the skill to walk smoothly and the assurance that comes with practice.

No definite date can be set for walking, but there may be a variation of months between the walking time for normal babies. Some babies walk before they are 1 year old; some cannot accomplish the feat until they are 18 months of age. By 2 years all will have mastered the skill to the point of running and even running away!

When the infant begins to walk he will need shoes that have a flexible sole and give support to an undeveloped foot. At birth the bones of a baby's feet are cartilaginous and incompletely formed. Because the child's foot is in the process of development, it is important that only well-fitting stockings and shoes be put onto his feet.

After the toddler learns to walk and run, he begins to experiment with climbing. In a short time he learns to climb up and go down stairs. If he is allowed to practice, he will also climb up onto almost anything that will offer some chance of success. He needs supervised opportunities to experiment and to discover his capacities. Overprotection by anxious adults leads to fear and inhibitions which slow the learning process.

Supervision should protect the child from trying feats that he is not ready for and should provide the encouragement that he needs to overcome difficult obstacles. Bumps and tumbles are inevitable during the experimentation period. They are a part of growth. The child takes them in his stride and learns to tolerate them if the adult refrains from offering sympathy and coddling except when he is hurt.

Learning to walk and climb is a complicated process. First the child develops gross motor power. Then nervous system growth and exercise produce the control which makes it possible for him to use his legs for walking.

Development of the muscles of the arms shows similar progression. At birth the infant has no control over the smaller, more delicate muscles of his hands. The newborn infant cannot reach out to grasp and draw things toward him. Only random movements give him the experience of making contacts.

After the 4th month of life progress in the use of his hands is rapid. At about 4 months of age, the infant holds a rattle and enjoys waving it about, but he cannot get it unless it is placed within his hands. With growth and experience he learns which movements bring him in contact with objects. He repeats over and over the activities which gave him pleasure. Exercise increases the size and the strength of his muscles. Soon he is able to grasp things within his reach. But when he gets the object he lets it drop from his hand with no realization of his part in the release process. The automatic grasp reflex present at birth has disappeared, but now he can grasp and reach more or less voluntarily.

Between the 4th and the 10th months of life the infant acquires new powers in the use of his hands. By 7 months the baby can reach for his bottle and hold it. He can also take it out of his mouth and put it in again, which shows how skillful he is in hand-mouth co-ordination. He revels in the sounds that he creates with noise-producing toys. He learns to bring thumb in opposition to finger—the "pincer technic," Gesell calls it—a definite advance over grasping with the whole hand. With mastery of this technic he is driven to pick up tiny objects. The undesirable as well as desirable objects will get into his mouth for investigation unless his mother is on guard to protect him.

From the 6th month onward the baby uses his hands constantly during his waking hours to master the skills of manipulation which are so important for work and play. He picks things up and puts things down; he pushes them away from him and draws them toward him. He puts one thing on top of another or into another. Over and over he does

these things, and his mastery of himself and things increases.

Play has purpose; it fosters growth of ego resources; it is not idling away time; it is his business. Through the use of toys and social play with his parents and siblings, he acquires motor skills, tests reality and learns its properties. He develops sensory perception and feels the joy of having others interested in his activities. With his siblings he probably will feel some measure of frustration as well. He will find that they are fun to have around; also he will discover that they can thwart many of his desires.

The adult with insight into the purposes of play selects the play equipment that furthers learning and provides opportunities for self-expression. Low shelves or cupboard space with toys easily accessible facilitate self-directed activity. The child is free to get his things when he wants them, and very soon he will also enjoy helping to put them away. Respect for this space for his things helps him to learn property rights. To learn property rights, he needs the experience of having his own things and his rights to ownership respected. The infant is not discriminating; his only requirements are equipment and freedom to experiment. If he is provided with play materials and is encouraged to use them he will discover the way he learns best. Not all children learn and play in the same way. Each child's play springs from inner needs. Therefore, self-directed play serves his purposes most effectively.

Use of Skills

There are many ways in which adults can help children to utilize their new skills to advance their powers of independence. If an infant's mother follows a general pattern of giving care, his powers of adjustment increase. Repetition of experience teaches him to expect to have his hands washed at a certain time, to be turned over at another time or to have a shirt held so he can put his arm through it. Between the 7th and the 11th months of life the infant uses his hands to get food into his mouth and reaches for the spoon in an attempt to feed himself. The infant of 11- to 12-months of age pulls at the toe of his sock and tries to take his clothing off. Simultaneously, he enjoys using the washcloth and soap to imitate his mother's technic of bathing him. In the second year he enjoys putting away his toys, getting into his clothes and hanging up his clothing.

Self-help clothing and well-placed equipment facilitate the child's growth in independence. Elastic waist bands, zippers and large buttons help him acquire independence in dressing and undressing. Hooks placed where he can reach them help him to get the joy of waiting upon himself. He loves learning to hang up his toothbrush, towels and clothing. He also delights in steps that help him get to the wash bowl, the toilet and the bathtub independently.

Utilization of the infant's signals which communicate interest in learning to do things for himself is ego-supporting. Each step that furthers his ability to meet more of his own needs brings more security and mastery of his helplessness. Learning to get pleasure through self-directed activity increases his power to tolerate frustration; it prepares him for weaning—the first crucial step in adaptation to the socialization process.

When a child's interest in learning to do for himself is not utilized, he is thwarted; his reactions will depend upon his nature and his past experiences with his mother. He may fight to use his powers, or he may acquiesce to his mother's desires to do for him and cling to babyish modes of behavior. Later, when his mother wants him to take over the responsibility of self-care, he resists. He does so because he has lost interest in learning and obtains so much pleasure from his mother's solicitation that he cannot bear to give it up. Readiness to learn often goes unrecognized. Sometimes this is because his mother's enjoyment of doing for him blinds her to his needs. Or it may happen because she feels that teaching is burdensome.

Self-feeding is messy. Teaching and waiting for the child to do things for himself takes time, but it is rewarding for the child and his mother. Observing the personality growth that comes with accomplishment brings special satisfactions. His mother needs wisdom in teaching, but it, too, comes with practice. Failure which incites the child to further effort is a wholesome experience; constant failure which discourages is not. In all teaching, the child's strengths and limitations must be noted. He needs opportunities to do that which he is ready to do and help to turn limitations into strengths.

WEANING

The child needs age-adequate frustration and support to master his instinctual drives. Age-adequate frustration implies frustration which the particular child's ego can reasonably be expected to master. It is a necessary factor in personality growth, for each successful mastery strengthens the ego. Appraising an individual child's readiness to adapt to frustration and providing ego-support protects his growth potentials. Giving the bottle or the breast beyond the stage when he is ready to adapt to cup-feeding is as depriving as withholding his bottle when he is hungry. If he is coerced into cup-feedings before he has had optimal gratification of sucking or becomes motivated in learning to use the cup, he responds with rage and resentment toward the person who has deprived him of that which he continues to crave. If these feelings are pushed out of consciousness with an unsatisfied craving, they increase the potency of the id (the primitive part of his personality) and exert their force on him not only in this period of personality development but also in those which are to come. If he is given the bottle beyond the stage when he is ready to learn to drink, he will become overly dependent upon it. This happens because his interest in finding a substitute pleasure was destroyed. Therefore, he clings tenaciously to the bottle because a prolonged period of sucking has come to have more significance emotionally than it ought to have at his chronologic age. He resists giving it up because he has not acquired other ways of getting the gratification that he needs. The situation is totally different if a child has readiness for weaning and help in mastering it. This child will make progress in weaning himself. There will be evidence that proves he is getting pleasure and inner strength from the experience—the satisfaction and the power that come when one surmounts a difficult task in growing up.

Appraising an individual child's readiness to adapt to frustration is not only important in the weaning experience but also essential for toilet-training, and for discipline which seeks to redirect aggression into socially acceptable channels. These experiences will be discussed later in this chapter.

The child needs preparation for his first crucial step in the socialization process. A period of fulfillment and rapid physical growth prepares the infant to adjust himself to the weaning process. Satisfying experience gives the infant feelings of trust in his mother and a desire to emulate her way of drinking. If he has been held for feedings, has been given ample opportunity to meet his need for sucking and has been talked to while eating, he will have acquired pleasant associations with words, smiles and gestures. Because words, smiles and gestures have come to mean love, interest and expression of his mother's pride in him, the infant will need less physical demonstration of affection. He will be ready to utilize substitute satisfactions in mastering a new experience. If he has had opportunities to use his developing skills, he will have acquired increased ability to obtain gratification from his own accomplishments. He will seek self-directed activity and prefer it to the confinement which bottle or breast-feeding necessitates.

After the 6th month of life the infant begins to show interest in learning to drink from a glass. Accustoming the infant to drinking water and sips of milk from a small glass from the 5th month onward is the goal toward which the mother should strive. Soon after he learns to sit independently, he begins to reach for eating utensils. He picks up a cup, brings it to his mouth and looks to the adult for help in learning. It signals his readiness to learn. His mother's delight in his developing ability and his own thrill of accomplishment heighten his interest in perfecting the skill. When he takes a goodly quantity from the cup, the bottle or the breast can be eliminated at that feeding. When he shows less ability to accept the cup, the breast or bottle-feeding can be resumed.

With the above method, weaning is a gradual process which is adapted to his individual capacity. He regulates the amount of frustration that he can tolerate; he is not abruptly or heartlessly deprived of something which has become one of his greatest sources of pleasure.

Readiness for weaning coincides with a period of seeking new play and social experiences. The infant is awake for longer periods of time and delights in social experiences with his mother. If this need is met, he will not feel deprived, even though he has his beloved bottle less frequently than he did before. He will have obtained substitutes which are more valued than the bottle or the breast—a feeling of being more grown-up and a new kind of social relationship with the person to whom he is becoming more attached each day.

When weaning is done gradually after a period of sucking satisfaction, many babies wean themselves by the end of the first year. Some babies continue to want a bottle at bedtime. If the cup has been used most of the day, there is no reason why he should not be allowed to regress to his first love at night as he struggles to help himself go to sleep. Eventually, he will give up his bottle; he will decide for himself that it is no longer necessary. Successful mastery of the weaning process marks the end of the period when the primary satisfactions come from the mouth and from physical closeness to the mother.

THE TODDLER
(1 to 3 Years)

About the time the infant is mastering the weaning process and developing skill in the use of his body he is getting ready to branch out into other learning experiences. *During this period the toddler will need help in acquiring language; in acquiring a healthy concept of himself as a person; in controlling body functions; and in developing the capacity to abide by the standards of his culture without self-injury or injury to others.*

LANGUAGE DEVELOPMENT

Growth must occur before the infant is able to communicate feelings of pleasure as well as discomfort with his organs of speech. At birth the infant can communicate only discomfort with his organs of speech. The welcome cry of the newborn develops fairly soon into sounds which express hunger, pain and anger. The babbling sounds of comfort, the coos, the laughs do not come until the infant is 3 or 4 months of age. The so-called "talking" increases with varying intonation. He squeals with delight in his bath, he crows, he responds with various noises when one talks to him. He becomes increasingly more aware that sounds come from his mother's mouth. He watches her as she talks, imitates the movement of her lips and attempts to "talk back" to her.

The child's speech development depends on various factors—on his ability to hear and retain what he hears and on his motivation to understand and to talk.

Social experiences with his mother give the infant a model and motivate him to learn to understand her and to speak with her.

Understanding of his mother's words precedes his ability to communicate with her verbally. Between the 9th and the 12th months of life the infant begins to understand his mother's verbal communications with him. At about 9 months of age the infant begins to utter sounds which seem to mean certain people or things. He has come through the cry-and-babbling stages of speech development and has entered into the third stage of imitative expression. Certain words are understood, especially those that name concrete things and have been associated with them repeatedly. By the time that he is a year old, he responds to his name and to simple directions. He also understands the words associated with certain activities. "By-by," connected with the pleasure of going outdoors, and "No, No," connected with inhibition, are understood by many infants before they are a year old.

In the 2nd and the 3rd years of life vocabulary increases rapidly. Because many factors influence learning, there are wide variations in the vocabularies of different children. Some children at 2 may have a vocabulary of 300 or more words; others may use less than a dozen. The child who is credited with a vocabulary of 300 words doubtlessly is using a much smaller number than that, but he has been recorded as having said that number. Some words may be said once, possibly in direct imitation, and then may not be used again for months. Without doubt, many of the words used are not spoken with the clearness of enunciation necessary to be understood generally, but to the adult caring for the child they are intelligible.

The child needs help in acquiring a vocabulary; he also needs an interested listener who strives to understand his verbal communications. If there is no hearing or mental impairment, learning to communicate verbally develops naturally when child and mother have consistent, mutually enjoyed experiences together. The interested mother talks to the child, helps him to associate words with things and activities and listens to the way in which he expresses himself. She soon discovers that he is "parroting" her words and attempting to use them in appropriate ways. She rewards his efforts with her responsiveness, and soon his quest for vocabulary begins.

The baby will have been exposed to countless words as people enter his life, not only the name words (nouns) but also the words describing action, space, time, relationships, feelings, etc. He will acquire an understanding of all those aspects of life. He will learn to reason and to solve problems. At first, his comprehension will be what might be called gross understanding. Through experience he will become more and more sensitive to meanings and be more discriminating in his choice of words. For example, he will understand "big" as a 2-year-old, and "bigger than" and "biggest of all" as a 4-year-old. "Gone" can only be "gone" out of sight. It will be months before the words "not here" become associated with the idea of "downstairs" or "downtown." As children are learning to talk, they necessarily must hear much more than they can understand. Such circumstances challenge them to greater understanding if their need for attention is not slighted.

The limited language of young children must be recognized. Unless directions are given simply and are accompanied with the act itself, understanding is often impossible. In times of stress the child's limitations in self-expression also need understanding. When the child is experiencing strong emotional feelings, he cannot communicate them verbally. He jumps with joy; he also screams in anger or in moments of fright. To say "Don't cry" or "Stop moving your arms about" indicates lack of understanding of his nature. The young child cannot say, "I am scared of the technician in the clinic. Why didn't you tell me she was going to prick my finger? If you had I'd be able to manage myself better." Nor can the young child control himself unaided when he is afraid or angry. He has not yet gained that degree of control.

In situations like the above the mother needs to be able to accept the way the young child expresses his feelings. "Don't cry" makes him feel misunderstood. "Of course you're scared, Timmy. All children are when it comes time for a blood count" recognizes the child's natural feelings and supports him in times of stress. The child not only needs understanding but also he requires help in holding himself still when he cannot do it himself. If he is held by a mother who understands his inability to control himself, he will welcome her helpfulness.

BOWEL AND BLADDER CONTROL

In this period from 1 to 3 years of age the toddler is ready to learn the toileting customs of his society. His mother is his guide and teacher. She should watch for signs which indicate readiness to learn. She must interpret the customs and make learning a satisfying, growth-producing experience.

When the weaning process is completed the child's interest shifts to himself, his body, its products and functioning. As he toddles about the house he views the toileting facilities and becomes fascinated with the way they work. He becomes keenly interested in all his mother's activities, including those which take place in the bathroom. He seems to be more aware of his body; he views and explores every part of it and delights in his excretory products. He sees nothing shameful about urine and feces. They are interesting substances because they are the products of his body and activity. Observation shows that he has a drive to examine his feces just as he has the drive to explore every other substance or object within his reach. He is not born with the idea that urine and feces are wastes and inappropriate play materials. He must learn this through carefully guided experiences with his mother.

The child needs help to find socially acceptable outlets for his natural instinctual drive to explore and to mess. If his mother understands his feelings about the products of his body, she will accept his interest. In addition, simultaneously she will help him to obtain instinctual satisfaction from play with appropriate materials such as sand and water and eventually clay and finger paint. His drive to explore and to mess is not "bad." It needs outlet and expression not in its original form but in socially accepted ways that satisfy him. If he is forced to put the drive out of his conscious thoughts, some of his energy will be consumed in keeping it in check. Such energy is lost to more constructive purposes. When he is given appropriate materials to use, he feels understood and lovable. The understanding mother knows that scolding, shaming or withdrawal of love produces fear, hostility and loss of self-esteem. He cannot understand this kind of management, and it leaves him feeling that his instincts are "bad." It also leaves him with destructive feelings toward the person he needs to love.

Readiness Essential for Mastery

The child must learn the customs of his society through experiences with his mother. Our customs place inhibitions on the individual and make definite requirements of him. The young infant is completely unaware of these expectations. He passes his urine and moves his bowels whenever the urge comes. He has no inhibitions and can exercise no conscious control over his sphincter muscles. He relieves himself irrespective of time or place—in the drawing room, in the lap of the haughtiest visitor, no matter how it may embarrass his mother. He does so because it is more comfortable to do so and because he has not learned that his culture expects him to relieve himself only under certain conditions.

The child can meet the requirements of his culture if both physiologic and psychological readiness for learning have been attained and if he is provided with ego support throughout the experience. After a period of pleasure from unrestricted soiling, wetting and exploration which gives him awareness of his family's toileting customs, he develops interest in excretory activity. He shows his readiness to master bowel control when he shows his awareness of his need to defecate. This usually occurs when nervous system growth makes standing possible. His signals of awareness of a full rectum are individual. Some infants make grunting sounds or strain; others communicate their interest in learning control by pulling at their diapers or saying self-formulated words which express the feelings that they are experiencing.

Learning excretory control is a social experience which should foster healthy personality development. When the child is ready to participate he will signal his interest in learning. The mother's responsibility is to interpret her expectations in a kind fashion, to respect his autonomy and to expect functioning on the toilet only when he is ready to co-operate. She also needs to provide rewards when he withstands frustration to meet her requirements. When he feels understood he will give in return for all he has received and will get satisfaction in return for his efforts. His satisfaction will come from his mother's pride and approval and from his own growing self-mastery. With this method of teaching there is no coercion and no deprivation that the child is unable to tolerate. As a result he *feels* good about himself, and his relationship with his mother is sustained at an optimal level.

Readiness to develop bladder control is equally essential for personality growth. When physiologic functioning has progressed to the stage where a child's bladder can retain urine for a 2-hour period, he is usually ready to learn that the toilet is also a place to deposit his urine. Preceding this stage of development (15 to 18 months) the child will show awareness that he has already urinated. He will point to his wet panties or show the puddle he has made. This is growth in awareness; it needs understanding. Just because he notifies that he has wet, it does not mean that he has matured sufficiently to warn *before* he urinates. This requires more growth and will come at a later date.

Helping the child to learn to use the toilet for urinating should be a gradual process. *Again his autonomy needs to be respected.* When his bladder has held urine for a 2-hour period, the chances are that he will be able to co-operate. Then it is wise to take him to the toilet, interpret the custom with simple words that are within his understanding and maintain faith in his capacity to function as best he can. The child will respond to his mother's confidence in him and will need approval for his efforts.

Successful functioning on the toilet will be influenced by the child's current emotional and physical state. Illness produces regression because it utilizes energy that he needs for adaptation. Anxiety does the same thing. When a young child is separated from his mother, the source of his emotional security, he regresses to infantile modes of behavior. If he is anxious about his mother's love, regression may also occur. This can happen when a new baby arrives in the family. It can also happen when his mother's interest becomes diverted away from him to a new apartment or to herself during pregnancy, for instance.

Gradually, the child will take his mother's standards into himself and desire cleanliness as she does. This is accomplished slowly, a step at a time. At first he will be able to function successfully only when his mother is with him. However, gradually control will come from within, and when it does he will have attained real self-mastery. In the interim accidents are bound to occur for they are the natural outcome of stress or absorption in play. They are nothing about which the mother needs to feel discouraged. If there is a good relationship between adult and child, if successes are commended and failures ignored and treated in a matter-of-fact manner, the goal of mastery will be attained eventually. Expecting complete independence before 3 years of age is demanding behavior which is incompatible with a child's nature.

After the child has attained mastery of excretory functioning during the daytime, he becomes ready to learn nighttime control. Usually diapers are worn at night for some time after they are discarded in the daytime. When daytime control is achieved, it is wise to discard the diapers at night. Discarding the diapers with teaching like the following interprets the standard and motivates his interest in his growth: "You don't need diapers at night any more. Soon you won't need to urinate while you sleep. You will wake up when you need to urinate. You can use the potty chair which is next to your bed."

Taking the child to the toilet during the night may keep the child's bed dry but it teaches little of lasting value. The child who has become accustomed to urinating into the toilet and is a bed-wetter at night may be taken up some-time between 10 o'clock and midnight and placed on the toilet with some de-gree of success. However, if he is not awakened, it is not valuable as an aid in learning. It may save wet beds—and that has its values, to be sure—but the important lesson of subconscious con-trol of the sphincter muscles of the blad-der is not achieved. The child is still continuing to urinate in his sleep. It is difficult to waken a soundly sleeping child, and if the attempt to do so creates antagonism or long periods of sleepless-ness, it is wiser to discontinue the attempt.

If there are neither physiologic ab-normalities nor disturbances in the par-ent-child relationship, nighttime control will evolve eventually with growth and with a better understanding of the social requirements of his culture. Sometime between 3½ and 4½ years of age, physi-cal and psychological growth makes nighttime control a reality. It will come about naturally if the standard is taught with understanding and if the family interpersonal relationships continue to foster personality growth.

Appropriate Clothing and Toilet Facilities

When a child develops readiness for learning control of bowel and bladder functioning, he needs to be kept dry and in training pants. This is necessary to accustom him to a feeling of dryness. Diapers are usually given up in the daytime, sometime before they are dis-carded at night. Daytime use of diapers should be given up as soon as the child has understanding of the use of the toilet. Diapers are infantile clothing and presuppose the infantile habit of empty-ing the bladder and moving the bowels without heed to time or place. The very fact of discarding the diapers helps in the learning process. The child feels more grown-up and is motivated to want to master himself.

Clothing which a child can manage easily is a help in a child's learning. For girls, there should be panties that slip down easily. Boys need trousers with few and large buttons and buttonholes, and with wide legs that can be pulled up for urinating. The trousers with zippered flies are intriguing to boys because they can manage them in-dependently.

A toilet chair is most advantageous from the child's point of view because eventually he can use it independently, without fear. Small seats placed on the adult toilet are also useful if movable steps with a good base are available. Any possible experience of fear by being placed for the first time on a large toilet should be avoided. Unless the noise of flushing is anticipated for children, fear reactions may be the outcome. When the toilet is accessible to the child, a boy of 2½ or 3 years of age can learn to stand for urination.

DISCOVERY AND ASSERTION OF SELF

The Concept of Self

The young child is an egocentric per-son who is concerned primarily with himself. At this stage he takes; others give. He says "Mine," clutches his toys and holds them away from the child who approaches him. He is selfish, pos-sessive and feels himself to be the most important person in his universe. It is the natural way for him to feel. *He needs to identify himself and his powers.* Before he can share and be concerned with others, he must feel the joy of pos-session, self-expression, personal power and the self-respect that comes when one is accepted as he is. He will become concerned with others, learn his limita-tions and develop into a socialized per-son after he has received bountifully and become motivated to have social experiences with other children.

In the years from 1 to 3 the child discovers himself and expresses his feelings, wishes and thoughts more potently than before. Between 12 to 18 months and 3 to 4 years he goes through a negativistic stage of development. It is so natural and easy to assert himself by saying "No" and "I won't" that one cannot be surprised that this occurs. After all, "No" probably was one of the first words that he ever came to understand.

Negativism, Dawdling and Ritualistic Behavior

A period of negativism is natural, desirable and important for growth toward maturity. The young toddler has tasted the joy of independent activity but simultaneously he continues to have dependent longings. Sometimes he wants both satisfactions simultaneously. When he does he gets confused and reacts with behavior that stems from conflict and anxiety. One minute he asserts his independence; the next he begs to be held and manifests the most infantile dependency. In this stage of development he has new-found powers, and he is aware of his capacity to assert himself. He does so in a negativistic way. He does it impulsively; it springs from a drive to be powerful, controlling and independent. Often it may be only by saying "No" and doing the thing which is asked.

This period is a short one if the child's nature is understood and his nurture includes ego-support which assists him in finding ways to use his new-found powers in constructive and socially acceptable ways. Overcoming negativism is never accomplished by opposition. Opposition merely increases his need to assert himself. It does not help him to acquire the satisfactions that he is seeking. He needs help to learn how he can participate: "It is time to go to bed now. You can bring Teddy with you and help

to open your bed." A 2-year-old needs a certain amount of physical direction as well as verbal. Taking him by the hand as the above help is given communicates expectancy of co-operation and gives the dependent gratification for which he is longing. Pointing out the fact that his mother recognizes his newfound powers of independence heightens his self-esteem and motivates him to co-operate. When a child is in good rapport with his parents, he is eager to please. When his mother expresses her pleasure in his helpful co-operation he gains status and self-importance. When his mother recognizes his ability and desire to learn to do things for himself, his adaptive capacity becomes strengthened. He acquires a wholesome concept of himself which is basic to his acceptance of others.

During this stage of development dawdling and ritualistic behavior are a part of the child's nature. These characteristics appear because the child is in a transition period; he does not know right from wrong; he cannot make one choice, so he makes two. His mother calls him and says: "It is time for dinner now." He dawdles; he does not know whether to come or to go so he does both. He needs help to know what is expected. When he learns this through consistent experiences, he can make a decision more quickly, and the dawdling will cease to be a predominant characteristic of his behavior.

Ritualism arises in response to the child's deep need for self-mastery. He formulates ritualistic ways of doing things because then he knows what to expect and can master himself and his environment more effectively. Ritualistic behavior is at its peak at 2½ years of age; it is less pronounced at 4 because the child is surer of himself and can adapt to changes in routine with a greater degree of ease. It is wise to utilize his self-devised rituals within a framework of the limits which he is able to tolerate and needs for growth. It saves time and energy and gives him the security that he requires during this phase of his development.

DISCIPLINE

Discipline is education; it is support which helps the child to reach his fullest potentials. It is concerned with the preparation of the child to live in harmony with himself and his fellowmen. Acquiring an integrated personality takes time. It is a matter of growth, development and continuous ego support which begins at birth and ends when emotional maturity is reached.

Discipline should help the child to achieve control from within. The toddler is ambivalent, uncontrolled, aggressive and has unbridled exploratory impulses. He feels kindly when he has what he wants and hates as violently when he is angry. When he is thwarted, he feels destructive and acts out his feelings toward the very person he accepted wholeheartedly a minute before. If he is angry because his mother takes a dangerous object from him, he strikes out at her if he is not stopped quickly enough. He cannot express his aggression verbally or check the overt expression of it. He is frustrated often because his wants are many, varied and forever changing. He wants to make himself understood with language, do for himself and get things from places he cannot reach. He plays intensely as long as his interest lasts; then he spies another toy or thinks of a project that he would like to tackle. He takes what he wants when he wants it without heed to ownership, value or the feelings of others. When he is with other children, he hurts them if he is not watched constantly. He not only pushes, bites, hits and scratches others but also he shows evidence that he enjoys it and obtains pleasure from hurting the very child with whom he was playing happily a few minutes before. In this period he is not only sadistic and without feelings of shame, disgust or pity but also

he is ambivalent. He has feelings of both rage and love. When his rage is over, love prevails until he is frustrated again. His feelings of love and hate are not fused into a pattern of constant friendliness. This will happen at the end of the period that is to come.

The toddler acts this way because he has no controls within himself to check his impulsiveness. He has no inner standards (conscience), and his self-ideal is unformed. He is governed by instincts that have no other object but pleasure. But within him there are feelings which make socialization a possibility. By 1 year of age his attachment to his mother has deepened, and because he is becoming increasingly aware of his inadequacy to get what he needs without his mother, he grows more dependent upon her. The emotions which link the child to his mother make socialization a possibility. He comes to feel that her love and approval are more important than the immediate gratification of his instinctual desires. With these feelings and consistent, understanding guidance which helps him to know what behavior his parents consider "good" and what behavior is considered "bad" or forbidden, he gradually adjusts to his parents' cultural standards.

At the beginning of this period, he does not *know* his mother's standards; he must acquire them through experiences with her or her substitute in this period and the next. Until he has acquired controls from within, his mother or teacher must act as his *ego* and conscience. She is the person who must teach him what activities are safe and appropriate and which ones are dangerous and unsuitable for his growth and the protection of other people and things within his environment. She must also help him find socially constructive outlets for his feelings. He cannot find them unaided. He cannot learn to postpone satisfaction unless he is given a substitute at the time he is feeling the tension of frustration. Stopping him from a destructive act is a part of the support he needs but usually it is not enough. He also needs distraction toward some acceptable way of releasing pent-up feelings. His mother's redirection communicates understanding of his feelings and his need to express them. This is the substitute satisfaction that helps him learn to tolerate increasingly larger doses of frustration. It also increases his independence. After he has had consistent experiences of help through the preschool years, he becomes able to find his own outlets. And what a sense of accomplishment and security this generates! He feels less inadequate; he can venture farther away from mother or teacher because he *feels* the controls he has within himself which will protect him from his own destructiveness and safeguard his relationships with other people. He is also mobilized to learn and get satisfaction from peer relationship.

Controlling asocial behavior is difficult for many young mothers because they can remember how they rebelled at parental discipline during their own childhood. Some mothers have experienced a punishing kind of discipline and have come to loathe the word. To them it connotes punishment, thwarting and loss of love. They have grown up determined to protect their children from that which they experienced. Some mothers do not curtail their children's activities because they are afraid of the feelings which result in themselves or in their children. It is hard for many mothers to help their children find emotional outlets because they never had experiences with their own mothers which taught them how. These mothers need understanding of their own feelings and help to gain insight into the true meaning of discipline and its value for the child and themselves.

Controls and redirection give security and freedom within bounds. The child feels loved when there is someone who cares enough to protect him from his own primitive, asocial nature at an age when he cannot do it himself. He wants to learn the ways of his world and remain safe in the affection of those upon whom he is dependent. He also desires approval from others in his society. Controls are not punishment; they are protective. They give freedom. If he has learned what the limits are from consistent discipline, he can express himself freely within their boundaries. These limits also provide security because he feels safe in his parents' affection if he meets his parents' standards. When he is certain there is someone close by who will protect him from doing that which will destroy what he needs the most, he feels secure. He does not need to be fearful lest he exceed his parents' patience or do something which will make him lose his self-esteem or the approval of a playmate.

Controls also help the child to channel his aggressive impulses into activities from which he can gain increased motor and mental skills—skills which give more pleasure than rampant expression of instinctive drives. A young child who looks as though he felt aggressive can be removed bodily from the situation or stopped temporarily. Then he should be redirected into an activity which will help him learn as well as discharge tension. He can be given a hammering board, bean bags to throw into a pan or a puzzle to take apart and put back together again. In this way he can become prepared to use his aggressive energy in learning at school.

Controls must change as the child grows and must be enforced in ways that foster healthy personality development. Emotional growth is fostered better by rewarding the child's efforts to meet parental standards than by punishment. Curtailing asocial behavior with *consistent,* firm, kind help is supportive. It protects the child's feelings of self-esteem and makes it possible for him to incorporate his parents' standards into himself. Consistency of kind support has been stressed throughout because of its importance in the adaptive process. Alternating between too much gratification of instincts which must eventually become redirected and too strict and harsh methods of discipline confuses the child and makes mastery of impulses nigh to impossible.

THE CHILD DURING THE EARLY PERIOD OF SOCIALIZATION
(3 to 6 Years)

Development from 3 to 6 years is a period of marked psychological growth. Gradually, the child acquires the ability to communicate with language his feelings, wishes and thoughts. His curiosity expands, and with questions and exploration he strives to understand the world of events which touch him personally. In this phase of development the child's relationships with his parents change. He also becomes more social and seeks friendships with children and adults outside his family. He develops increased security; he learns to do more for himself; he gains more inner controls; and he discovers many new ways of obtaining gratification through hours of important play each day. He tolerates separation from his mother, if there are no difficult problems with which to cope. *The child needs ego-supporting interpersonal relationships within his home and the outside world which help him to accept his place in his family, to understand and accept himself as a boy or a girl and to acquire healthy attitudes and feelings toward every aspect of life which he is experiencing.*

LANGUAGE AND UNDERSTANDING

During preschool years the comfortably adjusted child increases his vocabulary by leaps and bounds and probably averages about a yearly 600-word increase between the ages of 2 and 6. Children acquire vocabulary through "parroting" what they hear, through association and through the answers given to questions. The 2-year-old begins with the "what" question: "What's dat?" "What are you doing?" It is his way of learning about his world. At 2 years of age his vocabulary

is largely made up of nouns and verbs, with possibly a sprinkling of pronouns, adjectives and prepositions. But as perception, understanding and experience expand, they become reflected in his speech. Adjectives, descriptive and qualifying, appear; these are followed by more prepositions, adverbs, words indicating some understanding of time and space relationships, of human relationships, of cause and effect.

The 3-year-old uses longer sentences, and his questions become "when," "where," "why" and "how" questions as he seeks increased understanding of the complex life about him. The 3-year-old uses sentences like "I want to go outdoors after breakfast." His questions are often incessant and run something like the following ones: "Where's Daddy gone?" "Why you doing that?" "What's that for?" "When is my Daddy coming home?" "Why can't I do that?" *His questions reveal his needs and require answers which give him increased understanding of what is going on about him.* The child needs to have the events of life interpreted to him. From observation and the adult's interpretation, the child gleans feelings, attitudes and ideas which will influence his feelings about himself and others, about religion, sex, school, hospitals and the other aspects of life to which he becomes exposed.

Before questions are answered, the adult should try to discover the need which has motivated the question. There are many reasons why children ask questions. The most obvious reason is to obtain information or to discover how things work or how they may be used. However, many more questions are asked to obtain relief from anxiety. Some queries are bids for attention and companionship. The child feels lonely and is seeking a social relationship with someone who will be interested in him as a person. When questions are asked the mother needs to interrogate herself before she responds: "What is my child trying to understand? How can I respond so that his need will be fulfilled?"

The questions at 4 and 5 years are more complicated and require more detailed explanations. They want to know how things work: "What makes them do that?" "Where have the icicles gone that were hanging on the roof?" Often a parent is puzzled as to how to answer such searching questions. The one guiding principle should be to give the child the truth to the best of the parent's ability and as simply as possible. Often the question is so far from simple that this is difficult. If the parent does not know the answer he should acknowledge that fact to the child. It will not bring loss of respect. The parent who answers a child's question with "I don't know, Skipper, but let's find out together" will nurture an eager spirit of learning. Telling the child untruths and deceiving him undermines his sense of trust. It fosters suspiciousness and a sense of insecurity.

The 4-year-old child chatters as he plays. A vocabulary of 1,500 or more words is fairly adequate equipment for communication. As he plays house, creating all aspects of family experience —store, policeman, fire, hospitals, school, flying, even all the tragedies which are a part of life—he has at his command the language for each situation.

The 4-year-old child is also acquiring number concepts. When he was 3 years of age he knew number 2, but now that he is 4 he can count to 3. Within the next year he probably will learn to count to 10. A child often learns to say the numbers by rote before this, but that is a feat of memory and does not indicate an ability to make use of the numbers to count.

The 3-year-old, or even the younger child, is interested in color. He differentiates colors and puts objects of the same color together. The 4-year-old begins to name colors, and by 5 he can be counted on to be accurate in regard to the primary colors and even to some of the other colors. Some children may name colors at a much earlier age.

The concepts of time, size, space and shape slowly become more clearly defined. A 3-year-old child has little conception of present, past and future. "Today" has some meaning for him, "yesterday" comes to mean a time that has gone, "tomorrow" a time that is to come. When a 3-year-old child is with his mother, waiting until "tomorrow" is usually comparatively easy. But when his mother is in the hospital having a baby, "tomorrow" must seem like an eternity. It must seem endless to him not only because he misses the security he has when she is there but also because he feels uncertain of what a new baby in his home will mean to him personally. "Tomorrow" is a word that means a relatively short time to the adult, but to a young child experiencing the pain of separation anxiety "tomorrow" brings little comfort.

The understanding of gradations in time is slow in developing and far from perfected even for the 5-year-old. The 4- to 5-year-old becomes interested in "week" as a unit of time and is also desirous of learning the days of the week. A child of 4 years and 8 months at the nursery school was heard to say on a Friday in haughty reproof to a child who had said "I'll see you tomorrow," "No, I won't see you tomorrow, Janet, I'll see you Monday." The 4-year-old child can also tell how old he is; and if 4½, the ½ is as important as the 4.

The preschool child grows in understanding of space relationships. The 2-year-old, with no comprehension of size or shape, may try to put the big square into the small hole. An understanding of difference in size will come first, and later shape will be understood; the square and the circle first, and then the more difficult shapes. A 4-year-old enjoys simple puzzles but he must rely largely on the trial-and-error method of putting it together because his perception of shape is not yet accurate enough to be a completely reliable guide.

The 4- or 5-year-old child becomes increasingly interested in the matter of relatives. He has known his mother for a long time as "Mother," but now he comes to know that she may be a daughter, a sister or an aunt as well, and that he, too, stands in various relationships to other people.

SEX EDUCATION

Sex education is preparation for satisfying marriage and parenthood. The child's capacity to give and receive love begins to develop at birth and continues until emotional maturity is reached. Sex education is more than the transmission of the biologic facts of growth, reproduction and the sexual relationship. It is guidance which prepares the individual for satisfying marriage and parenthood. To be sure, specific knowledge must be imparted, but of even greater importance is the creation of wholesome attitudes and feelings toward the self and toward others as male and female personages.

Preparation for marriage and parenthood requires ego support which makes emotional maturity a possibility. It begins with acceptance of the child as a boy or a girl and is influenced by all the care and the experiences of the growing-up process. Well-guided experiences within his home and community foster self-respect, the capacity to give and receive love, and the acceptance of responsibility for himself and others. Wholesome sex education is achieved more readily when the child has two parents who respect each other, who are satisfied with their life together and are ready and desirous of sharing their life and love with him in ways which are appropriate for his emotional growth.

If the reader reviews the relationship experiences which have been cited on the foregoing pages of this chapter and thinks through the ways that they can influence the child's feelings about himself and others, it will become evident that preparation for marriage and parenthood begins even before the child is born. The feelings that the child acquires about himself and others during the growing-up process will become reflected in his marital relationship. For example, the woman who respects herself and those of the opposite sex will have better chances for marital satisfaction than will the woman who depreciates masculinity or feels inferior because she is a woman.

The feelings that the child acquires about himself and others during the growth process also become reflected during pregnancy and in his relationship with his children. The feelings that a girl acquires about herself and her mother will affect her response to pregnancy and the manner in which she adjusts to it and to the role of mother after her baby is born. Feelings that the boy acquires toward himself and his parents will color the way he adjusts to his supportive role during his wife's pregnancy and to his role as a father. When a woman is confronted with the task of mothering her baby, feelings that she had as a baby become reactivated and determine the way she feeds and guides her young child. The woman who has had her earliest needs gratified abundantly will take the feeding and the dependency of a helpless baby in her stride. A woman who has been deprived of the satisfactions that she needed early in life is apt to have a conflict in the feeding experience with her baby—a conflict between her feelings and the intellectual ideal of mothering that she formed during her pregnancy.

Curiosity

In preschool years the child's curiosity becomes heightened, and he seeks answers to the many problems which perplex him. The 3-year-old knows that he or she is a boy or a girl, and soon inevitably there will be an interest in the differences between boys and girls and between men and women. He also ponders about his origin, and eventually he will raise questions pertaining to reproduction and birth. It is right and natural that he should be interested in his body and find pleasure in it. Every child explores his body and experiments with masturbation. It need not cause any concern unless he consistently chooses it instead of play with others, or instead of interesting activities which are available to him.

It is also natural that the child should be curious about his origin and the origin of others and seek to understand what he is feeling, hearing and seeing. *The child needs to grow up with the feeling that sex is an important quality inherent in his personality and in the personalities of all other people.* He needs to grow up feeling that sex is something which is right to think and talk about. Only then will he get his fantasies or thoughts clarified and the understanding that he needs for growth. In each stage of growth new questions will arise. Sex education cannot be given in one lesson; it must be given a step at a time as growth creates a need for deeper understanding of life in a bisexual world.

When a child shows curiosity or verbally communicates his questions, he needs help in finding logical answers which will serve him in later life and avoid the anxiety which follows the mystery that surrounds unanswered questions. Before factual information is given to the child over 3 years of age, it is wise for the parent to encourage him to talk about his thoughts. This can be done with sympathetic listening and with attitudes that communicate acceptance of any thought he might have. Children fantasy answers to their queries and more often than not they are unrealistic. Erroneous concepts need to be expressed to an interested listener and corrected *before* factual information is given. A child who has pushed unrealistic fantasies out of his conscious mind because they were too painful to think about has a difficult time gaining emotional understanding of truths at a later time. For example, a girl who has been given factual knowledge of the birth process during pregnancy and comprehends it intellectually may be unable to accept such facts emotionally because she has purposely forgotten a fantasy that she had years ago which pictured birth as a gruesome process. Factual knowledge does not relieve her anxiety because it does not rid her of the feelings which were submerged into the unconscious part of her mind along with her erroneous fantasy.

Changes in Family Relationships

Growth during the first 3 years of life is accompanied by changes which make the child more strikingly masculine or feminine and influence his relationship with his parents. The little boy acts more manly; he imitates his father and strives to do the things that he does. The little girl delights in "playing mother and wife"; she dresses up in her mother's clothing and dramatizes her activities in her play. The boy's attachment to his mother becomes intensified and possessive, and he manifests rivalrous feelings toward his father and competes with him for his mother's love. He has aggressive feelings toward his father and wishes that he might destroy him. These feelings and wishes make him fearful lest his father suspect him of having them and retaliate against him. The girl shifts the center of her interest from her mother to her father.

She has similar feelings and wishes which make her anxious. It is obvious what losing a parent of the same sex might mean to a child in this stage of development. Because he has not had enough experience to learn that wishes cannot destroy, he might well conclude that he had been instrumental in bringing about the loss. He would need help in understanding the real cause of the loss. He would also need repeated experiences to learn that wishes are not the same as deeds.

This phase of personality development gives rise to conflicts, anxiety, disappointment, anger and confusion. The child has conflicting feelings toward his parent of the same sex. The boy not only hates his father and wishes for his banishment but he also loves him. The boy loves his father because he supplies pleasure and a model from which he can fashion himself. The boy hates his father because his father is bigger and gets what he covets from his mother. This makes the boy feel angry and inadequate, which destroys his peace of mind and administers a crushing blow to his pride. The same relationship pertains to the girl and her parents. She adores her father and wishes that she could take her mother's place, but at the same time she loves her mother and feels her great dependence upon her. In this period both the boy and the girl meet the painful reality of their immaturity. This gradually corrects any distortion that they may harbor concerning their powers. They discover their limitations. No longer do they feel that they are master of all they survey!

Meeting reality is painful and anxiety-provoking; the child cannot face it immediately; he has to deny it temporarily. His play reflects this denial. He talks and acts like his parent of the same sex. In fantasy he *is* the parent. If one observes the 3- to 4-year-old child at play he might think that he continued to feel that he was the king-pin in his family but this is not so. Much of his play

keeps him free from anxiety. In play he denies reality; he devises play which makes him feel powerful and loved. This is the age when it is not unusual to see twosomes ganging up against a third child with such comments as: "You can't play with us. You're not our friend." This is the period when boys show off, wear cowboy suits and carry guns. It is the period when girls strut, beg to wear fluffy dresses and talk of "*my* babies." This behavior says: "Look at me! I've a great deal that is desirable. I'm trying to make myself feel stronger and more desirable than I really feel."

The above kind of play serves many purposes. It gives the child experiences at playing father or mother, and it provides some insight into what it feels like to be a parent. Such play helps him to master the fear of bodily injury which besets all preschool children. It also helps him to tolerate the frustration that he feels. He adapts to the reality of his family situation as he can cope with it. As he gains ego strength from play and accepts the gratification that it is possible for him to get from his parent of the opposite sex, his limitations become less painful, and his need for denial in fantasy becomes less necessary. Through satisfying experiences with children, he also finds outlets for his feelings of love. This, too, helps him to renounce his desire for exclusive attention from his parent of the opposite sex and to accept his place in the family.

Supportive parental guidance during this phase of personality development is of paramount importance. The frustration that the child experiences is painful but necessary for growth. He cannot move ahead emotionally until he submerges his sexual feelings toward his parent of the opposite sex into his unconscious. He must also submerge his rivalry and hostility toward the parent of the same sex and identify himself with him. When this occurs his goal changes. Instead of wanting to *be* mother or father, he wants to *be like* his parent of the same sex. When this occurs, his love and hate will become fused into a constant pattern of friendliness toward both his parents. To accept his place in the family, he needs help to tolerate the frustration that he must experience in order to grow. He will get support from experiences which help him to feel cherished as he is—not as a love object but as a beloved child. When he has parents who love each other, accept his urge to love and respect his needs for growth, he receives the support he needs to solve his complicated problems in a healthy way.

SUPERVISED PLAY WITH OTHERS

By 3 years of age a child should be prepared to profit from play experiences with peers to help him solve the problems cited above. He should have acquired ego resources which make it possible for him to broaden his horizons and feel safe in the company of those outside his family. Continuity of a warm relationship with his mother gives the child trust in others and a goodly degree of security within himself. The 2-year-old is not ready to separate himself from his mother. He continues to need her as a constant companion. He may venture away from her into the next room for a few moments of play but soon he returns to her. He does this because he becomes anxious when she is out of his sight. He is dependent upon her for love and for protection from his own destructive instincts. He is lost and afraid without her. She gives comfort, protection from danger; she helps him to learn; and she makes it possible for him to master himself in ways that he could not if she were not there. The 3-year-old child feels safer in his world because his mother has helped him conquer the unknown that he met when his horizons broadened as he learned to walk.

A 3-year-old child can profit from a nursery school or play-group experience if he has gained security in his relation-ship with his parents; if he is familiar with the teacher and the school environment; if he knows why he is being placed there and what is going to happen while he is there; if he knows that his mother will return to take him home; and if he is sure that his needs will be fulfilled in her absence. These are the emotional requirements which are necessary to master any experience that requires separation from the security which the presence of Mother and familiar surroundings represent.

Motor Growth

In the years from 2 to 3, motor skills which show themselves in play and daily living are acquired and perfected. Learning to skip, hop and jump becomes engrossing activity. The 3-year-old will jump from a low height, e.g., a stair or a low stool. Between 4 and 5 years, he is ready to jump from a greater height, say, 3 to 4 steps. He learns during this year to skip and hop as well, and to run lightly on tiptoes.

Balance is acquired with growth and practice. At 2 he did not have sufficient control of body balance to stand on one foot. Before he is 3, he tries it for a brief second or two; and by the time he is 5, Gesell reports that he can do it for 8 seconds.

Learning to use a Kiddy Car and a "bike" absorbs the interest of the preschool child. The 2½-year-old goes about on a Kiddy Car with the greatest of ease. Soon he wants to try the 3-wheeled "bike" with pedals, and between 4 and 5 years of age he can ride around the playground with speed and dexterity.

Opportunity and encouragement to practice using his body during these early years promote self-confidence and prepare him to compete favorably with others. The 5-year-old usually has excellent motor control if he has been given opportunities to practice. The child who has been inoculated with adult fears ("Look out," or "Don't fall," etc.), probably will be slower in learning and possibly may never acquire skill in some of the more complicated and daring activities. All this practice in learning to use his body during the early years will help him when later he starts to skate, ski, etc. In the school-age period physical skills are necessary to compete favorably with age-mates. Especially is this true for boys.

Not only has the 5-year-old child learned to use his large muscles more but also he has become skillful in the use of his hands. He learned before 1 year to bring thumb in opposition to finger. Even before he was 2 he enjoyed making marks with crayons. The 3-year-old paints with great pleasure and begins to design with lines or masses of color. The 2-year-old cannot cut with scissors, although he is interested in learning. The 3-year-old begins to use scissors with some success. The 5-year-old has had a year or more of enjoying cutting, pasting, stringing beads, building with blocks and doing puzzles. The baby's banging with his rattle has slowly organized itself into the skill of "hitting the nail on the head." The 3-year-old is fairly accurate in hitting big pegs, and the 5-year-old learns to use a real hammer and nails and even a saw.

The child needs supervision to learn to use materials. Supervision should guide him in the use of paints, brushes, scissors, hammers and other equipment; and it should provide him with opportunities for free expression within the limits which are necessary to protect himself and others and the physical environment he is in. Supervision is not adult domination; it is leadership and support. Children need help in learning the use and the care of the tools of the craft. When the adult has completed the task of teaching the use of the tools and the places where they may be used, she should give the children freedom to express themselves in their own way. Setting standards of adult performance stifles creativeness. Children cannot compete with it or measure up to stand-

ards that adults inadvertently set when they do this. Children need opportunities to learn. Learning comes from within and should be a creative experience which produces feelings of accomplishment. Children feel no accomplishment if their activities are directed or interfered with by adults who "want to help" by doing the task for them.

Psychological Growth

Social and emotional development comes with growth and supervised activity with others. The 2-year-old wants to make friends but he usually does not know how. In addition, he has uncontrolled aggression that gets in his way. His aggressive methods of approach need redirection as has been cited in the section on Discipline. Two-year-old children cannot play together. They enjoy being together; they may sit side by side at the table in the playroom and do the same thing, but there is no co-operative play, and a friendly experience together does not last very long; it becomes interspersed with punching, pushing or hugging which is usually too violent for one of them.

The adult who understands that consistent guidance is necessary for growth does not vacillate between overindulgence and strictness or condemn the child who snatches as selfish or force him to give up all his toys. Instead, she consistently helps each child to find pleasure in being in the presence of other children. When this is accomplished she gives them help in sharing and in discovering that playtime is happier when this is done. She knows children are born selfish and need time to learn to share. They learn to share, to control their aggressive instincts and to consider the rights of others gradually. *This learning comes through their desire to please the mother or the teacher.*

It is obvious that a good adult-child relationship must exist for healthy psychological growth. Motivation must exist. Unless the child values the adult's approval and can identify himself with her, little self-mastery or growth will occur. He may inhibit his instincts out of fear but when he does, his control of himself continues to depend on the presence of an adult. When the adult is absent, he is afraid because he has no controls from within.

Between 3 and 6 years of age the comfortably adjusted child learns to play with other children. At 3 years of age children become motivated to play together. Their play develops into the imaginative play of the 4- to 6-year-olds. Playing together means that the child is old enough to co-operate with another child, each one doing his part in making play successful. In the early stages of playing together, only a short time of co-operation between two children can be expected. Between 4 and 5 years of age social and emotional growth emerges. The play of these children is more elaborate and continues for a longer period of time. They dramatize what they are experiencing at home in an attempt to understand and master all that they are feeling. Several children play together, and often new ones are permitted to join them. This denotes progress; it means they are making strides in acceptance of their place within the family.

Gradually, with understanding guidance the child grows more able to express his aggressive feelings in socially accepted ways. Methods of guidance which help the child direct his aggressive feelings into constructive channels have been suggested previously. Little by little he can be helped to find ways to work through his feelings in play and eventually to express his anger verbally. Being able to express anger verbally manifests growth. It is a constructive way and protects others from getting hurt.

Growth in the ability to handle anger constructively is observable in preschool children. The baby screams with anger if he is thwarted by having his hands held down. The 4- or 5-year-old says, "I hate you when you tell me I can't go over to Suzie's house. I'd like to smash you." The 5-year-old may be enraged by seeing another child knocked down. True, he may come to the rescue by first knocking down the culprit, but the reason for his anger is concern for another, not himself, and we know that psychologically he has grown.

Opportunities for learning to share, to take turns, to help each other, to make plans about their play, to modify the expression of their emotions all come as part of learning to play together. All the qualities that make for harmonious living may be guided and fostered in the play of preschool children. With understanding guidance the 6-year-old has become a co-operative, gregarious person who is beginning to recognize and respect the rights of others.

Through guided experiences in the home, the school and the community the child's personality becomes formed. His ego is strengthened, and he internalizes the standards and the ideals of his parents and teachers. By the end of this period these standards and ideals should have become a part of him. They are his super ego or conscience which is made up of inner controls and a self-ideal. He will not need his parents with him as much as he did before. Because he has made their standards and ideals his own they will function independently of the persons in his environment. They will tell him what is right and what is wrong. Guilt follows when the conscience is overridden. Fear of the conscience's punishment (guilt) will check the overt expression of his asocial instincts in order to obtain maximum pleasure in his social world. Fearfulness of guilt motivates him to act in ways that please both himself and his parents. Therefore, his conscience is an influencing factor in socialization. However, it will also be a source of conflict. He will not always be successful in pleasing himself and his parents but he will become gradually more self-directing during the early school years. In school he will want his teacher to be on the side of his newly internalized superego. She will represent an authority whose demands must be respected. He will be prepared to identify himself with his teacher and other authority figures in this outer world. Through these relationships with adults in the outer world his superego will become strengthened. His teacher's ideals will become his ideals, and his standards will become influenced by her and by his experiences with playmates and other important adults in his environment.

THE SCHOOL-AGE CHILD
(6 to 10 Years)

PREPAREDNESS FOR SCHOOL

The basis for the child's adjustment and success in school lies in the first years of his life. His relations with teachers and peers will be determined by the personality structure that he has acquired through interpersonal experiences with his parents and siblings. His adjustment in school will be determined by his feelings about himself, siblings and parents, by the degree of independence and security that he has acquired, by the degree to which he has gained control of his sexual and aggressive drives, by the extent to which his sexual curiosity has been satisfied and by the way he has learned to relate himself to his playmates.

Intelligence and the emotional climate of his school environment are factors which influence success in school, but more important is the way in which he approaches the learning process. His approach to his teacher and scholastic activities is not only determined by what he meets in the school situation; it is influenced by all that has gone before. Many normal and superior children fail in their first years at school because they are physically unfit or are unprepared emotionally to use school activities for growth.

Life in the school-age period arouses conflict and offers new and difficult developmental tasks to surmount. Physical growth slows down and frees energy for personality growth. *To succeed in this stage of growth the child needs emotional freedom to acquire intellectual and physical skills (ego), to break away from parental dependence and become a part of a group. He also needs energy available to gain increased control over his sexual and aggressive drives through strengthened inner controls. In addition, he needs to learn the laws of his society through play and school activities (superego).*

All of these tasks are difficult ones requiring perseverance and the capacity to give up many personal desires involving frustration. Surmounting these tasks requires an ego that can function on the "reality principle." *The goal of the reality principle is different from the goal of the "pleasure principle." Its goal is to postpone relief from tension (pleasure) until the individual attains what will satisfy his deepest needs most fully. It entails problem solving and thinking.* An example will serve to demonstrate one way the ego functions to maintain emotional equilibrium. A child may become frustrated by a legitimate demand of his teacher. When this happens the child experiences conflict between his drive to strike out against the situation which has frustrated him and his wish to keep his teacher's approval and to maintain his own feelings of self-esteem. The child's response to his frustration will depend upon the strength of his ego. If he has learned that greater pleasure comes from the approval of his teacher and of his own self-ideal than from immediate discharge of tension, his ego will act in a way that will maintain his security. In this situation his ego perceives that the teacher's demands are legitimate. Past experiences have taught him that the teacher's approval was worthwhile. His id says, "Get pleasure no matter what the cost." His superego says "Keep your aggression in check. If you don't, you'll get punished and hate yourself for losing control of yourself." His ego is the executive of his personality. Its task is to keep his id, his superego and his teacher (the reality world) satisfied. The healthy ego says: "Meet the teacher's demands. You will get more pleasure if you do. As soon as you begin to do what the teacher asks, you will feel less tension. Your aggression will be channelized into an activity which will give you satisfaction. If you still feel tense at recess, you can get rid of it by running."

If the child in the above situation has not had the experiences which are necessary to strengthen his ego's capacity to function on the "reality principle," he will express his aggressive instinct and get relief from tension immediately. He will not be able to wait; he will be dominated by his id instincts. It is obvious which child will have the greatest satisfaction. The child with the stronger ego will get the approval of his teacher; he will also get pleasure from mastering the teacher's demands and continue to feel at peace with himself. He will have taken another step in adaptation to reality. The child with the weak ego will get immediate relief from tension, but that is all the pleasure he will receive. He may get punishment immediately afterward. If he does, he will harbor feelings that make the next demand even more difficult to meet.

Mental Growth

So much of what might be called basic learning has been accomplished before the child enters formal school life that this latter seems to be a time of expansion in the fields of knowledge that he has already acquired. He can learn arithmetic because he has the number concept. He can learn to read because he can recognize the shapes of things. He can learn geography because he has a sense of shape and direction. He can learn history because he has a sense of time. He can acquire his own vocabulary and learn another language because he has one already.

He has learned to use his mind, to reason, to solve problems in his preschool years; and he can go on to more complex problems in this stage of development because of previous experiences and because growth of his nervous system makes him biologically ready to begin to learn to read and write.

Mental growth or the learning to function as an intelligent human being will take place according to a general pattern. The sequence of this general pattern and the approximate ages when mental skills are acquired can be outlined. However, widely varying individual differences must be expected, for they are as characteristic of mental as they are of physical growth.

Intelligence Tests

Standardized intelligence and personality tests provide understanding of a child's mental and personality development. These tests have come to play an important part in helping adults to understand the child in home, in school and at work. They are not infallible, but they are extremely useful tools when employed by those who are skilled in interpreting their results and in recognizing their limitations. Intelligence tests are divided into group and individual tests. The group tests are less reliable than are the individual ones. However, they are practical in school situations. They aid teachers in understanding the child's capacities for achievement and guide them in formulating plans for his education.

Intelligence tests are usually reported in terms of I.Q. (intelligence quotient), which is arrived at by dividing the mental age by the chronologic age and multiplying by 100. A child who has an I.Q. between 90 and 110 would be said to have shown the intelligence to be expected of a child of his age. The child's mental age is arrived at by listing his ability to perform those items in the test which have been found possible for most children of his age. If he can perform those at a higher age level, his mental age is correspondingly higher. It may be that he can perform some items at a higher age level and others at a lower. The system of scoring is such that the mental age can be computed in spite of the marked individual difference in performance.

One isolated test is of far less value in studying a child than is a series of tests given at different age levels. By doing this, it is possible to check the child against his own development as well as against the standardized picture of development. Tests for infants and those at the preschool level covering motor development rather than language, as well as tests for school-age children and adults, have been worked out.

PERSONALITY GROWTH

There are problems for the child to face in school, but there are also many opportunities for gratification. As the mental skills of the period are accomplished, the child feels strength in his personality. His feelings of confidence and self-esteem expand, and he revels in his new knowledge, and the things that he learns to do. In this period the child's curiosity expands from the subject of himself and his parents to other aspects of life about him. He is avidly interested in the activities of school and of the church and in learning about the world in which he lives. His interests take him away from home—to museums, airports, parks, clubs, playgrounds, to the country to fish, swim, hunt and to learn about birds, animals and vegetation.

His interests and desire for growth compel the child to seek friendships with his peers. No longer is he satisfied with the attention of his parents. After he has surmounted the task of adjustment to his teacher and the learning process, his interests expand. He feels a need to find security, satisfaction and a way of life from experiences with his peers. The groupings change in this period. The preschool child played with both boys and girls; the school-age child wants a "gang" of his own sex. They draw off into little groups and follow their particular interests. Through identification with those of their own sex, they acquire characteristics of masculinity or femininity. They also have opportunities to find their places in a group, to learn the laws of fair play, to respect the rights of others, to work through their feelings of rivalry, to find outlet for their aggressive feelings and to master their fears.

Growth during this period of development entails conflict and frustration. Parental standards are different from those of the child's group. He wants both parental acceptance and security and satisfaction in his life within the group. As a result, he experiences conflict and anxiety. If he succumbs to parental standards, he will remain dependent and be deprived of the experiences that he needs for growth. If he identifies with his group and follows their codes, he experiences anxiety because his newly formed conscience or inner voice says, "This is wrong." He feels guilty and he has a problem to solve. The way he solves it will depend upon past experiences with his parents and upon their attitudes toward him in this stage of development.

The child needs freedom to venture forth and become a part of the group outside his family. When his parents understand his needs for growth, they will provide this freedom. They will know that he needs their love expressed in new ways. They will continue to give him their undivided attention when life in school or within the group brings more frustration than he can bear; they will continue to give him security for his emotional needs. But they will also recognize that his teacher and peers need to become increasingly more important to him. They will accept the changes in behavior which come through association with his gang. They will let him wear the togs of which the group approve and will permit him to do most of the things that the other kids do. They will accept his moments of rebellion and devaluation of them as important people because they know that it is a necessary phase of his growth. If he continues to do as Mother says, his conscience cannot become modified by peer interaction. And he will miss experiences which help to turn his interest away from his parents and to learn to get along with his contemporaries.

Play with others provides opportunities for mental, social, physical and emotional growth. Through play the child learns new skills, gains knowledge and self-confidence. He learns to sacrifice his wishes for the benefit of the group; he learns to conform to their self-imposed rules and regulations; he learns to depend upon the emotional satisfactions that come from relations with contemporaries; he learns to adapt himself to the outside world—to discover the meaning of life in his own way.

Observation of school-age children at play shows what takes place as a result of interaction with peers. The play of school-age children is different from the play of preschoolers. They are concerned with skill and perfection, with rules and regulations and in learning to become self-directing individuals. They feel a need to learn to control themselves, to abide by the rules of the game and the group. Instinctively, they are trying to master their fears and gain control of their sexual and aggressive drives and to become increasingly less dependent upon their parents.

Personality growth is the outgrowth of parental and teacher guidance and group interaction. Parental and teacher guidance is necessary to help the child sublimate or redirect his impulses into constructive activities. With wise discipline the child's capacity to control impulses becomes strengthened in this period, and he develops increased independence and new powers of self-direction. *As a result he requires less direction and needs permission to be as self-directing as he is capable of being.* He enjoys and is proud of the independence that comes from being able to take care of himself. He feels depreciated when adults fail to recognize the many things he is able to do for himself. No longer does he need the directives essential for the preschool child who has not yet learned what is expected of him. The school-age child *knows* when it is time to go to school, time to go to bed or to get ready for his daily trip to the physiotherapy departments. And he feels respected when his mother recognizes the ego resources that he possesses.

Broadened social experiences also bring personality growth. Through group experience the child acquires new ego resources. He gains new physical and social skills which give him security and a place in the affections of his peers. He also acquires stronger inner resources which prepare him to accomplish the difficult developmental tasks of adolescence.

THE PREADOLESCENT
(10 to 12 Years)

GROWTH WITH A PURPOSE

Preadolescence, the 2-year period prior to the onset of puberty, produces changes in behavior. By 10 years of age the comfortably adjusted child has acquired superb mastery of himself and of his environment. He is sympathetic, well-mannered, courteous, diligent, co-operative and self-directing. These accomplishments make both the child and his parents secure and satisfied with themselves. However, this period is one of short duration. Parents no sooner relax and revel in their accomplishments than they begin to be aware that changes in behavior are occurring. His composure, control and thoughtfulness gradually diminish. His activity increases as he redoubles his efforts to master reality in preparation for the physiologic changes which he intuitively knows are going to come.

The change in behavior which comes in preadolescence has purpose; it loosens up the child's character structure, provides further opportunities to resolve old conflicts and problems that were incompletely solved before; and it makes growth and reorganization of personality during adolescence a possibility. *Preadolescence is a period during which the individual needs to gain the ego strength that he will need to make healthy solutions to the conflicts of adolescence.*

The preadolescent is filled with abounding energy. He is full of ideas and experiments with every conceivable project known to children. He is active incessantly and seems to recognize the behavior which annoys his elders the most. Part of his activity is the result of his driving need to assert himself and impress others with his independence. Part of it stems from the supply of energy that he has at his disposal. He uses most of his energy in constructive activities that help him to master reality. However, some of it spills over into finger-drumming, feet-tapping and impulsive behavior of one kind or another which relieves his tension.

There are other characteristics of preadolescent behavior which are often criticized because the purpose of the newly developing behavior is misunderstood. The preadolescent is preoccupied because he is absorbed in himself, his development and in the activities of his important "gang." Outwardly, he shuns his parents' interest in his growth and excludes them from his innermost thoughts. The controls that he formerly had seem to vanish; he becomes exhibitionistic, unsympathetic, greedy, annoying, sloppy and negativistic temporarily. Chores that he formerly enjoyed become bugbears—"the things his parents hate to do," "unimportant," "rot," "the result of the old-fashioned parents he happened to acquire." His interest in school work often diminishes, and he conveniently "forgets" to do those things that his parents desire him to do first and foremost. Old problem behavior reappears which his parents thought had been outgrown forever. He depreciates his parents. He seeks an adult friend of the same sex to identify himself with, emulate, idealize and use for satisfaction of his continuing dependent needs. He looks longingly on the family situation of his friends. He is unappreciative. Nothing his parents do seems to please him. His parent of the same sex is the object of most of his criticism.

ADULT-PREADOLESCENT RELATIONSHIPS

The changes in behavior produce anxiety in both the preadolescent and the adults unless the adults who live and work with him understand his needs for growth. It is infinitely easier to accept and work with the preadolescent if one realizes that he *needs* to assert himself, rebel and depreciate others in the process of working through his conflict between dependence and independence. He does not hate the adult he depreciates; he is merely trying to prove to himself and his world of associates that he is grown-up—that he really does not need them as much as he did before. He continues to have powerful dependent needs but he cannot tolerate having them satisfied in the same way that he could when he accepted himself as a child. Now accepting dependent gratification from his parent makes him feel infantile. His behavior manifests the way that he obtains his goal without accompanying anxiety. He hides his wish for satisfaction of his dependent needs by rejecting his parents; he gets them met through his relationship with other adults.

Sustaining adult-preadolescent relationships with democratic guidance is imperative to support the youngster in surmounting the developmental tasks of the period. His changing behavior needs acceptance. He continues to need limits and the strength of his parents' support. He cannot completely direct himself by any means. His impulsiveness is heightened in this stage of development. He needs help in accepting himself as he is and in finding ways to channel his feelings and energy. Recreational therapy provides outlets for his feelings, builds self-respect and provides a way to use the influx of energy that he has at his disposal. He accepts guidance which considers his new pre-adolescent status and helps him to handle himself more independently. He loathes the kind that he has experienced as a child and rebels at autocratic discipline which fails to recognize his personal powers. He is approaching adolescence. The more the adults in his environment can do to build up his self-esteem, the more adequately he will be prepared to solve the many personal problems that are a normal part of adolescence.

THE ADOLESCENT
(12 Years —)

Adolescence is the crucial stage of personality development which begins with the onset of physical maturity and merges gradually into young adulthood. During the space of a few years the adolescent must prepare to take his place as an interdependent member of society. *To attain emotional maturity, the adolescent needs to find and accept himself and his sexual role, resolve his conflict between dependence and independence and emancipate himself from his attachment to his parents. He also needs to choose and become prepared for his future role, be it in marriage and parenthood or in a profession or a vocation.*

The adolescent's past experiences influence the way he will approach and resolve his problems. All that he has experienced prior to adolescence will become reflected in his behavior. The adolescent who has trust in himself and others will approach his problems with courage, hope and confidence. He also needs a character structure that is strong enough to master the increased potency of his sexual and aggressive drives. If he has these personality traits, he will waste less energy on anxiety over the problems he faces and will be able to solve them in a manner more satisfying to himself and society.

The child who has been deprived of supportive relationships prior to adolescence will be less well-prepared to tackle new tasks. He will be encumbered with a multitude of old problems and conflicts and have excessive anxiety to master. He will have fewer inner resources to use in solving his problems. As a result he will need more understanding and support than the individual who enters adolescence prepared by growth-promoting relationships within his family.

THE NEW SELF

The hormonal changes which mark the onset of physical maturity stimulate physical and psychological growth. The adolescent has a rapidly changing body and new bodily functions to which he must become adjusted. He also has new feelings, attitudes and interests. His impulses are stronger, and old patterns of behavior cease to keep him in emotional equilibrium. These changes produce conflict, anxiety and uncertainty which are manifested in vacillating, unpredictable and oftentimes impetuous behavior.

The adolescent's anxiety, uncertainty and searching for mature patterns of behavior also become manifested in behavior which is paradoxic. One minute he is bursting with pride in his newly formed body; the next minute he is embarrassed with it. He desperately needs advice on all manner of things, but when it comes he flies into a rage. One moment he loves his parents deeply and values their way of life and their qualities of parenthood; in the next breath he loathes the ground they walk on and can see no good in anything they think or do. He is daring, brash and courageous; simultaneously, he is cautious, fearful lest his body is weak or abnormal. He is often hypochondriacal. He forges ahead toward those of the opposite sex and then runs away from them, denying any interest whatsoever in their persons. He criticizes with abandon but simultaneously conforms like an automaton and wants to be exactly like those he berates. His ideals express utopia. He wants to change the world, yet he wants it to remain exactly as it is. One minute he is abounding in energy, the next he is completely depleted and finds the easiest of tasks an insufferable burden. Is it any wonder that his parents say, "I just can't understand him"? And does not the teen-ager's behavior spell a mental state of emotional disequilibrium, confusion and turmoil?

The adolescent's behavior is not only trying to himself but it is also frustrating to his parents. It is not easy to live with an unpredictable, vacillating teen-ager. His parents never can anticipate his reactions, and 99 times out of 100 they get a response different from that which they expected. Parents of a teen-ager never can be right for long, no matter how hard they try. It takes secure, stable parents to maintain their equilibrium while they are living with an adolescent.

Many parents of adolescents need understanding as much as their children do. Many parents had adolescent trials, heartaches and bouts of rebellion which were too painful to remember. As a result they view their teen-ager's behavior with acute apprehension. Some are not emotionally ready to handle the problem of guiding their teen-agers. They get confused, anxious and uncertain. They need help in understanding themselves and their youngsters. Unless they get it they may inflict an unreasonably strict regimen of discipline on their teen-agers or give up in despair, leaving them alone and unsupported.

Learning to understand a new self requires self-examination, exploratory experiences, knowledge, parental acceptance and guidance. To solve his problems, the adolescent becomes absorbed in himself, daydreams and tests himself out in competition with others. He also seeks security through association with his age-mates and struggles to find solutions which relieve his anxiety and help him to feel more competent.

The adolescent needs acceptance as a growing individual and guidance which helps him to discover his powers and his limitations. He needs the help of strong parents and professional workers who understand his anxiety and support him with their strength. He needs interest in himself as a person and faith in his capacity to find solutions to his personal problems. The adolescent must find his own solutions to his problems. He will, if he is counseled in a way which increases his self-esteem, confidence and understanding of himself and others of both sexes. Those who guide the adolescent also need patience, tolerance and the intuitive insight which is necessary to appraise his capacity to utilize freedom constructively.

The adolescent continues to need

limits. The young adolescent's personality is disorganized from the changes of preadolescence. In addition, he has powerfully strengthened drives to master and an intense desire to become independent of his parents immediately; but he is not psychologically ready to be independent. He does not have inner controls which provide consistent mastery of himself. Until he acquires a new set of inner controls which permit socially acceptable and personally satisfying emotional outlets, he needs wisely chosen and diplomatically imposed limits. These limits on the one hand must be sufficiently flexible so that he has opportunities for growth. Yet on the other hand they must constrain him from actions which will merely serve to heighten his anxiety. For example, it is reasonable to encourage a 15-year-old to go to adequately supervised social parties, but it is unwise to subject him to the temptations of an unchaperoned house party.

The adolescent who is not confined within reasonable limits is left unsupported and unprotected. The unsupported adolescent may respond with impulsiveness which leads to excessive guilt, delinquency or other signs of mental ill-health. Or he may become so frightened that he overcontrols himself to the degree that he blocks his opportunities for legitimate satisfactions and further personality growth. There are adolescents who respond to unrestricted freedom as though it had given them license to express themselves fully. Such behavior neither meets their needs for growth nor considers the needs of others.

The adolescent needs limits which change as experience promotes growth in self-understanding and mastery. Guided experiences which foster feelings of success, self-esteem and security in his relationships with others prepare him to handle increasingly larger amounts of freedom. Unless he is given freedom to try himself out in increasingly more difficult situations, his opportunities to gain a new self-concept will be thwarted, and he is apt to wind up in unwholesome rebellion or equally unhealthy submission.

EMANCIPATION

Growth of the child's love life normally progresses through stages which begin with simple love of himself, in which full personality development ends with a love of humanity. The newborn infant is incapable of loving anyone else but himself. As he grows, the consistent satisfying relationships with his mother permits his capacity for love to extend so as to include her. Later, his father becomes an object of his affections. Then come the changes in his relationship to his parents which were described in the 3- to 6-year-old period of development. Solving his problem in a way which permitted identification with the parent of the same sex made it possible for the child to begin the long process of becoming a man like father or a woman like mother.

Rivalry with brothers and sisters within a family is a natural part of the growing-up process. Children within a family enjoy each other as playmates. However, they also find that the presence of siblings results in friction, rivalry and competition for their parents' love. Gradually, through discovery that each child in the family is loved for himself, the child outgrows his rivalrous and ambivalent feelings toward his siblings.

When the child acquires increased security in his relationships with his parents, his love interests expand to include those outside his immediate family. Playmates of either sex become the object of the preschool child's affections. His relationships with them help to wean him from the consuming love that he feels for his parent of the opposite sex. In the school-age period, the child turns his love interest to those of his own sex. These attachments provide security at a time when he has an urgent need for companionship but is as yet unready for friends of the opposite sex.

When puberty comes, the adolescent's love for his parent of the opposite sex is revived, and he has to struggle to emancipate himself from it. He must free himself of this tie in order to develop relationships with members of the opposite sex outside his family. In the process of weaning himself from his parent he becomes attracted to persons of the opposite sex who are often years older than he. The next step in development is general interests in age-mates of the opposite sex. He dates several persons. This experience gives him understanding of the opposite sex, brings security in his capacity for acceptance and should sharpen his powers of discrimination. After he has gained security in his capacity to be accepted by the opposite sex, he begins to focus on one person. He "goes steady," "gets pinned" or engaged and prepares himself for his role as a wife or a husband. After the individual has solved the developmental tasks of marriage, his love expands, and he wants children to nurture. When the developmental tasks of the child-bearing and child-rearing stages of development are mastered, his interests expand to the needs of humanity.

The above sequence in normal development takes place through wholesome relationships within the adolescent's family. During the child-bearing and child-rearing stages of development, help in growing also comes from professional workers. The adolescent's parent of the opposite sex is the object of his greatest attachment. He must free himself from his attachment to this parent before he has energy available for a mature heterosexual adjustment in marriage. The parent of the same sex is an object of conflicting feelings. These conflicts must become resolved as well, for their solution influences profoundly his marital adjustment and the way in which he will face and adapt to pregnancy and the parental role. Because growth has occurred within the framework of family interpersonal relationship, it is logical to assume that emancipation and personality reorganization must take place within the adolescent's home. Moderate degrees of rebellion are natural. He has to find fault, defend himself against his unconscious love for his parent of the opposite sex, resolve his ambivalence toward his parent of the same sex and search for standards and a philosophy of life which are his very own.

Emancipating himself and becoming emotionally free to develop mature adult relationships is an arduous task which precipitates a repeated series of advancement and regression to childish modes of behavior. The sequence of development outlined above may give the impression that progress is simple and that the individual merely moves from one level into the next. Progress in personality development is not this rapid or as smooth. Often there is forward movement toward the opposite sex, then withdrawal to the more comfortable relationships that he has experienced before. There are bursts of independence, braggadocio and exaggerated competitiveness—then periods of dependence which are more pronounced than during the preschool years.

The adolescent is in conflict; he desires both independence and the comfort that he has known before. One part of him calls for adventure, adult pleasures and responsibilities; another part wants to cling to childish pleasures and escape from the trials of adulthood. Conflict generates anxiety and uncertainty of his capacities. He moves forward to explore and test himself and then becomes fearful of the responsibility that growing-up entails. Anxiety makes him regress. Babyish modes of behavior make him feel inadequate. This feeling is less tolerable. To alleviate his anxiety he asserts his independence and tries again. Over and over this cycle of behavior repeats itself! Gradually his powers expand. As they do he experiences pleasure, security and trust in himself. He discovers that adulthood is more pleasurable than childhood. When he makes this discovery he is on his way to becoming an emotionally mature member of his society.

The adolescent is fortified when the adults in his world understand the reasons why he is erratic, rebellious, competitive, self-concerned and contradictory. The adolescent is in the process of becoming reorganized, integrated and directed toward certain goals. When his parents and professional workers believe in him and understand the many problems that he is facing in the process of growing up, he will have the strength that he needs for healthy personality reorganization.

His Career

It is obvious why an adolescent needs to know himself and identify the role that will bring satisfaction and productivity. When a person is fitted for his work, selects it independently and enjoys it, the possibilities of creativity and success are infinitely greater. *The adolescent needs help in appraising his abilities, and in learning about the opportunities presented by the different fields of endeavor.* He also needs freedom to make his own decisions concerning the role for which he wishes to become prepared. With careful help which neither directs nor leaves him uninformed, he will be able to think through his needs and plan his preparation wisely.

The healthy adolescent is emotionally ready for help in becoming prepared to meet the developmental tasks inherent in the young adult period of personality development. Logically, the major portion of this preparation should be provided in the home. When it is not, the school and the church must be ready to supplement preparation for marriage, and health workers must be prepared to provide ego-supportive care and guidance during the child-bearing and child-rearing stages of personality development.

SITUATIONS FOR FURTHER STUDY

1. How does prevention of disease protect a child's potentials for parenthood?

2. Why should pediatric nurses be concerned with preparation for marriage and parenthood?

3. How can support of an expectant mother affect her relationship with her child? What is entailed in this support?

4. What makes you agree or disagree with the concept that birth is a traumatic experience for a newborn? How do your feelings of agreement or disagreement influence the care that you give to a newborn infant?

5. What is the purpose of providing the young infant with care which prevents frustration of any need?

6. Observe an infant under 3 months of age in a pediatric ward and answer the questions which follow: How often in an 8-hour period did he show a need for food? Describe the behavior which signaled his need for food? How did he respond during feeding? How often did he cry in the 8-hour period? What care brought relief from anxiety? How did his physical condition thwart his basic emotional needs? What substitute satisfactions were you able to give him? Did they produce relief from anxiety?

7. Observe an infant between 3 and 6 months of age for whom you are caring and describe his reactions to all types of sensory stimulation. Which ones produced reactions which manifested pleasure? How were pleasurable feelings manifested? Did any stimulation show evidence of producing discomfort? How was it communicated to you?

8. If you were introducing food into an infant's diet, what principles would you try to use? Of what value would they be to the infant and yourself?

9. How do an infant's needs change during the first year of life? What produces these changes? What reasons do you see for adapting to his changes in behavior? What behavior would lead you to believe that the infant was not growing emotionally?

10. Observe infants of 1 month, 6 months and 1 year of age. Indicate some of the differences in their social, motor and emotional responses. Observe 2 or 3 infants of approximately the same age and indicate the differences in their responses, describing them as to personalities. Have you any clues as to the factors affecting their differences in behavior?

11. What types of toys do infants need during their first year of life? Why do they need the types that you suggest?

12. What might be the outcome of punishing sucking or restricting it during the first year of life?

13. If an infant under 6 months of age had a "nothing by mouth" order, what substitute satisfaction could a nurse provide?

14. What might some of the reasons be why a 4-year-old child sucks his thumb in the hospital? What would you do if this 4-year-old were your patient?

15. How does growth in independence affect personality development? Describe a situation in which you observed the effect of teaching in a child.

16. How does weaning affect personality development? What might be the effects of early weaning (before 6 months of life)? How can a nurse use knowledge of the effects of abrupt weaning on personality development?

17. What are the developmental tasks of the 1- to 3-year-old child? How can you use knowledge of the problems of the 1- to 3-year-old and of the way in which he can be helped to surmount them in your care of young children?

18. How is personality growth in the training period influenced by the guidance received during the first year of life?

19. Of what importance is toilet-training to the child?

20. How do you suppose a child who had mastered the toilet-training experience might feel if he were put into diapers in a hospital?

21. How might hospitalization affect a 3-year-old's bladder and bowel functioning?

22. Observe a convalescent 2-year-old during a 2-hour period and describe his behavior. How do you suppose he feels about himself? What evidence did you see which substantiates your answer?

23. How can the adult help the child pass through the negativistic stage of personality development?

24. Describe the ritualistic behavior you observed in a 2½-year-old child. How did you adapt yourself to his need for rituals? What ways did you discover to help him become secure about the hospital routines with which he had had no previous familiarity?

25. Of what importance is it for the child to acquire a good concept of himself? How can the adult help the child to acquire a feeling of power and yet learn his limitations?

26. How do the needs of the 3- to 6-year-old child differ from those of the infant and the toddler?

27. Why would death of a parent during preschool years be more potentially traumatizing than in a later stage of development?

28. What are some of the questions that children have asked you in the ward and what did they reveal to you as to the child's development and personality? How did you handle his questions, and what guided you in behaving as you did?

29. What is the significance of the preschool child's questions pertaining to sex? How do you think they should be

handled? What influences your thinking? Of what value is wholesome sex education?

30. What do preschool children learn from playing together? Observe a group of nursery school children playing together. List the things that you consider the children have learned during the play period. What did you learn that would assist you in planning for the play of hospitalized preschool children?

31. Why does the child of preschool years need help in learning to relinquish his parent of the opposite sex? What help does he require?

32. What behavior in the preschool child would lead you to believe that he was not making progress in emotional growth?

33. What makes a preschool child fearful of bodily injury? Observe preschool children in the ward to find evidence that they are fearful of body injury. What are their reactions to intramuscular injections? Are their reactions out of proportion to the real pain of the injection? Why do you suppose they are? How might the nurse help them master their fear of bodily injury? Give examples of your work with children in this area of guidance.

34. Observe a teacher in a nursery school. What attitudes do you think that she has toward the children? What do you think her philosophy of guidance is? How did she encourage independence, self-expression and sublimation of their aggressive impulses? How can you use the knowledge that you gained from observation in your care of hospitalized children?

35. How do you react to the word "discipline"? Write a paragraph which expresses your philosophy of discipline. Do you sincerely believe that setting limits is essential for security and growth? If you do, what problems do you have in setting limits and consistently helping the child to meet them? How do you suppose a hospitalized preschooler feels when you restrict an impulse and others who are caring for him allow the overt and unbridled expression of it? How do you suppose he feels when you vacillate between these two extremes?

36. What does emotional preparedness for school entail?

37. How does a child's conscience affect his adaptive capacities? What factors could prevent conscience formation? If you observed a consistently impulsive 8-year-old in the ward, how would you go about discovering the reasons why he continued to function on the "pleasure principle"? After study of the child and his problem, what conclusion did you draw concerning his needs?

38. What makes functioning on the "reality principle" a possibility? What would be the outcome if he never achieved the ego resources he needs to adapt to reality?

39. Observe an 8-year-old and a 3-year-old for whom you are caring. How does your guidance of the 3-year-old differ from that necessary for the 8-year-old? What adaptive capacities has the 8-year-old that are not developed in the 3-year-old?

40. How does the play of the school-age child differ from that of the preschool child? Observe the play of a 6-year-old and that of a 2-year-old and describe the differences you observed.

41. How do you imagine a school-age child would feel if you did not set limits on his behavior?

42. Observe a group of school-age children in the playroom. What did you see which showed their interest in rules, fair play, etc.?

43. What changes in behavior are seen during preadolescence? What are the purposes of these changes? Of what significance is knowledge of the child's nature to you as a nurse? Describe an experience that you have had with a preadolescent which aroused your feelings

of antagonism. How did you handle your own feelings and the experience with the child?

44. What behavior in the preadolescent would lead you to suggest that he was a disturbed child who needed psychiatric therapy?

45. How will an adolescent's past experiences be reflected in his behavior? What behavior in the adolescent would lead you to suggest that he was a disturbed individual and in need of expert guidance?

46. What are the common fears of the adolescent? How can a nurse help an adolescent master his fears? What meaning might illness have to an adolescent? How might they be reflected in his behavior?

47. Of what value are limits to an adolescent? Upon what factors are changes in limits based?

BIBLIOGRAPHY

Aldrich, C. A., and Aldrich, Mary M.: Babies Are Human Beings, ed. 2, New York, Macmillan, 1955.

Berlien, Ivan C.: Growth as related to mental health, Am. J. Nursing 56: 1142, 1956.

Blake, Florence G.: The Child, His Parents and the Nurse, Philadelphia, Lippincott, 1954.

Blanton, Smiley: Love or Perish, New York, Simon & Schuster, 1956.

Caplan, Gerald: The mental hygiene role of the nurse in maternal and child care, Nursing Outlook 2:14, 1954.

Dennis, Lorraine: Psychology of Human Behavior for Nurses, Philadelphia, Saunders, 1957.

Duval, Evelyn Millis: Facts of Life and Love for Teen-agers, New York, Popular Library, 1953.

Frank, Anne: The Diary of a Young Girl, New York, Pocket Books, Inc., 1953.

Gallagher, R. J.: Understanding Your Son's Adolescence, Boston, Little, 1957.

Gelb, Barbara: The ABC of Natural Childbirth, New York, Norton, 1954.

Gesell, Arnold, et al.: The Infant and Child in the Culture of Today, New York, Harper, 1943.

———: The Child from Five to Ten, New York, Harper, 1946.

Gruenberg, Sidonie: The Wonderful Story of How You Were Born, Garden City, N. Y., Hanover House, 1952.

Hartley, Ruth E., and Goldenson, Robert M.: The Complete Book of Children's Play, New York, Thomas Y. Crowell Co., 1957.

Hurlock, Elizabeth B.: Children need the masculine touch, Today's Health 35:62, 1957.

Hymes, James: Understanding Your Child, New York, Prentice-Hall, Inc., 1952.

Isaacs, Susan: The Nursery Years, New York, Vanguard, 1929.

Josselyn, Irene M.: The Happy Child, New York, Random, 1955.

Leimert, Mary Law: Presents and Playthings (pamphlet), Chicago, The Scholarship and Guidance Assoc., 1954.

Levine, Milton I., and Seligman, Jean H.: Helping Boys and Girls Understand Their Sex Roles (pamphlet), Chicago, Science Research Assoc., Inc., 1953.

Peto, Marjorie: Communicating with little children, Am. J. Nursing 57:602, 1957.

Piaget, Jean: The Language and Thought of the Child, New York, The Humanities Press, Inc., 1951.

Plagemann, Bentz: This Is Goggle, New York, McGraw-Hill, 1955.

Redl, Fritz: Pre-adolescents: what makes them tick, Child Study 21:44, 1943-1944.

Redl, Fritz, and Wineman, David: Controls from Within, Glencoe, Ill., The Free Press, 1952.

———: Children Who Hate, Glencoe, Ill., The Free Press, 1951.

Ribble, Margaret: The Rights of Infants, New York, Columbia, 1943.

Richmond, Julius B., and Pollach, George H.: Psychologic aspects of infants' feedings, J. Am. Dietet. A. 29:656, 1953.

Spock, Benjamin: Baby and Child Care, New York, Pocket Books, Inc., 1957.
——: The middle-aged child, Pennsylvania M. J. **50**:1045, 1947.
Staff of The Child Study Association of America: When Children Ask About Sex (pamphlet), ed. 3, New York, Child Study Association of America, Inc., 1953.
Swift, E. H.: Step by Step in Sex Education, New York, Macmillan, 1946.
Infant Care (pamphlet), Washington, D. C., U. S. Dept. of Health, Education and Welfare, 1955.
Problems of Infancy and Childhood, Tr. of the first, second, third, fourth, and sixth conferences, New York, Macy, 1947, 1948, 1949, 1951, 1952.
Proceedings of the Midcentury White House Conference on Children and Youth, Raleigh, N. C., Health Publications Institute, 1951.
Your Child from One to Six (pamphlet), Washington, D. C., U. S. Dept. of Health, Education and Welfare, 1956.
Your Child from Six to Twelve (pamphlet), Washington, D. C., Federal Security Agency, Children's Bureau, 1949.

Disease and Its Prevention

Medicine once concerned itself primarily with curing human ills, but in modern times this goal has been broadened to include the prevention of disease and disability. Pediatricians and others concerned with the welfare of children have led this trend during the last half-century by attracting attention to the benefits of preventive medicine and by contributing ideas and scientific discoveries to its rapid advance. The early successes were achieved in the control of infections—diseases which exacted their heaviest tolls among children. Stimulated by the dramatic results of public health measures and prophylactic immunizations in controlling smallpox, diphtheria, typhoid fever and infantile diarrhea, the medical profession has directed an increasing amount of its energies toward the prevention of diseases of all types. Pediatrics always will play a key role in preventive medicine, for "the child is father to the man," and whatever affects the health of children is of great importance to future generations of adults.

Of course, those responsible for the care of children must retain and perfect their curative skills. Fortunately, modern discoveries have simplified the treatment of many diseases. Thus time and energy are freed which can be devoted to forestalling these unfortunate interruptions of normal growth and development. To prepare a proper defense the nature of the enemy must be known. The first chapter of this unit describes the incidence, the severity and the special characteristics of diseases which affect children. The second chapter is concerned with the weapons currently available—specific technics for preventing physical disease and circumventing emotional disorders. The final chapter outlines one type of attack by which these weapons are put into use, carrying the protection derived from medical and psychological research to the parents and to the children themselves.

CHAPTER FIVE

Characteristics of Pediatric Disease

CAUSES OF DEATH—MORTALITY

The first obligation of medicine is to preserve life. Thus, a rough measure of its success is the rate at which deaths are occurring in the population under its care. Death rates among children have particular significance for they exclude those due to the inevitable consequences of aging. Experience has shown that the infant mortality rate (which is described below) provides one of the best indices of the health of a country or other population unit. Where health hazards are high, the infant mortality rate is high. As medical care and public health measures improve, the infant mortality rate falls. Because of this special significance and because a considerable fraction of all children's deaths occur during infancy, the mortality prior to 1 year of age will be considered separately from that of later childhood.

In addition to knowing the rate at which deaths are occurring it is desirable to know the cause. Only from this latter information is it possible to evaluate the effectiveness of preventive measures already in force and to identify the directions in which new efforts should be bent. Unfortunately, it is easier to gather reliable figures for mortality rates than to fix the causes of deaths. In the United States where communication is good and enforceable laws provide for the registration of all births and deaths, the rates are highly reliable. Figures for the cause of death are less exact, since even in regions where postmortem studies are usually made, it is not always possible to assign the cause of death accurately.

Infant Mortality

The Infant Mortality Rate

This is the ratio between the number of deaths of infants less than 1 year of age during any given year and the number of live births occurring in the same year. The rate is usually expressed as the number of deaths per thousand live births. If the infant mortality rate is 65, it means that for every 1,000 liveborn infants 65 will die before reaching the age of 1 year. The rate may also be expressed as a percentage, 6.5 per cent in this case.

If the births for any given area are not recorded accurately, the infant mortality rate cannot be computed exactly. It was not until 1933 that all 48 of the United States required registration of births.

102

At the beginning of the 20th century the infant mortality rate for those states reporting was approximately 200. In 1930 it had decreased to 64.6, and Figure 12 illustrates how it has continued to fall to 26.1 for 1955. In this latter year the rates for individual states ranged from 20.2 to 36.1.* The high rate for nonwhite infants is falling at a similar rate, lagging about 15 years behind the rate for white infants. The United States compares favorably with other countries, although several report even lower infant mortality rates. Some countries which are less favored by climate and economic resources still contend with infant mortality rates of 150 to 200 or even more.

In 1954 approximately 35 per cent of all babies who died during the first

* Provisional vital statistics for the United States, Annual Summary for 1956, Monthly Vital Statistics Report, U. S. Dept. Health, Education and Welfare, Vol. 5, p. 13.

year succumbed before they completed 24 hours of life; 72 per cent of them died before the age of 1 month. Such figures emphasize the tremendous importance of the newborn and neonatal periods in any program which is designed for further reduction of infant mortality. Figure 13 shows that over the past 40 years most of the reduction in infant deaths has been accomplished in the age period from 1 to 12 months with less dramatic salvage of those under 1 month and almost no improvement in the death rate during the first day of life.

Causes of Infant Deaths

The main causes responsible for infant deaths in the United States during the year 1954 are given in the first column of Table 3. Since it has been pointed out already that about two thirds of these infants now die before the age of 1 month, it is not surprising to find that 15.8 out of the total 26.6

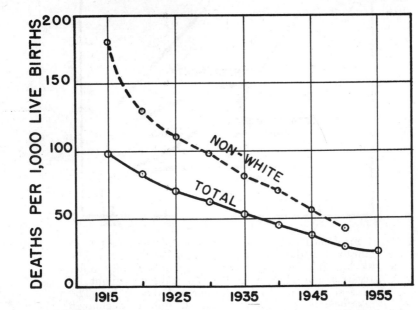

FIG. 12. Infant mortality rates in the United States, 1915-55, showing the total rates and the rate among non-white infants. (Children's Bureau, U. S. Department of Health, Education and Welfare, Statistical Series, No. 42, 1957)

per thousand live births were due to "diseases of early infancy." Before analyzing further this category which now dominates infant mortality it is interesting to look back over the first half of the century. Figures for New York City are used for this comparison, since no complete records are available for the country as a whole. In 1905 the total rate was nearly 5 times that reported for 1950. The great excess of deaths in the former year was due to infections, with diarrhea leading the list and respiratory infections such as pneumonia and bron-chitis, pertussis, diphtheria, measles and tuberculosis contributing an important share. It would be easy to assume that the over-all improvement in the prognosis from infections was due to the introduction of antibiotics. But an examination of the figures for 1935, a year in which the very first antibacterial agent was scarcely known, show a tremendous decline in fatal infections. This change must be ascribed to general public health measures which rendered formulas safer and limited the interchange of infectious diseases. To be sure, the

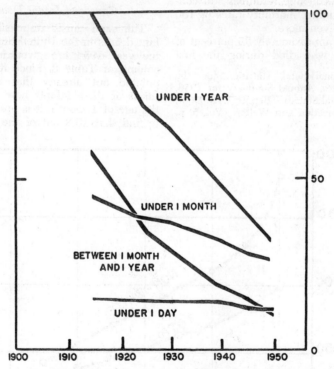

Fig. 13. Trends in age segments of the infant mortality rate in the United States from 1915 to 1949. The top line shows the rapid decline of total mortality under 1 year of age. The bottom line shows the very slight decline of mortality for infants under 1 day of age. The intermediate lines show a moderate rate of decline in deaths under 1 month and a very steep fall in deaths among infants of 1 to 12 months of age. (Children's Bureau, U. S. Department of Health, Education and Welfare, Statistical Series No. 9)

TABLE 3. CAUSES OF INFANT MORTALITY

	U.S. REG. AREA 1954	NEW YORK CITY 1950	1935	1905
Diseases of Early Infancy	15.8	15.5	24.0	31.0
Infections—Total	3.0	4.5	15.0	72.0
(Respiratory Diseases)	(2.1)	(3.5)	(6.5)	(22.0)
(Diarrhea)	(0.9)	(0.5)	(5.5)	(39.0)
(Other)	. . .	(0.5)	(3.0)	(11.0)
Malformations	3.8	3.5	4.0	2.0
Miscellaneous and Unknown	4.0	1.5	5.0	15.0
Totals	26.6	25.0	48.0	120.0

Figures are the deaths per 1,000 live births in the area within the year. Figures for United States Registration Area from Children's Bureau Statistical Series No. 42, U. S. Department of Health, Education and Welfare, 1957. Figures for New York City adapted from Holt and McIntosh: Pediatrics.

discovery of antibiotics has worked a further reduction in infections, but it would be wrong to give major credit to these new therapeutic agents. Improvements in obstetric and newborn care are reflected in the progressive decrease in deaths due to the diseases of early infancy. Notable is the failure of any real change in the rate due to malformations.

In Table 4 the focus is sharpened to a consideration of deaths occurring during the first 4 weeks of life. In 1954 these made up 72 per cent of the total infant mortality. Prematurity by itself is the largest single cause and is associated with enough of the deaths from other causes to make it a factor in well over half of the cases. A significant fraction of the total is due to malformations which are errors in the formation of the infant during pregnancy; to injuries occurring during the birth process; to asphyxia, which is really a variety of birth injury; and to atelectasis which implies a failure of the newborn to establish and maintain respirations. Thus, birth is the focal point of danger. Small wonder that obstetricians and pediatricians are joining their efforts in programs of maternal and child health to make pregnancy and delivery safer.

Associated Factors

The above analysis of infant mortality is that of the pathologist who tries to assign the immediate cause of death. Many fatalities in the United States could be avoided if all infants were to benefit from the best available care.

TABLE 4. CAUSES OF DEATH OF INFANTS LESS THAN 28 DAYS OF AGE
(NEONATAL MORTALITY IN U.S., 1954)

	TOTAL RATE	CONTRIBUTION BY IMMATURE INFANTS
Certain diseases of early infancy		
Immaturity alone	5.4	5.4
Postnatal asphyxia and atelectasis	4.3	2.9
Birth injury	2.7	1.5
Pneumonia	0.8	0.3
Erythroblastosis fetalis	0.6	0.1
Hemorrhagic disease	0.2	0.1
Diarrhea	0.2	0.1
Maternal toxemia	0.1	0.0
Other, including nutritional	1.1	0.9
Congenital malformations	2.4	. .
Other conditions, specified and unknown	1.3	. .
Total	19.1	11.3

Rates are given in deaths per 1,000 live births. (Children's Bureau, U.S. Department of Health, Education and Welfare, Statistical Series No. 42)

Some of the elements of this care will be described in following chapters. Sociologists look at infant mortality in a different light, seeking factors which interfere with optimal results. Such economic factors as low family income, poor housing, ignorance and employment of the mother away from home can be shown to have a direct bearing upon infant mortality. They interfere with the desire or the ability of parents to obtain adequate care before, during and after delivery of the baby.

CHILD MORTALITY

Rates of Death Beyond Infancy

After the first year of life the mortality rate decreases very rapidly. Whereas

26.6 infants out of each 1,000 under 1 year of age in the United States died during 1954, only 1.2 per 1,000 of those between 1 and 4 years succumbed, and the older group of 5 to 14 years had only 0.5 losses per thousand. Figure 14 illustrates how the rates have declined progressively during the last 50 years. As with the infant group, the most dramatic fall has occurred in the rates for younger children. Children in the years just prior to adolescence enjoy the most favorable mortality rates of any age period in the human span.

Causes of Child Mortality

The important causes of death among children of the United States Registration Area for the year 1954 are listed in

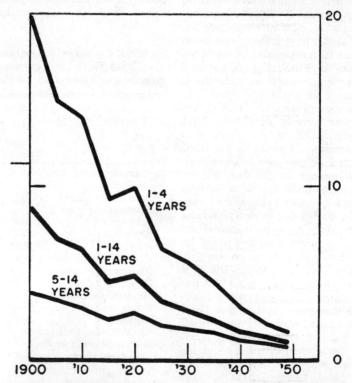

FIG. 14. Trends in mortality rates of children of various age groups in the United States, 1900-49. (Reproduced from Children's Bureau Statistical Series No. 9, U. S. Department of Health, Education and Welfare)

TABLE 5. CAUSES OF MORTALITY AMONG CHILDREN IN THE UNITED STATES FOR THE YEARS 1954 AND 1944 (Ages 1 to 14 Years)

CAUSE		1954 RATE	1944 RATE
Accidents		0.247	0.372
Motor vehicle	0.110		
Fire, explosions, burns	0.047		
Drowning	0.039		
Falls	0.013		
Other	0.038		
Malignancy		0.082	0.064
Influenza and pneumonia		0.069	0.171
Congenital malformations		0.059	0.047
Heart disease		0.019	0.068
Diarrhea		0.015	0.054
Poliomyelitis		0.013	0.022
Meningococcal infections		0.012	0.028
Other		0.209	0.555
Total		0.725	1.381

Rates given in deaths per 1,000 population of this age. (Children's Bureau, U.S. Department of Health, Education and Welfare, Statistical Series No. 42)

Table 5. The rates are given in the same form as those for infants.

A study of the table shows how with his expanding environment the preschool child faces a completely new set of hazards. His increased range of locomotion within and outside the home and his natural drives to climb and investigate set the stage for accidents. His movement out of the home environment into neighborhood and later school groups increases his opportunity to pick up infections which are not always controlled adequately by native resistance or by medical treatment. Those congenital malformations which have permitted temporary survival continue to exact a toll of lives which dwindles during the later years of childhood. In the preschool period the neoplastic diseases (cancer and leukemia) begin to contribute to mortality, gaining slightly in importance among the school-age children. Unlike most of the other causes of death this figure is showing an absolute increase during the last few years. Rheumatic fever appears also as a significantly lethal illness during the school-age period. For both groups, however, accidental death is distinctly the most frequent hazard.

Associated Factors

The same sociologic factors which influence infant mortality operate in determining the mortality among preschool children. In the older children accidental death, rheumatic fever and tuberculosis are influenced to a degree, but the differences in rates among privileged and underprivileged children is less striking.

CAUSES OF ILLNESS—MORBIDITY

WHAT AFFLICTS CHILDREN

The amount and the kind of illness among children is not reflected accurately in the mortality figures. Nearly every child suffers from measles and chickenpox, but very few of them die of these disorders. Conversely, rabies and leukemia are uncommon, but their victims inevitably enter the mortality tables. An accurate notion of the prevalence of nonfatal diseases in a community is not easy to obtain, for most of them are not reported to a tabulating center. Except for some of the major contagious diseases such as measles and poliomyelitis, usually it is necessary to rely upon the general impressions of those who care for children in hospitals, doctors' offices and clinics.

Pediatrics is general practice before the age of maturity. It is possible for children to have almost any of the troubles that assail adults. However, the degenerative, neoplastic and metabolic disorders are much less common among the young, while infections, nutritional disorders and problems related to adaptation and growth consume the bulk of pediatric time. As previously intimated, the pediatrician is attuned to the anticipation of serious illness and devotes a high percentage of his time to prevention and to the consideration of incipient or relatively minor disorders. The medical problems of child patients, in offices and hospitals is bound to reflect this prophylactic attitude.

How Children's Disease Differs

Congenital Anomalies

Defects in the physical formation of the body may be noted at birth or later during the periods of infancy and childhood. In general, the recognition and the treatment of such conditions is the responsibility of pediatrics. A few disorders may lie dormant or unrecognized until adult life (polycystic kidneys, Meckel's diverticulum, for example). The severity of anomalous development covers a very wide spectrum from the trivial to the type which does not permit survival for more than a few hours. Improved diagnostic and surgical methods now make it possible to correct or ameliorate many disorders not only of the heart but also of the nervous system,

the digestive system, the urinary tract and the lungs.

Disorders of the Newborn

The special problems of the newborn infant are also unique to pediatrics. Their importance has been indicated above in the discussion of mortality among infants. More detailed consideration is given in Chapter 10.

Nutritional Abnormalities

Rapid growth makes greater demands upon nutrients than does the static state of the adult. Thus, deficiencies are most likely to occur in the infant, less so in the child and least frequently in the adult. Failure in growth is sometimes an indication of a more fundamental disorder of genetic origin.

Infectious Disease

Adults, of course, suffer from infections too, but for children they are particularly frequent and important. Diseases which produce permanent immunity are suffered only once in a lifetime, most commonly during the early years. Respiratory infections which result in only transient immunity are the bane of pediatric practice, presumably because the child is unable to suppress them as readily as the adult who has had a longer experience with them. Exposure to many of these infections is inevitable and to a degree is desirable for the stimulation of immunologic defenses. However, the particularly vulnerable small infant or sick child must be protected in order to avoid serious consequences.

Neoplasms

Neoplasms are not nearly as common during childhood as in adult life. Those that do occur tend to have distinctive features. Leukemia, for instance, is seldom seen in either myelogenous or chronic form but is usually of the acute stem-cell or lymphatic variety. Carcinoma and sarcoma are seen occasionally. The most common tumors of childhood affect the brain, the extensions of the sympathetic nervous system and the kidneys. Many of these appear to be derived from embryologic rests which have grown slowly for a time and then suddenly enlarge under the influence of unknown stimuli. The primitive nature of many of these tumors makes it difficult to recognize them before metastatic or irreparable local growth has occurred.

Psychological Disorders

Behavior which is judged to be inappropriate for the child's age is an extremely common phenomenon. A large fraction of these disorders are due to unusual intensity or persistence of infantile forms of behavior and correct themselves without long-term effects upon the child. Other deviations result in neurotic traits, conduct and behavior disorders, anxiety states and psychosomatic disturbances. The more severe disorders are not common among children, or at least are not frequently recognized. Psychosis is unusual.

Surgical Conditions

The surgical procedures performed upon children are directed in a large measure at the correction of congenital malformations and the restoration of tissues injured in accidents. A few disorders such as intussusception and pyloric stenosis are found only in the pediatric age group.

EFFECTS OF DISEASE UPON THE INDIVIDUAL CHILD

SYMPTOMS

Acute illness in the child usually begins abruptly and dramatically. Before he or his parents recognize that he is sick the onset is announced by a sudden change in disposition or activity. In the early stages of infection a sharp rise in body temperature to 102-104° F. or even higher is common. Other early symptoms commonly seen are refusal of food, vomiting, abdominal pain, and diarrheal stools. These do not necessarily give any exact clue to the location of his disease. For example, sometimes tonsillitis is ushered in by abdominal pain and vomiting. Chills are an infrequent counterpart of illness in children. Those who are so disposed may suffer a convulsion during the initial period of rising fever, an alarming event which may appear out of the blue before it is suspected that anything is amiss.

The dramatic onset of acute illnesses understandably stimulates anxiety among parents, particularly when they have had little experience with childhood disease. Often they are rendered temporarily incapable of providing the reassuring support which should be available in order to control the child's own anxiety about his symptoms. Children react in different fashion. Some suffer complete physical and emotional disorganization during illness; others accept it in spartan fashion. The manner in which a particular child reacts is likely to be repeated during succeeding upsets. This is true not only in respect to his emotional state but also to the sharpness of his febrile rise and the pattern of his associated symptoms.

The younger the child the more labile is his temperature-regulating mechanism. Fevers rise to greater heights than they would in adults with the same disease, and diurnal swings in temperature are characteristic. Usually the child's powers of physical adaptation are good, and he accommodates to fever which would exhaust an adult completely or precipitate delirium. The resilience of the young body is also apparent in the speed with which children recover from acute illnesses. Once the crisis has been reached and temperatures are back to normal it is common to find the child ready to take up activity where he left off. His caretakers may have a hard time convincing him that full recovery has not yet been achieved.

PHYSICAL EFFECTS

Illness places the child's fluid balance in jeopardy. The relatively high water requirements of the infant and the young child have been noted in a previous chapter. When illness strikes, fever, vomiting and diarrhea increase the rate of water loss from the body, and his inability or unwillingness to take food may curtail the intake. Serious depletion of body water cannot be permitted without having an adverse effect upon the progress of the disease itself. Thus, therapeutic measures to prevent dehydration are employed more commonly among sick children than they are among sick adults.

Nutrition always suffers, at least briefly, during acute illness. The effects are more noticeable during the rapid growth of infancy. They are inevitably reflected in irregularities in weight progress and sometimes in temporary cessation of longitudinal growth. Permanent scars of old illnesses can often be seen in roentgenograms of the bones where dense transverse lines reflect a period of growth failure, and in the enamel of teeth which may show grooves and pits due to the effects of disease which occurred at the time when this portion of the tooth was being formed.

Chronic illness or recurring acute illness may have more serious consequences for nutrition and growth. The mechanism is sometimes obvious in the persistently poor intake of food or the loss of nutriments and minerals through chronic diarrhea. But in addition subtle changes in the function of the endocrine organs occur during prolonged inactivity which interfere with the rate of new tissue formation. Chronic major disease may be responsible for growth interferences which are so serious as to result in permanent dwarfing.

Some acute illnesses leave behind permanent defects which saddle the child with a handicap for the rest of his life. For instance, the brain may be irreparably damaged by birth injury, by encephalitis accompanying some of the contagious diseases, by meningitis or by vascular accidents within its substance. Poliomyelitis too often leaves muscular weakness in its wake; rheumatic fever carries the threat of permanent functional damage to the heart; deafness is an occasional sequel of mumps and of protracted infections of the middle ear. Apart from the need to adapt himself to a body which is incomplete in its functional capacity, the child must also be helped to accept and deal with the psychological reactions which his handicap stimulates.

PSYCHOLOGICAL EFFECTS

The full effects of illness in childhood are by no means reflected by the mortality and morbidity tables. Acute, chronic, crippling or frequently recurring illness can affect the child's psychological development adversely. The normal growth from dependent, egocentric infancy to emotional maturity may receive severe setbacks through the experience of being physically handicapped or ill. The way in which illness or a physical handicap affects the child's personality growth is determined by his parents' attitudes and feelings toward him and his physical condition, and by the quality of care that he receives when hospitalization becomes necessary. A sense of insecurity from the very presence of the illness or the handicap itself cannot help leaving its imprint upon the mind of the child. In addition, he may be confronted with hospitalization which results in separation from his parents, fear-provoking experiences, and a dearth of the kind of experiences that he needs for personality growth. Preventing the traumas that affect the ill child adversely will be developed in subsequent chapters.

SITUATIONS FOR FURTHER STUDY

1. What are the reasons why a nurse needs to know the causes of death and illness?

2. What are the factors which have prevented marked decrease in mortality rates of newborns? How does the nurse function in preventing death of newborn infants?

3. What are the most outstanding causes of ill health during childhood?

4. Disease has different effects on the child than on the adult. What are these differences? How do they affect your attitude toward pediatric nursing?

5. How may illness affect a child's physical development? His psychological development?

6. Observe a child that you believe has been affected adversely by illness and hospitalization. Describe his behavior and indicate why you feel that his personality growth has been affected by his current experience. How might it have been prevented?

BIBLIOGRAPHY

Children's Bureau Statistical Series No. 42, U. S. Dept. Health, Education and Welfare, 1957.

Holt, L. E., Jr., and McIntosh, R.: Pediatrics, ed. 12, New York, Appleton, 1953.

National Office of Vital Statistics, U. S. Dept. Health, Education and Welfare, Monthly Vital Statistics Report, vol. 5, no. 13.

CHAPTER SIX

Preventive Measures

Toward the end of the 18th century, Jenner, an English practitioner, introduced the first specific measure for preventing a contagious disease—smallpox vaccination. During the century that followed, preventive medicine focused on the control of contagion, attempting to limit its spread through quarantine and isolation regulations. With the birth of the new science of bacteriology just before the present century began, knowledge about infectious agents advanced rapidly and with it vaccines began to appear which were effective against many of the old-fashioned scourges. In addition to smallpox it is now possible to exert good control over diphtheria, pertussis, typhoid fever, and probably poliomyelitis by this means. Parallel growth in the field of biochemistry and nutrition fostered the development of safe formulas for infants and preparations capable of preventing vita-min-deficiency diseases. In recent decades preventive pediatrics has outgrown the narrower concept of prevention of specific disease and now takes in all measures that are designed to improve the physical health and the emotional adjustment of children generally. With this larger goal in view physicians and nurses are extending their responsibilities and now find themselves collaborating with workers in such diverse fields as public health, education, psychology, sociology, research and even genetics and law-enforcement. This chapter surveys briefly the protections which may be placed around the child before and after birth to avoid or ameliorate later troubles. The nurse who understands the implications of these protective devices will be prepared to utilize and perhaps to improve the resources of her own community.

PREPARATION FOR BIRTH

Even before his conception, society attempts to shield the child from undesirable parents. In addition to laws which set a minimum age for marriage, many states now require from all applicants for marriage licenses at least a cursory physical examination and blood tests for syphilis. Social, moral and religious forces regulate marriage in a less direct way by setting cultural standards to be met. On occasion, professional advice given by doctors, psychologists, social workers and others who engage in marriage counseling plays a significant role in molding the quality of a marriage relationship. Where undesirable hereditary traits are known to exist in the antecedents of either partner, genetic counseling is useful in evaluating the wisdom of bearing children.

Once pregnancy has begun, a number of precautionary measures can be invoked to shield both mother and child. Unfortunately, the quality of such care varies with socio-economic circumstances. Comprehensive prenatal care of the mother should include the following: complete medical examination and appraisal of her capacity to adapt to her pregnancy, gynecologic examination, Rh-typing, screening for tuberculosis and syphilis, regulation of diet, protection against certain infectious diseases, and education and support of both parents which helps them to adjust to pregnancy, labor, delivery and their parental roles. When physical defects or lack of progress in adjustment to pregnancy are noted, referral to sources of medical and psychological therapy is not only indicated but essential. It is imperative to prevent physical complications and disturbed mother-child relationships in the neonatal period when mutually satisfying experiences are of crucial importance for each person within the family. This is a large program if properly done, but experience has demonstrated that it pays dividends in decreasing maternal and infant mortality and morbidity and in minimizing the problems of child-rearing in the first crucial weeks of life.

Careful physical and laboratory examination of the mother early in pregnancy protects not only her own interests but also those of the fetus. The detection and the prompt treatment of diabetes, anemia, tuberculosis, and cardiac and renal disease has a direct bearing upon infant mortality by decreasing the chances of premature delivery, toxemia and anoxia. Similarly, careful pelvic measurement and periodic gynecologic examination permits accurate planning of the delivery in order to minimize birth trauma and anoxia from mechanical causes. Rh-typing of the mother's blood segregates the negative reactors so that they may have additional tests and be delivered under conditions prepared to handle an infant with erythroblastosis fetalis. States which require all pregnant women to be screened for syphilis can expect almost complete control of the congenital form of the disease, since, when detected during the first half of pregnancy, treatment of the mother can be accomplished before she infects her infant. The detection of tuberculosis in the mother not only permits better protection of her health during pregnancy but also warns of her infectious danger to the infant after his birth. Ideally, screening should be extended to include fathers and others who will be in the child's close environment after his birth.

Vaccination of pregnant women against poliomyelitis is designed to protect them from the extensive paralysis to which they are particularly prone. At the same time the infant is shielded from prenatal or postnatal transfer of the disease from his mother. Rubella with certainty, and perhaps some other infectious diseases, may be responsible for congenital malformation of the fetus when the mother becomes infected during the first 3 months of the pregnancy. Pregnant women should be shielded from virus infections whenever possible. Gamma globulin or hyperimmune serum may have some benefit in protecting those who have had a known exposure to rubella.

Supervision of the food intake of pregnant women is desirable to make sure that sufficient protein and vitamins are being ingested. Severely deficient diets are known to increase the rate of premature delivery, which in turn increases the hazard to the child. Experimentally, it has been possible to produce congenital anomalies in the young of pregnant animals deprived of vitamins such as A and riboflavin. Although there is no conclusive proof of a relationship between vitamin deficiency and congenital malformations in man, the supplementation of diets during pregnancy is undoubtedly desirable.

Supportive care during pregnancy is given through group educational programs and within the context of a constructive relationship with a health worker. Education of the prospective parents in the rudiments of obstetrics fosters better co-operation with the doctor and the nurse, an intelligent approach to the coming delivery and security in their ability to function as parents. Today the pendulum has swung back from scientific rigidity, and young couples are showing enthusiasm for a return to natural methods of child-bearing and rearing. The increased popularity of educational programs, natural childbirth, breast-feeding, rooming-in and self-regulatory schedules are manifestations of a desire to recapture some of the instinctive emotional forces which have become submerged in the artificiality of scientific medicine. Today's parents are not as familiar with young children as they were in the days of large families. Fifty years ago there was always a young child around the house. Our current educational system neglects the teaching of the practical aspects of child-bearing and child-rearing. As a result of this lack many expectant parents are concerned and anxious about their ability to deliver a child and to function as parents. Classes for expectant parents which are conducted as a question-and-answer period provide a popular device for giving some guidance before difficulties arise. Discussion periods have the advantage of permitting the audience to ventilate their anxieties either directly or vicariously through others who have the same worries. Many parents have said that they accepted with equanimity those aspects of labor and delivery and of their infant's behavior which had been forecast for them in classes for expectant parents. Principles and attitudes which are discussed beforehand are accepted more readily in guidance of the child after birth.

In addition to the group educational program cited above, the expectant mother needs continuity of personal relationship with a health worker who understands the psychology of the reproductive cycle. Continuity of relationship not only gives reassurance but also provides the milieu that is necessary to help her with those problems in her personal adjustment which cannot be aided in group discussion. Every pregnant woman needs an opportunity to share her feelings, fears and doubts with an understanding person. Many individuals who need the help of an expert will never be detected unless there is continuity in relationship which helps the woman to feel safe enough to disclose her true feelings. Ideally, this relationship should continue throughout the maternity cycle. When it does, the mother has the advantage of having a health worker who understands her individual needs for help in making a healthy adjustment to motherhood.

PERINATAL SAFEGUARDS

The analysis of infant mortality rates presented in the preceding chapter emphasizes how birth and its aftermath constitute the most dangerous period of a child's life. Not only the saving of lives but also the saving of cerebral function is at stake. While arguments can be offered to urge the safety and the psychological advantages of home deliveries, the fact remains that infant and maternal mortality rates are lowest where the percentage of babies delivered in hospitals is highest. The concentration of expert professional skills and resources in the hospital setting gives the infant who is destined to have trouble during delivery his best chance of a happy outcome.

Public health and professional organizations are striving continually to render the conditions of delivery as safe as possible for each infant. The quality of obstetric judgment which monitors his birth is often critical to his welfare. State and local health departments, hospitals and certifying boards set standards of professional training which must be met by physicians, nurses and midwives. In many large cities all fetal and neonatal deaths are subjected to critical review by a maternal and child-care panel in an effort to determine the factors responsible for death and to suggest ways in which care could be improved. Rules for asepsis in the delivery room or the home and for the control of infections within hospitals have been promulgated by many interested bodies. Most states have laws which require the prophylactic use of silver nitrate or antibiotics in the eyes of the newborn baby in order to prevent gonorrheal ophthalmia. Detailed consideration of the many ways in which a newborn baby can be protected against mishaps is given in Chapter 10.

The persons who successfully usher the infant into the world have responsibilities which extend beyond the physical care of the mother and the child. The postpartum period is of crucial importance for each member of the family. Every effort must be expended to help the parents adapt to their parental roles. This includes ego-support which helps the mother to become united with her child emotionally. She also needs help in understanding her own physical and emotional postpartum requirements. She needs help to become familiar with her baby's nature and to feel confident of her capacity to give him care. Feeding is the first and all-important activity which a new mother faces. Feelings of triumph arise when she is successful; feelings of failure are generated if her baby does poorly. Around the anxiety over this primitive lifeline, important relationships develop—that between the mother and her child, that between the mother and her doctor and that between the mother and her nurse. If the nurse helps the mother and the infant to work out a mutually, satisfying relationship during the feeding experience, the foundation has been laid for intimacy and rapport in later infancy and childhood. Similarly, if the mother finds in her nurse a source of understanding and noncritical judgment she will be increasingly more able to talk over her problems with her and to utilize constructively the help that she offers. In addition to the support that the nurse gives to enhance the mother-child relationship, the nurse must be sure that the mother has instruction which ensures the protection that is obtained from guidance, evaluation and immunization offered by the personnel in a child-health conference or by a private physician. Fathers also need consideration during the postpartum period. When they are recognized as a part of the family, adjustment to the father role can be acquired more easily.

PREVENTIVE MEASURES AFTER BIRTH

PUBLIC HEALTH

At birth the infant becomes a member of a society which assumes a considerable amount of responsibility for the prevention of disease and death among its members. Many of the public health protections from which he profits are discharged so automatically by local and national health agencies that their benefits tend to be overlooked. Supervision of the supply of water, milk and foods is carried out so successfully by community health departments that they seldom act as purveyors of disease.

Sewage and garbage disposal, street cleaning, isolation of contagious disease, investigation of epidemics and inspection of housing are some of the other functions which operate locally to protect the general health. At the state and national level protection is afforded by laws which require licensing of physicians and pharmacists; by the Pure Food and Drug Act which regulates medicines, poisons and the purity of foods; through disaster relief; through programs for the care and the rehabilitation of handicapped children; and through the multiplicity of educational devices used to encourage people to protect their own health and that of their children. Many of these governmental activities are being supplemented by privately financed organizations. The regulation of motor vehicles by state licensing bureaus and by law-enforcement agencies should be included as a form of protection which is assuming increasing importance with the rise of street and highway accidents toward the top of the list of causes of death among children.

PARENT EDUCATION

One of the most important aspects of preventive pediatrics is the education of parents. Until those who have immediate responsibility for children are informed and convinced of the need for protective measures, results will be disappointing.

In the early part of this century efforts were directed toward the reduction of the infant mortality rate, and success was achieved. Education was focused upon the provision of a safe milk supply, for much of the infant diarrhea was due to ignorance about the preservation of infant formulas. Prophylaxis against smallpox and diphtheria was soon added as another objective of parent education. Later, the emphasis shifted toward improving the nutrition of infants and children, with specific campaigns against rickets, scurvy and anemia. The results of these efforts are gratifying, for the diseases enumerated have been virtually abolished in communities which have good programs of parent education.

But the task is never finished, for new generations of parents are continually arising to be instructed in the established technics of prevention, and the scope of activity continually broadens. As the task of saving lives and preventing physical disease becomes simpler with modern facilities and a better informed group of parents, more time and energy can be devoted to considerations of physical and emotional growth and development and the manner in which they affect the individual child's adjustment to his environment.

Periodic Examination

New parents are usually receptive to the idea of submitting their infants to periodic examinations in order to measure growth and solve feeding difficulties. Such well-baby visits, if properly conducted, can foster an appreciation of the benefits to be derived from periodic evaluation. The desire to continue will depend in part upon the parents' own desire to give the child optimum opportunities for health, but to an even larger degree continuation depends upon the quality of advice and sympathetic encouragement they receive from the evaluators.

During infancy, visits should be fairly frequent, for growth changes are rapid, and a number of aspects of infant care need continual modification. The scope of activity can be enlarged from evaluation of weight and feeding to include the search for incipient disease or abnormality, protection against specific diseases, developmental guidance, accident prevention and mental health measures. As the child grows the frequency of visits may be decreased from the monthly rate of early infancy, but even at school age an annual visit is desirable. Of course, children with diffi-

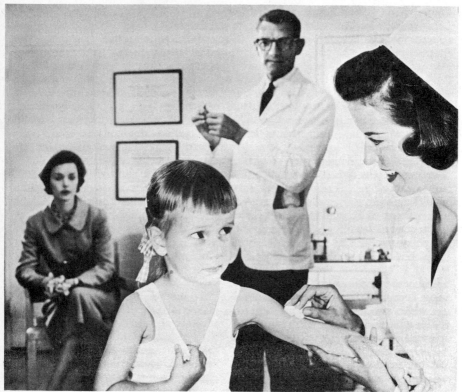

Fig. 15. With adequate preparation of mother and child immunizations can be accomplished with minimum discomfort to all parties. (Parke Davis Co., Detroit, Mich.)

culties will have to be seen more frequently. In many communities school health programs attempt to encourage at least minimum health supervision. Programs vary in their extent. Sometimes the parents are requested to submit the results of annual medical examinations made elsewhere; sometimes the school system itself provides a medical staff which makes periodic surveys of the students; sometimes evaluation is restricted to special items such as nutrition, sight, hearing or dental hygiene. The concept of periodic examination which originated in the well-baby clinic has spread to encompass well-child and school health programs and is now taking roots in adult medicine where the benefits of periodic health examinations are becoming appreciated.

Nutrition

The nutrition during each period of infancy and childhood is important for general health, not only during the period under consideration, but also for all later periods as well. Good prenatal nutrition produces more vigorous infants. Good infant nutrition gives the baby a better start into childhood. Some of the defects which are discovered later at school, which may persist through life, may be contracted in infancy and the preschool period, often to a degree which affects the stamina and the learning capacity. Dental caries is as yet an uncontrolled human scourge and is caused in large measure by improper diet.

Specific Protective Measures

An important part of the periodic consultation is the protection of the child against the serious infectious diseases which he may encounter in later life. Practices differ somewhat, depending upon the health circumstances of the community. It is almost universal practice to give all infants protection against smallpox, diphtheria, whooping cough and tetanus as a minimum. Smallpox vaccination is usually given during the latter half of the first year of life. It is ineffective if the procedure fails to result in a "take," i.e., the production of a blister and a scab. For the other 3 diseases a triple toxoid is now in general use which permits simultaneous administration. A basic course of 3 injections spaced about a month apart is required. Although the immunity produced is somewhat better if this procedure is delayed until after 6 months of age, many physicians feel that it is preferable to establish some degree of protection earlier in life. Frequently, initial immunizations are begun at 2 to 3 months of age and sometimes even earlier. Booster injections are added at the age of a year or 18 months when early immunizations are given. Periodic stimulation of the immunity should be continued through childhood about every 3 or 4 years.

Vaccination against poliomyelitis is gaining general acceptance since extensive tests with the Salk type of vaccine indicate that a significant degree of protection is conferred and that adequate checks have been devised to assure the safety of commercially produced vaccine. Infants should be immunized during the early months with 2 injections about 2 to 4 weeks apart, followed at an interval of at least 7 months by a booster injection. It is pos-

sible that later booster injections throughout childhood may be required and that poliomyelitis vaccine can be incorporated into the triple vaccine now in general use.

In countries with a high prevalence of tuberculosis, infants are vaccinated regularly with BCG (Bacillus of Calmette and Guérin). Like smallpox vaccination, this consists of purposeful infection with a known attenuated strain of organism in order to produce immunity to the more virulent types. The effectiveness of BCG vaccination appears to be definite among populations which cannot hope to control tuberculosis by isolation and treatment of individual cases. In the United States it is used to protect some infants who must live in environments where tuberculosis is prevalent.

Protection against other diseases is also available. In regions where typhoid fever is prevalent, active protection by the administration of vaccine during the first year of life is desirable. Under special circumstances, active protection against typhus fever, Rocky Mountain spotted fever, mumps and rabies may be desired. Effective treatment with penicillin has made vaccination against scarlet fever obsolete.

In certain instances it is desirable to give a child or an infant temporary protection against a disease to which he has been exposed recently. Immediate but transient protection is available for many infectious diseases through the administration of preparations of convalescent serum or adult blood products. This type of protection is called passive immunization and should not be confused with the previously mentioned immunizations which are designed to give long-lasting protection. Passive protection against measles is desirable for infants and children between the ages of 6 months and 3 years when known exposure has taken place. Gamma globulin is the most widely used preparation for this purpose. Convalescent serum is desirable for protection of unimmunized infants who are exposed to whooping cough within the family. Tetanus antitoxin must be given following certain injuries if the child has not been immunized previously.

Of the preparations used for passive protection against disease, those which are manufactured in animals such as the horse or the rabbit carry the disadvantage of serum sickness and the induction of sensitization to animal proteins. Human convalescent serum and gamma globulin do not have this disadvantage.

Accident Prevention

The increasing prominence of accidents as a cause of death and disability among infants and children has emphasized the need for better safety education of parents and of the children themselves. Such a program requires a concerted attack from several directions with an emphasis which shifts according to the age of the child. According to figures of the Children's Bureau for 1949, accidental deaths among infants are due most commonly to the inhalation or the ingestion of foreign materials. The potential danger of small objects, medicines and poisons which may be reached by the exploring infant can be discussed profitably during the sessions of a periodic examination or a well-baby conference. Fire constitutes the second most frequent hazard for the infant. The preschool child who is beginning to explore beyond the confines of his home runs his greatest risk from motor vehicle accidents, with fire and drowning next in order of importance. Within these age groups accident prevention is primarily a problem of parent education and of establishing safe habits in the child through parental discipline.

Among children of school age the hazard from motor vehicle accidents increases with age until within the teen-age group 1 out of every 4 deaths is due to this cause. In addition to parental influence, the school can exert some constructive effort through driver-training and safety programs for older children. The major campaign for reduction of deaths through traffic accidents must be a broad one, striking at all age groups striving for better self-discipline and safer operation of motor vehicles.

Drowning is the second most common cause of accidental death among children of school age. The school, the camps and the youth organizations can assist in accident prevention by offering instruction in swimming and water safety.

Mental Hygiene

The nurse's role in parent education is changing with the newer concept of health which considers not only physical disease but also the child's social and emotional adjustment as well. Previously, the nurse's role in parent education was largely concerned with the physical health and care of the child. Now she is participating in preventive health programs which function to prevent physical disease, to prepare expectant parents for labor, delivery and parenthood and to assist parents in understanding themselves, their children's nature and nurture and in handling the developmental problems of growth.

Detecting physical and emotional deviations from normality and referral to appropriate sources of help is a fundamental ingredient of preventive health work. The developmental tasks which the child must master to achieve self-respect, security and the approval of society were described in Chapter 4. The factors that promote optimal physical and personality development were also cited. Early detection and treatment of physical defects and personality distortions gives greater assurance that the child will be ready to master the tasks of development. Identification of incipient behavior problems at the earliest possible time is fundamental to the treatment of behavior disorders. Because the nurse spends more time with children and parents than any other health worker does, she can play an important role in identifying emerging patterns of antisocial behavior, in giving psychological first-aid, and in interpreting the manner in which the child-guidance specialist can help the troubled mother and child. If deviant behavior is noted early before it has developed into fixed patterns of behavior, there is a much greater chance to help the child become psychologically ready to progress further emotionally.

The nurse's role in mental health programs is one which requires keen observation, understanding of the self and others, the capacity for teamwork and an ability to interpret children's developmental requirements without being judgelike or authoritarian. Functioning in preventive health programs requires preparation to do what Levy calls "anticipatory guidance."

Anticipatory guidance prepares parents to understand their childrens' needs for growth and development. It gives parents understanding of the changes in behavior which are produced with growth and assists them in recognizing their children's readiness for new growth-producing experiences. It also helps them to prepare themselves to support their children so they can master the tasks of development with comfort and a feeling of accomplishment and self-satisfaction.

Providing anticipatory guidance requires understanding of oneself and parents as well as children. The nurse's success in guiding parents is dependent upon her attitudes and feelings toward them as persons. It is also dependent upon her ability to appraise their readiness for guidance and upon her skill in interpreting knowledge to them. Self-understanding, objectivity and clear recognition of her own limitations are equally essential, for a nurse's efforts may do more harm than good if she permits herself to become involved too

deeply in the complexities of emotional disturbances of parents or children. She can interpret the findings of those who have studied the basic needs of children; she can utilize her knowledge in her relationships with children; she can be alert to symptoms which manifest emotional distress, but the serious disturbances must be left to someone with training in this area. Emotionally disturbed parents and children need the help of someone who has special training in the dynamics of human behavior and in the use of therapeutic measures which are required to restore individuals to mental health—a physician, a child-guidance worker, a social worker or a psychiatrist. If the nurse continues to work with the child or the parent after the referral to a specialist has been made, teamwork will further the disturbed individual's return to health.

Helping parents of children who are chronically ill or handicapped is another facet of preventive mental health work. Physical handicaps and chronic illness may thwart the child's progress toward maturity. If the child's limitations are not faced by those who nurture him, and if he suffers deprivation of love and opportunities to use the strengths that develop from growth, he will be handicapped psychologically as well as physically. The parents of these children and the children themselves require the help of all persons on the health team. Their problems are complex and difficult to surmount. When each member of the team pools his knowledge of the child and his family and uses the recommendations which are formulated from group participation, the family will make better progress in adjustment to the realities that they face. This subject will be discussed further in Chapter 8 and in other chapters that deal with children who are handicapped.

Preventing maternal deprivation during periods of illness of the mother or of the child is a further area in which preventive work must be done. Helping he family to obtain the services of a homemaker during periods of illness or strain within the family protects the child from experiencing pain when he should be obtaining pleasure from his relationship with his mother. If the child must be hospitalized, protection from traumatic experiences must be provided. Separation from the mother during the earliest years of a child's life can injure the mother-child relationship upon which his personality growth depends. Young children who have been hospitalized frequently show disturbed relationships with their mothers.

Illness and hospitalization can be a constructive experience or they can leave the child with residual feelings of anxiety, anger and revenge which hamper his opportunities for optimal personality development. One of the most important determinants of the effect of illness and hospitalization is the quality of care that the child receives in the hospital and at home after he is discharged. The nurse's role is to prevent emotional deprivation during hospitalization. This requires support which recognizes the child's need for a continuing warm relationship with his mother and for protection from experiences which are beyond his capacity for mastery. This subject is discussed further in Chapter 8.

Protection of the child from further illness and periods of hospitalization is another supportive measure of great import. When visiting hours are liberal and they are used to help the mother to develop understanding and competence in the care of her child, subsequent difficulties can be eliminated. Mothers of premature infants and of babies with such conditions as eczema *need experience in caring for their babies before they take them home.* Mothers not only need to give their infants care under the direction of understanding guidance but also they should have an opportunity to share with a helpful person their feelings concerning the child and his care. When such a person has real interest in the feelings of a woman who gives birth to a child who deviates from normality and requires a special kind of care, the mother gets strength to face reality. Experiences of this kind are imperative for those mothers who have had to face separation from their babies immediately after delivery. Separation produces conflict and anxiety which must become resolved before the mother can be united with her baby emotionally. Keeping the mother in touch with her baby during periods of separation through reports concerning his progress and helping her to establish emotional unity with him before discharge from the hospital can have far-reaching effects in enhancing the mother-child relationship. A mother who takes a baby home from the hospital feeling fearful of her capacity to care for her child will have little energy available to develop motherliness. This is also true for the mother of a normal newborn.

Obtaining referral to a community agency that can provide home service for the mother who needs continued support after she takes her child home from the hospital is a preventive measure that warrants great consideration. When referral is indicated, the family will profit if the agency has the benefit of the knowledge which hospital personnel have acquired from their work with the family. Lines of communication between the hospital and workers in community agencies must be kept open if families are to obtain the help they need.

SITUATIONS FOR FURTHER STUDY

1. How does comprehensive prenatal care safeguard the mother and the baby physically and emotionally?

2. In the days that follow the birth of a baby the mother needs opportunities to feel united with her child emotionally.

How can the nurse function to satisfy this maternal need? Of what importance is it to members of the family?

3. What protective measures must be instituted at the time of delivery of a baby?

4. What preventive health measures exist in your community?

5. How does the hospital you are associated with function to protect the health of the family in its community?

6. How can the nurse function in programs of accident prevention? Are there ways you can function while you are working in the pediatric ward? Cite these ways if they exist.

7. Observe a mother who had been separated from her baby at the time it was born. What does she do when she comes in to visit her baby? After a period of observation give her an opportunity to talk with you. What did she talk about? How do you think she felt about her baby and his care? What makes you think so? What opportunities did you find to help her feel more comfortable with herself, her baby and with you? Do this daily until the baby is ready to be discharged and report the results of your efforts.

8. In what instances would you suggest referral of a family to a community agency? Cite a situation you observed which led you to conclude that the family would need further help after the child had been dismissed from the hospital.

BIBLIOGRAPHY

Auerbach, Aline B.: New approaches to work with expectant parents—a report on a pilot leadership training program, Am. J. Pub. Health 47:1184, 1957.

Holthaus, Louise S.: Cooperation to prevent home accidents, Am. J. Nursing 56:1160, 1956.

Lemkau, Paul: What can the Nurse do in Mental Hygiene? Pub. Health Nursing 40:583, 1948.

Rodgers, Kenneth D.: Preventable accidents in preschool children, Nursing Outlook 4:552, 1956.

Health Services and Juvenile Delinquency, Washington, D. C., U. S. Dept. Health, Education and Welfare, Social Security Administration, Children's Bureau.

CHAPTER SEVEN

The Child Health Conference

GOALS, PERSONNEL AND FUNCTIONS

The forerunners of the Child Health Conference were the milk stations which were started in New York City just prior to the opening of the 20th century. These were opened to provide safe, properly prepared formulas for babies in an attempt to reduce the high mortality and morbidity from gastro-enteritis or summer diarrhea. The milk stations became centers to which mothers could bring babies for examination and advice. As mothers' needs were felt, gradually they were met more and more adequately. Today there are Baby Health Stations, Well-Baby Clinics or Child Health Conferences in many areas of the country. The Child Health Conference is the name which probably best expresses their goal—study of the family as a basis for helping the parents obtain what each member needs for optimum mental and physical health.

The Child Health Conference functions primarily for the children who are not directly under the supervision of a physician elsewhere. Many mothers bring their children to the Child Health Conference for health supervision even though they may have a private physician when the child is ill. The Child Health Conference may be voluntary in its organization and financial support, or, as it becomes recognized as a necessary public health function, it may be taken over by the tax-supported or official agencies. In either case, the personnel requirements, functions and goals are the same.

Planned health supervision of the child begins with good prenatal care and continues indefinitely. The importance of the earliest periods in the child's life are emphasized repeatedly by specialists who deal with problems of maladjustment in later childhood. Parental guidance during these early periods is especially productive from the standpoint of prevention and early correction of physical defects and emotional disorders. Before 6 years of age, neurotic tendencies have not yet been internalized into the child's personality structure and therefore are modified more easily through changes in parental handling. Thus, every health worker who guides the mother in the care of her young child can play an important role in the ultimate improvement of the mental health of the community. As the scope of pediatrics has enlarged more time is required for health supervision. Dispensing milk, vitamins and immunizations can be done in an assembly-line manner for large numbers of babies, but physical examination and the application of mental hygiene principles take such large amounts of time that the physician is unable to meet all the needs of mothers who bring their young children to the conference for health supervision.

The nurse has many functions in the Child Health Conference. The nurse in charge of the Child Health Conference should have had work with children and a broad public-health experience. The physician, when possible, should be a pediatrician, or at least one who has had experience with mothers and children. The nurse is the person who screens for problems and sees that routines are carried out. In doing so she saves the doctor's time and has an opportunity to function as his substitute either before or after the mother has her conference with him. She also supplements his activities by a follow-up conference. Ideally, the mother should see the same doctor and nurse each time she comes for a visit. When such a plan is in effect, the benefits for all concerned are multiplied.

In addition to the above duties, the nurse has the responsibility of working with all other personnel in the Child Health Conference. If students are assigned to her she will have the responsibility of interpreting to them the goals of the Conference. Today there is a social worker, a nutritionist, a child guidance worker and a dental hygienist available for consultation or for treatment purposes in many centers where Child Health Conferences are held. Many doctors use these specialists to save themselves time and to give mothers and children the benefit of their special knowledge and skill. Other doctors use them only when they discover that a family has a problem which requires the help of a specialist.

It is also the responsibility of the nurse in charge to plan for the public-health nursing visits which follow the work of the conference. In some agencies it has been found possible for the nurse who makes visits in a certain district to be in charge of the Child Health Conference when the mothers and the children from her district are given their appointments. This has proved to be of inestimable value.

In many Child Health Conferences volunteers are used to relieve the nurses for the functions requiring their professional skill. Usually they are trained by the nurse in charge to carry out certain procedures during the conference. The well-planned use of volunteers serves also to interest and educate the community in the functions and the work of the Child Health Conference.

The Conference is introduced to mothers in many different ways—during prenatal care, in the hospital when the baby is born or by the public health nurse who delivers the baby's birth certificate and invites the parents to the conference at the same time. Many parents are not aware of the help they can get in child-rearing in the Child Health Conference. Once a mother has attended a well-planned Child Health Conference, she usually discovers how much help she can find for the many problems which confront her as she begins to assume the responsibility of mothering. Once she has made this discovery, her use of the conference broadens.

It is the responsibility of every nurse to know the facilities of the community for well-baby health supervision so that she can interpret such services to mothers. The nurse caring for newborn babies needs this information. A nurse caring for sick babies needs equal preparation. The mother whose baby is discharged from the hospital is receptive to suggestions because she is doubly aware of the need for keeping her baby well. Hospital personnel need a well-worked-out plan whereby any baby discharged from the hospital inpatient or outpatient service, who is not going to have the health supervision of a private physician, is referred automatically to the most accessible Child Health Conference in order that health supervision may be uninterrupted.

CONDUCTING THE CONFERENCE

The waiting room must be large and equipped in a way that is comfortable for all who attend at one time. The waiting room is not only for adults but also for well children for whom play space needs to be provided. Small furniture is very desirable. Most young children like to move about rather than be held on their mothers' laps during the waiting period. The waiting room is also a room where learning can take place. Posters, charts, exhibits and demonstrations can be utilized if they are well presented. People waiting are more likely to observe and absorb new material than people who are in a hurry.

A friendly, pleasant atmosphere is more important than elaborate equipment. Mothers should want to come. The hostess, a volunteer or a nurse, ought to be ready to help them feel welcome. The value of the visit, or even future visits, may depend on the first contact. A "play nurse" or a "play teacher" is invaluable in making the waiting period pleasant for the children and their mothers. A "play nurse" gives mothers an opportunity to take advantage of the educational exhibits and makes it possible for them to have an opportunity to talk with each other.

Mothers will have many questions at the time their children are being weighed and measured. They will be interested in height and weight tables and will want to know how their children stand in relation to others. They will need to know that height and weight tables are interpreted with caution; that a steady rate of growth is more important than the total height or weight; that growth and development show wide variation in different babies, but that the patterns are similar. The mother may learn a new skill from watching a skillful nurse—how to lift the infant onto the scales, how to take his temperature or how to utilize safety measures in handling him, etc. Mothers will ask many questions. Some the nurse can answer by interpreting the knowledge that she has gleaned from specialists. Others she will refer to the doctor.

During the examination the doctor and the nurse have an excellent opportunity to observe the mother-child relationship as well as the child's physical status and behavior. As the doctor makes his general physical examination he notes growth and development and points out significant aspects to the mother. He observes the child's state of nutrition and his general health status and looks for any abnormality, defect or evidence of disease. Any immunization or test which is needed is usually done after the physical examination. The nurse prepares the child and gives him support while the needle is being inserted. The mother should be the provider of comfort as soon as the procedure is completed. Blood for a serologic test for syphilis may be taken. After a tuberculin test, some arrangements must be made for the return of the child for reading of the result.

After the examination most doctors like to confer with the mother. They interpret the findings of their physical examination and make comments concerning their observations of the child's behavior with his mother. The mother is given suggestions for any changes in the baby's care, such as addition of new foods into the diet, readiness for help in learning bowel control, etc. The doctor also encourages her to tell her story, to express her concerns if she will, and to describe the way she has already attempted to solve her problems.

The effectiveness of the conference will depend on the confidence that the mother has in the person who is conferring with her and the degree to which she feels that the personnel are trying to gain understanding of her as a person. The mother's ease in asking questions, in suggesting her need for amplification of the doctor's suggestions or in revealing her feelings and problems will depend largely upon the doctor's and the nurse's approach to her. An inhibited, anxious mother will find additional frustration if she is permitted to describe only the superficial aspects of her problems and then is presented with didactic advice which she probably has tried already and found that it does not work. The approach used to obtain her story is of great importance in the establishment of a constructive relationship with the mother. Mothers who are not yet acquainted with the doctor or the nurse may feel as though they were on trial at their first visit. A request such as "Tell me about your day with the baby" is preferable to "Are you nursing your baby on a self-demand schedule?" Questions often put mothers on the defensive. This question implies that she probably *should* be nursing in accordance with her baby's demands, whereas the request provides opportunities to learn more about the mother's feelings and methods of care. Guilty feelings can often be relieved by a question which implies that it is reasonable for the mother to have negative feelings toward her baby or her new role on occasion. "How often have you wished you might send the baby back to the nursery for care?" or "How has the baby disrupted the pleasures you had before the baby came?" are questions which may be resented by a mother who believes that she has accepted her role fully, but these queries indicate to many other mothers that being human is acceptable.

If a mother is anxiety-ridden, fearful or frustrated, she may exaggerate what is actually happening in the care of her baby. When this occurs, discrete pursuit of details will help the doctor and the nurse to discover what is worrying her. Sometimes a mother reports that her baby is vomiting at each feeding. If examination shows no evidence of disease, it is important to get further information to know how to relieve her fears. If the doctor or the nurse accepts her story as reality and suggests corrective measures, they will do nothing more than reinforce her groundless anxiety. Many of the accounts that mothers give doctors and nurses are bids for reassurance. If the listener gets trapped into agreeing that the condition must be corrected, he increases anxiety rather than lessens it. If the listener has evidence to prove that nothing abnormal is occurring, his matter-of-fact attitude toward the situation provides the reassurance that the mother is seeking.

One important purpose of the Child Health Conference is to meet the mothers' needs and in so doing to bolster the confidence of the anxious mother. If the mother is approached with interest and nonautocratic attitudes, it will be easier for her to disclose the problems that are troubling her. They may be in relation to some aspect of development or behavior which she does not understand. Or they may be in relation to the confusion that she feels about the widely divergent attitudes toward child care which are expressed in the magazines she reads and in the advice she gets from friends, relatives and casual acquaintances. When a mother discovers that her doctor and nurse are interested in her problems, eventually she will look to them for help in understanding her child or herself in relation to him. In the meantime the personnel begin to see the mother as a person and to understand her and her situation. As a result they are in a better position to help her.

Mothers come to the Child Health Conference seeking satisfaction of varying kinds of needs. Many times a mother is only trying to find reassurance and security in knowing that her judgment is sound. Some come seeking information; some only to have their children examined medically; and others because they feel that it is the thing to do. There are mothers who use the Child Health Conference as a social experience. They enjoy meeting other mothers, sharing their problems and dressing their youngsters up for inspection. Many mothers come feeling discouraged, perplexed and fatigued. *A sincere interest in the feelings of a distraught mother concerning herself or others in her family is emotional first-aid in the mental health of the family.* An opportunity to talk with someone who does not jump to conclusions, judge or evaluate often helps mothers through a period of confusion which is having emotional repercussions on each person within the family. If mothers find understanding they will leave the conference more relaxed and with increased strength to solve their problems more effectively. Some mothers come with realization of their mistakes. They feel guilty, inadequate and insecure. These mothers need help to feel competent in the mother role. The mother who fails to discharge her duties well is probably a person who in turn has received insufficient mothering during her own childhood. She may have had a poor model from which to fashion herself, or she may have had a change in mothers at a point in her early life when continuity of maternal care was necessary for acceptance of her femininity. The ill-prepared mother needs respect, help and approval. Direct teaching is not an essential element of a Child Health Conference. Often the greatest contribution lies in alleviating anxiety and guilt and giving mothers the understanding that they crave. This will be the inevitable outcome if the mother finds acceptance, generosity, interest and objectivity in the personnel of the Conference.

A mother may come to the Child Health Conference feeling hostile toward her child and yet be exceedingly guilty because she feels that way. All mothers get angry at their children sometimes. There are also times when they resent their responsibility, feel overburdened and wish to be dependent themselves. These feelings are natural and inevitable when women are adjusting to the mother role or to an increase in responsibility which the arrival of an additional child produces. Adjusting to the mother role takes time and energy. Child-rearing 24 hours a day, 365 days a year is a responsibility of great magnitude. It is also a tiring and perplexing job for many mothers. It is especially so in our society which is facing rapid change and an uncertain future. Negative feelings which arise upon occasion are inevitable, normal and understandable. Mothers need help in accepting such feelings when they arise. They will not only feel better themselves but also will accept their children's angry feelings and the "I hate you, Mother" which bursts from the mouths of their offspring in moments of frustration. When mothers can express their hostile feelings and air the burdens and the confusion that they feel, pleasanter relationships with their children are usually the outcome. Feelings which are kept suppressed generate guilt and tension. Energy, which should be available for loving, is used to keep the unacceptable feelings under control.

Mothers also come to the Child Health Conference with questions concerning thumb-sucking, negativism, rivalry, masturbation, etc. There are no formulas which will solve the mother's problem. The cause of prolonged thumb-sucking, for instance, varies in different children. Helping the mother think through possible causes of the "problem" behavior is infinitely more helpful than giving a formula. Often in talking about the problem with an understanding listener, the mother's anxiety becomes dissipated. If the listener can reflect the mother's feelings and restate what she has said in a way that she can accept, the mother not only feels understood but she also has an opportunity to look at her problem and begin to think of ways to do something about it. In many instances the mother is worrying about behavior that is common to all children during the age period which her child is traversing. Often the mere knowledge that certain behavior is found universally in children of her youngster's age helps the mother to gain perspective. Such understanding decreases the emotional tension which has contributed to the child's insecurity and hence has increased his problem.

Anticipatory guidance is a preventive measure. It prepares parents to understand the developmental process and the changes which arise with growth. When the nurse-mother and doctor-mother relationship are constructive, the mother welcomes preparation to recognize and to handle the developmental phases of growth and feels free to express her feelings about them. Interpreting the growth changes and helping the mother to gain insight into the way children feel about new socializing experiences prepares the mother to recognize the normality of change and to understand its purpose for personality growth. The mother will be freer of anxiety because she has been helped to feel competent in guiding her child toward mastery of his difficulties. Her understanding prevents problem behavior from developing.

Many serious problems arise because parents are unaware of the behavior changes which must occur if the child is to become an increasingly more independent person. Often a parent interprets a child's natural behavior as abnormal. The parent communicates this anxiety and increases the child's burdens. It also robs the child of the energy he needs to solve his current developmental task. Behavior which

might have been transient becomes exaggerated and fixed. Instead of support which helps him through a particular stage of his development, the child receives criticism, rejection or punishment which have their effect upon the production of personality distortions.

Another of the major objectives of the Child Health Conference is to help mothers obtain satisfaction in their relationships with each member of the family. The ability to interpret growth changes and developmental needs in a nonauthoritative way fosters more constructive relationships with mothers. Knowledge is necessary for work with mothers. Skill in interpreting it in a way so mothers can accept and use it is equally essential. Guidance which makes the mother feel that the health worker is a transmitter of knowledge rather than a supporting helper blocks the health worker's opportunities to be of service to families. Mothers need to apply knowledge in their own way to the individual needs of their children. This privilege must be granted in wholehearted, supportive ways. The goals of the conference cannot be accomplished if the personnel assume a superior role and give mothers little freedom to make their own decisions and develop their own inherent capacities for self-direction and motherliness.

It is in the realm of anticipatory guidance that the nurse can and should function, for she has a real contribution to make to preventive health programs. Her effectiveness can do much to alleviate the mother's anxiety so she can enjoy and feel confident in her role and provide her child with what he needs for sound physical and mental health.

When serious problem behavior is observed, the nurse must provide emotional first-aid, recognize her limitations and be prepared to help the parent to accept the services of a health worker who is specially trained in the treatment of troubled children. She can interpret the function of the social or child-guidance worker. She can also alleviate the fears that arise when a mother recognizes that her child has a problem which requires psychological therapy. The mother who has a disturbed or troubled child usually feels frustrated and incompetent. She is often fearful of psychological therapy because she expects condemnation from the therapist or from the community in which she lives. In referring a mother to a social worker or to a child-guidance clinic, the nurse and the doctor need understanding of these natural feelings. When a mother learns that social workers and therapists in child-guidance clinics have special skills which enable them to help parents and children solve their problems, her fears are often dispelled. As a result, she becomes motivated to seek help. This is especially true if the nurse helps the parent to transfer her relationship to another person and continues to provide the support that she is competent to give.

From this Conference, plus the entire report of previous conferences and home visits, the health team plans for the future needs of the family. When careful records are kept of the child's physical and developmental progress and of the parents' responses to their parental role, there are observational data which are available for future reference.

FUTURE GOALS

The Child Health Conference movement has spread rapidly, in cities and in rural areas. In some rural areas there are clinics which go from place to place, stopping long enough to hold a Child Health Conference and then moving on. Child Health Conferences have proved their value in reducing mortality and morbidity. Good attendance illustrates the value that mothers have found in them. However, more than half the counties in the United States still do not have Child Health Conferences available. To remedy this, more work is required: better education of the public, favorable legislation, financial support, and constant effort on the part of those who realize the value of health supervision of infants and children to the nation's well-being.

Not only is there need for more facilities and for health supervision but also for more effective use of those already in existence. Many fathers would come with their wives if they knew it would be helpful to the family. An unattended conference ceases to have value. Those in the health professions need to recognize an outstanding trait in human nature: people tend to do things the easy way, the way they are accustomed to doing them and the way that gives them pleasure. If attendance at Child Health Conferences can be made easy, pleasant and helpful, the habit is formed. Parents who get constructive guidance and support when they need it will continue to come, even though they may never comprehend the far-reaching effects of the whole movement. One unpleasant visit, a few uncertain, uncomfortable moments may be enough to discourage a parent and prevent return. The more health workers can help parents feel that they want to return because it has been a valuable experience for them, the greater will be the benefits derived from it.

SITUATIONS FOR FURTHER STUDY

1. How is infant health supervision provided for in your community? How are appointments made?

2. What play equipment would be practical and useful in the waiting room? How much play supervision is desirable?

3. Arrange an exhibit for a Child

Health Conference waiting room on any pertinent subject you choose. Explain your choice and methods of presentation. If possible, present it and observe results.

4. If attendance is falling off in the Child Health Conference, what might be some of the reasons for it?

5. Describe a conference between a mother and a nurse which you observed. How did the nurse approach the mother? Did she encourage her to talk about her problems? How did she do it? Was she successful? Why? If she failed, what do you think were the reasons? What questions did the mother ask?

6. Describe a conference that you conducted. What were your feelings concerning it? What did you learn about the mother, the child? How do you think the mother felt about you? Did you feel adequate in giving the mother the help that she required? If not, what further preparation do you feel that you need?

7. Describe a conference that you observed between a doctor and a mother. Did he show interest in the mother's problem? How did he show it? How did he approach the child? What technics did he use to gain the child's co-operation? What specific help did he give the mother? What was her attitude toward him and his teaching?

8. Describe a situation in which you observed a nurse offering anticipatory guidance. What was the mother's reaction to it? Had she anticipated the change in the child's behavior that the nurse described? What were her questions concerning it? Do you think that the mother received enough insight into the behavior and her feelings concerning it to be able to handle it wisely when it arises?

BIBLIOGRAPHY

Amann, Anna, and Williams, Allie M.: A study of child health problems, Nursing Outlook 4:109, 1956.

Foster, Mary L.: Reasons for attending child health station, Pub. Health Nursing 44:123, 1952.

Gilbert, Ruth: The Public Health Nurse and Her Patient, ed. 2, Cambridge, Harvard, 1951.

Ginsburg, Ethel L.: Public Health Is People, New York, The Commonwealth Fund, 1950.

Greenhill, Maurice H.: Interviewing with a purpose, Am. J. Nursing 56:1259, 1956.

Hawley, Eleanor: Our stake in the future, Pub. Health Nursing 44:447, 1952.

Korsch, B. M.: Observing, interviewing and advising parents—an attitude study, Pediatrics 18:467, 1956.

Lemkau, Paul: Mental Hygiene in Public Health, ed. 2, New York, McGraw-Hill, 1955.

Levy, D. M.: Observations of attitudes and behavior in the child health center, Am. J. Pub. Health 41:182, 1951.

Levy, Julius: An experiment in training nurses to help mothers in preventive mental hygiene, Ment. Hyg. 23:99, 1939.

Richmond, Julius: Health supervision of infants and young children, Am. J. Nursing 52:1460, 1952.

Wandett, Mabel A.: Teaching is more than telling, Am. J. Nursing 57:625, 1957.

Wishik, S. W.: Parents' group discussions in a child health conference, Am. J. Pub. Health 43:888, 1953.

Health Supervision of Young Children, New York, The American Pub. Health Assn., Inc., 1955.

UNIT THREE

General Nursing Care

CHAPTER EIGHT

The Nurse-Child and
Nurse-Parent Relationship

Comprehensive care includes support which fosters the growth and the development of the individual. Before the student progresses very far in this section she will become aware that both physical and emotional support contain elements that affect the individual's whole being. It is difficult to think of any detail of physical care that does not affect the individual's feelings as well as his body. Feeding a patient nourishes his body; it also has emotional significance for him as well. It lessens hunger tension; it gratifies and supplies physical and psychic energy. The effects of having her needs recognized can be easily comprehended if the student recalls some of her own experiences of being observed, listened to and understood and compares the feelings she had then with the feelings she had in situations where she was unobserved, unheard and misunderstood. When she feels that her needs have been perceived, her feelings and thoughts respected and understood, her energy is abounding. She has interest in other people and in new experiences; she has hope that helps her through difficult situations. But when she thinks that her

point of view and feelings have been disregarded, she reacts quite differently. Until she drains off the tension that such a situation evokes, she has few interests outside of herself; she is discouraged; she feels inadequate in making herself understood; she feels under par physically and has little surplus energy for giving. Feeling misunderstood affects her whole being. During illness such a state of affairs could lead to a relapse or emotional regression because the patient's energy becomes consumed in handling the resentment that he feels instead of being available for recuperation and for mastery of the personal problems which are always associated with illness.

Another example will serve to illustrate further the interrelatedness of the physical and the emotional elements which are intrinsic in supportive care. If the student thinks back again into her own experience she will recall that different feelings were aroused in each of the following three situations: (1) when she was told to accomplish a task for which she was unprepared and was given no help to do it, (2) when someone did a task for her that she was ca-

132

pable of doing independently, and (3) when someone recognized her strengths and limitations and provided the support that she needed to accomplish the task. When the reader was asked to do something for which she was unprepared she probably felt put out and resentful. Such feelings left her feeling helpless and incompetent. She could not do the task as it needed to be done. She used what skills she had and fumbled through as best she could, but her feelings were those of dissatisfaction with herself and with the person who had been unaware of her needs for personal growth. When the reader was deprived of doing a task that she was able to do, she undoubtedly felt depreciated as well as angry. When she was supported in doing a task for which she was unready, in all probability she felt that the helping person believed in her and recognized her capacity to develop further. The outgrowth of experiences like the last conserves energy; it strengthens the individual's ego resources; it helps her feel that she can succeed again and leaves her with healthy, warm feelings toward the helpful persons.

The children and the parents with whom the nurse works have similar feelings and needs in circumstances similar to those cited above. The mother who is expected to leave her child in the hospital for an emergency operation and must adapt to the news unaided will show evidence of rebellious and anxious feelings. The child with cerebral palsy who is taken care of by a nurse who is not sensitive to his need to do the things he is capable of doing loses opportunities to feel his worth as a person.

The adolescent who has had a background of wise nurturing has many ego strengths to face long-term hospitalization for rheumatic fever. He can utilize preparation for going to the hospital. He has a background of memorable experiences that he can draw upon in periods of loneliness and discourage-

ment. He has had a multitude of experiences that have taught him that people can be trusted. He has acquired manual and mental skills which he can use to keep himself occupied. He has many other personality strengths, but he also has limitations. Therefore, he needs support to adapt to reality. Illness produces change in his life and confronts him with a reality situation that he is unprepared to meet independently. Many of his personality limitations stem from the fact that he continues to be in the process of mastering the developmental tasks of adolescence. Some of his limitations come from painful childhood experiences that he has not fully digested or integrated as this emotional process is often called. No child has *all* his needs fulfilled in childhood. Parents are not infallible! They, too, are human; they make mistakes, as do all human beings. Raising a child is a complex process. To come through the growing-up process without some personality limitations is unrealistic. Likewise, it is unrealistic to expect an adolescent to adapt to the realities of illness and hospitalization without a helping relationship. To demand this of him would create more anxiety than he could handle in a healthy fashion.

The adolescent hospitalized with rheumatic fever needs more support than a healthy child of the same age because the reality he faces includes not only the usual problems of adolescence but also the implications of hospitalization and of his disease. He will need the support that a normal adolescent requires. He will also need help to adjust to changes in his mode of living and to understand his disease and himself in relation to it. The meaning that the disease has for him personally will need to be taken into account because it will color the way he adapts to the reality limitations that it imposes. The adolescent who feels supported during hospitalization will be strengthened by the experience. Because he has acquired kind feelings toward those who have helped him during a period of stress, he will be ready to profit from their advice in the care of himself at home. Also, he will know that he can turn to them again whenever he feels insecure about himself or his relationship with other people.

PHYSICAL SUPPORT

To provide the physical support that the growing, ill, handicapped or convalescent child requires, the nurse needs special training and skills which increase her judgment and prepare her to study the patient's physical condition and needs and to supply care which supports his body. This is life-sustaining and supportive emotionally as well as physically. Carefully given physical care helps to restore the sick person's body to health; it also brings the patient comfort and reassurance that he is cared for, protected and loved. It conserves his energy for it decreases the high rate of consumption which occurs when he is fearful lest his bodily needs be fulfilled incompletely.

PHYSICAL SKILLS

There are special skills which the pediatric nurse must acquire because she works with a smaller and more delicate individual and uses smaller tools. Gentleness of touch and performance is necessary. Certain diseases are peculiar to childhood. Among the diseases which are common to both adults and children, there are some which have implications of greater severity and poorer prognosis for the child. These circumstances make necessary special pediatric nursing knowledge which is the subject matter upon which the principles of physical care are based.

When pediatric nursing procedures are analyzed, certain fundamental principles emerge which are accepted by the personnel in all hospitals. However, the actual performance of the procedures will vary somewhat in different hospitals. The maintenance of a sterile field may be the basic principle in one procedure; absolute accuracy, the essential factor in another; continuous administration of a liquid at a given temperature may be the requirement in a third.

The purpose of setting up procedures and working out routines and technics for the care of children is to ensure safety and maximum comfort. Ensuring safety requires adherence to the principles underlying the procedure. To succeed in bringing comfort to children, the nurse needs manual skills. She also needs imagination to find ways to make the procedure acceptable and a profitable experience. In this textbook, specific nursing procedures will be discussed as they relate to the care of children with specific diseases.

OBSERVATIONAL SKILLS

Observational skills are a vital part of nursing care. Each day as the pediatric nurse goes about her work with children, she needs to exercise her powers of observation not only through her sense of sight but also through her sense of hearing and touch. Listening is an art and a natural response to interest in human beings. The school-age child or the adolescent can talk about his feelings if the nurse communicates respect, tolerance and interest in seeing the problem from his point of view. The young child cannot talk about his feelings; nevertheless, he communicates them in ways that can be heard as well as seen. Listening to the child's mother and observing the interaction between her and her child provides valuable information. This information assists the health team in appraising their needs and in planning ways to give them the ego support that they require. In addition to using her sense organs, the nurse needs to use that subtle sense of "feeling"—that discerning quality which somehow tells her of changes in her patients and in their mothers which are not observed by the eye, the ear or the hand.

The child, unlike the adult, cannot detect and report verbally every change in feeling to the minutest detail. The adult identifies pain, chilliness, nausea or a feeling of uncertainty and reports his discomfort. This the young child cannot do. He *feels* changes in his physical and emotional status and reacts to them with behavioral changes. Frequently, however, he cannot locate his physical pain or identify the feeling which is changing his behavior. Through crying, restlessness, tempestuousness or the opposite type of response—withdrawal from emotional contacts or objects within his environment—he signals discomfort from physical changes in his body. Through behavioral responses he also tells us of his need for someone who is alert to his wants and ready to restore his feelings of emotional and physical security. Unlike the convalescent child who may express a dozen wants, loudly and lustily, the acutely ill child will do little to announce his change in symptoms. The nurse must be able to note the first evidence of a rise in temperature, a drop in blood pressure, a rise in intracranial pressure, the behavior that warns of an insulin reaction. She must be constantly alert to notice changes in her patient's physical condition, for they take place quickly and often without warning.

EMOTIONAL SUPPORT

To provide the emotional support that the ill, handicapped or convalescent child requires, the nurse needs knowledge, attitudes and skills which prepare her to supply care which strengthens the child's ego so that he can make a healthy adjustment to the reality of his new experience. (1) She needs awareness of herself and others. (2) She needs the capacity to help the child at the time of admission to the hospital. (3) She needs competency in maintaining a constructive relationship with him and his parents during the period of hospitalization and with others of the health team who are helping to meet the complex needs of the family.

Ego support which is the heart of nursing can be given only within the context of a constructive relationship. It cannot be given without it, for strength comes only from persons who have positive emotional meaning to the individual. Experience must have taught the individual that the helping person was a person whom he could trust and rely upon to understand his needs. This knowledge created the impetus for the case method of care. Today we know that children need continuity in their relationship with nurses. This is especially true for the infant and the young child who is deprived of his mother during prolonged periods of hospitalization. Unless he has daily periods of concentrated care by one person his need for attachment to and trust in his mother may be injured to the degree that his opportunities for healthy personality growth may become thwarted. It is also true for the care of the older child and the adult. It is difficult to discover a person's strengths, limitations and needs without continuity of experience with him. The child's needs change as he grows; the sick child's needs change as he progresses through the stages of his illness; the handicapped child's needs change as he adjusts to his limitations and learns to use the strengths that he possesses; the disturbed child's needs change as he works through his problems and masters his fears. Care must be modified as the child makes progress in adaptation to reality and becomes ready for new learning experiences.

Continuity of care has been found to provide greater assurance that individual and changing needs will be met.

AWARENESS OF SELF AND OTHERS

A pediatric ward needs an emotional climate which communicates feelings of hospitality to children and to parents. Equipment and an attractively decorated pediatric unit are helpful aids in the care of children but they are no substitute for emotional satisfactions. Most of us would infinitely prefer a sparsely furnished room in a residence that is permeated with friendly feelings and respect for our need to be ourselves than a lavishly furnished room in a dwelling which is managed by individuals who constantly expect us to meet their demands, regardless of our need for self-expression. When a child is ill and separated from his parents, he needs a relationship which gives comfort, security and proof that he has not been abandoned but will be taken care of and receive the understanding, the protection and the support that he needs in a strange, fear-provoking and painful situation. His parents need to *feel sure* that they are welcome in the hospital and will be understood and respected. The nurse is an important part of her patient's environment. Her health—mental, physical and spiritual—influences her patients and their families. This is especially true when the patient is a growing, impressionable, dependent child and his parents are meeting reality problems that they never have met before. Sometimes in the pressure of our work we forget that we have the power to use ourselves therapeutically. Children and their families look to the nurse for knowledge, emotional strength and comfort. The nurse's contacts with children and parents must give more than a pill, a treatment or a bit of information; they must communicate her understanding of them as persons.

The capacity to give fully of herself will not exist when the student begins her experience in pediatric nursing. She, too, needs time to adjust to the tensions that are produced when working with children and parents. The student will be exposed repeatedly to situations that are emotionally draining. Assuming responsibility for the care of sick children is taxing. Because children are in the process of growth, they need pleasure and support in abundance. When children are ill and separated from familiar surroundings, they react in ways that evoke feelings that take time for nurses to learn to handle comfortably. The reality existent in pediatric wards is difficult to face. The sight of deformed and acutely ill children arouses disquieting feelings. Adjusting herself to giving them care takes far more time than a fortnight.

Working with frightened, angry and grief-stricken children and parents calls heavily on the nurse's store of patience and energy. Because the nurse is a human being she has her share of limitations as well as strengths. She should not expect herself to react with poise perpetually. There will be many experiences that evoke conflict and anxiety. At these times she has to cope with her own feelings as well as the child's, and this is not easy. It is natural for an inexperienced nurse to feel aggressive and hurt when a child directs feelings of hatred toward her or has a temper tantrum just as the doctor or her teacher arrives. It is equally natural for her to feel her anxiety mounting when she is faced with a panic-stricken child. Grieving children and parents evoke feelings in the sensitive nurse. These, too, are difficult feelings to handle. They may stir up feelings that the nurse herself had in similar situations. Or they may make her feel inadequate or uneasy because she has not had sufficient experience to know how to give comfort. Or she may not have the time to ease the person's distress. Sometimes the nurse protects herself from anxiety by shutting out the sight of the anguish. She might do this by closing the door to his unit, by leaving the situation or by developing a blind spot in her own perception. This solution meets her immediate needs, and she may need to do this temporarily while she is adjusting herself to the realities of pediatric nursing. To make it a permanent defense against anxiety would be unfortunate for her because it would limit her opportunities for learning ways to comfort others. It would also be harmful to the child or to the parents for it would leave them with a problem that they would have to bear alone.

Acquiring serenity and poise in the face of all the trying situations that a nurse faces in a pediatric ward requires time and motivation to develop further. Gaining understanding of her feelings and learning to handle them in ways that are constructive for others as well as for herself takes time. Acquiring patience, tolerance, understanding and objectivity does not come quickly. Before knowledge can be used in relationship with others, it must be integrated or digested. This is a slow process. The knowledge that individuals bring feelings from the past into their relationships with others does not automatically confer instant objectivity. Anger directed at the nurse is felt and reacted to until she has experience which teaches her that what she did or said triggered off feelings from the past. It is not unusual for children to displace the feelings that they have toward their mothers onto a nurse, even as they can displace all their anxious feelings onto a specific treatment—intramuscular injections for instance. The nurse should be patient with and tolerant of herself while she is learning. If she is, she will learn more rapidly, experience fewer conflicts and have more energy for giving. Also, she will be more tolerant of other peoples' feelings.

Pediatric nursing offers many opportunities for personal and professional growth. If the student is motivated to develop awareness of herself in relation to her patients, their families and her co-workers, she will discover that she has some feelings and attitudes which prevent her from meeting her patient's needs as fully as she would like to do. Sometimes she will find that increased knowledge of the child's background of experience will help her to acquire more accepting attitudes toward him. Self-inspection also reaps results. With it the nurse can discover the situations which make her anxious and the way she reacts to them. She can discover the personal biases, the intolerance and the tendency to make value judgments which exist in varying degrees in all of us. However, discovering the foibles of her own personality is not enough. She also needs to accept them as fringe results of her own upbringing. When the nurse discovers through experience that all persons, including herself, behave in the light of their past experiences, she will undoubtedly be motivated to search for new relationship experiences which will help her to change and to grow. She may not be able to eliminate the feeling or the attitude completely, but bringing it into the open and looking at it by herself or with a helpful person will assist her in handling it in a way that safeguards her relationship with her patients, with parents and with co-workers.

Awareness and acceptance of oneself as a person who needs new helpful relationship experiences for growth prepares the nurse to acquire awareness of children's feelings and to identify herself with them. Awareness of feelings and the capacity to respond with understanding and recognition of the patient's needs are the basic elements of ego support. The nurse must be able to identify herself with the listless newly admitted child who sits without touching the food on his tray. She must know that his behavior may spell homesickness, fear and loss of personal identity. She must have insight to know that his behavior most likely means that he is missing his mother—the most important source of his emotional security. When the nurse is able to experience imaginatively how a child feels when he is in a new place without any important emotional ties that ensure love, protection and care, she becomes ready to give—to use herself in ways that are therapeutic. She will help the child to feel that he *is* Johnny or Susan or Mark, as the case may be, and an object of her concern. She will make herself available to him and watch for cues that help her to understand him further. When his feelings of personal identity are restored, changes in his approach to food will become increasingly more evident.

The nurse also needs to be able to identify herself with the child who is using great portions of his energy in coping with conflict and anxiety which are beyond his capacity to master unaided. She must be able to detect and feel with the child who is angry, fearful or grieving for a mother who is gone but he knows not where. She also needs to detect and identify herself with the child who has withdrawn not because he is a quiet, "good" child but because he imagines his hospital world so scary or threatening that he dare not remain in contact with it. She must be able to feel the threat of an acute illness so she can anticipate wants of the child of which he himself is barely aware. She needs to be able to allay the fears that he cannot express and find his special sources of comfort and pleasure. Furthermore, she needs to be able to feel with the child who is loaded with feelings that are ready to explode and is scared to death lest he let them loose in ways that have brought punishment in the past. When the nurse can feel with such a frightened child, she will appreciate his need for constructive play activity through which he can express himself, relieve tension and master his fears. The third section of this chapter serves to increase the nurse's insight into the feelings and the needs of children in pediatric wards and outpatient departments. Insight that will further the nurse's capacity to feel with mothers follows subsequently.

Parents as well as children need a nurse who can identify with them because they are under stress and need support to make a healthy adjustment to the painful reality that they are facing. The nurse cannot assume that everyone feels as she does about a child's illness, deformity or handicap. The nurse may be able to take illness and hospitalization in a casual, matter-of-fact way because she knows that the condition is not serious or because she knows from experience that an operation can correct the deformity. She may have knowledge that tells her the mother has no realistic cause to feel guilty, frightened or angered. However, this does not mean that the mother feels the same way about it. Her reasons for feeling guilty or afraid may be irrational from the nurse's point of view but to the mother they are real or she would not be under stress.

Emotional reactions to a child's illness or deformity and his need for hospitalization show wide variation. Guilt is almost a universal reaction. Some parents resent the financial burden. Some mothers feel rivalrous with nurses and fearful lest their child transfer his affections to a nurse. Some mothers are in terror lest hospitalization arouse the child's hostility toward them. Others are anxious about leaving their child in the hospital. Some resent the fact that they are not permitted to stay and take care of their child. This is particularly true of mothers of infants and young children. Most mothers of school-age children have mastered their fear of separation from their offspring, but this is not true of many mothers of young children, who suffer acutely from separation anxiety. Mother and child have a mutual interdependency which meets the needs of both. When a mother is separated from her young child some of her needs will be frustrated. Until she adjusts constructively to this change, she will be in conflict and have anxiety. Self-pity is another feeling that exists in some parents. They see the child's illness or deformity as something that is catastrophic to themselves. Some of these parents are resentful because illness or deformity has befallen them. Others feel ashamed of the child's deformity; others feel stigmatized by the attitudes of society and anticipate being ostracized. Others are grief-stricken because they realize the seriousness of the illness and dread the pain that the child must endure.

A large proportion of mothers have strong egos which help them to face the reality of illness and hospitalization. Even so, they will be anxious until the child's condition improves and he evidences comfortable adjustment to the illness. Then their anxiety will subside, for although intense at first it is limited to the duration of the illness. The nurse must recognize this as normal anxiety that is appropriate to the situation. During the mother's period of acute anxiety, she may talk of problems concerning many other facets of her life. This is to be expected. When a mother is anxious about a sick child, every other problem that she would ordinarily solve comfortably is magnified and seems to be insurmountable. She talks about the collateral problems in order to get understanding, reassurance and relief from tension.

If the nurse can listen to expressions of anxiety or anger without making the mother feel guilty or becoming anxious herself, she will note that the mother becomes increasingly more comfortable. *Passive acceptance of her anxiety as normal is therapeutic to the mother.* When the child's condition improves most mothers solve their other problems easily because they have energy to handle them. But if the anxiety continues unabated after the child's condition has improved, the nurse should

begin to suspect that it has wider implications than legitimate concern over the immediate illness. The mother, for instance, may wish to use her child's illness to solve other problems. Such a mother may try to use her child's illness to foster an abnormally dependent relationship with him. In such instances, the nurse should report her observations to other members of the health team. The way in which a social worker can help a mother solve her problem more constructively for the child and herself is illustrated in the discussion of the care of the child with diabetes in Chapter 23.

The manner in which a mother handles her anxiety during acute illness of her child depends upon her past experiences and the way she has handled other stressful experiences during her lifetime. If the nurse had a complete understanding of the mother's background, the reasons for her type of behavior would be readily apparent. All behavior has purpose for the individual. It is an attempt to solve a problem that is disturbing his peace of mind. It is easy to conclude erroneously that he is creating a problem when in reality he is merely using the only ego resources that he has and the environment offers to solve one. The mother who previously has taken flight when faced with stress probably will do so again. Another mother will strike out at the situation. A third will cover conscious or unconscious feelings of guilt in oversolicitude or fearsomeness. Still other mothers project their guilt onto hospital personnel, blaming them for everything that goes wrong instead of facing the suspicion that in some manner they themselves are at fault. Such mothers cannot face their own guilty feelings without the risk of some measure of disorganization of their personalities. If the nurse is able to accept the critical tirades, however unjust they may be, she will do much to relieve the mother's anxiety. Much to her surprise, she may find that in a short time the parent who has been unreasonably critical is warmly praising her competence and care of the child. This is due to the fact that the nurse protected her from facing feelings that she could not master. As a result, she is able to see her as a helpful person. The examples that follow illustrate how a mother's past experiences explain her behavior and how the nurse through her patient listening and observation can gradually acquire information that enhances her understanding.

When Mrs. A. brought Ann into the hospital for cataract extraction, she was "jittery" and completely unable to support her child in the early part of her hospitalization. She fled from the ward as soon as Ann's history was taken, without heed to Ann's need of her for a longer period of time. When the operation had to be postponed because of a respiratory infection in Ann, she vented angry feelings on hospital personnel and on Ann. When she came for visiting periods, she could not tolerate Ann's tears of rebelliousness. She said that she could not wait to get out of the hospital because, as she said venomously, "It makes me jittery. I can't stay put. The quicker I can get out of here the better." Mrs. A.'s discomfort motivated the nurse to want to understand her. She discovered that Mrs. A. had had cataract extractions from both eyes when she was 4 years old. She remembered little about hospitalization, but from conversation it seemed evident that she never had made peace with the childhood difficulties that concerned her eyes and their treatment. She expressed resentment because she had to wear thick glasses constantly and felt herself to be unattractive in them. She felt guilty about having what she called a "defective child." After her first child, Billy, was born, she sought medical advice and made sure that his eyes were perfect before she became pregnant again. "I'd never have had another child if I'd known it would have cataracts," she said. When her second child's eyes were found to be imperfect, she expressed guilt and resentment. Mrs. A.'s brother also had had congenital cataracts during early childhood, but his children had normal vision. She expressed resentment toward her brother's successful achievement.

Postoperatively, Ann cried and expressed angry feelings toward her mother when she arrived late in the ward. Ann's response to discomfort and disappointment increased Mrs. A.'s guilt. It also made her anxious and intolerant of frustration. She reacted with anger and inability to see anyone else's problems but her own. Her behavior was understandable when the facts of her past experiences were known. It is highly probable that Mrs. A.'s own painful childhood hospital experience made her vulnerable to her current life-situation with Ann. When an adult meets a situation that is similar to one which scarred his developing personality, the turmoil and the anxiety originally associated with the childhood wound is stirred up. Or, in other words, her current problem with Ann aroused old feelings that she never had fully mastered. As a result she felt "jittery," which is a common way for lay people to express anxiety verbally and she acted in a way that was inappropriate to her current situation. She knew that she felt miserable but she did not know why she acted as she did. In addition to feeling responsible for Ann's visual difficulties, she felt guilty about her impulsive behavior.

It is also possible that Mrs. A. was misunderstood when she was hospitalized as a child. If her crying and anger were punished and she had not made peace with the resentment that she felt then, she would be especially vulnerable to similar expression in Ann. Deep down inside her she might have wanted to punish Ann as she had been punished. If she could not let herself do this she would be in conflict and have more tension to handle. If this were true it is understandable why she came late, fled from the ward before visiting hours were over and had to leave Ann repeatedly for a smoke.

When Mrs. G. brought her child, Joe, into the hospital for cataract extraction she reacted very differently from Mrs. A. Her background experience did not include an operation in childhood. She had felt guilty when she learned that her child had a visual defect. But she was more fortunate than Mrs. A. Her feelings were observed by the clinic nurse and reported to the ophthalmologist. He suggested that the nurse refer Mrs. G. to a social worker because he recognized her need of help to solve the problem which was interfering with successful social functioning. Because the nurse had already established a constructive relationship with Mrs. G. she was able to help her accept the help that the social worker could provide and move into a relationship with another member of the health team. This did not mean that the nurse's support ended with the referral. She continued to help her during clinic visits. The social worker not only helped her to feel the irrationality of her guilt feelings but she also helped her handle her feelings concerning her child's impending operation. The nurse and the social worker shared their experiences with Mrs. G. and prepared the head nurse in the ward for Joe's admission to the hospital. During Joe's hospitalization Mrs. G. was supportive. She visited as often as she could. She understood the feelings that Joe had in relation to his hospital experience and helped him to handle them in play.

The pediatric nurse needs understanding that will prepare her to identify herself with many kinds of parents. She needs to understand how abysmal ignorance can be and to be ready without any note of scorn in her voice to explain in the simplest of terms. Fear of the unknown is a terrific fear! And many mothers as well as children are in the throes of this fear when they enter the clinic or the hospital. Some mothers are guided more by superstition than by reason. Some have had unhappy experiences in hospitals. They assume that all hospitals are alike. Some mothers have been forced to bring their children to the hospital. They have irrational fears that block their capacity to learn. The mother who is frightened needs to know that her child is in kind, gentle and wise hands. Her fear will decrease gradually when she gains faith in hospital personnel.

There are, on occasions, women who are terrified of the unknown, and sometimes they are hysterical or belligerent as well. These women are trying. They tax the nurse's ingenuity to the utmost. They will leave her feeling frustrated, antagonistic and critical unless she understands the reasons for emotional instability and can identify herself with a panicky person who has lost control of herself.

In instances like the above, time and the help of a social worker prove to be advantageous. The nurse must protect the child by establishing rapport with him. She needs to be ready to give him the support that his mother is unable to give him. The terrified, hysterical mother needs calming, support and kind, firm, positive and consistent treatment. She needs help to meet the unknown. She is like a child—in need of a sense of security. If she had had it in her childhood, she would be ready to give it to her child. Before she can give it to him, she must receive it in abundance from hospital personnel. It will take time and the help of an additional person, but it is the only human thing to do. She, too, is a sick person who needs understanding.

Then there is the mother who recognizes the true seriousness of the situation. She knows that her child is seriously ill. She has observed his change in behavior and recognized the onset of more ominous symptoms. She is acutely anxious. And there are rational reasons why she feels this way.

The mother who recognizes the seriousness of her child's condition needs the support that comes from understanding of her concern and from skillful sympathetic care of her child. Denials of the seriousness of the child's illness will not alleviate her anxiety but rather will increase it. Denials will make her feel that the nurse is an incompetent observer. They will also make her skeptical of her capacity to care for her child. In addition, she will feel misunderstood because her feelings have not been accepted. A mother gets relief from anxiety when hospital personnel recognize the seriousness of the situation and share their concern with her. In addition, she needs to know that everything possible is being done by sympathetic, skillful persons. Words alone will not convince her of this. She must *see* and *feel* that everything is being done. She will gain this feeling not only from seeing her child cared for scientifically but also from the attitudes and the feelings that are communicated to her and to her child. It cannot come from efficiency or scientific treatment alone. It comes when the hospital personnel's skillful work stems from a capacity to feel with other people and from a genuine concern for their needs.

Words, attitudes and feelings that convey understanding and explanations that assist people in adjusting healthily to stress are essential parts of nursing care. They are not a waste of time; they are timesavers. They ease the mother's mind, give her strength, win her confidence and prepare her to be supporting to her child. A friendly greeting and an opportunity to talk to someone who can share her burden will do much to allay the mother's anxiety. In doing so the child is also benefited, for he will be protected from the contagiousness of his mother's anxiety. The mother is the child's source of security and strength. If she is secure he will have more strength to adapt to the painful reality that he will meet.

Admission to the Hospital

The nurse who supports the child and his parents through the admission period of hospitalization is confronted with a responsibility of great magnitude. When she goes into the waiting room she will find a child and one or both parents who need her understanding help. Both the child and his parents may have been helped to face the experience at the time hospitalization was recommended. But in many instances, unfortunately, this probably will not be true.

The way the admitting routine is carried out is of great significance to the child and his parents. It can be a supporting experience which lessens anxiety or it can be one which heightens existing feelings of apprehension. During admission the parents' and the child's feelings and attitudes toward hospitals, their personnel and procedures are influenced. Being noticed and listened to immediately upon arrival heighten self-esteem and give strength. When the child and his parents arrive at the ward feeling that they are in the hands of understanding people, the child's adjustment to his illness and hospitalization is better ensured.

Even though the child and his mother have been prepared verbally, adapting to the new experience will be a difficult process. *Preparation is essential.* It assists the child in preparing himself to meet the situation. *However, of equal importance to his adjustment at the time of admission is the understanding guidance that is available to help him understand and accept all that is happening to him.* The nurse must be emotionally ready to supply the support that the parents and the child require. Often the admission procedure is a routine experience to the nurse. It is anything but routine to the child and his parents. In most instances they do not know what is going to happen to them. The admission procedure is only one of the many things to which they must adjust themselves. In addition to the illness and the anxiety that it generates there is the thought of separation which looms large in the mind of almost every parent and every child if he is old enough to comprehend that is what hospitalization requires.

Each child will have his own individual way of handling the anxiety which arises from anticipation of a fearful situation, even as each mother has hers. Each child acquires an individual pattern of behavior in response to conflicting feelings which produce anxiety. Because the young child is so identified with his mother it is not unusual for him to handle anxiety in ways similar to hers. If a mother handles her anxiety about impending hospitalization by denying the reality of it, her child will have difficulty in handling his feelings concerning hospitalization in a healthy way. If his mother denies the reality of it, the child gets little help in preparing himself to meet it. If he questions to discover what the doctor said about hospitalization, the mother who denies the reality of this situation probably will communicate her need to keep the thought hidden from her mind.

Children utilize preparation for hospitalization in many different ways just as their parents do. Some children will come ready for the experience. However, there will be others who have been unable to assimilate the preparation. It may be that they were too young to see into the future and anticipate what it would hold. Or it may be that the thought of hospitalization was so painful that they had to put it and the feelings that it evoked out of their conscious minds. Some must produce fantasies that make the experience different from what they will meet in reality.

Jessner and Kaplan studied the emotional responses of children to tonsillectomy and adenoidectomy. They concluded that preparation for hospitalization and operation was necessary. They also made the following statement pertaining to the child's use of information:

The factual information is sometimes not accepted by the child, but is replaced or remodelled by fantasies. Fantasies are often indicative of the fact that earlier anxieties or anticipations are mobilized by the operation or expectation of the operation. On the other hand,

fantasies may also represent another method utilized by children to assimilate the new experience, to translate it into their own picture language and to integrate it into their former experience and body conceptions.[*]

Before the admission routine is carried out the nurse will need information which will prepare her to support the mother through the experience. *The child needs protection from hearing what he cannot understand.* He should not be within hearing distance when his personal history, disease or treatment is being discussed. Nor should he hear his mother talk about her feelings pertaining to his illness or deformity. In fact, it is better if he does not hear any conversation about himself that he cannot understand. The unknown so often means fear to the child. Matters of everyday occurrence to nurses and terms that fall easily from their lips are strange to the imaginative child and full of portent to him. "A shot" means a hypodermic injection of healing medicine to a nurse but to a child it might have quite a different meaning.

When a mother attempts to discuss her child's personality and habits of behavior within his hearing, the nurse can suggest that she wait until she can get someone to attend the child during the conference. Curiously enough, in some instances, the mother's comments about her child are derogatory. When a child hears his mother criticizing him, he may become frightened lest he start a new experience handicapped by a reputation that he feels he does not deserve. Information about the child can be obtained while the child is being examined by the doctor. When it is possible, both parents should be encouraged to bring

[*] Jessner, Lucie, and Kaplan, Samuel: Observations on the emotional reactions of children to tonsillectomy and adenoidectomy, in Problems of Infancy and Childhood, Transactions of the Third Conference, New York, Josiah Macy, Jr., Foundation, 1949, p. 115.

the child to the hospital. Then he will not need to be separated from a parent so soon after he enters the hospital. There will be another advantage. The father will be there and become involved in plans which concern him as well as other members of the family. The importance of the father's participation in plans for the child's care is illustrated in the discussion of the care of the child with diabetes in Chapter 23.

In addition to listening to the mother talk of the things which are of concern to her, the nurse can obtain information that will help others to understand him. Wilkins[*] constructed the following form to collect data about preschool children:

[*] Wilkins, Gladys: The Role of the Nurse in the Admission of Preschool Children to Hospitals, Unpublished Master's paper, University of Chicago, Dept. of Nursing Education, 1950, p. 61.

NAME OF HOSPITAL

Name . . . . Age . . . .
Date of Admission . . . .
Birthday . . . .
By what name does the child like to be called? . . . .
Are there other children in the family? . . . .
    Brothers: Ages . . . .
    Sisters: Ages . . . .

Eating Habits

How is the child usually fed?
    Bottle? . . . . Cup? . . . . Spoon? . . . .
Feed self independently? . . . .
Feed self with help? . . . .
Food disliked? . . . .
Favorite foods? . . . .
What is his appetite like? . . . .

Elimination

Is the child independent in toileting? . . . .
. . . . To what degree? . . . .
What is the term used to refer to urination? . . . .
    Bowel movement? . . . .
Is the child accustomed to a toilet chair? . . . .
    Bathroom? . . . .
What is the approximate time of daily bowel movement? . . . .
Is the child taken to the toilet at night? . . . .
If so, at what time? . . . .

Sleeping Habits

Does the child take a daily nap? . . . .
What is his usual bedtime hour? . . . .
Does the child sleep alone? . . . .
    If not, with whom? . . . .
Does the child sleep in a bed with sides? . . . .
Adult bed? . . . .
Does the child have a prayer that he says at bedtime? . . . .
Does the child have a special bedtime routine? . . . .
If so, what is it? . . . .
. . . .

Play Interests

What type of play does the child like best? ....

Is the child accustomed to playing alone? ....
   With other children? .... With adults? ....
   Does he have a favorite pet at home? ....
   If so, state name and kind ....

Favorite type of toys? ....

Personal Habits

Does the child brush his teeth? ....
   Comb his hair? ....
   Bathe himself? ....
   Dress himself? ....

Miscellaneous

Does the child know why he is being admitted to the hospital? ....

....
What information did you give him? ....

....
How did he respond to it? ....

....
When was he told? ....
Has the child fears, such as fear of unfamiliar adults? ....
.... People in white uniforms? ....
   Needles? .... Surgery? ....
   Other? ....
Do the parents live together? ....
   If not, divorced? ....
   Deceased? .... At what age was the child when the parent died? ....
   Have any new experiences occurred in the home recently such as birth of a sibling?
.... When? ....
   Other? ....
Has the child attended nursery school? .... Kindergarten? ....
   Grade school? .... Sunday school? ....
Mother's remarks:

[Record on the reverse side observations which describe the mother-child relationship, the child's and the mother's response to admission, and the kind of adjustment that he made in the ward initially.]

After the nurse has learned more about the mother and the child from her conference with them she is in a better position to know how to prepare the mother to participate in the admission experience. Describing the details of the routine prepares her to interpret the steps of the procedure to her child. Mothers need to know that the nurse understands how difficult the experience is for both of them. When a mother recognizes that the nurse does not expect complete compliance from her child, her anxiety is often lessened. The nurse can also explain visiting hours and interpret the child's need for them. She can anticipate and help her to understand the possible responses that may come at visiting hours and at the time of her leave-taking. Some mothers may express dread of parting from their children. It helps a mother to know that she will be able to go to the ward and remain with her child until he begins to become more comfortable in his new surroundings.

Many mothers need help in knowing how to carry through leave-taking. Many mothers cannot face telling their children the truth about their leaving. They may fear the anger that is produced when a child is irritated with his mother's behavior. Or they may not know that children need a truthful explanation of why they are being left in the hospital. Explanations that give mothers understanding of the impact of the experience on the child usually help them to be supporting. Many mothers will need help in learning that their children will be helped most if they truthfully prepare them for their leave-taking and for the time of their return and then quickly leave their bedsides. Mothers should know that at this point nurses will be there to support their children.

Information collected on a form like the one above and from a conference with the mother can be used to provide individualized care. It should be readily available for the nurses who are assigned to the child's care. It is not enough to report the admission of Johnny Smith, aged 3, diagnosis—hydronephrosis—and follow it with a reading of the doctor's orders. *Each nurse caring for Johnny Jones needs to know the history of his disease, its symptomatology and treatment. She also needs information that helps her to understand him.* The nurse receiving Johnny as a patient can report the observations that she has made pertaining to his reaction to her, to his mother, ward mates, treatments and the adjustment that he is making in the ward. In this conference the nurse assigned to Johnny could report the plan of nursing care which she has formulated from the knowledge that she already has acquired about him.

Need for Mother

The child needs the help of his mother throughout the admission procedure to support him in adjusting to change. In the conference with the mother, the nurse can evaluate the mother's capacity and interest in assisting. She can use these clues in planning ways to meet both the mother's and the child's needs at this time. The mother can help undress, bathe, weigh and reclothe her child. With help she can also take his temperature and obtain a specimen of urine. At such times most mothers have a great need to do for their children. It gives them a tensional outlet and helps them to handle guilt feelings if they are felt. If they are fearful lest they lose their child's affection to a nurse, they will get some reassurance if they note that the nurse is cognizant of the importance of sustaining the mother-child relationship.

A co-operative project increases the child's security. He has his mother near-by for support and can adjust to strangers more slowly. The child's comfort is increased when he observes friendly feelings between his mother and the nurse. If he recognizes that his mother accepts the nurse, he will be more ready to do so. In addition, he will be less apt to feel guilty if he likes the nurse. A co-operative project can give the child a "we" feeling. It will foster his trust in nurses.

A co-operative project also gives the nurse time to observe the mother-child relationship and their response to the total situation. The newly admitted child needs help in adjusting at once. Observational material is helpful in understanding his immediate needs.

Hospital routines need to be flexible enough to allow for changes in procedure when they are indicated. There will be times when a child is unready to co-operate in some of the admission procedures. Forcing a child into having a bath, or in being weighed, for instance, may condition him negatively to nurses and to the hospital. When a child indicates a need for variation in procedure, his feelings should have thoughtful consideration. Nurses need to ask themselves the following questions: Is this procedure absolutely essential for this child's safety? Would the child be benefited if the procedure were postponed until he has become more familiar with his surroundings and gained confidence in the personnel? Are there ways in which the procedure could be modified to gain the child's interest and cooperation?

The child needs to have his mother accompany him to his room or ward and remain with him until he begins to feel comfortable with the nurse to whom he has been assigned. The time will vary with different children. Only when rules are flexible can they be of service to children. Parting at the bedside does much to foster a sense of security in both the mother and the child. If they have not been able to find security in their new situation, for their sakes and the sake of other patients in the ward, they may have to be separated temporarily before the child is taken to the ward. Then the mother and the child should be helped independently. They should be reunited after better equilibrium has been attained. To send the mother away before she sees where her child is located is an inhuman thing to do. The child needs to see that his mother knows where he is. Otherwise he may live in dread lest she not find him. Feelings of being lost are minimized after he sees that his mother knows where he is.

Establishing a Relationship

The child must be admitted to a nurse rather than to a hospital unit or ward because he needs the security of knowing that he has support and protection in a strange world. When a mother and a child enter the ward, they should be introduced to the head nurse, who has the responsibility of introducing the patient and his mother to the nurse whom she has assigned to the child's care. Children know the people in their homes and neighborhood by name. It is also important that they have that added sense of intimacy which comes from knowing their nurse's name. When the nurse meets the child, an interpretation of her role will help to relieve his anxiety concerning his welfare. When a child knows that he is going to be separated from his mother he wonders who will take care of him. It is one of the first questions that a child usually asks. He may say "Are you my nurse?" Or he may express his uneasiness more directly by asking, "Who is going to take care of me?"

After the nurse has interpreted her role to the child, she should proceed by proving through all she does that she *is* the person who will take care of him in his mother's absence. Telling him that she is going to take care of him will be of little value to him unless *he finds through experience that it is true.* When his nurse goes off duty it is her responsibility to inform the child whom he can turn to for help and care. Until the young child is assured that there is someone who is his own protector, he will be uncomfortable and afraid. He knows that he needs help in controlling his inner drives. He also senses that he needs support in meeting what is to come in a new situation. The child is not an independent being. When the young child's mother is not with him, mastery of himself and his environment is often an insurmountable task.

The newly admitted child, sick, or arriving in the hospital for some operation, is forlorn and afraid. This is especially true if it is his first experience in the hospital. He has had to part from his parents, perhaps for the first time in his life. He has come into a room, the like of which he never has seen before. The student nurse's first night alone in a hospital ward may not hold one tenth the terror that hospitalization does for the child. Perhaps recollection of the way the student nurse sought the support of her classmates in new situations will serve to help her identify herself with the newly admitted child's feelings.

There is no sounder way to establish a relationship with a child than by relieving whatever physical or emotional discomfort he may have. Separation from mother evokes conflict between the young child's need for pleasure and his need to strike out against painful situations. By discovering his needs and meeting them, he gets pleasure and is protected from using his energy destructively. When the nurse gives him relief from discomfort, he recognizes her as a comforting person. To establish a relationship, the nurse must meet him at his current emotional level. This means she must be ready to accept his individual pattern of response to stress. He may fight tempestuously because he wants only his mother and because he is afraid that he has lost her forever or he may withdraw and reject her approaches toward him.

The child needs an opportunity to become familiar with his surroundings and with his nurse. A tour about the ward and the playroom affords the child this opportunity. A child is less fearful if he knows what is down the corridor and behind closed doors. He also needs to know that there is a place in the ward which belongs to him. The following introduction to the ward gives the child increased feelings of belonging: "This is your unit, Johnny. This is your bed and table. This is where you can keep your toys and the things you brought from home. Inside the table are the things I will use to take care of you when your mother cannot be here with you." When a child enters nursery school, the teacher shows him his locker and explains its use to him. His locker is important to him! It is not unusual to hear a child saying, "This is mine. It's my special place."

In this period when the child is becoming oriented to the ward, the nurse can watch for clues that will tell her how to establish a relationship with him. The more the nurse can follow his lead, the more successful she will be. If the child does not need to be put to bed at once, freedom to investigate his surroundings as he so desires will facilitate adaptation. If the nurse is interested in him, he will sense it. Gradually, as he becomes adjusted to her presence, he will reach out toward her emotionally. He will show her in words or actions what he needs from her. Because she is an unfamiliar person to him, he will observe her intently and possibly test her out in many ways. In this way he will discover her responses to his behavior. The child who discovers that he dares express what he really feels will be fortunate indeed because he will not have to use his energy to bottle up feelings that are legitimate in his circumstances.

Knowledge of the child's preparation or lack of preparation for hospitalization is helpful in orienting the child to his surroundings. Often the child does not know why he has been brought to a strange place or why he has been put to bed before nighttime. Often a question like the following brings information that helps the nurse to know how to help a child understand his current situation: "Johnny, why are you here?" or "Children stay in their beds here. Do you know why?" If the nurse discovers that he does not know why he is in the hospital, she should explain the reason for it just as she explains everything else that is new to him. Such explanations should be given gradually so that he can assimilate them.

The child will also require help in learning the routines of the hospital. This is as important for the infant as for the older child. It is also as important for the child who comes in for a tonsillectomy as it is in the case of a child who enters for a prolonged stay. The way children go to the toilet, summon the nurse, have meals, rest hour and playtime in the hospital are all things about which the child needs information. Hospital routines are different from those that he has known before. The infant will observe every move the nurse makes. It is his way of saying: "What is this new world all about? Nothing seems the same. Give me time to know what is coming next." Many older children question incessantly during their earliest days in the hospital. They need to know what the nurse is going to do, what is expected of them and what they must anticipate in the immediate future.

A child's need "to be in the know" is no different from the nurse's need. Nurses probe new situations to discover what is expected of them. Perhaps the nurse can remember how she felt the day she went to the pediatric ward. She probably can also remember how she felt when a doctor arrived in the ward ready to do a treatment for which she was unprepared. She may remember thinking, "I don't understand what he wants. Why didn't he call the head nurse and tell her he was coming? I wonder if I will know what instruments he will want. I wonder how he will expect me to assist him?" The hospitalized child is in a similar predicament. He, too, wants to be ready to participate. He, also, dislikes being caught unawares. He wants to feel competent and accepted. But he does not have the past experiences to draw upon as does the nurse!

The principles involved in approaching the child who must be put to bed immediately upon arrival are the same; methods of carrying them out will require modification. The child's adjustment will be facilitated if his nurse is permitted to postpone painful procedures until he begins to become more secure with her. In the meantime the nurse can give him toys, sit beside him quietly and attentively and wait until he approaches her. Presenting play materials tells the child that the nurse is a friendly person who understands his need for play. Merely placing toys on his bed is not sufficient because he needs more than toys. A child requires emotional gratification before he has energy available for play. Through play with

his nurse a relationship can be established, after which the child will be more prepared to co-operate to the best of his ability. The following situation serves to illustrate one way in which a relationship can be established.

Billy was 18 months old when he was admitted with cystic fibrosis of the pancreas. When his mother left, he stood in his crib, shook it and went into a rage. He tossed all his toys onto the floor and protested in every way he knew how. When the nurse entered the room he bellowed more loudly and turned his back on her. When the nurse showed her willingness to hold him, he ran into the opposite corner of the crib like a frightened, angry animal. He seemed to be both panic-stricken and furious, which is the loved toddler's first response to separation from his mother. The nurse sat quietly by his bedside to give him an opportunity to become familiar with her and to discover the way he needed to use her most. Billy's screaming continued for many minutes during which he alternately looked at the nurse and away from her. Then tempestuously he tore a rubber washer from the cribside and threw it onto the floor. The nurse picked it up and put it back in place. Billy repeated the performance not once but a dozen times. Each time the nurse replaced the washer on the cribside to communicate her acceptance of his angry feelings.

Gradually, Billy's behavior began to change. His tears vanished; he relaxed and began to smile. Then the nurse placed a ball on his bed. He used the ball exactly as he had used the washer. Then a pyramid of wooden rings was placed on his bed. Again the nurse watched for clues which would indicate ways in which Billy needed her. Billy began to play *with* the nurse. He removed the rings from the stick, handed one to the nurse and then held out his hand to have it returned to him. Was this his signal of need for a give-and-take relationship or was it his way of trying to master his fear of separation from his mother? It is interesting to note that this type of play is seen repeatedly in hospitalized children under 3 years of age. During the first 3 years of life mastery of separation anxiety is one of the child's most important tasks. Hospitalization cannot help but inhibit progress in mastery of this fear. It may be the reason why this play is seen over and over again. (One 17-month-old hospitalized child in the writer's acquaintance played at dropping a toy and picking it up every day she was with him during the 3-month period he was hospitalized. His play never changed. Hospitalization prevented him from solving his current problem. He was stuck emotionally and could not move ahead because he was deprived of the continuous maternal care that he needed.)

Before long Billy moved closer to the nurse. Soon he scrambled to the edge of his cribside and made known his wish to get onto the nurse's lap. In a few minutes Billy's need for closeness lessened. He reached for the toy and began to play. Soon he indicated a desire to be put back onto his bed.

Later when the nurse said, "Billy, I must go now. I'll be back," she left a child who was more at peace than he was when she arrived. And his nurse did go back very soon. In the period when she was away from his cribside, she watched constantly for signs of anxiety. When he signaled his need for her, she went to him immediately because she wanted him to *feel sure* that there was someone nearby who had interest in him personally. When she went to him she said, "Billy I came back. I'll always come back when I tell you I will." A relationship had begun and Billy had made a start in his struggle to master his new situation.

MAINTENANCE OF A SUPPORTING RELATIONSHIP

Billy had made a start in adjusting to the realities of his new situation, but that was all. He had found a person who probably helped him anticipate kindness again, and for a period he had pleasure which minimized his conflict. The reality demands of Billy's new situation were beyond his ego capacity to deal with them without support. This is true of all children entering the hospi-

tal. *For this reason the child needs ego-supporting relationships throughout the period of his hospitalization.* To maintain a constructive relationship with a child the nurse will need the knowledge, the attitudes and the skills which have already been cited in this chapter. There are other skills that she will need, one of which is the capacity to adapt her knowledge of the nature and the nurture of personality to the care of her ill, handicapped or convalescent patients. An example or two will illustrate the meaning of this concept. All babies need to learn the properties of objects in their environment. Most babies learn them from kinesthetic and visual experiences. The baby with congenital cataracts has no visual perception. Unless objects are brought to him or he is taken to them and is helped to associate touch experiences with words, his capacity for testing and learning the properties of his reality world will be grossly limited. In addition, he probably will feel unloved because he does not get the stimulation that his nature craves and the relationship experiences that he needs to discover himself. A blind baby has limitations. However, he also has strengths. He has the capacity to learn from other perceptive experiences. He also has the capacity to respond to loving relationship experiences. If his limitations are faced and he has the intimate experiences that he needs for ego growth, he can learn to use his growth potentials equally as well as the sighted child. A normally intelligent preschool child with cerebral palsy has a drive to do and express himself equally as much as the normal child, but methods of teaching must be modified to meet his requirements for learning. To learn to feed himself, for example, he may need specially designed utensils, dishes that are heavy enough to stay put when he pushes against them and patience far beyond that required to teach a child with normal muscle co-ordination. A baby who is fed intravenously continues to need to suck to get the pleasure that relief from tension produces. He also needs kinesthetic stimulation for comfort. Unless substitute satisfactions are provided, observation will show that he becomes increasingly more apathetic and withdrawn. Fondling the immobilized baby, providing a pacifier to suck upon and giving him the pleasure that comes from the presence of a person who communicates concern for him as a person will lessen his feelings of frustration and make the treatment bearable. Traumatization is lessened when he does not have to bear the experience alone.

To maintain a relationship with a hospitalized child the nurse must also (1) understand the child, his health problem, the meaning it has for him personally, the past experiences which have produced the strengths and the limitations in his adaptive capacities; (2) appraise his needs in the light of study of him as a person; (3) construct and predict the effects of a tentative plan of care which provides him with the experience that he needs currently; and (4) implement the plan, observe the child's response to it and redesign her plan of care as the child shows progress in adapting to his disease or handicap and to hospitalization. Further concepts pertaining to emotional support will be presented under the following 5 headings: (1) factors influencing adjustment, (2) relief from anxiety, (3) preparation for and support during new experiences, (4) play and social experiences, and (5) anticipating changes in behavior at home.

Factors Influencing Adjustment

Not all children enter the hospital equally well prepared for the experience. Age, the severity of his health problem, past family and cultural experiences and the quality of care he receives during the experience and at home after the period of hospitalization will all have a bearing on the way the child adjusts to the changes that ill-ness and hospitalization produce. Age influences the child's adjustment profoundly. The infant and the young child are immature physically and emotionally and dependent upon a continuing, constructive relationship with their mothers or permanent mother-substitutes for personality growth. They *need* to be positively attached to their mothers to gain the ego strength which is necessary to venture away from mother into the world where the wider social experiences essential for emotional growth are obtainable. If they are subjected to psychic pain (conflict and anxiety) before they have the ego strength to master it, residual feelings of fear, anger toward mother and a wish for revenge are inevitable. Because of their ego limitations they need support that contains elements different from those needed by the school-age child who has had relationships which fostered healthy ego development.

The severity of the child's health problem has a bearing on the child's adaptive capacities. The acutely ill or disturbed child has less ego strength to cope with strange surroundings and new experiences than the healthy child who enters for elective surgery. They already are consumed with anxiety and have little tolerance for the reality frustrations they will meet. The blind preschool child cannot see what is happening about him. He hears screams and crying and strange noises, but his eyes cannot help him understand them. The sighted child sees the nurse approaching with his intramuscular injection. In the interval between her appearance and her arrival at his bedside, he can often mobilize his powers to withstand it or to express his feelings about it. Unless the blind child is given time to prepare himself for it, he is caught unawares. Interpreting it as a hostile attack is not out of the realm of reality!

Of all the influences that affect children's capacity for adjustment to change, past experiences probably have the greatest bearing. In the pediatric ward there will be children who have not been well fed, others who have had little wholesome discipline, some who have been deceived, and some who are filled with rage and fears which are the outgrowth of disturbed relationships with their parents. However, the majority of children will come from homes where they have been cherished and have received thoughtful nurture. They respect authority because it has been reasonable. They trust others because they have received in accordance with their needs and have not been deceived. They expect friendliness, protection and care because they have had it. These children are the fortunate ones in times of illness. If they are young children they will protest initially and feel intense grief when they are separated from their mothers, but they will approach the new situation with less anxiety, with trust and belief in the friendliness of others. These ego resources will help them adapt to the treatment and the care which they require to become restored to health.

Relief from Anxiety

Common Fears of Childhood. The quality of care that the child received during hospitalization is another important determinant of his adjustment. *The child's first emotional need is for a relationship which minimizes his anxiety.* He needs energy to combat his disease and also to master all that hospitalization entails. The nurse's task is to minimize his anxiety. *To do this she must first know what is making him fearful.* Insight into the emotional life of the child increases the nurse's sensitivity to the things of which children are afraid. Fear of the unknown is universal at all ages. The child under 3 years of age is predominantly afraid of separation from his mother, of disapproval, of punishment and of his own aggressive impulses. In addition to being fearful of his aggressive impulses and of punish-

ment, the preschool child fears bodily injury. The school-age child has a conscience. He fears punishment from it. In addition, he fears the disapproval of his peers. The adolescent fears the increased intensity of his sexual and aggressive drives. He also has anxiety concerning his physical and psychological adequacy. He persistently questions himself: "Am I normal? Will I measure up to my own standards and those of society?" Until he proves that he is normal and capable of meeting the responsibilities of adulthood he has concerns which drain his energy.

Many of the child's fears are irrational. The nurse can help him discover that they are unreal by standing by to prove to him that the world he is in now is less frightening than he imagines it to be. Trying to explain irrational fears away with words is useless. It is the nurse's protectiveness, interest and understanding of his need for personal reassurance that gives relief from irrational fears. The hospital is an unknown. All children are anxious when they come to a new place. Until they meet the experience and discover that their needs are recognized, they will be anxious and uncomfortable.

The child needs protection from fearful sights and sounds to relieve irrational fears. Every ward should have a room where children can be taken for treatments which are painful or for experiences which could easily be misinterpreted by other children in the ward. Children need to be shielded from sights that are disturbing. Things that hospital personnel take for granted are often fear-provoking to the imaginative, anxious child. If he sees another child having a paracentesis, for instance, he may well wonder if that will also be done to him. Likewise, children should be protected from seeing children who are critically ill or dying. Furthermore, they should be protected from hearing discussions that might arouse fears. Children are keenly sensitive to everything that is going on around them. They are especially aware of conversations that concern them. When they cannot understand all of what is being said, they become anxious, as adults do.

When a child cannot be protected from the experiences cited above, he will need help in understanding what he has seen, heard or felt. The nurse must be alert to signs of anxiety. She also must discover the child's interpretation of the event or the conversation that he has seen or heard. Often he has interpreted it erroneously. Sometimes he suspects that the event he witnessed will happen to him also. Reassurance given before the nurse has discovered the child's fears is rarely effective. It must come *after* she has helped the child feel comfortable and safe enough to verbalize his fear.

The hospitalized child needs his parents to protect him from conflicting feelings which evoke anxiety and from building unhealthy defenses against them. More and more hospital personnel are becoming sensitive to the effect of separation on young children who have not yet developed the ego strength to understand why hospitalization is necessary or to tolerate the frustration that it produces. As a result of their understanding, hospital personnel are increasing and lengthening visiting hours. In some hospitals they are also permitting mothers to give care to their children while they are with them. In a few instances mothers are also permitted to bring food from home.

Visiting hours are important for the child and his parents. The daily arrival of his parents relieves the child's anxiety lest he has been abandoned. It also helps to assure him that he has not been placed there as punishment. The child feels hostile because he is deprived of the security to which he is accustomed. Visiting hours give him an opportunity to ventilate his feelings. They also provide the comfort for which he longs and which he deserves to have.

Crying at the time of his mother's arrival and leave-taking is not damaging; *it is therapeutic*. It does disturb the peace of the ward. It also makes the nurse's task more difficult. However, it provides an emotional outlet which the child apparently needs. If he did not need it, the presence of his parents would not evoke a tempestuous response. Repressed hostility, anxiety and grief disturb the child's relationship with his mother. Many little children are so grieved, anxious and angry that they have to deny their need for their mothers. Many also are forced to deny their need for mothering to alleviate unbearable anxiety. Some must forget the image of their mothers because remembering them makes their longings too intense to bear. Failure to recognize the mother after a period of separation is frequently observed. It is an ominous sign. The child who "forgets" his mother needs more frequent visiting hours, not fewer. The example that follows serves to illustrate the reasons why some children reject mothering.

Bill was 4 years old when he came into the hospital with leukemia. He sat in a big chair hour after hour, but his mind was elsewhere. A nurse attempted to establish a relationship with him. She told him that she wanted to play with him. Then she sat down to give him an opportunity to relate himself to her. Almost immediately he yelled, "Get out of here. I don't want you here. I want to be alone." The nurse said, "Billy, I want to stay with you and take care of you." Billy's screaming "Get out," etc., continued. It was evident that Billy did not want a nurse to stay with him.

During the remainder of the morning the nurse acceded to Billy's request. However, simultaneously she made herself available to him. She placed him in the doorway where he could see her sitting at the desk. She said, "Billy, I'm going to be at the desk. I want to help you; when you need something you call me." But Billy never called her! He sat watching—yet he did not seem to see what was going on about him. After lunch, he permitted the nurse to put him to bed. However, he rejected the nurse when she expressed her wish to read him a story. Again he screamed, "Get out of here. I don't want you here." Why did Billy want the nurse to leave? Why did he reject her offer to care for him?

The next morning Billy's resistance to the nurse was equally pronounced. To discover the meaning of Billy's behavior, the nurse said, "I wonder why you don't want me to stay with you." His response was revealing. It was as follows: "Do you know why? It's because you make me lonesome, that's why. Get out." The nurse said, "You want your mommy here. You need her so much, and she can't be here. All children want their mommies in the hospital. When a nurse is here, it makes you want mommy more. That's the way lots of children feel." Billy's response was filled with longing. He said, "My mommy is the *goodest* mommy in the whole wide world." Then his feelings broke through. He cried piteously and was able to accept comforting in the arms of the nurse. It began a constructive relationship which helped Billy accept the care that he needed desperately. At first he resisted the nurse's offers of help. However, gradually he became more receptive to her nearness and care.

When an adult is frustrated because his most valued friend does not visit him, he also reacts to his disappointment. He either expresses his feelings to the person who created his discomfort or to some sympathetic friend. Or he may brood and take his anger out on himself; or he may be hostile to a nurse who has not provoked his anger. He may say or think, "I don't ever want to see that person again. The quicker I can forget him the better." It will not be difficult for the nurse to remember how relieved she felt when she vented her feelings after she had been disappointed or hurt. Or if she suppressed her feelings of disappointment, undoubtedly she can remember the misery that she experienced.

The child responds in the same way

as an adult, but his need for a continued relationship with a loved object is urgent because his growth is dependent upon it. If a child rejects the person who has disappointed or angered him, his personality cannot grow. The adult's personality is formed. He can continue to grow without the interest of a valued friend. It will be a painful feat but it is within the realm of possibility. The child cannot grow if he represses his hostility and anxiety and denies his need for his mother or for mothering. He continues to need his mother because his ego is too undeveloped to make it possible for him to be an independent person.

Parents have needs as well as children. It is not easy for a mother to leave her child in the hospital. Nor is it a simple matter to turn the care of her child over to someone else. Bringing food and toys to her child has emotional significance for her and her child. A bit of mother's food is infinitely more delectable than the food that comes from the hospital kitchen. And taste is not the only reason why the child feels this way! His mother's food has emotional meaning to him. Associations pertaining to comforting experiences with his mother come into play; the taste is of minor significance. Perhaps the nurse can recall her feelings when she received a box of food from home during the first weeks of her experience in the school dormitory. Was it the taste that stimulated her feelings or was it the idea that someone important had remembered her?

Nurses can use visiting hours to great advantage. During visiting periods nurses have an opportunity to develop relationships with parents. Nurses can learn much from parents which will help them to become better nurses. They can also observe parent-child relationships and use what they see in planning the care of their patients. They can also do something for parents in this period. If a mother finds that the nurse is in-

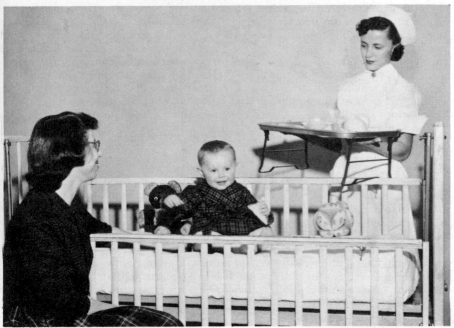

Fig. 16. A nurse who recognizes a child's needs for his mother minimizes the discomforts that are associated with hospitalization.

terested in her child and herself, she will be more ready to seek guidance that will increase her understanding of her child's needs. Parents who feel welcome in the ward and are allowed to care for their children will look to the nurse for help when they need it. Sometimes the most effective teaching is done indirectly. When nurses are skillful and understanding in their care of the child, the parent sees the effect that it has on the child. Often more is accomplished this way than through methods which involve direct instruction.

Preceding or following visiting hours, parent discussions can be held by nurses or by social workers. In such conferences different aspects of child care can be presented. Parents can have an opportunity to learn from each other. Many parents need help in understanding the reasons why their children react as they do to hospitalization. Insight can help many parents understand how a child feels when he is separated from them. With insight they will understand why children withdraw from them—and sometimes even forget them. They will also understand the child who turns to the nurse for affection rather than to his mother. It is not because the child does not love his mother; it is because he feels that she has punished him. As a result he is angry and hurt. He has to have substitute satisfactions. To obtain them he turns to the nurse as a possible source of satisfaction. Many a mother feels rivalrous with the nurses. She demonstrates her anxiety in her behavior toward them. Her anxiety will be relieved if she can be helped to see the situation from her child's point of view.

Children manifest and protect themselves from anxiety in many different ways and therefore are in need of nursing care which is based on understanding of their behavior. This subject will be discussed under the following headings: (1) the child with separation anxiety, (2) the rebellious child, (3) the depressed child, (4) the helpless child, (5) the provocative child, (6) the denying child, (7) the acutely ill child and (8) the chronically ill and handicapped child.

The Child With Separation Anxiety. Crying is one of the young child's ways of showing his feelings; he cries when he is afraid, feeling hopeless or angry. Naturally, he cries when his feelings or body are hurt. It is the only way that many children can express their feelings. Many children regress and utilize self-comforting methods to alleviate their anxiety. Some suck their thumbs, masturbate, bump their heads or rock their bodies to and fro. In addition, they may pick their noses, scratch their fingers or faces or sit fingering a lock of hair or clutching a toy in their arms. They are anxious and getting what comfort they can by themselves. This kind of behavior is symptomatic of excessive distress.

Clinging is another symptom of separation anxiety and is commonly observed when the loved young child has continuity of individualized care. The child under 3 years of age goes through characteristic stages as he relates himself to a new person. At first he accepts care quite passively because he is so needful of it. However, the situation changes after he has had repeated satisfying experiences that have made him feel his nurse is his protector and the person who provides pleasure. At this point it is not unusual to see him growing clinging and tempestuous when his nurse prepares to leave him. Some people interpret this behavior to mean that his nurse has "spoiled" him. Others interpret it as separation anxiety. Observation of the change in behavior which understanding management produces will support the theory that his behavior manifests separation anxiety.

He has experienced one separation already—perhaps even more. When repeated pleasurable experiences have made it possible for him to displace his dependent needs from his mother onto his nurse, his fear of separation looms up again to disturb his emotional equilibrium. Experiencing one separation before he is ready to cope with it makes him vulnerable to all subsequent ones. Unmastered feelings from the first experience are stirred up, and he protects himself from another loss by clinging as tightly as he can. This stage in the development of a relationship is trying even when the nurse understands the genesis of his demanding and irascible behavior. Clinging, demanding behavior evokes aggressive feelings in many people. Their instincts (id) say: "I've got to strike out at this child who is making me uncomfortable. I need pleasure, too." Their conscience says, "You must not. If you do, your self-esteem will become injured, and I'll punish you with guilt feelings." Their ego says, "There's a reason why this child acts this way. If I scold or reject, his anxiety will mount, and his clinging will become more persistent. If I use my intelligence I can find ways for both of us to get pleasure. If I sit down to reassure him I am going to stay, his anxiety will lessen, and he can use his energy in constructive activity. I'll help him learn to get pleasure from his play. Then he will have less need of being held and will grow less demanding of my attention. If I postpone the pleasure I could get from hitting or screaming at him, I will get infinitely more. I will get the pleasure of seeing him grow. In the meantime I'll relieve my tension with constructive activity which will give us both pleasure."

The Rebellious Child. Some toddlers and preschool children respond to anxiety by screaming, kicking and fighting rebelliously. Some come into the hospital ready to fight because they expect the worst, having been deceived on many previous occasions by their parents. They assume that they are being deceived again. Some have been threatened with hospitalization as a punishment. Such children are fearful and suspicious of every unknown they meet. They look upon the nurse as an enemy. They are ready to use their fists at the slightest provocation or without any. *But there has been provocation,* even though the nurse has not been a party to it. Already these children have been threatened or deceived; their reaction is understandable, even though it is difficult for the nurse to handle.

The child who comes into the hospital mobilized to fight needs an immediate experience which shows him that the situation he is in is not as fearful as he imagines it to be. If the mother is threatening the child, the nurse should help her to see that such a course is unnecessary. Usually her threats become ineffective in the face of the nurse's statement that they never would be carried out in the hospital. Following this, the nurse might add: "Sometimes mothers do not know that nurses and doctors want to help children. I will tell you and your mother exactly what I am going to do. Then you both will know all about it. And you can help me."

The Depressed Child. Some children withdraw into themselves like frightened little animals and become depressed. Many of these children have experienced excessive frustration and rigid discipline in the earliest years of their lives. Past experiences have made them feel that anger was "bad," and punishable either by physical means or by loss of love. As a result they have acquired a punishing conscience and often at a much earlier age than is healthy. Destructive past experiences have made them fearful of people and of their own aggressive feelings. And in addition they are filled with rage! They defend themselves from anxiety by withdrawing and becoming depressed.

The strictly disciplined child who is unprepared for separation from his mother is often unable to express his hostility overtly. Lack of preparation may be due to inability to understand because of his age or to failure to anticipate for him what going into the hospital entails. Feeling hostile toward someone he is supposed to love is often unbearable. If he thinks that it is his fault that he is ill, his anger at his mother is not justified. Therefore, he feels it is "bad." If it is "bad," he cannot direct it at her. Instead, he keeps it bottled up inside of himself. In doing so he punishes himself instead of his mother.

The depressed child often behaves as though he thought that his treatment was punishment. Often he also acts as though he thought he was deserving of discomfort. Each time the nurse came to give Timmy his intramuscular injection of penicillin, he whimpered quietly and said, "I be sorry. I be good." Timmy seemed to think he had done, felt or thought something "bad" or wicked. The needle and the syringe seemed to represent punishment to him. When asked why they are in the hospital, some children say, "I naughty" or "I bad." The depressed child often goes unnoticed for he is quiet, withdrawn and outwardly accepting of everything that is done to him. Unconsciously, some of them want punishment. If they feel guilty, punishment relieves it.

The withdrawn child is not as comfortably adjusted as many people think he is. Closer observation discloses abject misery and unhappiness. He does not smile, eat or play. Nor does he relate to children or adults because he hates them. Instead, he sits or lies still. His facial expression betrays the depth of his inner turmoil. Much of his energy is being used to keep his hostile feelings and anxiety under control. As a result, he has a smaller quantity of energy available to combat his illness, to play or to relate to others.

The depressed child is in urgent need

of sympathetic understanding and interest in spite of his rejecting attitudes toward others. Usually the depressed child is not overtly demanding in any way, but this does not mean that he needs nothing but physical care. His behavior says: "I hate everybody in this world. I'm scared to death. I have to watch every move you make because I'm suspicious of you and expect punishment. I'm a regressed baby. Please give me what I need because I can't ask for it with words." At first the child may reject the nurse completely and pull away from any physical overture of affection. His need to reject needs acceptance with behavior that communicates the feelings expressed in the words which follow: "You don't like me because I symbolize persons who have brought you psychic pain. You have a right to pull away from me. I'm glad you can tell me how you feel. Even though you hate me I am going to stay here with you. I know you're a scared, angry child but I want to help you when you are ready to let me." When a child responds to treatments as if they were punishment, his interpretation of them needs correction. "I wonder what Timmy thinks he did that makes him feel scared," often gives rise to a response which furthers the nurse's understanding of his behavior. If the child cannot verbalize his fantasied misdeeds, something like the following communicates understanding and encourages expression of feelings: "Sometimes children think injections are given to punish them. They aren't given to punish you, Timmy. They are given to make you well. And when you are better, you will be able to go home again. Your mother is coming back." *The nurse must be ready to accept a tempestuous response from the depressed child.* If he has continuity of understanding care, he will gradually acquire courage to test the nurse's capacity to tolerate his aggression and the demandingness he has been hiding from

himself. If his words and deeds have communicated acceptance of him as he is, he will grow gradually less afraid of his aggression and become ready to vent his feelings in play. He will need his nurse close by in play to protect him from expressing his rage too flamboyantly. If it comes out too fast, he will become afraid and retreat into his protective shell again.

When the child is able to express his anger and discovers that his illness is no fault of his own, depression symptoms begin to subside. Gradually, a change in behavior becomes observable. He has energy to play because his hostility has become released and accepted. His anxiety is relieved. He begins to eat, demand attention and resist things he formerly accepted in a compliant way. *This is progress; it is not undesirable behavior.* The following example serves to illustrate the above principles.

Sally was 3 years old when she was brought from the South for surgical repair of exstrophy of the bladder. She never had been away from home before. She found herself surrounded by a multitude of strange people and subjected to experiences that she never had had before. Her malformed body was viewed repeatedly. She had many treatments which were painful and restricting. She complied submissively. She showed no overt response to pain, restraint or to the unknown.

The day after her operation, Sally was more silent and withdrawn. She never whimpered when the doctor changed her dressing or inserted the needles for intravenous therapy. She did not relate to her nurse who was in constant attendance each morning. The third day her dressing was changed again. The doctor probed her wound and inserted a drain. Pain and anger were stronger than her controls. She shrieked at the top of her voice, "No more, I hate you. Go away." Simultaneously, she reached for the doctor's hands. Sally's face was contorted with terror. She looked as if she expected to be demolished.

Instead of being punished, Sally got immediate understanding and praise. The nurse looked at Sally, smiled acceptingly and said, "It does hurt, Sally. It hurts terribly when the doctor uses the instrument. I'm glad you can tell us how you feel." Simultaneously, the nurse stroked the hand that reacted to her aggressive feelings. Sally looked up at her nurse and nestled her hand into hers. It was Sally's first personal contact since admission. Previously, the nurse had held her hand and stroked her head, but Sally's hand was limp. There was no response that indicated that she even had felt the nurse's interest in her.

Sally's nurse encouraged expression of feeling. She provided reassurance which proved that her interest would not be withdrawn because of tempestuousness. A bond was established between them. Later, Sally continued to express her anger. She became more resistant to treatments. Temper tantrums also began to appear. Expression of feeling was welcomed. Her nurse knew that pent-up feelings would retard her physical progress and disturb her relationships with others. Gradually, Sally's anxiety and depression lifted. She began to play and became interested in all the activities that were going on around her.

The Helpless Child. Not infrequently the nurse meets children who have been deprived of experiences which help them master their feelings of helplessness and begin to learn to tolerate frustration. These children strike out at everything that displeases them because they do not know how to handle frustration in any other way. Since they never derived this kind of help from their mothers, experience has taught them that direct expression of their primitive aggression paid dividends. It got them what they wanted. Furthermore, this form of behavior had received the tacit stamp of approval from the parent whose responses the child was merely imitating. Consequently, they regard it as a successful method of overriding the unfamiliar or unpleasant.

The mother of a child who reacts in this way is usually trying to control his behavior by guilty overaffectionate kissing, soothing and by the proffer of bribes and promises to take him from "the horrid hospital soon." Observation of this kind of maternal behavior leads inevitably to the conclusion that the mother is unprepared to help her child learn that temper tantrums are an ineffective way to handle frustration. She may well be responding to guilt from her own helplessness in handling her own aggressive feelings. Such feelings usually give rise to inconsistent guidance. The child is punished because the mother has not learned to express her own aggression in any other way. If this produces guilt feelings in the mother, she may react with overindulgence to relieve her guilt. Such circumstances make the child confused and fearful of his own helplessness. He responds tempestuously, whenever his wishes are not met instantly, because he has not acquired any ego resources with which to act differently. *He needs help to develop inner resources to handle frustrations and to obtain increased mastery of his helplessness.*

In a situation of emotional tension the calm, firm, positive voice carries weight. There are voices, low rather than high in pitch, full rather than thin in tone which can express kindness and understanding at the same time that they communicate expectancy of reasonable behavior.

The mother who, with promises of candy, begs her child to stop crying or kicking, needs her own anxiety alleviated. She requires help to see that blandishments are an ineffective way to help a child meet the reality of unpleasant situations. But first her cooperation must be won. Undoubtedly, she is anxious and frustrated. In most instances temporary separation of the mother and the child is indicated.

The first approach to the child should be one that helps him to know that the nurse is friendly, honest, understanding and unperturbed even in the face of a temper tantrum. If a few friendly gestures are not effective, it is wise to sit down beside him and wait until he has become calmed. If nothing happens for a few minutes, a frightened child has time to realize that there is little to be afraid of. When he re-establishes his equilibrium, friendly words will assure him further that his interests are being considered. Familiarizing him with his new surroundings will also provide reassurance. The nurse's behavior should demonstrate that she respects him as a person; that she will be honest in her dealings with him; that she can be depended upon; and that she will not make him the victim of her moods or become the victim of his. This type of guidance increases his sense of security and prepares him to learn to tolerate gradually increasing amounts of frustration.

The Provocative Child. Some children defend themselves against anxiety with provocative behavior. It may be a way of testing out the limits of the adult's tolerance or of relieving their fears of their own consciences. The child who has not had consistent discipline at home is insecure. He does not know the limits of his environment. He is constantly afraid lest his behavior precipitate physical punishment or loss of love. To get the security of knowing the limits of his environment, he persists in irritating his mother until he learns her tolerance. He gets relief from anxiety because he discovers how far he can go without being punished.

A child may also use provocative behavior to get relief from fear of his conscience—in other words, from guilt feelings. The child who is provocative is often unable to sublimate his aggressions into constructive channels. He cannot channel his aggressions because he has not had the help of consistent, unwavering discipline. Instead of getting help in channeling his aggressions, he re-

ceived condemnation which made him feel that he was a bad child. Experience taught him that punishment relieved him of discomfort.

If a pattern of behavior like either of the above has been established at home, the child undoubtedly will use it in the hospital, both because it has become a habitual way of relieving his tension and because his illness often serves to intensify his feelings of guilt. In the ward there are often children who literally ask for punishment—not in words because their need for punishment is unconscious—but in behavior. Johnny used provocative behavior to rid himself of guilt feelings.

Johnny was 7 years old and in the hospital with rheumatic fever. Every time the nurse came to give him care, he would knock the equipment off the table. When she pulled up his cribside he would leap over the side of the bed. He did not wait until she had left the room; he did the jumping in her presence.

Punishment merely serves to encourage the child with provocative behavior to repeat his misdemeanors. Punishment relieves his guilt and gives relief from anxiety. Under these circumstances he naturally does the things that he is forbidden to do. When he is not punished for his provocative behavior, he will be less apt to repeat it because it brings no satisfaction. Instead of punishing him, the nurse should use her energy in trying to help him discover that he is not the bad child that he believes himself to be.

The child who defends himself against anxiety with provocative behavior requires *consistent,* kind and firm guidance. He should know what is expected of him and what he can and cannot do. Only then will he have the security which comes from knowledge concerning the limits of his environment. The child who is under compulsion to provoke adults to anger is a difficult child with whom to deal. He is the way he is because he has been made that way. When he discovers that his behavior brings a response different from the retaliatory kind he previously has been accustomed to, his behavior will show signs of change. If it does not change, it probably indicates his need for psychological therapy.

The Denying Child. Denial of fear is another way some children handle their anxiety. Sometimes they cover it with aggressive, overly brave behavior. Vander Veer[*] cites the case of a boy who used a pocketknife to try to outbluff a person he fantasied to be an attacker. As the child entered the doctor's office, he drew a pocketknife from his pocket and opened it up. When the doctor asked him what he was doing, he said, "I'm going to cut the doctors before they can cut me." Vander Veer interpreted this behavior as a defense against his fear of being injured.

The situation described subsequently serves to illustrate denial as a method of handling anxiety. It also describes the nursing care which is essential to help a child face a situation of which he is fearful. Davy was prepared by his parents for hospitalization and for operation. However, his behavior showed that the details of preparation were too scary to think about. Davy needed further verbal preparation by his nurse. He also needed support both before and after the operation to face what he wanted to deny would ever happen.

Davy was a 5-year-old, red-haired, well-built and unusually bright and vivacious youngster. He entered the hospital for surgical repair of squint. Outwardly, Davy seemed to be quite self-contained. He was sociable and friendly with his nurse and the children in his

[*] Vander Veer, A. H.: The psychopathology of physical illness and hospital residence, in Personality Development and Its Implications for Nursing and Nursing Education, Springfield, Ill., Dept. of Public Health, 1948, p. 65.

4-bed unit. He co-operated well when he was permitted to express his ideas and suggest how things should be done. He resisted breakfast in bed. He could not wait until he could be out of bed. His nurse anticipated that he would be reluctant to have a bath in bed. She suggested using the bathtub. He was delighted with the suggestion. He bathed himself and talked constantly while he was doing so. He mentioned his red hair and showed pride in having hair "just like Daddy." He talked more about his father than about his mother. It was his daddy who was going to do things for him. He would bring him things, etc.

The nurse and the doctor met resistance when they attempted to discover how Dave had used the preparation that his parents had given him. When the nurse asked him why he was in the hospital he said, "To get a patch on my eyes to fix them up." He ran away from the nurse when she began to prepare him for some of the forthcoming events of the day. The doctor arrived and said, "Dave, do you know that today is the day you are going to sleep and have a patch put over your eye like you had put on in the clinic?" Dave answered, "Yes" and went immediately out of the door. Davy acted as though the subject of surgery was anathema to him.

To prevent Davy from being overwhelmed with the event, the nurse continued to help him understand the treatments which were forthcoming. She told him about the medicine she would give him with a needle. She explained its purpose. She also told him that it would hurt and that it was scary to many children. He said, "I don't want it." Then he ran away again to his play. To prepare him further, she showed him how hypodermics of medicine were given. She used a doll to demonstrate the procedure. His interest became stimulated. Independently, he took the syringe and the needle and returned the demonstration on the doll. He handled the equipment skillfully and seemed to have observed every detail of the technic. However, one experience of hypogiving was not enough! Davy gave hypos to every toy in the room that had arms, legs or tails. He even went down the corridor to the playroom in search of the huge elephant that he said had "great big ears." He stuck the elephant in the hip and in the ear. His face was serious while he manipulated the syringe. When he finished, his face became transformed with a glow of self-satisfaction.

The nurse used an alcohol sponge and a clown doll to show Davy how a mask and medicine would be used to put him to sleep. Davy paid no attention. He looked as if he were not hearing a word that she was saying. She told him that he would be unable to drink or eat until after he had been put to sleep and his eyes had been fixed. Again his facial expression was blank. He appeared as if he were thinking of other things than the current subject of conversation. His only verbal response was "I am thirsty." Then he ran away again.

Davy was active constantly. His attention span was short, and he did not concentrate on any activity for long. Once he wanted a playmate's toys. He proceeded to take them away from her against her wishes. When she clung to her possessions he said, "You ought to be ashamed of yourself for not giving them to me." Later in the morning the nurse again tried to help him face the forthcoming events. He would not listen. He changed the subject or ignored her completely.

At noon Davy's parents arrived, bringing him a record player, a new gun and holster and bedroom slippers. The nurse told him she would play the records for him the next day. He responded with, "No you won't. I'll play them myself." (Davy continued to deny that an operation was a reality which he must face.) When the nurse brought the hypodermic of medicine his anxiety was evident. His daddy said, "It won't hurt." (Davy's defence was like his father's.) His father's words seemed to redouble Dave's efforts to control himself. He submitted complacently. He did not seem to hear the nurse when she said, "All children are scared when they have hypodermics. Lots of them get angry, too. They tell us that it hurts." Immediately, he wanted to show his parents how well he could give a hypodermic. This time he gave a toy kitten a hypo in its tail.

Until it was time to go to the operating room Davy sat with his parents in the playroom watching television. When it was time to leave the ward, he waved good-bye to his parents. But first he said, "Give me my gun." En route to the operating room Davy shot every person in sight. During the waiting period, Davy continued to shoot. As he shot he talked incessantly about gangsters, cops and robbers. His nurse stood by supporting him with her presence and interest. To try to help him face his fear, she said, "Davy, soon the doctor will come. All children get scared when they know that they are going to be put to sleep. They don't know that the doctor and the nurse are going to tell them everything that they are going to do. I am going to stay here and help you go to sleep."

When the anesthetist arrived, she explained every step of the procedure to him. She also suggested that they play a game together while he went to sleep. He asked about the smell in the room and said, "I 'spose it's alcohol." He was also curious about the purpose of the tanks which were beside the anesthetist. Just before the mask was put over his face he said to his nurse, "Tomorrow you play my records for me, will ya?" The nurse assured him that she would. She also told him that she would be beside him when he awakened. He was more receptive at this point. He listened when she said, "Your eyes will hurt when you wake up. And you won't be able to see because there will be patches over your eyes. Your mother and I will be there to help you. In a day or two the doctor will take the patches off. Then you will be able to see again."

Davy's tension was evident, but his powers of control remained intact until he was anesthetized. Restraint was not necessary until the excitement stage.

The Acutely Ill Child. The acutely ill child manifests his anxiety in any number of ways. He is often apathetic to his surroundings. He is too sick to reach out to the nurse to indicate the ways in which he needs her. He has pain, anxiety and a feeling of helplessness which brings marked regression. Immediate transportation to the operating room or the ward is often indicated. Frequently, danger is imminent. Both the acutely ill child and his parents feel intensely the danger in the situation.

The sick child must get immediate physical support and emotional security because his survival depends upon the energy that he has available to fight his disease. Every word and act needs to communicate strength to him and his parents. Many times the nurse must work quickly and deftly. Combined with efficiency, there should be sensitivity to the fact that the child *feels* even though he is unable to make any overt behavioral response to the care that he is receiving. The sick child's relief from anxiety will come from medical treatment that supports his body in its fight against disease. It will also come from gentleness, sympathy and the strength that he feels in the touch of the nurse's hands, in the tone of her voice and in the manner in which she regards his parents. Both he and his parents need to feel confident that he will be cared for; that he will be made more comfortable; and that his pain will be eased. Both medical treatment and understanding care are imperative in promoting emotional security; one without the other leaves the child unsupported in his struggle for survival.

Conservation of energy is the foremost principle in the care of the acutely ill child. He should receive quiet, consistent supportive care which anticipates his every want. The nurse needs to be alert constantly to symptoms which indicate physical or emotional distress. She should plan her care to avoid interruptions in rest. This will require careful timing of feedings, medication and treatment, as well as consideration of his parents' need for help in handling their anxiety.

Most of the serious illnesses of childhood are acute. The child is usually desperately ill during the acute phase of an illness. He reacts to disease intensely. He is a sensitive little person who has not yet developed the physical or psychological stamina to withstand disease without being grossly threatened. The balance may tip quickly in one direction or another. For this reason every detail of care which conserves energy and helps him toward recovery needs to be provided.

One aspect of many acute illnesses is a high temperature. A temperature of 104° or 105° F. (40° to 40.5° C.) from an illness that is ordinarily of short duration, such as tonsillitis, usually requires no interference. However, the same temperature in a child with a more serious and protracted illness may require that something be done to lower the fever. The high fever should be reduced if it causes irritability, restlessness and loss of sleep. These symptoms are incompatible with rapid recovery. The presence or the absence of these signs is more of a guide than the degree of temperature in deciding whether or not to interfere. Hydrotherapy and antipyretic drugs are the most satisfactory method of combating fever.

All legitimate measures should be used to reduce the amount of pain that children are called on to endure. In caring for adults there are doubtless many situations in which the patient has something to say about the amount of pain that he can endure. However, in caring for children, this is seldom the case. An adult says that he cannot tolerate a treatment without something to alleviate the pain. His feelings are considered. A sedative is administered unless it is contraindicated. A child has nothing to say about what he can or cannot withstand. He probably has not had experiences which make him competent to judge.

Those who have the matter to decide need to consider the child's needs from his point of view. If a sedative or an anesthetic can spare the child unnecessary anxiety (pain) without causing complications, it should be given.

The Chronically Ill and Handicapped Child. There are children in the hospital who will go through life with some physical handicap. There are those whose lives will be circumscribed by a disease that sets them apart from the normal life of childhood. Many of these children will spend much of their time in hospitals or convalescent homes. These children lose their childish look and grow pathetically old before their time. They rarely laugh, express destructive feelings overtly or develop deep, warm feelings toward other people. They become the little old men and women who are seen in many children's hospitals. What produces their appearance and behavior? Part of it can be traced to physical causes but not all. Psychological study of these children will disclose the dynamics which produce their flat emotional tone, superficiality and hopelessness. It will disclose the fact that they have developed unhealthy defenses against their anxiety.

Even though the above-described children are not physically able to do all that well children can do, effort should be directed toward making personality growth possible during hospitalization. Everything possible needs to be done to help them look out rather than in upon themselves and their symptoms. This is no easy task. The chronically ill child's needs for normal personality development are difficult to satisfy in a hospital or a convalescent home. This is especially true of his deepest need of all—a continuous relationship with a warm, giving mother or a permanent mother substitute who recognizes his physical and psychological readiness to master new development tasks. *A plan of nursing care which includes continuity of care with persons who recognize his need for growth-producing experiences is essential if he is going to be helped to make a healthy adjustment to life.*

Another group of children who need help in growing more capable and secure are the handicapped. These children have physical or mental limitations. Many times they have severe personality handicaps as well. Many tests have been devised and used to discover whether or not children with a designated handicap have a special kind of personality. All tests have failed to prove that they have. The crippled child who has a personality handicap was not born that way. He was deprived of emotional satisfactions and of opportunities to use the powers he possesses.

The parents of a child who is born with a deviation from normality face problems which are difficult to surmount. Giving birth to an abnormal child or discovering later that the child is blind, deaf or incompetent mentally is a painful, emotionally disrupting shock. It takes months and sometimes years for parents to recover from the frustration, loss of hope and the blow to their pride. Every parent longs for a normal child. In addition to disappointment parents often feel afraid of the responsibilities that the child's care entails. They are often frightened of their own feelings and of society's attitudes toward the handicapped child and those who produce him. Producing a child who deviates from normality gives rise to painful, energy-sapping conflict. Hostility and anxiety are natural and understandable to professional workers with insight, but these feelings often conflict with the mother's ideals of motherliness. It takes superb ego strength to master this major disappointment and solve the conflict to the point where parents can mobilize their resources to participate in planning for the child's care and in providing him with the nurture he requires for growth of his personal endowment. Raising a handicapped child requires wisdom, skill and parental security. *The multiple problems involved prevent each member of the family from getting what he needs the most—intimate, mutu-*

ally satisfying relationships with each other. Until the parents master their feelings, they will be preoccupied and anxiety-ridden. The sight of the handicapped child evokes feelings of pain, inadequacy and frustration which must be handled in a healthy way before the family security can be restored.

The way the parents handle their disruptive feelings depends upon the inner resources that they possess. They may deny the existence of the handicap to defend themselves from anxiety. They may hide their negative feelings by developing overprotectiveness or they may escape from the painful feelings that are evoked from the sight of the child by neglecting his most basic psychological needs. When parents are upset when in contact with the child, they are unable to respond to his overtures to get the emotional satisfactions and the experiences that he requires to grow physically and emotionally. The child tries to explore his world and get the responsiveness that his nature requires, but he is often thwarted because his parents are unready emotionally to accept him as a person. As a result, his cues of readiness to learn are not seen, or he is pushed to achieve in ways which produce resistance to learning. When his cues for learning remain consistently ignored or he is not permitted to learn in his own natural way, regression is inevitable.

The parents of an infant who deviates from normality are in great need of a health team which functions harmoniously together to restore their security. Many parents cannot accept emotionally a handicapped child without the help of a social worker or a psychiatrist. The nurse working with the family needs knowledge of the developmental process, of the basic principles involved in the learning process and of the specific needs of each child. She needs understanding of the problems and the anxiety which parents of handicapped children face. She needs the capacity to support parents in ways which strengthen their confidence to meet the needs of the child. She can help parents to understand the normal aspects of the child's development and his special needs. In addition, she needs skill in timing her guidance to the emotional readiness of parents to receive it and the capacity to support parents in ways which help them achieve their goal. Help in timing and in learning ways to support the particular parents must be obtained from the health worker who is helping the parents to accept the reality of their problem.

Recommending that the parents teach the infant skills which are unrelated to his daily living *before* the parents have had help in handling their feelings concerning the child and his handicap merely adds to the parent's feelings of incompetence. Parents are already afraid of the responsibility that raising a child with special requirements entails. If teaching is emphasized *before* the mother has mastered her fears concerning her ability, she either gives up and wants to turn over her responsibility to experts or she conscientiously tries to do what she has been told is best for the child. Conscientiously followed recommendations which are implemented without spontaneity of warm feelings rarely reaps results for the baby or for the mother because their use does not take into account the basic principles involved in the learning process.

In order to learn, the child must feel secure, enjoy mutually satisfying experiences with his mother and be given freedom to explore with all the senses and the powers with which he is endowed and in the way which is natural for him. Given this emotional climate, the handicapped child will reach his learning potential if his specific needs are taken into account. For instance, the blind child cannot explore unless objects are brought to him and he is given the interpersonal experiences he needs to learn to use his body so he can reach the world which he must explore in order to master it. A blind baby who is left in his crib because contact with him arouses painful feelings cannot learn to use his body. Nor will he learn to use his body and master his world if his mother follows instructions *before* she has worked through her conflicting feelings and is able to accept the child as a *child with a handicap*. When a mother conscientiously carries out recommendations before she feels giving and responsive to her baby, he gets insufficient emotional satisfactions to gain ego strengths. The mother is also deprived. When she sees no progress, her discouragement, anxiety and feelings of incompetency are heightened, not lessened.

Parents who do not make progress in their relationship with their handicapped child are torn with conflict which becomes reflected not only in their relationship with the child who deviates from normality but also in their relationship with each other and with the other offspring. Anxiety-ridden parents who overprotect the child to hide their true feelings or neglect him because contact with him produces unbearable pain are troubled people who need help from experts and support from nurses not only to restore their feelings of self-confidence and security but also to protect their relationships with other members of the family.

The nurse who has faith in the parents' capacity to build an intimate relationship with the child can be of great help in periods of discouragement. If she understands the parents' feelings of disappointment, guilt, frustration or resentment against the tremendous responsibility they are forced to carry the nurse can be of real support to the family. Helping the parents to feel that they are not alone with their problem is of immeasurable value to many mothers and fathers. Discovering that someone understands their frustration and feelings of being overburdened prevents guilt feelings. It also often helps parents acquire more constructive attitudes toward the child, gives them hope and motivates them to use the resources that the nurse helps them to know are available to them.

After a 5-year study of the preschool blind child, Norris, Spaulding and Brodie have presented insights and knowledge concerning the blind child and his developmental patterns and an analysis of the environmental factors that foster or thwart his optimal development. Their findings have implications not only for the nurture of the blind child but also for the guidance of the child with other types of handicaps. The approach of the research staff which carried out the project "was twofold— first, to strengthen the family's confidence in their ability to meet the day-by-day needs of the child; second, to help the family understand and appreciate [the child's]* behavior within the framework of sound principles of child development."† In writing of the child's need for learning opportunities in contrast with direct teaching, they say:

Freeing the parents from their anticipated responsibility for teaching specific skills unrelated to daily living is often the first step in helping them to think realistically about the blind child and to be comfortable in their relationships with him. If this can be accomplished within the first few months of the child's life, his responsiveness gives assurance to the parents that they are on the right track. Their resulting confidence in their ability to meet the child's needs and their pleasure in his achievement then become primary factors in encouraging his further progress. Major developmental problems are avoided, in contrast to those situations where fail-

* The words in the brackets are the authors.

† Miriam Norris, Spaulding, Patricia J and Brodie, Fern H.: Blindness in Children, Chicago, University of Chicago Press, 1957, p. 95.

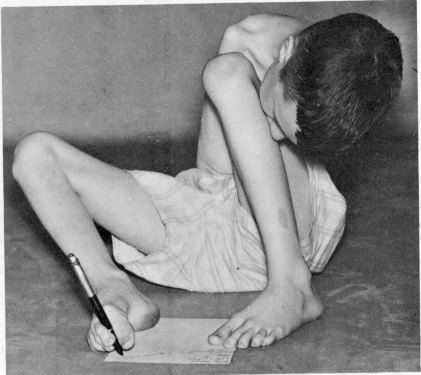

Fig. 17. A handicapped child who is making the most of his assets. This 7-year-old-boy born with complete absence of arms has learned to feed himself, put on his clothes and manipulate objects with his feet. Although not easily visible in the picture, the foot-writing when magnified is very legible.

ure to understand and meet the child's needs in the early period has created difficulties which are discouragingly slow to respond to treatment.*

Many of the handicapped children the nurse will see in the hospital and in the community have not had the benefits of growth-producing experiences. Because the child's parents have not had the benefits of teamwork, they were unable to supply the nurture their children needed. The handicapped child feels and reacts to the impact of his parents' feelings toward him and the problems that his handicap has created. He cannot help sensing their frustra-

tion and anxiety and feeling as if he were a disappointment to them. His adjustment to his anxiety and to his limitations was the outcome of the emotional interplay between his defect and the parental and social attitudes that he felt in his relationships with his parents and society early in his life.

The handicapped children whose parents have not been able to accept them have coped with their anxiety and limitations in the only way that they were able to do. Some, who felt unloved, have withdrawn into a world of fantasy. They never learned to use the strength with which they were born. Some have compensated for their diffi-

* Ibid., p. 72.

culties and fought to overcome their limitations. Some have denied their limitations to solve their problems. Some feel pity for themselves. They expect solicitude without any feeling of responsibility toward others. Some have grown discouraged concerning their capacity for social relationships and deny their need for love. They often try to hurt others as they have been hurt. Then there are others who unconsciously seek punishment because their hostility makes them feel guilty.

The handicapped child whom the nurse meets in hospital wards needs nurturing that will help him toward a realization of the powers which he possesses. He needs ego support that helps him learn to feel competent, self-satisfied and acceptable to others. The nurse needs to know the outcome of the health team's examination. She needs to know his strengths and limitations and the health team's recommendations for his guidance. Then she should give him every opportunity to develop whatever powers he possesses. Some of these children, the mentally retarded, for instance, will need patient, consistent repeated help to learn to master the care of themselves. Children over and over again measure up to what is expected of them. *Success is the result of the faith that others have in them.* Many of these children learn to do because they feel that others have confidence in their capacity to learn. They depend upon their judgment and absorb the deep faith that others have in them.

The handicapped child does not want or need pity; he craves understanding which helps him adapt to the reality within himself and in his world and become secure in his relationship with others. Like the normal child, he, too, has a drive to develop his capacities for self-direction and competence unless he has met defeat so often that he has given up in despair. Understanding carries no taint of pity; it recognizes and accepts his differences and permits a wholesome relationship toward him as a person. The person with understanding *accepts the implications of his handicap.* He directs his energy toward helping the child use the powers he possesses in his own way to build inner strengths which give him security, self-esteem and the recognition of his society.

In working with a child who is mentally or physically handicapped, the nurse needs to be aware of her feelings toward him and his parents. Feelings of fear, pity or repugnance are not "bad," unusual or anything of which the nurse needs to feel ashamed. Most people have them until they face them. When the nurse accepts her feelings, often she can change them because awareness makes it possible for her to discover how unrealistic her fears and unwholesome attitudes really are.

Many a nurse who reacts most comfortably to quiet, withdrawn and emotionally bland chronically ill children in the ward or is prepared to meet the nursing challenge of the care of the critically ill children feels utterly lost and often anxious when she enters a ward of convalescent or orthopedically handicapped children. There she finds an amount of surplus energy with which she is unprepared to cope. Many times she resorts to a type of discipline to which she as a child and as a student nurse may possibly have been expected to submit. She lays down rules. She is restrictive beyond actual necessity and resorts to "don't" instead of "do." The results are usually disastrous. The older boys lead the younger ones on to pranks. The nurse is often totally distracted, and ward order is reduced to chaos.

Restrictive discipline produces no growth; it brings order out of chaos but none of the qualities that a child needs to become self-directing. The child who is subjected to rigid, autocratic discipline becomes an obstructive factor in a social situation instead of a co-operative one. He submits because he must but with no spirit of co-operation.

Situations like the above probably arise because the nurse has not had sufficient experience to meet the children's need for constructive activity. Many convalescent and orthopedically handicapped children are bursting with energy. They cannot be expected to lie quietly in bed with nothing to do. Democratic guidance produces growth. It, too, can bring order out of chaos, but the results produce different feelings from those acquired from autocratic discipline. Children need adventure, fun, opportunities to practice their skills and to learn. The pediatric ward is for children. The nurse needs to help them know that this is true. The older children can be won readily by a nurse who enlists their help and shows them that she actually needs that help. They will revel in responsibility because it gives them a feeling of satisfaction and importance. It wins them to the side of law and order rather than to opposition. If the nurse finds the ring-leader, wins his co-operation by acknowledging his powers and encourages him to work with her, she will be on her way to establishing peace and comfort for her patients. Positive direction tells children what they can do. Consistently enforced limits give them the help they need to control themselves.

The example which follows serves to illustrate the application of some of the concepts presented in this chapter in the care of one child.

Mickie, aged 5 years, was admitted to the hospital for study to determine the etiology of the cataracts which were first observed by his parents when he was 18 months of age. A nurse reported that Mickie was a "queer" child. During rest hour he walked constantly about his bed with a blanket over his head and mumbled incoherently. When he was out of bed and came upon a nurse who was sitting on a low chair, he tickled her face and arms and literally burrowed himself into her arms. The tickling annoyed the nurse. She said that she felt like running as far away from

him as she could. She reported his behavior in an effort to get help to change her attitudes toward him. The nurse reported further details concerning his behavior. Soon after arrival in the hospital Mickie was taken for skull roentgenograms and had blood tests. Because his behavior betokened intense anxiety during these diagnostic measures, he was sedated before a catheterized specimen of urine was obtained. Although Mickie was asleep when the doctor arrived to do the catheterization, Mickie became aware of what was happening to him and shrieked and struggled to the extent that firm, strong restraint was necessary.

After listening to the account of the nurse's observations, it seemed apparent that both she and Mickie needed help immediately. Neither person had a relationship with the other, and they were obviously troubled. To help the nurse understand Mickie so she could establish a relationship with him, an observational study was made to get answers to the following questions: (1) Was Mickie psychotic, mentally retarded or disturbed because he had no one to help him to feel secure in a strange world that he could not see or understand? (2) Would recognition of his visual defect provide the key that would open the door to a relationship with Mickie? (3) What strengths did Mickie bring to the experiences which would help him solve his problems? (4) What was Mickie so desperately afraid of? After thinking through the observational data which had been presented, the observer predicted that rapport could be established if she could use her eyes to discover when Mickie needed her to help him learn what he would learn by himself if he had perfect vision and the help of a person who accepted him as he was.

When first observed Mickie was in the playroom crawling on all fours. As the observer entered the room, Mickie crawled into the playpen, put a blanket over his head and began to mumble quietly. At this point the observer was called away. She saw Mickie next in the otolaryngology clinic of the hospital. His respirations were 60 per minute, his face was immobile, his pupils dilated, and he stood rigidly as if he were frozen with fear. Mickie got into the examination chair, permitted the ear and nose examination but clenched his teeth tightly when the doctor tried to examine his throat. After the doctor left the room, Mickie was given a tongue blade and a nasal speculum to handle. He handled them gingerly without a word or aggressive gesture. A second doctor came in to try his hand at examining Mickie's throat. He was jovial and positive. He was successful in getting Mickie into the examining chair. Mickie's respirations decreased; he permitted the doctor to look into his throat but resisted the use of a tongue depressor. Immediately after this examination he was scheduled to visit first the eye clinic and then the dental department. He cooperated with the eye examination but was silent and partially immobilized during it. When it was over he burrowed himself into his nurse's lap. It seemed as if he could not get close enough to her.

In the dental clinic Mickie's feelings erupted. He drew back and screamed. Instead of forcing him to have the examination, another attempt at preparation was done after Mickie's control of himself had been regained. Mickie, the dentist and the nurse conferred and decided that a visit the following day would be more profitable for Mickie. Outside the dental clinic there were pictures that could be illuminated. Mickie felt these with his hands and put his face close to them in order to see. Because the observer noted that Mickie managed himself better when helped by a man, she received the dentist's help in familiarizing Mickie with the dental x-ray procedure. She knew that Mickie would feel safer if he had become acquainted with the person who would direct the study on the following day. The dentist promised Mickie that he would be there the next day. Before Mickie left the dental department, he showed evidence that he had felt the dentist's friendliness. Upon his return to the ward Mickie uttered his first intelligible words since admission 4 days

before. He said, "I want to go to the playroom."

Mickie was taken to the playroom at once, and for 20 minutes he played as a 2-year-old child plays. He ran to the toy shelves, fingered toys, found a wind-up truck with his hands and set it in motion. Then he began to play with vehicles. He ran one across the floor and followed the noise it made. When his hands landed on another toy he began to play with it. He used pull toys as toddlers do. All of a sudden, he picked up a pull toy, ran to the observer and said, "Lady, what's this?" The observer told him it was a toy caterpillar. "Give me your hand Mickie. This is the caterpillar's ears. This is its tail. This is its body. This string is used to pull it about," she said. He ran off and played with intensity. He put a small car in a truck and raced it across the floor. Often he pulled the small car out of the truck, put it close to his eyes to look at it and then replaced it in the large truck and banged its door closed. Next he tried to wind a mechanical toy and was unsuccessful. Immediately the observer went to him and said, "Mickie, I'll show you how to make it go. Let me have your hand. Feel the winder. I'll teach you how to use the winder." Mickie learned at once and repeated it over and over again. During the next 15 minutes Mickie did not contact the observer. He talked as he played, and his speech became more and more intelligible. The observer watched for opportunities to help him the minute he showed a need for it. He had communicated his urgent need for recognition of his inability to see when he brought the caterpillar to her and requested help to identify it, and the observer perceived his signal of need.

Twenty minutes after he had requested help in learning about the caterpillar, he came to the observer with a tiny wooden train in his hand and said, "Lady, how do you put this together?" The observer said, "Mickie I'll show you how. Feel the metal at the end of the train car. It is a hook. One end is open so the hook of another car can be placed into it. The hook keeps the cars together." She helped Mickie to feel the parts and learn how to put them together. In her desire to help him learn to connect the cars, the observer had not noticed that one car was upside down. Mickie had felt it to be so and said, "Lady, it's upside down." "So it is, Mickie. I'll help you fix it. Thank you for telling me. When boy's can't see very well, they need help to learn. Your nurse and I can help you learn, Mickie." Mickie looked up at the observer and smiled a smile that looked as if it had come from deep down inside of him. His whole being seemed to say, "I feel understood. Now I don't have to try to hide my blindness any more." Later when the dinner hour was anticipated for Mickie, he said, "You mean lunch hour, don't you?" In the next few minutes, Mickie learned how to put away toys.

From this observational study the observer learned that Mickie was neither psychotic nor mentally retarded. He could relate, and he learned rapidly when he was taught. She concluded that meeting his need to learn was a way to communicate feelings of friendliness. She interpreted his needs to his nurse and functioned during the meal period which followed the play period in a way which would help him transfer his beginning relationship with the observer to the nurse who had sought help in understanding him.

At the lunch table Mickie tried to cut up his orange salad. He held the knife so the blade was away from the orange. This evidenced his need for help in learning how to use eating implements. After being taught, he used the knife over and over again not only on the orange slices but also on other foods. In the middle of the meal he held his hands close to the nurse's face and mentioned the smudge of dirt on them. The nurse said, "You're right. I didn't show you how to turn on the faucets so you could wash your hands." Mickie said, "Let's do it now." The nurse took him to the sink and helped him to learn how to manipulate the faucets. He washed meticulously. During the process, he wiggled on one leg and then the other. When his nurse said, "Mickie, I think you're telling me you need to go to the

toilet," he looked up at her, smiled and said, "Yeh, I do!"

After Mickie had eaten an enormous meal, he was called to the dermatology clinic for skin tests. "Mickie, the nurse is going to put medicine under your skin with a needle. It will sting for a minute. I'll help you hold yourself still," the nurse said. Mickie's respirations increased immediately. The nurse took him in her arms where he cried and squirmed vigorously. His motor power increased tremendously. Half way to the clinic, the nurse had to stop for rest. Because Mickie was crying so hard, a clerk brought out a drum, drumsticks, and beads to string. Mickie began to play at once. His crying ceased, but his respiration rate continued at a high level. He pulled himself together in an amazing fashion for a 5-year-old. He beat the drum in a beautifully rhythmic fashion and chewed chocolate mints as fast as the nurse could give them to him. He began to string beads and learned how to tie a knot in the cord to keep the beads from falling off. Then he said he had to go to the toilet. The nurse got down to his level and said, "Mickie, it's so scary to go for skin tests. I will stay with you and help you." Mickie put both his hands on the nurse's face and caressed it. As she rose from her squatting position, he closed the door of the toilet. When he finished they walked toward the clinic. Then he stopped and shrieked. His nurse picked him up, and he fought to prevent himself from being taken through the door. He spread his legs and put a foot on each side of the doorway in an attempt to protect himself. He acted as if he expected annihilation. He mobilized every resource he had to escape. Mickie's anxiety was inappropriate to the situation. Preparation increased rather than lessened it. Therefore, it seemed advisable *to help Mickie learn as quickly as possible that nothing was as bad as he imagined it to be.* She predicted that experience would help him master his irrational fear.

A doctor came and held Mickie firmly during the procedure which necessitated 5 intradermal injections in each forearm. He screamed at the top of his voice: "I hate you. I'm dying. I'm going to die." It was interesting to note that his screaming and respiration rate lessened with each injection. As soon as it was over, Mickie pulled himself together, enjoyed sitting on the kind doctor's lap and munched chocolate cookies that the doctor gave him. Mickie showed evidence that he was listening as the doctor talked. He made no attempt to withdraw himself from his lap, but he did not burrow himself against the doctor's body as he had into the nurse's lap. After a few minutes, the doctor put him down.

Upon return to the ward Mickie went willingly to bed but he was unable to sleep. He kept putting his forearm close to his eyes and asked, "When will they go away?" The nurse said, "In a few days you won't be able to see them any more. The nurse put medicine in your arms. The doctor is trying to find out what keeps your eyes from seeing well. They stung and you were scared as all boys are. I'm glad you could tell us how angry and scared you were. Did you think you were going to die, Mickie?" His reply substantiated the nurse's hunch; Mickie had expected the worst. The nurse said, "The nurses and the doctors wouldn't kill you, Mickie. They want to help you so you can see again. Those were tests. They do them to find ways to make you see again."

The next day Mickie walked hesitantly and silently to the dental clinic. At the door of it, he stood still and refused to enter. His respirations mounted as they had in every other anxiety-ridden situation, but he did not shriek as he had done the day before. The dentist whom Mickie had met the day before came out to greet him. He told him the technician was going to take pictures and he interpreted every step of the procedure to him. When the dentist invited Mickie to enter, he followed him into the room. Slowly he climbed into the chair and laid his head on the film as he was directed to do. Mickie smiled when he was given a film to hold. His co-operation was elicited by such comments as: "Mickie, you can help us by holding your head still on this plate." When it came time for the teeth roentgenograms to be taken, Mickie not only

opened his mouth widely for the insertion of a film but also he opened it in between times over and over again. He was able to do what he had not been able to do the day before when the doctor wanted to put a tongue blade into his mouth. After the film was placed in his mouth, he concentrated on holding it in place. With the first two films, the technician told him when he could remove it. He must have associated her words with the vanishing sound that occurred when the machine was turned off. After she had said, "You can take it out now," twice, he responded to the silencing of the machine by withdrawing the film from his mouth. When the doctor said, "You can tell your boy friends that you had pictures made of your teeth," Mickie replied, "But I haven't any boy friends."

When the x-ray pictures were completed, the dentist invited Mickie into the next room, having first forewarned him that he needed to examine his teeth. Mickie walked directly into the room, climbed into the dental chair, opened his mouth widely and showed that he had mastered his fear of having something put into his mouth. Mickie left the clinic clutching in his hand the films the doctor had given him. On his return trip to the ward, there was no halting. He skipped ahead of the nurse. He carried himself more erectly and kept saying, "It was fun." He seemed to have acquired some new feelings about himself and the world which had been so scary to him before.

Mickie's situation when first observed was a precarious one. He could not see unless an object was held close to his face. He came into a strange world unprepared for all that he would experience. He could hear the cries of children and feel the anxiety in the air. Yet he could not see to gain understanding of the world about him. Nor could he question or reach out for help in any other ways than he did. Painful things had been done to him when he was under the influence of a drug which made him unable to control himself. He reacted to the situation with panic and disorganization. When the observer first saw him he seemed to be in a world of his own. His behavior in the play pen showed that he wanted to hide and get protection. Mickie's behavior spelled a need for help to master his feelings concerning the situation he found himself in. When he was given help to discover that tests were different from what he imagined them to be, he gained a measure of mastery of his fear. Throughout the period of restraint for skin tests, he expressed verbally his aggression and his fears with abandon.

The manner in which a child is restrained determines his feelings toward the measure and toward the person who carries it out. Youngsters can tolerate restraint when it is done protectively and they are allowed to express their feelings about it. The young child knows he cannot restrain himself during painful and fear-provoking situations. He welcomes aid in holding himself still.

Mickie showed unusual personality strengths for a blind boy of his age. With support he could pull himself together and channel his aggression into activities which gave him pleasure. He was able to use the doctor's friendliness and help. He showed evidence of trust and a desire to co-operate. Experiences that originally provoked panic became "fun." Other signs of increased mastery became manifested. His play became more productive; he was able to rest; he became capable of communicating by the use of words; his need to burrow himself into the lap of the nurse vanished; and he found pleasure in a relationship with 7-year-old Johnny.

There was an additional factor beside Mickie's ego strengths that contributed toward his progress in adjustment to the hospital. Mickie's signals for help were respected. When there was a period of freedom from tests, the observer provided a play period not only to give Mickie an opportunity to release tension and to obtain some therapy for himself from self-directed play but also to learn more about Mickie as a person. It was not long before Mickie approached the observer and showed her the way she could help him. Bringing the caterpillar with the question, "Lady, what is this?" could well have been Mickie's way of communicating the following feelings: "There is so much in this world I don't understand. I cannot see well enough to identify the elements in it. I need to know. I'm turning to you to help me learn." When the observer faced his visual handicap and used ways of teaching that took his limitations into account, Mickie's behavior seems to manifest that he felt understood and worthwhile. His capacity to think was respected. When he told the nurse they had connected a car that was upside down, she welcomed his helpfulness. His body language showed that his self-esteem had been heightened. His response to understanding manifested itself in a desire to co-operate with her when it was time to leave the playroom. It was an experience that taught the nurse the importance of facing a child's handicap. Without the capacity to face Mickie's visual handicap, the nurse would have been unable to help him learn that she was a helpful, friendly person. Had she not had awareness of his handicap and met his needs, he might have felt rejected. Such feelings can prevent a child from relating with a nurse.

Preparation for and Support During New Experiences

Support During Treatments. The child's need for a nurse who is concerned about the emotional upheavals created by hospitalization and about sustaining her relationship with him has been cited above. As important as these factors are, the nurse must be careful lest overidentification with the child and her compassion for helpless, hospitalized children blind her to the reality of their physical state and their urgent need for diagnostic studies and treatment measures. Diagnostic procedures are *protective. They ensure accurate diagnosis and curative therapy and often must take precedence over the nurse's desire to keep her patient free of pain.* When a conflict arises between a doctor's order and the nurse's concept of what is emotionally desirable for the child, she must feel obliged to follow the order. If an order arouses antagonism, the nurse ought to use some introspection to discover why she is reacting as she is and to think through the possible reasons why the doctor deems his order necessary. The doctor carries the major responsibility for the child's life. If he feels that painful studies and treatments are necessary, the nurse must rely upon his judgment and do everything possible *to maintain the child's trust in his doctor and to help him understand the reality of the protective value of the treatment. Children can tolerate much pain if they are prepared for it, if they interpret its value realistically and if they are supported by a person who has energy avail-able for giving.* A nurse who feels antagonistic toward a doctor's order is in no emotional state to help the child understand its protective significance. She is to busy handling her own negative feelings to perceive the child's need to trust his doctor and to supply the support he needs to handle his own uncomfortable feelings. The example which follows serves to illustrate (1) the child's capacity to tolerate discomfort when he is supported, (2) the ways substitute pleasures can be provided to prevent the child from feeling that he is being punished and (3) the way appraisal of the child's limitations and strengths can provide the basis for determining needs. In this situation the child had ego limitations imposed by age. His strengths were observable in his capacity to relate to the nurse and in his response to her manifested trust. When the intravenous therapy was discontinued, the nurse redesigned her plan of care because change in the child's behavior and health status indicated a need for it.

Frank, aged 8 months, was admitted to the hospital with anemia. Five days after admission he developed signs of a gastro-intestinal infection. He vomited, had many loose, green stools and became dehydrated rapidly. At the time the following observational data were collected, Frank was receiving fluids intravenously. His left leg was immobilized to an arm board which was fastened securely to the bed. Prior to the time Frank began receiving intensive nursing care, he spent most of his waking hours sucking his thumb. When a nurse approached his cribside, he whimpered; his pupils dilated; his brow became wrinkled. He looked frightened and as if he wanted to say, "Go away. I can't stand the sight of people any longer. Every time they come, they give me pain. My thumb is my only source of satisfaction."

OBSERVATIONAL DATA	INTERPRETATION
F = Frank N = Nurse	
N: "I wonder if you're ready to eat. You're always ready."	The nurse recognized Frank's thirst and talked with him about it.
F: (He followed the nurse's hands and watched intently as she put the nipple onto the bottle.)	He responded to her words. His behavior proved her assumption that he was longing to ingest fluid.
N: "Do you like this? Do you want to give up your thumb for the bottle?" (She gently removed his thumb and put the bottle in his mouth.)	The nurse observed the comfort he obtained from his thumb and wondered if he would be reluctant to remove it. She removed his thumb gently out of respect for his interest in it and put the nipple in quickly to prevent frustration.

OBSERVATIONAL DATA	INTERPRETATION
F: (He whined and tossed his head as she removed his thumb. His brow puckered and he rolled his head back and forth. Then he calmed as he got the nipple onto his tongue. He sucked vigorously and drained the bottle.)	His response to frustration was natural. When his avenue of comfort was removed, he sought another. He rolled his head back and forth to release tension and get pleasure. Head-rolling ceased when he got the nipple to suck upon.
N: (She removed the nipple from the bottle, gave it to him to suck, held his hand and talked to him.)	The nurse did this because Frank manifested an urgent need for comfort.
F: (He kept his hand in hers and began to vocalize as he looked directly into the nurse's eyes. Then he whined, removed the nipple and replaced it and began to chew.)	He wanted closeness. The touch of her hand gave him momentary pleasure, and he focused on the person who gave it. Because of inner discomfort, he could not feel happy for long.
N: (She put her arm under his head and back and soothed him as she talked tenderly to him.)	The nurse sensed his need for relief from tension. He appealed to her motherliness, and she responded with an impulse to love him. She provided all the physical closeness that she could and communicated her feelings with words and caresses.
F: (He chewed, whined, clung to her finger, wrinkled his brow and looked into her eyes. Then he removed the nipple from his mouth, looked at it and reinserted it backward. Simultaneously he looked at the nurse and whined.)	His behavior manifested discomfort, yet simultaneously his facial expression communicated some positive feelings toward her. His behavior as he reinserted the nipple backward seemed to say, "You help me. I know you will."
N: "I'll help you get it in so you can suck."	The nurse did for Frank what he could not do for himself. She understood his need to fidget, chew, whine to get relief from painful tension.
N: (She positioned herself so the child's head was against her arm. She caressed his back with one hand and held her other hand against his tummy and arm.)	The nurse responded to his appeal for help and gave as bountifully as his restrained body would permit.
F: (He looked up at her as he sucked and vocalized. Periodically, his eyes drooped; then he looked up at the nurse before he closed them again.)	It almost seemed as though he were driven to see if she were still there or he needed the pleasure the sight of an interested person provided.
N: (She talked to him with gentleness. She moved her arm to get closer to him.)	Again the nurse tried to position herself to give Frank maximum comfort.
F: (He cried and pulled his body away. Then he brought it closer to her. When he found her arm there, he relaxed against it.)	For a moment it may have seemed as if the nurse was about to remove herself. He reacted to his fear of loss of her. Quickly, however, he relaxed when he found she had not removed herself.

OBSERVATIONAL DATA	INTERPRETATION

F: (As the nurse presented a bottle of fluid, he cried. Then he drank avidly. When the bottle was removed, he sucked on the nipple, vocalized, pulled it partially from his mouth and put his thumb into his mouth. Then he began watching the family in the next room. After 5 minutes his eyelids began to droop.)

His behavior seemed to say, "Give it to me quick, I can't wait." Some tensional outlet was imperative for Frank because his need for physical comfort was frustrated. When he got comfort from his thumb, his interest moved away from himself to others.

N: (She drew him closer, stroked his head, talked to him, and he fell asleep. After 5 minutes she gently removed her arm.)

The satisfaction he derived from sucking, visual stimulation and closeness relieved his anxiety and he went to sleep.

F: (He looked at her, then he closed his eyes. When she stroked his head and held his hand, he went soundly to sleep; he did not stir when the nurse removed her hand and pulled up the cribside.)

Did he open his eyes to reassure himself that she was still there?

The nurse held Frank's hand because she wanted to make it unnecessary for him to have to look to see if she were still there. During the time Frank slept, she kept close watch of him not only to check the flow of i.v. fluids but to make sure he saw her when he awakened.

When the nurse arrived Frank showed signs of anxiety. He demonstrated a need for oral fluids and for sucking. His positive response to the physical closeness the nurse could provide seemed to show his intense need for her. He seemed to look to her for help and vocalized in return for what he was given. Relaxation came because his urgent need for mothering was provided. He was able to tolerate his physical discomfort when he was given support by a motherly person. This experience seemed to support the theory that babies can withstand and master the anxiety which is created from physical suffering and the treatment that disease requires if they are provided with the emotional security that their nature requires and if they are given substitute satisfactions for those they would enjoy if they were well.

Some of the child's fears will be realistic ones which can be alleviated by preparation, by support and by freedom to express the feelings which are stimulated by new or painful experiences. Preparation *before* the child must meet the experience helps him to mobilize his energy to master it. It also provides the basis for the maintenance of a trusting relationship. If he is approached for a treatment before he is prepared, he cannot help distrusting and being angered at his nurse, his doctor and perhaps even his parents for permitting him to be subjected to it. *Support during the procedure and permission to express the feelings which are aroused are equally as important as preparation in preventing psychic injury.* Explaining each step

of the procedure, helping him know its purpose and finding ways to help him co-operate are ego-supporting measures. These technics make him a participant and help him master it. There are always parts of the procedure that the child can do, and there are choices that he can make. Knowing it will hurt is also ego-supportive because it maintains his trust in the nurse and mobilizes him to adapt to the procedure. Knowing that expression of feeling is expected and legitimate relieves the child's anxiety lest he lose control and be punished. Helping him to know that being afraid is natural makes him feel understood and encourages him to voice his fear. Approaching the child with faith in his capacity to help gives him strength.

Something like the following approach brings reassurance to many children. "Diane, it's time for your hypodermic now. It hurts and I know you were scared when you saw me coming with the medicine tray. It will prick when I put it in. Here you hold the cotton ball and tell me where to put it in. I'll help you hold your arm still. You tell me when it pricks—loudly if you want to. You can help me get it done quickly."

Many hospital experiences evoke hostile feelings which need outlet in words and constructive aggressive play. Providing outlet of destructive feelings protects the child's ego development. It helps to sustain his relationship with his mother and mother figures. Hostility which is submerged in the unconscious part of the child's mind because the nurse communicates disapproval of it injures the child because it arouses conflict between his two basic instinctual drives and produces anxiety against which he must defend himself. The child who is forced to inhibit expression of hostility has residual feelings of hostility, anxiety and revenge. It is natural to want to retaliate when one is hurt and misunderstood. Observation of a child's play after a painful treatment during which he has had no support provides evidence to prove the existence of destructive feelings. Some children respond with immobilization and withdrawal; they have no energy to play. It is consumed in the erection of defenses against anxiety. They are afraid of their impulse to strike out against the person who has inflicted pain. They are afraid because they dare not lose the love they are dependent upon. Other children strike out at their dolls or other toys. They give their dolls not one treatment but a succession in an attempt to master their rage and rid themselves of feelings of revenge. Residual destructive feelings produce unhealthy adjustment because the defenses children erect to handle anxiety are most often the kind that prevent maintenance of constructive relationships with their mothers and subsequent mother figures.

Support During Operations. The child who enters the hospital for an operation needs care which is adapted to his special requirements. For the time being he is not a sick child whose illness requires special attention. It is easy to forget the child who has been admitted for diagnosis or future operative procedure. He is not sick and needful of symptomatic treatment. Nor is he convalescent and so much at home that he has no inhibitions about making his wants known. However, undoubtedly he has a sense of insecurity, for he is in a new situation. He cannot help but sense that something unusual is going to happen to him.

Before operation, the child should become familiar with the nurse who is going to help him through the critical experience which he is to meet. After a relationship has been established the child needs gradual preparation for everything that he will experience before and after operation. A 2-year-old will not understand everything that he hears but he will catch the nurse's feelings as she talks. He will recognize that she is trying to help him. When he meets new experiences bits of her preparation will have its effects. He will know that she had forewarned him. Therefore, his trust in her will be sustained.

If the nurse knows that the child has been prepared for operation by his mother, she should attempt to discover his concept of what is to happen to him in the hospital. Children interpret explanations in the light of their own needs. Often a child's ideas are unrealistic. If he has interpreted his mother's explanations erroneously or dressed them up with fantasies of his own making, the nurse should help him understand what is really going to happen to him. Often what he imagines is more gruesome than reality. When he knows the truth, his anxiety is relieved. A way to help the child who handles his fear with denial has been presented already. There are physicians who would not operate on a child unless he showed evidence that he was ready to accept the realities of what he is to meet. There are others who do not feel that acceptance is necessary. Therefore, many times the nurse will be confronted with children who obviously have put the painful thoughts out of the conscious part of their minds or denied knowledge of what is to occur. When she does she should explain what she is doing and tell him what is to come, even though her words go unheard. The child who has purposefully forgotten or denied the event to handle his anxiety needs more support because he is unprepared to meet the situation in which he finds himself.

After operation the child needs an opportunity to master the anxiety which was evoked at the time of the experience. His nurse should help him know that she is interested in all that he is feeling. If he feels her interest, he will be encouraged to talk. Many times his concept of what occurred is unrealistic. Again she can help him understand reality. Everyone, including children, needs to talk about disturbing events to understand and to digest them. The young child who cannot communicate his thoughts and feelings verbally will disclose them in his behavior. He needs play activities as soon as he is physically able. Through play he will be able to master his anxiety. The following situation describes one child's response to operation. It also shows the way he was helped to master his fear and to cooperate in the process that was necessary to make him well.

Jimmy, aged 7 years, had just experienced a pneumo-encephalogram and was lying in a tiny room waiting to be anesthetized for a craniotomy. He was strapped down and alone; he was in anguish! He knew that he was going to be operated on, but there was no one present to help him meet the painful frightening reality. He knew that "operation" meant anesthesia because he had experienced that before. He also knew that they were going to do something to his head because it had been aching constantly for days and days. His conversation ran as follows: "I don't want to go to sleep. I don't want a mask. I want to go back to my room. Why isn't my mother here? Don't people around here know that I need her? My mother and doctor said I could go to sleep from a needle or by taking deep breaths from sweet-smelling stuff on a cloth and blowing it out again. How will they put my head back together again? They are going to cut through the bone, aren't they?"

Jimmy was in no condition to be anesthetized. He was unready to meet the experience before him. He needed honest answers to his questions, as well as reassurance that his head would be put back together again after the doctor had fixed the inside so his headaches would cease. In addition, he needed to know that his head would be bandaged and painful when he awakened; that he would have fluid running into his veins; and that he would be just as he is now after new hair has grown on his head. The following questions showed the problems which were concerning Jimmy: "Where will I be when I wake up? Why do I have to go to sleep to have the operation?"

Relieving a child's fears, reassuring him that he will not be alone in moments of stress takes time, but it is time that the child has a right to and needs. In a half hour Jimmy had relaxed. He accepted the idea that the operation had to be. He knew exactly how the anesthetic would smell. He also knew that the nurse and his mother would be with him when he awakened. Jimmy had been helped to meet a fear-ridden experience. At the same time his confidence in nurses was strengthened, and he was better prepared to adjust to the pain of the postoperative period which was to come.

Helping the child to maintain positive feelings toward his mother is the heart of ego-supportive care. How would Jimmy have felt toward his nurse and his mother had he been left alone and unsupported? Would he have had the energy he needed to recuperate from brain surgery? Could he have drawn strength to adjust to postoperative discomfort from a nurse and a mother who had left him in the lurch when he needed them most? How much trust would he have? Could he relax and *know* he would get what he needed? There is further support that children need to master the natural feelings that hospitalization produces. This support will be discussed in the last section of this chapter.

Play and Social Experiences

Placement of the Child in the Ward. This is a significant determinant of adjustment to hospitalization. Placement should be based on the child's psychological needs as well as his physical ones. Protection from cross-infection must be considered. Dissemination of additional disease to the relatively well or convalescent child may prolong his hospitalization, and the seriously ill or debilitated child may be unable to tolerate such an insult. At the onset of acute illness the exact nature of the disease may not be immediately apparent. Isolation must be imposed to protect others until the illness is understood. Infants under 6 months of age have little need for the company of other children and should be placed in separate units to protect them from overstimulation and from infections that may circulate.

Each hospital unit makes general rules for the protection of its children, rules which must be adapted to the physical facilities and to the nature of the patient clientele. On the other hand, it must be recognized that for many children isolation is psychologically undesirable for it exaggerates the adverse effects of separation from the family and makes it difficult or impossible to provide adequate substitutes for it. Isolation should be regarded as a generally undesirable procedure which ought to be imposed only by medical necessity and should be kept as brief as possible. The nurse is obligated to abide by the decisions of the medical staff, for they have the ultimate responsibility for the patients' welfare. However, the nurse can do much to ameliorate the lot of the homesick isolated child if she comprehends his need.

The infant over 6 months of age and the toddler are least able to tolerate isolation. They primarily need the company of their mothers. Of all children hospitalization poses the greatest psychological threat to children between 6 months and 5 years. The school-age child is better able to cope with hospitalization and isolation if it is required. There are many ways in which he can amuse himself. He has ego strengths to use, but for him, too, prolonged isolation becomes dreary, boring and the producer of anxiety if emotional outlets are not available to him. Special methods must be employed to sustain his interest. Radio and television keep him in touch with the outside world and provide vicarious gratification and emotional outlet for some children but they never take the place of family, friends and continuing constructive relationships with members of the hospital staff.

The need for the company of other children varies with the character of the child's illness and with age. The acutely ill children, who need quiet and rest, may be grouped near each other. The sociable convalescent children should be in another section where they can visit and play with each other without harm to the sicker children. Unless a child is so ill that he is unaware of his surroundings, he will adjust with greater ease if he is placed near children who have become familiar with their new environment. Introductions help children to become acquainted with each

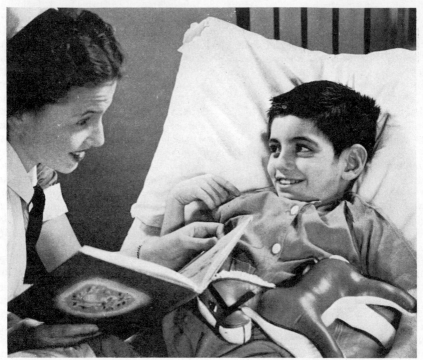

Fig. 18. Nurse reading to a child in response to his request for a story.

other; they also help them to feel recognized and important in their new environment. The children in the ward can assist the nurse. They can help her make the newly admitted child feel more at home in the hospital. The atmosphere in a ward should be that of a friendly neighborhood where each child has status and is a member of a group.

Play and Social Experiences Are Therapeutic. They are essential for physical recuperation and for mental, social and emotional maturation. Activity programs do more than divert and amuse children and keep the ward peaceful and quiet. Play is an essential part of nursing care and as much the responsibility of the nurse as the play director. It is as important for the nurse to see that her patients are occupied constructively as it is for her to provide them with nourishment and treatment. When the nurse provides play activities she is telling the children that their need for play is understood. This helps to assure them that friendliness and consideration govern life in the hospital even though the situation in which they find themselves is bewildering and often painful.

Play provides the child with opportunities to master his anger and fear and induces relaxation. Erickson* says "to play it out is the most natural self-healing measure childhood affords." The adult talks about painful, anger- and fear-provoking situations to master his feelings concerning them. The child cannot do this, but *he can work through his problems in play if adults permit him to play undirected. He will need an*

* Eric Erickson: Childhood and Society, New York, Norton, 1950, p. 195.

adult close by to protect him from fear of his own instincts and from destroying property or hurting adults or other children. With the exception of these limits he should have freedom to use play for self-curative purposes. Play with other children provides opportunities for mental and social growth. Furthermore, it fills the time between visiting hours—time that would seem endless and near to unbearable to the homesick, frightened child if he were left unoccupied and alone. Without satisfying play, regression increases. If the child has no way to release tension and master angry and anxious feelings, regression is inevitable.

Prolonging dependency, or infantilization as it is often called, also encourages regression. When a child is acutely ill, he needs the gratification that comes from comforting, dependency. He needs it not only because he is physically ill but also because illness and hospitalization make him anxious and uncertain. However, when he recuperates and his anxiety has been relieved he requires guided experiences which help him to meet reality. The child who has been acutely ill needs help in discovering that independent activities are more satisfying than complete dependency. Vander Veer° says:

Everyone, at every age, has some secret longings to escape from the responsibilities of the present into the less-demanding existence of earlier years. Bed rest tempts the individual to yield to his backward-looking trend because it legitimizes his dependency on other people. The longer the rest, the stronger the temptation.

Nurses need awareness of this tendency in children so they can relinquish the satisfaction which they derive from having children dependent upon them. They need to learn ways to get gratification through the help that they give children in growing in their capacity for in-

° A. H. Vander Veer, *op. cit.,* p. 62.

creased independence. With experience nurses can learn to help children find satisfaction in play with other children. When they develop skill in teaching they will obtain satisfactions which exceed those they obtained from routinized care.

Play helps the child who has been acutely ill to regain his independence gradually. First, he must discover that being with other children for play and meals is enjoyable. When he finds group experiences are fun, he will grow from the regressive state that his illness produced. At first he may want only to play with his nurse; but gradually, if the nurse gives him freedom to grow less dependent upon her, he will find more pleasure in activities with children in the ward. The preschool child will continue to need his nurse close by. However, his need of her will be different from that which he experienced before he found pleasure in play with peers.

Continuation of school work during convalescence helps the child to learn to take responsibility while he is in the hospital. Learning to do through doing is the child's job. Children like to take responsibility, and they need opportunities to use the strengths they possess. Nurses must see that children do not shirk from this responsibility. From the hospital school they will get the satisfaction that comes from ego-growth and from keeping up with their classmates.

Encouraging the child to help in the ward also helps him to acquire skills, confidence and recognition. The nurse who knows the value of ego resources will help him get pleasure from accomplishment. The ambulatory child enjoys sharing in the process of "picking up" in the playroom. It gives him activity and the feeling that he is a responsible, helpful person. Children enjoy putting away supplies, stamping ward stationery, helping to pass fluids and making cotton swabs and balls. Many school-age children will delight in reading stories to or playing with the younger children in the ward. It gives them a feeling of worth and thereby helps to restore their self-confidence.

Meal hours are an important social activity. Providing food that the child needs to maintain the body in condition to combat disease and to grow and an atmosphere that helps the child to feel like eating requires teamwork between nurses and dietitians. Food has deep-rooted significance to the child. Often its significance is connected with religion and race. Nearly every race has developed its characteristic dishes and diet. It is not happenstance, therefore, that nourishment of patients is often a problem to hospital personnel. Nurses should communicate their patient's likes and dislikes to the dietitian, just as symptoms are reported to the doctor.

The acutely ill child's lack of appetite or refusal to eat needs to be accepted and handled in a way that encourages co-operation. Lack of appetite is the usual response to an acute illness. It may be a protection against his lessened digestive capacity or a response to the emotional distress that he feels. The acutely ill child cannot digest the amount of food that a convalescent or well child can. The amount of his feeding should be lessened; he should be fed at shorter intervals; but he should receive those food components which the tissues of his body require. He should be given amounts of food that he can take easily. The food should be made tempting and should be served as attractively as is possible. Dishes of attractive design and color, or special dishes set aside for a special child are often intriguing to him. The element of surprise also makes an appeal to children. It is an excellent device for making the meal hour pleasant. The acutely ill child should not be expected to feed himself. He needs every ounce of energy, and self-feeding is a difficult process for a small child. On the other hand, if the child resists the nurse as she tries to feed him and expresses a desire to feed himself, he should be allowed to do so unless all physical effort is forbidden. Enough time should be devoted to meal periods to give the child sufficient help and encouragement and the company that he requires.

The child who has learned to eat a well-balanced and varied diet is far better equipped to fight his illness than the child who has endless food prejudices. Discovering the child's reactions to food at home is helpful knowledge for the nurse to acquire. Does the child refuse his food because of loss of appetite due to illness and hospitalization, or is it his usual reaction to food? The cause of poor appetite needs to be found and rectified. If his disinterest in food is the result of his illness, patient waiting until he feels better is necessary. If he is lonely and grieving or filled to overflowing with rage because he has been left in the hospital, the nurse's efforts should be directed toward supplying him with the comforts that he requires. Until his security is re-established, he probably will express his feelings of resentment by refusing to eat.

When a child enters the hospital with many food prejudices, he will require help to learn to accept an increasingly larger variety of food. The nurse will be more successful if she serves initially only those foods that she knows the child likes. Gradually, she can introduce *minute morsels* of disliked food with an approach that communicates her expectancy of co-operation. He probably will say, "I don't like it." This the nurse needs to face with him by saying something like the following: "I know it isn't one of your favorite foods. Lots of children do not like it when they first taste it. I know you'll try it. I'd like to help you try it." Each bit of co-operative effort should be encouraged. Learning to eat new foods is a difficult process for the child who has missed experiences in learning during the first year of his life. Therefore, it is wise to indicate understanding of his problem by commending his willingness to participate in a new learning experience.

A small amount of food eaten without friction and with a certain degree of pleasure is better than large amounts forced on an unwilling and tearful child. Forced feedings never are justifiable with a sick child or a well one. Some children who come into the hospital have already been in combat with an adult over food. Such children may even have resorted to vomiting a disliked food and so have convinced an unsuspecting adult that he cannot digest food. There are many children who come into hospitals whose inner conflicts are expressed by behavior problems in relation to food. Forcing food will not solve these problems; it will only increase the child's resistance toward food and his need to refuse.

The nurse can help the child if she does everything possible to make mealtime a happy period of the day. Conflict and the expression of resentment when the child refuses food slow the learning process. The child needs to feel that the nurse wants to help him learn to eat even what he thinks he does not like. If the relationship between the child and the nurse is constructive, and if she understands the reasons why he has refused food in the past, the food situation will cease to become a major problem. Serious cases of refusal to eat, having no physical basis, indicate some deep emotional difficulty. These children usually require intensive treatment by a psychiatrist or a child-guidance worker.

When the child is acutely ill and is not taking enough to sustain him, fluid and nourishment must be given either by gavage or by the intravenous route. The emotional trauma resulting when an acutely ill child is forced to eat probably has more long-lasting psychologically damaging effects than the technic of gavage or intravenous fluid administration. The acutely ill child's need for fluids is urgent. Consideration of the administration of fluids is given in Chapter 9.

When a special diet is prescribed, the nurse has the problem of helping the child to accept it. Any diet that is different from the one a child has been accustomed to may evoke feelings of deprivation or rejection because what he had been used to had become deeply meaningful to him. The older child is helped if he can feel free to complain and relieve his feelings of deprivation. If he is able to put his feelings into words and feels his nurse's sympathy, it will help him to accept frustration. The young child, who reacts as if he felt deprived or rejected, needs help and encouragement. Serving foods that he likes and avoiding those that he dislikes helps the child know that his nurse understands the meaning of food to him and is putting forth effort to find ways to give him greater satisfaction. Substitute satisfactions are also in order. If the nurse extends herself and provides pleasurable shared experiences, the child probably will take his changed diet in his stride.

The nurse who understands the therapeutic value of a special diet and has faith in the child's capacity to adjust to the unpleasant will approach him expecting that he can adapt himself to a new dietary regimen. She will understand feelings of disappointment and a desire for food that is different from what he has been served. Understanding his feelings will help him to accept his diet, even as it helps him to adjust himself to other therapeutic requirements which are necessary to restore him to health.

The school-age child and adolescent can use knowledge imparted by the nurse and the dietitian to help plan their own menus. If the child is going home on a special diet, both of his parents will need help in understanding the reasons for his dietary requirements. This should be a co-operative project involving the family and those who are

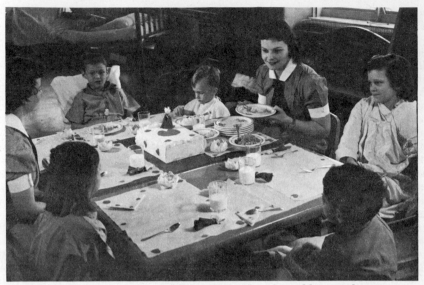

FIG. 19. Nurses eating with children to provide a homelike social experience.

participating in the therapeutic regimen. When children and parents have an opportunity to participate in plans for their care, they are infinitely more co-operative.

All children who are physically able to participate in a group meal period should have an opportunity for the growth that such social experiences can provide. If the playroom is large enough, bedridden convalescent patients can be moved in to enjoy it. Children like to set the table and play host or hostess. A nurse or two can share the meal period with them. It can also provide a happy, satisfying experience for the children. More and more hospitals are instituting this form of meal service because they have found that both the children and the nurses profit from it. The children's appetites improve, and the spirit of good-will and comradeship is furthered when children share an enjoyable ex-perience together.

Activity Programs Provide Learning Opportunities for Nurses and for Parents. Observing play helps the nurse to understand her patients as persons

and to be more successful in meeting their needs. She can discover whether or not they are making progress in ad-justing to hospitalization and to other children. She can discover the quality and the intensity of the child's feelings and get clues to help her modify her original plan of care in light of new observational data. She can learn how children use play to acquire increased mastery of their feelings. She can learn something of what a child's illness feels like from his point of view. She can learn what happens when she directs his play and compare these results with his response and progress in adjustment when he is given freedom within bounds to express himself freely. From observ-ing her patients at play the nurse will get information which will be helpful to other members of the health team. Many of them welcome observational data concerning their patients' re-sponses to play and to the group.

Parents also profit from a play pro-gram. They not only feel relieved to have their children pleasantly occupied but also they see that the children no longer need the kind of solicitous care that they required during the acute state of their illness. Parents of handicapped children can profit immeasurably from observing their children at play. Often mothers of handicapped children need help to provide their children with learning experiences. Their eyes can be opened to the children's potentialities for learning if they are permitted to observe the activity program.

Space, equipment, and a co-operative spirit which centers interest on the child's needs are fundamental requirements for a successful activity program. Ambulatory and convalescent children require a playroom for play, recreational activities and meal service. In the playroom they will not be subjected to necessary restrictions of a ward where doctors are making rounds and treating patients. Nor will they be interfering with the rest needs of acutely ill children.

With an understanding of a child's growing skill, knowledge, interests and needs, it becomes a comparatively easy task to select toys for hospitalized children. Play equipment should promote the development of motor and mental skills, sense perception, and encourage self-expression, mastery and social play. Much discarded household equipment makes excellent play materials. The toys that children like best are those which make possible independent and group dramatic and "pretend" play. They seek materials which they can use to master the feelings within them. It is interesting to note the frequency with which hospitalized children choose the equipment that is available for dramatic hospital play and the use they make of it. Nursery-school children who are struggling with feelings concerning their place in the family spend a goodly portion of their time with equipment for dramatic house play.

Raw materials encourage expression of feeling most fully. A square of cloth may become a bandage, a sheet to restrain a doll, a dress, material that can be torn into shreds, a mask or something that is merely pleasant to touch. Even then its possibilities are not exhausted. Small, simple toys light in weight are better for a bedridden child than are mechanical toys. Suggested play materials for the young child are as follows: tin pans, small saucepans, a set of measuring spoons, small wooden bowls, a string of spools and napkin rings, clothespins, boxes—these will give the baby as much delight as the expensive silver rattle, or one of the commercially made educational toys. Bathtub toys are also a delight to the baby and incite him to reach out and splash. As the baby learns to walk, things he can push or pull about will interest him. Large blocks, a small wagon or doll carriage, animals on wheels or other pull toys will stimulate pushing and pulling activity. Nests of blocks, or cans which have been made safe with can-openers designed to remove cutting edges, sand toys which can be filled and emptied over and over again are other toys that the child will enjoy and profit from before he is 2 and for many months afterward as well.

The list of equipment which appears below includes those things that would be desirable in a hospital playroom. Low shelves which make toys accessible to children encourage freedom of choice.

Blocks, big and little
Simple puzzles
Sand box on wheels, pail, shovel, etc.
Galvanized tub on wheels for water play, or rubber wading pool
Inflatable water toys
Wagon, kiddie car, tricycle
Teeter-totter, seesaw
Record player and records
Hanging blackboard
Books
Piano
Costumes—policeman, Indian, baseball players, etc.
Large wooden beads for stringing
Packing box, planks, sawhorse, ladder
Balls, large
Toys for dramatic house play—wood

people dolls, baby dolls, doll buggy, doll bed, toy cooking set, tea set, telephone, toy cleaning equipment, toy laundry equipment, bottles and nipples, overnite cases, adult clothing to dress up in

Equipment for dramatic hospital play —baby crib, rubber dolls, bedside table and equipment, doctor's kit, bandage, bandage scissors, adhesive tape, equipment which could be used to play doctor and nurse

Toys for dramatic transportation play —trains, trucks, automobiles, airplanes, fleet of boats, fire engines, toys for store play, farm and barnyard animals

Pounding toys

Painting easel for brush, paints and crayons

Raw materials for creative self-expression—crayons, paint, chalk, clay, finger paint, scissors, construction paper, bells, rhythm sticks, tambourines, cymbals, xylophones and drums

Pets—birds, rabbits, hamsters, fish and turtles

In addition to the play materials listed above, the following equipment is needed to meet the play needs of the older child:

Puzzles of graded complexity

Construction equipment for making buildings

Construction equipment for making airplanes, space ships, vehicles and mobiles

Tinker toys, erector sets, etc.

Materials for pottery, leather, papier-mâché, jewelry, block printing, crepe-paper crafts

Materials for making doll clothes

Materials for scrapbooks of collector's items

Paper dolls

Marionettes

Card and table games, including Anagrams, Animal Lotto, author and travel games

Adult standards of order and tidiness cannot be maintained when a play program is in operation. Orderliness which facilitates work and cleanliness which safeguards health are essential. However, they can be maintained without inhibiting children's interest in and need for play activities. Requiring beautifully smoothed bedclothes, absolute alignment of beds and chairs and military precision in the placement of furnishings and equipment tends to center the staff's interest on equipment rather than on the child's needs for activity. Such order may be restful and beautiful in the eyes of visitors and hospital administrators but it contributes nothing to the child's peace of mind.

A children's ward is for children, and *their* interests and needs must be the subject of the health team's greatest concern. A ward without the children's own toys could hardly be called child-centered for it would be without one of his important sources of comfort—not the most important by any means but one which helps him keep in touch with the persons who are important to him personally. Toys are an emotional tie to all that has given him comfort previously. As the child's stay lengthens, his number of cherished possessions will increase, and he needs a place to keep them. Toys and objects from home are precious possessions. (If they are not we had better ask ourselves why they are not!) None of them should be thrown away without the owner's permission. The sharing of toys is an important social experience for those who are socially developed enough to do so. A ward that keeps children segregated from each other is not child-centered either. Children will want their beds moved closer to other children or moved into doorways where they can view the activity of their nurses—or watch hopefully for their mothers to come. They will drop things on the floor and not bother about them. The ambulatory children will use play materials and then suddenly be diverted to a new interest which catches their attention.

What seems like disorder to the adult is orderly and satisfying to children. They cannot keep their beds and bedside tables tidy and play in a way that brings satisfaction and release of tension. A nurse who is perpetually tidying up a child's surroundings brings him little comfort. Inadvertently, she is telling him that play is not acceptable to her. Children should learn to take care of their play materials. This learning can become a part of preparation for meal and rest periods.

Children need play directors, schoolteachers, doctors, social workers, auxiliary personnel and nurses who work together in providing an environment that is suitable for those who require a period of hospitalization. In some hospitals play or occupational therapists direct the activity program. Nurses and auxiliary personnel need opportunities to assist in the program because it is a valuable training experience. They also need it to learn ways to co-operate in making the program successful for all the children in the ward.

Anticipating Changes in Behavior at Home

Observation shows that young children who have been hospitalized frequently show symptoms of disturbed relationships with their mothers after they are discharged. Some young children who have gone through the anxiety which follows separation from the mother during hospitalization become clinging, demanding and resentful. Others have put their feelings out of consciousness and express their hostility indirectly. They withdraw from their mothers and reject efforts to mother them because they have lost trust in people generally. Thumb-sucking, night terrors, soiling, enuresis, negativism, eating and speech disturbances and increased aggression are other forms in which the emotional effects of hospitalization may be manifested.

In addition to the care which has been cited previously in this chapter, *the child needs a mother who understands the emotional impact of hospitalization on him and is prepared to accept whatever residual destructive feelings he may harbor within him.* Many mothers need help to anticipate their young child's reactions when he is taken home. Insight will prepare the mother to accept him as he is and to handle the child's rejection or tempestuousness. It will also prepare her to understand the reasons why he may cling, regress or display feelings of hostility, directly or indirectly, when he arrives at his home. When she understands the genesis of his behavior, she is better prepared to help the child to re-establish a healthy relationship with her.

SITUATIONS FOR FURTHER STUDY

1. What does competency in providing physical support entail? What is your concept of emotional support?

2. What experiences in the pediatric ward distressed you most?

3. Talk with a mother immediately after she has left her child's bedside on the day of admission. What did you observe during your conversation with her? How do you think she felt?

4. Familiarize a newly admitted child with the ward and describe your way of helping him learn and his response to it.

Did you see evidence of fear? How did he handle it?

5. Select a child under 3 years of age who is going to be admitted to the hospital. Read the section which pertains to his nature and nurture. Read discussions in other books listed in the references at the end of this chapter. Observe the child daily from the time of admission to the time he has readapted to life at home and record what you see, hear and feel. Use the questions which follow to guide your observation and study.

A. Describe your patient's and his mother's behavior when you first observed them. How did his mother handle herself in the situation? Do you think it was a stressful one? What makes you think so? What feelings did the child show? How did he handle them? How did his mother function with him? Describe what you observed about their relationship.

B. What is the child's background of experience within his family?

C. After you have interpreted your nursing role to this child, sit beside him and observe what he does. How did he react to your words and behavior? What were the first things he did after you interpreted your role? How long did it take him to signal his need of you? Describe how he used you during the period you were with him. Did you find the waiting period long? Do you think that you learned more about him by waiting? How do you think he feels about his illness? His situation?

D. What is this child's health problem? What physical support does he require at this stage of his illness? How did you conclude that he needed this support?

E. What are the needs of a child in this stage of development?

F. How does his behavior differ from that described in the texts you read? What factors do you think have influenced these differences? What are his personality and physical strengths and limitations?

G. Using the knowledge that you gained from the above observational study, construct a plan for his care which includes the emotional support he requires.

H. Implement your plan and observe the child's response to it. When physical and behavioral changes occur, record these and indicate the way in which you modified your original plan of care. Include the changes in behavior that occur in relation to you, to treat-

ments and to his play materials and to activity.

I. Describe the changes which take place in his relationship to his mother and father.

J. If you were not able to implement any detail of your plan of care, think through the factors which might have prevented you from doing so.

K. At the time of discharge, think through the child's experience and answer the following questions: What kind of adjustment do you think the child made to his illness, treatment and separation from his family? Did he make a healthy adjustment to hospitalization? What makes you think so? If you concluded that he made an unhealthy adjustment, discuss what you based your conclusions on.

L. Visit the child's home after he has been discharged from the hospital for 3 days. In the home observe the following:

a. How did the child and the mother respond to you as a visitor in the home? Describe their behavior toward you.

b. How did the child respond to returning home? What changes in behavior did his mother observe? What changes in behavior did you observe? What do you think evoked these changes? What do you think these changes in behavior mean? How do you think they will influence his relationship with his mother? How do you think his mother feels about the changes in behavior that she has observed? What did she say and do which indicated her feelings toward the child and his change in behavior?

6. What are the factors which influence a child's adjustment to hospitalization?

7. What fears are characteristic of children at different age levels?

8. What is your interpretation of a "spoiled" child?

9. What are the different ways in which children manifest anxiety? Re-

lieve a child's anxiety and report answers to the following questions? What symptoms of anxiety did you observe? What did you do to relieve it? What results did you get? How did you react to the experience?

10. Do you agree that children should be prepared for hospitalization? Support your decision with the reasons why you agree or disagree.

11. Of what value are visiting hours to children and parents? Observe 2 children during visiting hours and describe what you saw, heard and felt. What did you observe that gave you a better understanding of these children?

12. Describe a situation in which you prepared and supported 2 children during a painful treatment. Include in your description the methods you used to prepare and support the child and the child's response to your care.

13. Prepare a child for operation. Describe your approach, your technic and the child's response to the experience. Accompany the child to the operating room and describe the child's response to each phase of the situation. What were his needs during the experience?

14. Of what value is an activity program in a pediatric ward?

15. Observe one of your patients and describe his response to the activity program of the ward. Of what value was it to him personally?

16. To study children and the usefulness of a nursery school type of food service, place the ambulatory children at tables for meal period. Group them according to age and sit with them to serve and eat with them in order to observe the following: What contributed toward making the meal period successful or unsuccessful? Of what did premeal preparation consist? Did it contribute to the success of the meal period? Which children needed guidance? Why? Describe situations encountered and discuss ways of handling them. Which foods were eaten most readily? Which ones were refused consistently? What comments were made when children were served small servings of food that they disliked? When comments were made, what was your response? How did your servings to individual children vary? What influenced variations in serving? Did the placement of a good eater next to a poor eater bring a change in the acceptance of food by the latter? Was this meal period more successful than the ones served in the traditional service style?

17. Observe a child at the table with poor food habits. Does his physical condition influence his disinterest in food? What is his response when no attention is paid to his unfinished plate of food? What is his response to minute servings of all food except that which you know he particularly relishes? Does he enjoy pouring his own milk and helping himself to "seconds"? Does he eat and drink more when he is given opportunity to increase his independence? Observe the child when his parents are with him. Has their relationship influenced the development of his poor food habits? Talk to the mother to determine methods of management during the period prior to hospitalization. If his food habits improve during the period of hospitalization, what responsibility would you feel toward the child and his parents? What would be your approach to the mother? How would you counsel her?

18. Observe one of your patient's play. Describe what you saw, heard and felt. How did you communicate your readiness to protect him from expressing aggression destructively? Of what value was this play to him? Did he show signs of anxiety during play or relief of tension? What problems did you meet in curtailing your impulse to direct his play? Did you see or hear anything which gave you clues as to the meaning which hospitalization and illness had to him? Did this observation period cause you to make a change in your plan of care?

BIBLIOGRAPHY

Albee, C. I.: Group work with hospitalized children, Children 2:217, 1955.

Arthur, Jean: The child with abdominal surgery, Am. J. Nursing 57:1038, 1957.

Axline, Virginia M.: Play Therapy: The Inner Dynamics of Childhood, Boston, Houghton Mifflin, 1947.

Baer, Ruth Frank: The sick child knows in Should the Patient Know the Truth, p. 100, New York, Springer, 1955.

Bakwin, Harry: Loneliness in infants, Am. J. Dis. Child 63:30, 1942.

Bird, Brian: Psychological aspects of preoperative and postoperative care, Am. J. Nursing 55:685, 1955.

——: Talking with Patients, Philadelphia, Lippincott, 1955.

Burlingham, Dorothy, and Freud, Anna: Infants without Families, New York, Williard, 1934.

Cobb, Beatrix: Psychological impact of long illness and death of a child on the family circle, J. Pediat. 49:746. 1956.

Cooley, Carol H.: Social Aspects of Nursing, Philadelphia, Saunders, 1951.

Erickson, Eric: Childhood and Society, New York, Norton, 1950.

Frank, Ruth: The frightened child, Am. J. Nursing 51:326, 1951.

Fuller, Alberta: A Withdrawn Hospitalized Boy's Responses to Self-Directed Play Experiences (Master's paper), Chicago, Dept. of Photographic Reproductions, Univ. of Chicago Library, 1957.

Glantz, Evelyn: Scrap Fun for Everyone, New York, Larch Book Co., 1944.

Goulding, Peter C.: Babies return to the pacifier, Today's Health 35:28, 1957.

Hagemann, Virginia P.: An Infant's Response to Concentrated Periods of Supportive Nursing Care (Master's paper), Chicago, Dept. of Photographic Reproductions, Univ. of Chicago Library, 1957.

Harris, Martha R.: Mary's doll had a gastrostomy, Am. J. Nursing 57:486, 1957.

Hartrick, Paulette: You and Your Child's Health, New York, Harper, 1955.

Jessner, Lucie, and Kaplan, Samuel: Observations on the emotional reactions of children to tonsillectomy and adenoidectomy in Problems of Infancy and Childhood, p. 97, New York, Macy, 1949.

Killilea, Marie: Karen, New York, Prentice-Hall, 1952.

Kobes, Herbert R., and Ford, Mary: Children with long-term illness, Nursing Outlook 3:662, 1955.

Mead, Margaret: Understanding cultural patterns, Nursing Outlook 4:260, 1956.

Moss, Muriel H.: A Study of a Four-Year-Old Hospitalized for a Herniotomy (Master's paper), Chicago, Dept. of Photographic Reproductions, Univ. of Chicago Library, 1957.

Newkirk, Louis V., and Zutter, La Vada: Your Craft Book, Scranton, Pa., International, 1946.

Norris, Catherine M.: The nurse and the crying patient, Am. J. Nursing 57:323, 1957.

Norris, Miriam, Spaulding, P., and Brodie, F. H.: Blindness in Children, Chicago, Univ. Chicago Press, 1957.

Philbrook, Anna L.: Emotional Problems of the crippled child, Child 18:22, 1953.

Podolsky, Edward: How the child reacts to his physical defects, Ment. Hyg. 37:581, 1953.

Prugh, D.: Study of emotional reactions of children and families to hospitalization and illness, Am. J. Orthopsychiat. 23:70, 1953.

Robertson, James: Young children in long-term hospitals, Nursing Times 51:1072, 1955.

Robertson, Joyce: A Mother's Observations on the Tonsillectomy of her Four-Year-Old Daughter in Psychoanalytic Study of the Child, vol. 11, New York, Internat. Univ. Press, 1956.

Rodgers, Carl R.: A counselling approach to human problems, Am. J. Nursing 56:994, 1956.

Ross, Helen: The handicapped child

and his family, The Crippled Child 30:10, 1953.

Sever, Josephine A.: Johnny Goes to the Hospital, New York, Houghton, 1953.

Sittig, Nancy J.: Mealtimes on the pediatric ward, Am. J. Nursing **55**: 551, 1955.

Spence, Sir James: The doctor, the nurse and the sick child, Am. J. Nursing **51**:14, 1951.

Stevens, Leonard F.: Understanding ourselves, Am. J. Nursing **57**:1022, 1957.

Stevens, Marion: Parents are welcome on the pediatric ward, Am. J. Nursing **49**:233, 1949.

Vander Veer, Adrian: The psychopathology of physical illness and hospital residence *in* Personality Development and Its Implications for Nursing and Nursing Education, p. 50, Springfield, Ill., Dept. of Public Health, 1949.

Wallace, Mildred V.: Feeding the hospitalized child, J. Am. Dietet. A. **29**: 449, 1953.

Wallace, M., and Feinauer V.: Understanding a sick child's behavior, Am. J. Nursing **48**:517, 1948.

Ware, E. Louise: Mental Hygiene of the Orthopedically Handicapped Child (pamphlet), New York Assoc. for the Aid of Crippled Children, 1947.

———: Parents of the Orthopedically Handicapped Child (pamphlet), New York Assoc. for the Aid of Crippled Children, 1950.

Weng, Lorraine. Group feeding for hospitalized children, J. Am. Dietet. A. **25**:620, 1949.

Wessel, Morris A.: The pediatric nurse and human relations, Am. J. Nursing **47**:213, 1947.

Wilkins, Gladys: The Role of the Nurse in the Admission of Pre-school Children to Hospitals (Unpublished Master's paper), Depart. of Nursing Education, Univ. of Chicago, 1950.

Wineman, David: When a hospitalized child must be disciplined, Am. J. Nursing **56**:568, 1956.

———: "Booster Shots" for childhood controls, Am. J. Nursing **56**:768, 1956.

Doctors, hospitals, nurses and children, Child Study, New York, Child Study Association of America, Winter 1956-1957.

CHAPTER NINE

Pediatric Therapy

In her care of sick children the pediatric nurse participates in many varieties of treatment. While she rarely has the responsibility for determining the type of therapy to be used or the exact details of dosage, her care of the child will be enhanced if she comprehends the general principles that she is serving and is successful in helping the child understand and accept it. Some of the medications and technics have rather limited usage and are described with the particular diseases to which they most commonly apply. It is the purpose of the authors in this chapter to consider therapeutic measures which have common application to many sorts of illness in childhood.

In dealing with child patients, the factor of size always must be considered in regulating doses of medicine, amounts of fluid to be administered. and in determining the variations that are necessary in certain technical procedures. With adult patients it is possible to use fairly standard dosages and technics, for the differences in size among patients is not very great. A large fraction of the nurse's adult clientele will weigh between 100 and 200 pounds, and all but the very unusual will be encompassed by the range from 75 to 300 pounds. The maximum discrepancy here is 4-fold. But in her pediatric experience, commonly her patients will range over a 30-fold difference in weight, from 5 to 150 pounds. If we include small premature infants and obese adolescents, the discrepancy may be as much as 100-fold. In some instances dosages may be computed on the basis of age, which is a rough guide. However, in most instances the calculations are more nearly accurate when they are referred to weight. Sometimes a more precise method of comparison through calculation of the surface area of the individual is used, but it has not found general favor because of its complexity. Size differences also dictate variations in certain technical procedures, such as transfusions, where the diameter and the accessibility of veins create special problems in the very small child.

FLUID ADMINISTRATION

Physiologic Considerations

Water

A continuous supply of water is a more urgent requirement for life than a supply of food. Martyrs have been known to starve themselves for a month or more and still survive, but life will not go on for more than a few days if the body is denied water. The essential processes of the body not only require water for their continuing operation but also they gradually exhaust the internal supply. During healthy existence there is a continuous loss of water in stools and urine, from the evaporation of sweat from the surface of the body, and with the air exhaled from the lungs. Disease not only aggravates these losses through such changes as fever, diarrhea, vomiting and increased urine output, but also it may increase the water requirement by speeding up some of the body processes through increased metabolic rate. At the same time the individual may be unable or unwilling to ingest even his normal quota of fluid. If the process continues, he uses up the reserve fluid stored in his tissues and begins to show the symptoms of dehydration—dry mouth, thick secretions, hollow eyes, loosening skin, concentrated urine and loss of weight.

The child, and more particularly the infant, reaches a stage of dehydration faster than the adult. In part this is due to the fact that he is less able to recognize and satisfy his needs for water, and in part it is because the smaller he is, the greater is the proportional quantity of water in his body and the more rapid is the rate at which it is used. This rapid use of water becomes apparent when we remember that it is not difficult for some adults to get along indefinitely on a pint and a half of fluid per day. Yet the newborn infant, who may weigh only one twentieth as much, usually cannot manage on much less than a pint of fluid per day.

When viewed under a microscope the various organs and tissues of the body are seen to be composed of tiny units, the cells. It is upon the activity of these small units that the body depends for its vital activities. Although cells differ widely in their appearances, in the functions they serve and in their chemical contents, they have certain general properties in common. Each is surrounded by a semipermeable membrane which ordinarily retains the protein and other large constituents of the cell. Water, oxygen, nutrient materials and certain salts and minerals can enter through this membrane, while the waste products and substances which the cell is designed to produce diffuse out through it into the surrounding space. Cells in general are distinguished chemically from the surrounding tissue fluids by their heavy content of protein and by the predominance of potassium and phosphate salts.

Intracellular Water. In both adults and infants about 45 per cent of the body weight represents the water contained within these vital units. It is called the intracellular water. To function properly, each cell must be supplied not only with the oxygen and the nutriment that it requires, but its water and salt contents must be kept from varying beyond certain narrow limits. The body tends to defend the integrity of the cells during health and disease.

Plasma. The blood vascular system, consisting of arteries, veins and capillaries, is a closed system of tubes reaching to all the recesses of the body which serves as an avenue of fluid communication among the various organs. The arterial side of the vascular tree carries oxygen and nutriments to the cells; the venous side removes their wastes and the soluble substances which they have fabricated for general use by the body.

The fluid portion of the blood (plasma) contains protein which cannot pass out of the walls of the vessels, and water and mineral salts which can freely leave the vascular bed and enter the surrounding tissues. To function properly the fluid volume of the vascular bed must be kept within certain limits. If it becomes too small, due to loss of blood or to extreme dehydration, shock will result; if it becomes too large, the heart may be unable to move it along at the normal rate, and fluid will ooze from the vascular bed to produce edema of the subcutaneous tissues or, more seriously, of the lungs. In health both the adult and the infant have about 5 per cent of their total body weight as plasma or intravascular fluid. In addition to its characteristic content of proteins, the plasma has mineral salts in concentrations which are quite different from those of the intracellular water, since the predominating components are sodium and chloride. As in the case of the intracellular fluid, many mechanisms in the body tend to keep the composition of the plasma within a narrow range.

Interstitial Fluid. Around the cells and between the blood vessels there is a third type of fluid—the interstitial fluid —which has a composition very similar to that of plasma except that it is practically devoid of protein. Interstitial fluid represents the reservoir within the body which responds most easily to the shifting conditions of disease. When it increases, edema results; during dehydration it is depleted in preference to the plasma or intracellular water supply. Unlike the latter two fluid compartments, its relative magnitude is greater in infants than in adults. The adult carries about 15 per cent of his total body weight as interstitial fluid; the small infant begins life with 25 per cent of his body weight in this form but approaches the adult proportions as he passes beyond the age of 2 years.

Electrolytes

Changes in the fluid content of the body during disease are relatively easy to visualize and understand. The infant with diarrhea and vomiting obviously is losing more fluid than he can take in. The consequent loss of weight due to exhaustion of his interstitial fluid is readily apparent. Conversely, the edema of the child with anuria and a persisting intake of fluid is easy to comprehend.

Unfortunately, however, these changes involve not only shifts of water alone but much more complex alterations in the concentrations of the various mineral salts (electrolytes) within the fluid compartments. The complexities of these changes are not entirely understood by biochemists. Without special knowledge of chemistry, it is difficult for the nurse to understand the details of such changes. However, a few of the mechanisms which operate should be understood in general terms.

As the body must take in water continually to replace the losses through normal metabolism and excretion, so too it must have access to a continuing supply of minerals, such as sodium, potassium, calcium, magnesium, etc., and of their salts, the chlorides, bicarbonates, phosphates and sulfates. Under normal circumstances there is an ample supply of these materials in the food from which the body can select to replace losses through metabolism, excretion or normal wear and tear. In the various fluid compartments mentioned above the concentrations of each of these substances (called ions) is kept within definite limits. The kidney plays the most important role in regulating these concentrations, for it has the ability to hoard or discard them selectively, depending upon the needs of the moment.

Acid-Base Balance

The relative concentrations of the various ions within the tissue fluids influence the acidity of these fluids. During health the plasma maintains a very constant slightly alkaline reaction. In chemical terms this is measured and expressed by the concentration of hydrogen ions or pH. An exactly neutral fluid has a pH value of 7.0; an acid fluid has a pH value which is below 7.0 and an alkaline fluid has a value which is greater than 7.0. The normal range for body fluids is from 7.35 to 7.45. Life is seriously threatened when the pH value of the plasma falls below 7.0 or rises above 7.7.

In maintaining the acid-base balance of the blood and tissue fluids, the kidneys and the lungs play major roles. The kidney helps to maintain normal equilibrium by its differential excretion of unwanted ions and other substances and by its ability to form ammonia, which greatly enhances its capacity to excrete the acid products of metabolism. The lungs assist in maintaining equilibrium by varying the rate at which carbon dioxide is blown off, hoarding this slightly acid substance when the plasma is getting too alkaline, and blowing it off at a faster rate when the plasma is getting too acid. During health normal body activities result in the production of an excess of acid substances which must be excreted. Thus the usual productions of the body metabolism (urine, sweat and expired air) are essentially acid in character in order to maintain the balance.

Disease (with a few notable exceptions) tends to aggravate the production of acid substances and places an increased demand upon the lungs and the kidneys. This demand must be met if the acid-base balance is to be maintained. Ordinarily, these organs are equal to the task because of their great reserve capacities. When a study of the chemical constituents of the blood reveals that kidneys and lungs are being placed under stress but are meeting the challenge successfully and preventing the blood pH from shifting out of the normal range, a condition of compensated acidosis or alkalosis is said to exist. When the stress has become so great that they can no longer prevent the blood pH from descending below 7.35, uncompensated acidosis is present. If the pH rises above 7.45 the condition is called uncompensated alkalosis. (It should be emphasized that in clinical usage the terms acidosis and alkalosis refer to deviations from the normal range of blood pH and are not determined by reference to chemical neutrality. Even in severe clinical acidosis with pH values of 7.0 to 7.2 the plasma is still chemically slightly alkaline.)

In clinical pediatrics most of the disturbances of acid-base balance are due to metabolic disorders. Under such circumstances the blood concentration of bicarbonate usually indicates the severity of the process. When facilities for more nearly complete chemical determinations are not available, the values of the CO_2 content or CO_2 combining power of the plasma are commonly used to guide treatment. These levels (which are essentially the same as the plasma

TABLE 6. EXAMPLES OF ACID-BASE DISTURBANCE

	pH	CO_2 CONTENT (mEq./L.)*	CO_2 COMBINING POWER (VOLS. PER 100 cc.)	CHLORIDE (mEq./L.)
Normal infant	7.35-7.45	22	49	98-106
Normal child	Same	25-30	55-65	Same
Mild metabolic acidosis (diarrhea)	7.25	18	40	112
Severe metabolic acidosis (diabetes)	7.10	9	20	95
Mild metabolic alkalosis (pyloric stenosis)	7.50	35	75	90

* This abbreviation is read "milliequivalents per liter." It means that the serum contains so many thousandths of a chemical equivalent in each liter. The concept of a chemical equivalent cannot be described in simple terms.

or serum bicarbonate) decrease during acidosis so that in a rough way a mild acidosis is usually present when the values are ⅔ of the normal, and a severe acidosis is present when they have fallen to ⅓ normal. In alkalosis the levels rise, and an increase by ¼ ordinarily indicates mild alkalosis; an increase by ½, a severe disturbance. Convenient as these relations are, they do not always indicate the chemical changes accurately. In certain types of acid-base disturbances which originate in respiratory abnormalities, the relationship is actually reversed. For illustration of these statements see Table 6. Additional discussion of acid-base changes will be found with the specific disease entities and in Chapter 20.

Calories

During the course of disease there is usually an increased need for calories because the metabolic rate has been increased by fever; but at the same time several factors commonly conspire to reduce the child's ability to ingest and digest food—vomiting, loss of appetite, weakness, disturbed digestive processes. Consequently, his caloric requirements are usually unmet during the acute stage of an illness, and he must live on reserve stores within his tissues. To an imperfect degree some of his caloric deficit may be met by including calories in the form of glucose in the oral or parenterally administered fluids which are given to combat the more immediate danger of excessive fluid depletion. Calories given in this form also spare body protein and combat the tendency toward the accumulation of some of the organic substances (ketone bodies, acetone and diacetic acid) which play an important part in the causation of acidosis. When fluids can be given only by the parenteral route, the ability to provide calories from glucose or plasma is limited by the amounts of plasma and the concentration of glucose which can be administered safely.

Replacement Therapy

Fluids by Mouth

During many illnesses the loss of fluid and electrolytes is slight, and the child is able to replenish his deficit gradually by taking *fluids by mouth*. The daily amount of fluid required varies with the degree of disturbance and with the size of the child. For infants the daily intake must exceed the normal requirement of 125 cc./Kg. of body weight if they are to catch up. Older children require less per unit of weight, so that intakes of 1,500 to 3,000 cc. per day are ordinarily sufficient. It can be assumed that the electrolytes will be restored if mineral containing fluids, such as milk, fruit juices and soups, are included as part of the intake. Enough fluid to produce a copious flow of urine is desirable in order to give the kidneys the optimum chance to correct minor changes in the electrolyte composition of the plasma and hence of the interstitial and the intracellular fluids. If the volume of urine is small, the opportunity for renal correction is handicapped.

Parenteral Administration

When illness is complicated by vomiting, by loss of consciousness, by refusal to eat, by the necessity of resting the gastro-intestinal tract, or by a severe loss of water and electrolytes which requires rapid correction, fluids must be restored by routes other than the oral one. Such *parenteral administration* may be given under the skin, i.e., directly into the interstitial fluid compartment from whence it will be taken up by the blood and distributed in time to the other tissues of the body; or it may be given directly into the vascular system by injection into a vein. A third route which is used occasionally is the injection of fluid into the peritoneal cavity, from whence it is absorbed in a fashion similar to that which follows subcutaneous injection.

Fluids which are to be given parenerally must meet certain requirements. They must be prepared sterilely and must be protected from bacterial contamination until the injection has been completed. Otherwise, the direct insertion of bacteria into one of the fluid spaces may result in local or generalized infection. Parenteral fluids must have a nearly neutral chemical reaction or they will be irritating and painful to the subcutaneous tissues or to the veins into which they are injected. In exceptional circumstances this requirement is broken with respect to intravenous injections, but it cannot be broken for subcutaneous injections. A third requirement of parenteral fluids is that they have approximately the same osmotic activity as the interstitial fluid (isotonicity). Osmotic activity is the capacity of a fluid to attract water from or dispense water to the surrounding medium. It is determined by the concentration of ions and molecules. An isotonic solution of sodium chloride (commonly called normal saline) is a 0.9 per cent solution; glucose is isotonic in a concentration which lies between 5 and 10 per cent and in practice is used in either of these dilutions. Other fluid mixtures, too, must be constructed so as to meet the requirement of isotonicity in order to avoid undesirable shifts in the distribution of water in the tissues into which they are injected. *Distilled water is never an acceptable fluid for either intravenous or subcutaneous use.* (Given intravenously it may cause hemolysis of the red blood cells which results in a serious or even fatal reaction. Given subcutaneously it is quite painful and may damage the tissues into which it is injected.)

Subcutaneous Infusion (Clysis)

When fluids are given by subcutaneous infusion or clysis the total quantity used is adjusted according to the size of the child and his needs. The rate at which the fluid is administered usually is governed by the speed of absorption from the subcutaneous space, the flow being adjusted so that painful swelling of the tissues is avoided. There is little likelihood that too rapid injection of fluid will cause any disturbance other than local discomfort when subcutaneous fluid is used, for the blood stream accepts what it needs at the moment and leaves the remainder unabsorbed. In some instances an enzyme (hyaluronidase) is added to increase the rate of absorption. Then care is required in adjusting the rate of flow.

Intravenous Infusion (Transfusion)

When fluids are given by intravenous infusion or transfusion the total quantity administered and the rate of injection must be calculated very carefully. Such fluid is passing into a closed space which is distensible within certain limits, but if it is overloaded it may lead to serious or even fatal embarrassment of the circulation. The normal intravascular space may be visualized as a partially inflated balloon. During a dehydrating illness the balloon collapses somewhat, due to loss of its fluid content. Filling it with fluid to distend it back to normal size is desirable in order to promote good circulation; however, if it is overdistended and tense the circulation will be hampered, and if pushed to the bursting point life will cease. Fluids which contain only water and nonprotein solutes are relatively safe because they can ooze through the walls of the blood vessels at a fairly rapid rate and relieve the mounting internal pressure if necessary. However, there is a limit to the speed at which they can diffuse out of the vascular bed. For nonprotein-containing fluids it is probably safe to administer 30 cc./Kg. at one time to an infant. When continuous infusion of such materials is being given, the daily volume should not exceed 150 cc./Kg./day.

Caution is imperative when protein-containing fluids (blood or plasma) are being used, for these substances cannot ooze out, and whatever increase in distension of the vascular space is produced will remain for a period of hours or days. The hazard is particularly great in infants. As a general rule, it is unwise to give more than 20 cc. per kilogram of body weight to an infant in a single dose. It is usually wise to allow 12 to 24 hours to elapse before the procedure is repeated. (The technic of exchange transfusion, which will be described in Chapter 10, involves simultaneous withdrawal of blood so that these rules do not apply to it.)

NURSING CARE

Oral Fluids

A skillful nurse can play an important therapeutic role by encouraging the child to accept an adequate amount of fluid by mouth. In doing so she may be able to help him avoid the discomfort of parenterally administered fluids. She will be more successful if she can adopt an attitude of patient and pleasant encouragement than if she displays demanding exasperation at the child's failure to co-operate. Too much urging may result only in overfilling the child's stomach with the induction of vomiting. In most instances some latitude of choice in the selection of the particular fluid to be given is permitted. Offering the older child a choice or trying the infant on several types of liquid may provide the answer to a problem of obstinate refusal.

Accurate record-keeping is always important in order that the necessity for parenteral fluids can be judged by the physician in charge. Estimates of the volume of vomited fluids should be subtracted from the intake administered. Truth and accuracy in such records promote the best interests of the patient. Observation of the frequency and the volume of urine production of a child who is in need of fluid therapy is also important. If urine is being produced freely, it probably means that the kidneys are able to perform their corrective work; if urine is scanty or absent, the fluid intake is probably insufficient.

Venipuncture

Measurement of the chemical constituents of the blood is usually desirable in the presence of important degrees of dehydration. With older children the technic of obtaining blood is the same as that used in the adult. However, infants and small children seldom have a vein of adequate size in the antecubital fossa, so that blood must be obtained from the external jugular vein, the internal jugular vein, the femoral vein, or in rare instances from the superior longitudinal sinus. Since failures are frequent, and the risk of reinjection of blood into the vein is a real one, only sterile syringes should be used in venipunctures on infants and small children. When the specimen has to be obtained under oil, sterilely prepared mineral oil is required. In spite of the small size of the child, a No. 20 gauge needle is usually necessary. Blood will flow slowly through a No. 22 needle, but the risk of clotting is increased.

Positioning of the infant for these procedures is important in order to afford the operator the best chance to obtain his specimen rapidly and with minimum discomfort to the child. Positioning of the infant for puncture of the external or the internal jugular vein is illustrated in Figure 20. The restraint most commonly employed is designated as *mummying*. A child is "mummied" by securing a sheet or a receiving blanket about the body in such a manner that the arms are held to the sides, and flexion of the lower extremities is relatively difficult (Fig. 21). The upper edge of the wrapping should be low enough to leave the tops of the shoulders out. The head is turned to the side so that the chin touches the shoulder. Then the neck is extended over the edge of a table or a small pillow so that the sternocleidomastoid muscle is well stretched. The nurse holding the infant must control the head and keep it in position without hampering the operator's ap-

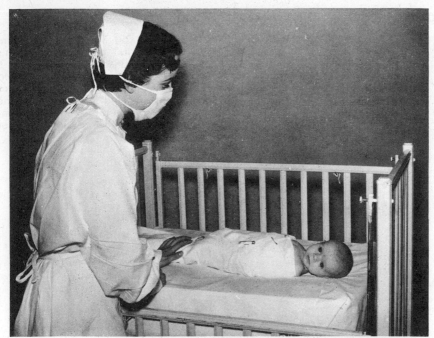

Fig. 20. An infant "mummied" for puncture of the external and the internal jugular veins.

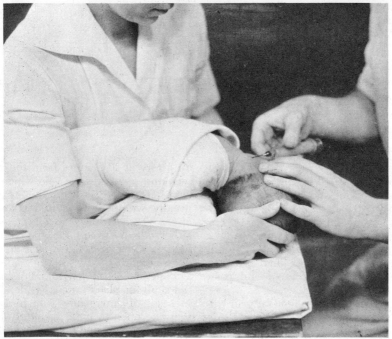

Fig. 21. Method of using the external jugular vein for venipuncture.

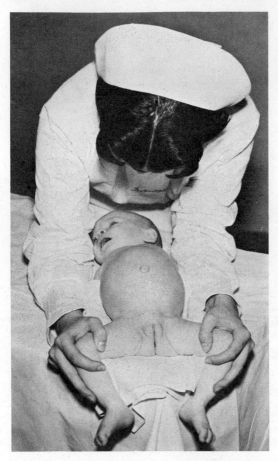

FIG. 22. Method of restraint for femoral puncture. The arms are restrained at the sides with a diaper. The child's body is placed diagonally across the table. Her legs are held in flexion over the edge of the table. The nurse immobilizes the trunk with her forearms.

proach to the vein. When the external jugular vein is used it will become visible during crying and will collapse when the infant inhales. Blood flows most readily if the infant continues to cry during the procedure. The internal jugular vein is not visible beneath the muscle and must be approached blindly. If it is punctured accurately, rapid and easy removal of blood is achieved.

For puncture of the femoral vein the infant's groin is exposed, and the leg is extended on the abdomen and held firmly. The operator palpates the femo-

ral artery as it emerges from the abdomen and punctures the vein which runs along its inner surface. The infant is usually wrapped so as to restrain the arms. Then the legs are abducted on either side of the corner of the table and held with the knees flexed over the table edge (Fig. 22).

Puncture of the longitudinal sinus of the skull for blood samples is done only in cases of emergency. The fontanelle must be open in order to afford access to the sinus coursing in the leaves of the dura mater. A special short needle is

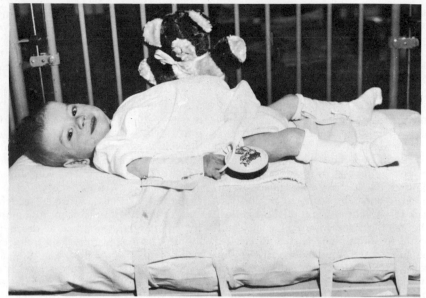

Fig. 23. Illustrating arm and ankle restraints and application of the diaper for hypodermoclysis into the thigh.

used and is inserted exactly in the midline, first through the skin and then through the dura. The infant is wrapped as for other procedures, and the nurse holds the head firmly with the face straight upward, the operator usually standing behind the infant's head. This procedure looks and is easy to perform, but the hazards of thrombosis of or hemorrhage from the cranial sinus are too great to permit its common usage.

Subcutaneous Infusion or Clysis

This is the most frequently used method of parenteral fluid administration. Several sites are available, but the anterior or lateral aspects of the thighs are generally the most serviceable. The child must be restrained on his back in such a way that he will not be able to reach his legs and remove the needles. For a prolonged procedure arm and ankle restraints are necessary (Fig. 23). The equipment for a subcutaneous infusion or hypodermoclysis, as it is sometimes called, consists of a graduated

bottle, or a container of ready-mixed solution, tubing, a Y-glass connector, 2 adaptors, 2 needles of gauge No. 19 to 21 and 2½ to 3 in. long, 2 stopcocks, cotton and iodine, Merthiolate or Zephiran for cleansing the skin, restraints, safety pins, 4 strips of adhesive tape ½ by 3 in., an irrigating pole and the solution.

First, the apparatus and the tubing are filled with the fluid to be infused, and air bubbles are washed or milked out of the tubing. Then clamps are tightened on each rubber tube, and the needles are firmly attached to the adaptors. After careful cleansing of the skin of the outer part of the anterior portion of the thigh, a needle is inserted into each thigh. After insertion of the needles, the tubing is secured to the thighs with adhesive tape. Then the clamps are opened so as to allow a flow of fluid which will not result in uncomfortable distention of the tissues.

The precautions to be observed are that careful sterile technic should be used throughout and maintained until the apparatus is finally removed; that the needle points should lie between the skin and the muscle layers of the leg and not within the substance of either; that the needles should not be near the course of the femoral or the saphenous vessels along the inner aspect of the thigh; and that restraint should be maintained adequately so that the needles do not come out before the treatment is concluded.

Other places into which clyses may be given are the pectoral region and the back. If the pectoral region is used, the arms must be pinioned behind the back to prevent removal of the needles. The needles are inserted below and lateral to the nipples, and fluid is permitted to distend the loose space of the axilla. Frequently, the back is used as a site for single injections of fluid into premature or small infants, in which case a large syringe is used rather than the cumbersome apparatus mentioned above. Sometimes the back is used in older children when the thighs are not accessible. A child who is restrained on his face must be watched carefully to prevent suffocation.

Close observation is necessary to prevent the solution from running too rapidly; blanching of the skin from internal pressure is to be avoided. At the completion of the procedure, the needles are removed, and the injection sites are covered with small dressings. Undoubtedly, the young child will need to be held when the treatment is over.

Intravenous Infusion or Transfusion

Older Children. The same sort of apparatus and method of immobilization which is used for the adult is satisfactory for the older child who is able to co-operate and has a good vein in the antecubital region. The arm is immobilized by taping it to a padded splint or a sandbag. With adequate taping the child will not have to concentrate on maintaining a fixed position while the fluid runs in. Pressure on the arm proximal to the point of needle insertion must be avoided, or flow through the vein may be hampered. Veins on the back of the hand, the flexor surfaces of the wrist or the medial side of the ankle may be used in similar fashion.

When fluids are injected directly into the venous system, careful observation of the patient, the apparatus and the rate at which the solution is flowing into the vein is essential. Between the graduated funnel or a container of ready-mixed solution and the needle adaptor a glass-enclosed dropper is inserted so that the speed of flow can be watched and measured from moment to moment. By counting the number of drops per minute the nurse can make a quick estimate of the rate of flow. She must also watch the rate at which the level is descending in the graduated cylinder and adjust the screw clamp or the height of the graduate accordingly. The doctor must designate the speed of infusion which he desires. If the level is descending too rapidly, the drop rate must be slowed down; if it is descending too slowly, the rate must be increased. If an infusion is turned off completely, even for a few minutes only, it may be impossible to start the flow again because of the formation of clots in the needle. If the nurse finds that the infusion will no longer run or that so much has gone in that she thinks it should be turned off, she should consult the doctor at once. Air bubbles must not be permitted to enter the vein. Bubbles above the dropper are of no consequence, but any in the tubing or the adaptor below the dropper are potentially dangerous and should be called to the doctor's attention. Pain accompanied by swelling at the point of insertion of the needle usually means that the needle point has slipped out of the vein and that it needs to be reinserted.

When blood is being administered, the nurse has additional responsibilities. The rate of flow must be adjusted to the speed determined by the doctor. If the

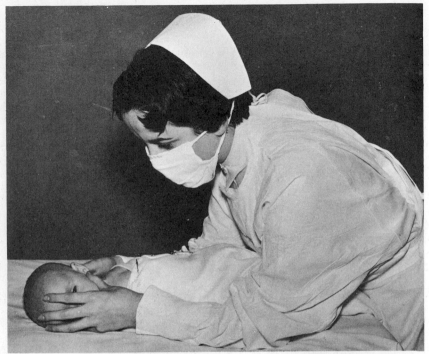

Fig. 24. Method of holding an infant for scalp vein technic. The nurse cups her hands over the occiput and the face, and holds the infant's head rotated at 90° and immobilizes his trunk with her forearms.

child complains of generalized discomfort, chilly sensations or backache, it may be a forewarning that he is going to have a transfusion reaction. The young child, who cannot verbalize the above discomfort, will manifest his feelings in his behavior. He grows restless and cries, and close observation probably will show changes in color, in respiration and heart rate. Whenever any of these symptoms are noted, the flow should be stopped, and the doctor should be notified.

Infants. The smaller the child the more difficult and potentially dangerous is the technic of intravenous fluid therapy. Special problems are created by the infant because he is harder to immobilize, his veins are smaller and less accessible, and often there is a very narrow margin between a safe speed of infusion and one that will keep the channels open.

In addition to the veins commonly used for infusions in the older child, the infant presents relatively large channels over the temporal region of his scalp which offer the best opportunity for successful entry. When such veins are to be used, first the scalp is shaved, and the infant is mummied as in the procedure of venipuncture of the neck veins. The nurse or other assistant then holds the head firmly turned to one side (Fig. 24). By pressing the head steadily and firmly against the table top it is possible to prevent slight movements of the head which may disturb the operator's aim or dislodge the carefully placed needle point. Care must be taken to allow the infant ample breathing space while he is being restrained. Sometimes

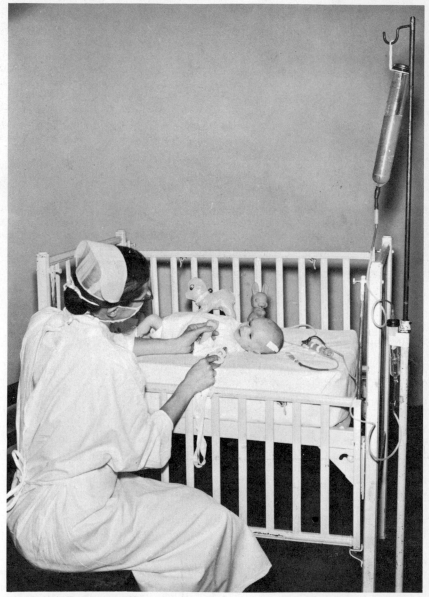

Fɪɢ. 25. Equipment for a continuous infusion into a scalp vein. A tongue depressor is taped to the polyethylene tubing which encloses the connecting needle to keep it straight to avoid puncture. A nurse is with the child to help him tolerate his discomfort.

it is possible to tape a needle in place and permit the slow continuous infusion of fluid into a scalp vein from the same type of apparatus as described above. Usually the needle which must be used is so small that prolonged flow cannot be expected, and a system of pumping syringes is arranged in the tubing so that a third person can slowly pump the fluid or blood through the small needle (No. 22 to No. 27 gauge). Thus a single dose of fluid may be injected in a period of 20 to 30 minutes if the volume restrictions previously outlined are observed carefully. There is a psychological danger of giving too much when the team is flushed with the success of completing a difficult maneuver. Other veins may be used in this same fashion, but the difficulty of immobilizing a hand or a foot is somewhat greater and calls for a strong and steady grip.

When it is anticipated that prolonged intravenous fluid administration will be necessary for the infant, often continuous intravenous infusion is used (Fig. 25). The scalp vein technic is satisfactory in instances where it is possible to maintain good immobilization of the head over a long period of time, or, as illustrated in the figure, when a length of polyethylene tubing is used to connect the scalp needle with the adaptor and the needle from the infusion set. More often a vein at the ankle or in the antecubital fossa is exposed by surgical dissection. Then a length of ureteral catheter or plastic tubing is inserted and tied into the vein. A tightly fitting needle adaptor then connects the vein catheter to the conventional type of intravenous infusion apparatus used for older children.

When the above technic is used, the flow rate must be carefully regulated and recorded. Prolonged stoppage of flow will necessitate a repetition of the tedious surgical dissection which is not only a nuisance but also results in the loss of one of a limited number of serviceable veins. On the other hand, permitting the fluids to enter the vascular system too rapidly may result in serious overloading or even fatal heart failure. The nurse who is charged with watching a continuous infusion in a small infant has a very important responsibility which demands accurate recording of the fluid level, frequent observation of the rate at which the fluid is dropping, and prompt notification of the doctor when the rate cannot be adjusted in a satisfactory manner.

Sometimes intravenous infusions or transfusions are given to infants through an adaptor temporarily tied into an exposed vein, usually at the ankle. The quantity of fluid and the rate of injection must be watched in this technic also, but the responsibility is primarily that of the operator who controls both.

DRUG ADMINISTRATION

GENERAL CONSIDERATIONS

It is the physician's responsibility to determine what kind and what amount of drugs are to be used in the treatment of a child. Determination of the proper dose of drugs is the legal and moral responsibility of the doctor and is usually converted into a written order so that there will be no misunderstanding. The dose of a number of drugs is calculated routinely on the basis of body weight rather than on age, although the age and the weight are related to each other in childhood. For example, in childhood the sulfonamides usually are given on the basis of weight, regardless of age. In some instances, the dosage varies with both age and weight.

All the drugs in common use are well borne by children when given in the proper dosage and dilution. Children are more susceptible to morphine and its related alkaloids than adults are, and a relatively smaller amount is prescribed.

Certain drugs, for example, chlortetra-cycline (Aureomycin) and salicylates, although otherwise well borne, act as irritants in the alimentary tract and so disturb digestion. Salicylates preferably should be in a soluble form and well diluted. Chloral, when administered orally, should be given in milk. Because of its irritant effect it is often given by rectum.

It is well to remember that certain drugs have a therapeutic limit beyond which they cannot be increased with safety. This limit is manifest by clinical signs peculiar to each drug. To this group belong all the drugs that are known (and labeled) as poisons. The important drugs of this class are bella-donna or atropine, digitalis, morphine and its derivatives, and thyroid extract. The signs of excessive dosage of these drugs are the same in children as in adults.

It is impossible to place too much emphasis on the grave responsibility which the nurse carries when adminis-tering drugs to any patient. However, when dealing with a child, that responsi-bility is all the greater because of the fact that drugs are being administered to a person who is often unable to com-municate verbally signs of distress that indicate overdosage or idiosyncrasy. The young child cannot say, "Have you not made a mistake? I never have received this amount of medication before." He has to rely upon the nurse's accuracy and on her ability to detect undesirable effects from the drugs that need to be reported to the physician.

When the nurse is familiar with the dosage of a given drug and believes that an order is erroneous, she should call it to the doctor's attention before proceed-ing to the administration. Occasional errors and misunderstandings will creep into the best systems of order controls. The alertness of the nurse in discovering them may spare her patient a serious episode. It is better to question and be embarrassed about being wrong than to miss an opportunity to rectify an error. In pediatric care this is especially im-portant because many drugs are not used in standard dosage and must be regulated according to the size of the child, as has been mentioned previously.

There are further responsibilities that the nurse has in relation to the adminis-tration of medicines. From her knowl-edge of pharmacology, the nurse should have some general understanding of what the treatment is intended to ac-complish and what an appropriate dose of the drug should be. Some of the drugs commonly used in pediatric prac-tice will be considered below. Others will be described in relation to specific diseases. The nurse also needs to find ways in which to make the unpalatable and the more uncomfortable medica-tions more acceptable to the child. Medi-cations are treatment. Giving them in a way that establishes and maintains a constructive relationship with the child is nursing care and is as important psy-chologically as the drug is important therapeutically.

Oral Medicines

In administering medications to an infant, the nurse's chief responsibility lies in getting the prescribed amount into his stomach with the least possible discomfort to him. Many medicines can be made more palatable by mixing them with a small amount of syrup. They can be given from the tip of a coffee spoon or with a medicine dropper. The baby's head and shoulders should be elevated as a few drops of the medicine are placed well onto his tongue. Giving medicine slowly enough to be swallowed and to prevent choking is a measure of great importance. If too much is given at one time, the infant will spit it out or choke. Choking is uncomfortable and negatively conditions him to the expe-rience of taking medicines.

The nurse's approach in administer-ing medicine to the toddler will be a potent factor in determining his capacity for co-operation. The toddler's nature has been described in Chapter 4. It explains the dynamics which are operating when he says, "No, I don't want to" or attempts to push the medicine away or closes his mouth to avoid the unpleasant. Because medicines are necessary for the child's recovery, the option of taking it or not taking it cannot be left to him. A child cannot comprehend the value of medicines so the nurse must function as his ego. She must help him to know *they must* be taken; that she understands his dislike of them and his wish to control her and the situation. Poise, expectancy of co-operation and faith in the child's ability to learn support his ego. This approach gives the child the help he needs to get controls from within. At first he may need to be held because he has no inner strength to control himself. After the nurse has helped the child to take it, saying something like the following prepares the child for further learning: "Someday you will be able to take your medicine all by yourself. I know you'll learn to do it by yourself." Soon the child will show interest in holding the glass by himself or in choosing between a spoon, a straw or a glass. Often with this simple device, the medicine is taken willingly. It is accepted willingly because giving a choice recognizes the toddler's struggle to assert his powerful new concept of himself which may well have been shattered by the feelings of helplessness engendered by illness and hospitalization. In the sick child's shaking hand a few drops of the solution may be spilled, but the progress made in helping the child recapture his feelings of self-power and in developing a constructive relationship with his nurse outweighs any loss of medicine that first time it is given. A good relationship solves the problem in regard to all medicines that are to follow.

Force in giving medicines is never justifiable because it communicates hostility instead of helpfulness. Besides, it accomplishes nothing because the child always can have the last word. Usually he can vomit the medicine that has been forced upon him—and he will unless he gets support in controlling his basic drive to remove the unpleasant.

In order to approach the child in the confident expectation that he will take his medicine, the nurse needs faith in the child's capacity to learn to adjust to disagreeable things. The acquisition of these feelings requires *experience* which helps the nurse feel that she has been *successful* in helping children master their feelings. Understanding the naturalness of the instinct to strike out against unpleasantness with verbal or behavioral resistance helps the nurse view the expression of feeling without becoming anxious about it. When the nurse acquires this ability she is bound to have the success she needs in order to build up confidence in herself and faith in the capacity of children to tolerate frustration of their instinct for perpetual pleasure. This takes time, of course. Success does not come instantly. If the nurse accepts her need to learn the individual way her patients resist the unpleasant, she will discover that she is growing in her capacity to take their behavior in her stride. She will wait calmly while they express their feelings and she will support them with her understanding of their need for help in tolerating frustration. The nurse who has faith in her patient communicates her feelings to him and thereby supports him. But the nurse who is anxious about his performance also communicates her anxiety and lessens the child's capacity to handle his feelings constructively since she reinforces his own anxiety about the situation. When the nurse has sufficient experience to become a supportive person, she will note that children take in her strength and make it a part of themselves. When a nurse has succeeded in helping a child accept the unpleasantness involved in taking his medicines, she will notice signs which indicate that he has gained ego strength.

His behavior will manifest pride in himself. It will also communicate his wish for his nurse's recognition of his accomplishment.

There is no one absolute technic that can be given to nurses for winning a child's co-operation. Each child manifests his uniqueness at medicine time just as he does at every other time. If the nurse thinks of children as persons who are in the process of learning, she will take more understanding into her relationships with children. She will also become motivated to study her patients as a basis for finding ways of teaching which increase each child's capacity to learn and to co-operate in getting well.

Injected Medicines

The psychological principles of giving subcutaneous and intramuscular injections of medicines are the same as those cited for administration of oral medications. The child's need for preparation, support and permission to vent his feelings in relation to painful treatments has been discussed in Chapter 8. Intramuscular injections are painful; they are also frightening to the vast majority of children. The sick child's threshold of pain and fear is lower than that existent in the well child. Therefore, every possible measure must be taken to help him master his feelings about the experience.

Previous mastery of the technic of giving injections of medicine gives the nurse the confidence and the poise that are required in working with children. The nurse needs not only skill but also good equipment, which includes sharp needles of appropriate length and gauge (1½ in. long, gauge No. 22 for the older child; 1 in. No. 22 gauge for the infant). Antiseptic treatment of the skin at the site of injection with aqueous Merthiolate, alcohol or green soap and saline must precede the injection. Maximum effect of the drug is obtained and discomfort is minimized when the tissue at the site of injection is held firmly, when the site of injection is varied, and

when the syringe and the needle ar held in a perpendicular position and in serted to the hilt quickly and deftly After testing has been done to make sur that the needle is in the muscle rathe than in a vein, the medication can b injected rapidly. Care must be taken t get the medicine into the muscle. If th drug is injected into the subcutaneou tissues, discomfort results; absorptio into the blood stream is less rapid; an there is greater danger of abscess fo mation. The nurse, who is skillful an plans her approach to the child though fully, can do much to minimize th panic which so often becomes a part c intramuscular treatments.

The first intramuscular injection is c great importance because it patterns th child's feelings and behavior for subse quent treatments. If the child's first ex perience with intramuscular injections emotionally traumatic, his days will b heavily weighted with anxiety, for h will dread medicine time thereafter. Th infant has fewer fears than the preschoc child. He is less sensitive to pain and ca be pacified easily at the completion c the procedure. Holding him a few min utes usually eases his discomfort.

Toddlers and preschool children hav the greatest difficulties in accepting pr longed treatments with intramuscula medicinal therapy. Preschool childre are in a period when fears are charac teristically more numerous, pronounce and difficult to handle. Understandin the reason for intramuscular therap and for being subjected to pain is im possible at this age level. However, th child can understand that it is medicin that is given in his buttocks or his arn and that it will hurt like the sting of bee or a mosquito. A preschool child ca help also by choosing the site of injec tion if it is a single dose and by cleansin the area if it is accessible to him. Ever effort to avoid forcibly restraining th child should be made. When two nurse are available, restraint is usually unnec essary. One nurse can distract and su

ort; the other one can give the injection swiftly and skillfully as a means of lessening anxiety arising during a period of fearful waiting. The nurse should remain with him until his equilibrium becomes re-established. Providing play materials and encouraging self-directed activity serves to communicate the nurse's acceptance of his individual way of responding to a difficult and painful experience and to make it possible for him to gain some degree of mastery of his feelings.

The school-age child and the adolescent can understand explanations and will become less fearful when they are helped to comprehend the nature of the medicine and the treatment. The nurse's approach should communicate her awareness of the youngster's capacity for control and co-operation. It should also recognize the fact that he probably has a variety of feelings concerning his treatment. Offering him the opportunity to talk about such feelings so he can discover that they are natural to all youngsters will help him to maintain a healthy concept of himself.

CHEMOTHERAPY

Sulfonamides

The sulfonamides are a group of chemically related substances that have the property of interfering with the operation of essential enzyme systems of bacteria. In general, they do not kill the bacteria but render them more susceptible to the usual defense mechanisms of the body. Treatment must be continued over a period of several days as a minimum because the germs are not completely destroyed early in therapy. As with any other chemotherapeutic agent, the bacterial strains may become resistant to a particular sulfonamide and learn how to exist in spite of its presence. This circumstance can be discovered by appropriate laboratory studies of the sensitivity of organisms that are infecting a given patient.

Historically, the earliest sulfonamides discovered were sulfanilamide, sulfapyridine and sulfathiazole. These particular sulfonamides are not often used any more because they have undesirable toxic reactions.

The more commonly used substances at present are sulfadiazine, sulfamerazine and Gantrisin (sulfisoxazole). To be effective these substances must be given in such a way as to maintain a minimum concentration in the blood, the urine or the spinal fluid, depending upon the variety of disease under treatment. Usually doses are repeated every 4, 6 or 8 hours. Under most circumstances an adequate level can be maintained if 0.1 Gm. of the sulfonamide per kilogram of body weight is given during each 24-hour period. Infants require somewhat more per unit of weight, and under special circumstances the level of dosage may be increased temporarily above this level. Excretion of these drugs is accomplished mainly by the kidneys, and unless an adequate flow of urine is being maintained, the drug may accumulate in the blood to undesirable levels because the expected fraction is not draining away in the urine. In addition to the dangers from the toxic effects of high blood levels, sulfonamides that are being excreted in highly concentrated and acid urine have a tendency to crystallize in the tiny tubules of the kidney. In mild concentration such crystals can be detected only by microscopic examination of the urine; in moderate concentration they irritate the tubules and produce bloody urine; in heavy concentration they may completely plug the tubules so that urine cannot be excreted from a part or even the whole of the kidney.

During the administration of sulfonamides the nurse then has two responsibilities: (1) to see that an adequate volume of fluid is consumed (usually at least 1,000 cc. per day for a child of 2 years); and (2) to watch carefully for the appearance of red or chocolate-brown urine which indicates renal irritation from the drug. In addition to maintaining a large urine output and consequently a dilute urine, sometimes two other measures are used to decrease the tendency toward crystalluria. One measure is to administer alkali in the form of sodium bicarbonate or sodium lactate in order to maintain an alkaline or neutral urine. This method may fail because the child resists taking the additional pills. The second method is to administer several sulfonamides simultaneously. With the total dose the same, the tendency toward crystal formation in the urine is reduced when two or more slightly different compounds are being excreted.

Other adverse reactions that the nurse can observe are the appearance of skin eruptions—either generalized or single spots—or the occurrence of ulcers in the mouth. Occasionally, the white blood cell count becomes lowered during sulfonamide therapy, but this reaction can be detected only by microscopic examination of the blood. Unexplained fever in some instances may be due to the sulfonamide.

In the treatment of gastro-intestinal disorders, two sulfonamides—sulfaguanidine and sulfasuxidine—are used frequently. These particular sulfonamides are so poorly absorbed that the dangers of renal irritation or other toxic reaction do not exist. Of course, they are unsuited for the treatment of any disease which requires the distribution of drug to other parts of the body than the intestinal tract.

Penicillin

Penicillin, one of the first antibiotics discovered, probably is used the most commonly. This distinction is merited because of the wide variety of infections against which it is effective and because of the relative infrequency of sensitivity reactions. It is universally effective against beta-hemolytic streptococcus infections and is usually effective against pneumococcus, gonococcus, meningococcus and some staphylococcus infections. It is the drug of choice in treating syphilis. It lacks the ability to inhabit the growth of the intestinal bacteria and the influenza bacillus.

Penicillin is most reliable when given by intramuscular injection. Crystalline penicillin dissolved in aqueous solution must be given either frequently (every 3 hours) or in very large dosage (2 or 3 times a day) in order to maintain an adequate blood level. Penicillin for injection is also prepared in combination with procaine and other materials which delay its release from the tissues. Procaine-penicillin in the usual pediatric dosage of 300,000 units continues to release an effective amount of drug for about 24 hours. Other preparations delay the release of drug for periods as long as 4 weeks. In this latter type of penicillin the quantity available to the body at any one time is relatively small so that the effectiveness of the drug may be insufficient to combat an acute infection.

Penicillin in pill and liquid form is also available. This method of administration is less reliable than the injection method, because absorption is more variable. Orally administered penicillin should be given on an empty stomach in order to provide optimum absorption. At least one half hour before the next meal should be allowed. Doses must be given 4 or 5 times a day. The quantity must be at least double the minimum dose used for parenteral administration.

Exact dosage with penicillin is not a consideration so long as enough is given. None of the toxic effects of penicillin are due to excessive blood levels. They occur only in a certain few individuals who have acquired sensitivity to the drug. Hives, peeling skin, swollen fingers and toes and painful muscles and joints are the common manifestations of penicillin sensitivity which may not appear until days or even weeks after the last administration of the drug.

In general, until a given individual has demonstrated sensitivity to the drug, no restrictions on the quantity administered need be imposed for any reason except expense. In sensitive individuals (fortunately a rather rare occurrence among children) no penicillin at all can be used safely.

Streptomycin and Dihydrostreptomycin

These two closely related antibiotics are useful primarily for their ability to combat infections with the tubercle bacillus, secondarily for their effectiveness against influenza bacilli and some of the organisms commonly found in the intestinal tract. They are also effective against many of the organisms that are susceptible to penicillin. Were it not for two serious disadvantages these drugs would compete with penicillin for preference in antibiotic therapy. One disadvantage is the toxic effects upon the eighth cranial nerve which follow prolonged usage. The other disadvantage is the apparent ease with which many strains of bacteria become resistant to the effects of streptomycin and dihydrostreptomcyin.

Streptomycin administered by mouth has no effect except upon bacteria within the intestinal tract, for it is not well absorbed. It is used in this form to treat some types of diarrhea and to sterilize the intestinal tract before operative procedures. No toxic effects result from oral administration.

For general treatment streptomycin must be injected intramuscularly. The daily dose for infants is usually about 40 mg. per kilogram of body weight. Older children receive amounts of 0.5 to 1.0 Gm. per day. If treatment is not continued beyond a period of 1 week the likelihood of toxic reactions is small. With many acute infections such brief treatment is adequate. In tuberculosis treatment must be continued over periods of several months. The hazards of loss of equilibrium must be faced if streptomycin is used, or loss of hearing when dihydrostreptomycin is the drug selected. Since the total quantity of drug used seems to be the main factor that determines the appearance of toxic symptoms it is hoped that by using the two drugs simultaneously the incidence of the two types of eighth-nerve damage will be reduced.

The emergence of resistant strains of tubercle bacilli can be prevented in most instances by giving large doses of para-aminosalicylic acid or promizole to the child during prolonged streptomycin treatment. Viomycin and carbomycin are newer antibiotics which may have a place in the treatment of tuberculosis.

Chloramphenicol and the Tetracyclines

These substances are sometimes called broad-spectrum antibiotics because they combat most varieties of bacteria (with the notable exception of the tubercle bacillus) and are somewhat effective against infections of viral and rickettsial origin. Unfortunately, they are not universally effective against bacterial disease for individual strains of organisms may show resistance. Thus, although *most* pneumococci are inhibited by tetracycline, laboratory tests may show that the *particular* strain isolated from a patient under treatment is not adequately affected. Laboratory checks of the effectiveness of drugs against individual strains of organisms are always necessary in the management of staphylococcal infections and in cases where the anticipated therapeutic response does not occur within a reasonable time.

Chloramphenicol (chloromycetin) has certain advantages over the tetracyclines. Its range of activity is wider; the appearance of resistant strains of bacteria is less frequent; and it seldom produces gastro-intestinal disturbances in the patient. However, its acceptance has been hampered by the occurrence of aplastic anemia in a group of patients treated soon after its discovery. Although a clear cause-and-effect relationship has not been established, many physicians reserve chloramphenicol for patients in whom the tetracyclines are ineffectual. It is given orally in a dose of 30-50 mg./Kg./day divided into 3 or 4 doses. Its bitter taste must be disguised in syrups or contained within a capsule. Intravenous preparations are available for severe infections and may be used in doses which are approximately double the oral dose.

The tetracycline compounds include chlortetracycline (Aureomycin), oxytetracycline (Terramycin), and tetracycline (Achromycin). The last is also marketed under a number of different trade names. Therapeutically, these drugs are almost interchangeable. They have the same bitter taste as chloramphenicol and must be disguised. Oral dosage is 20-40 mg./Kg./day in 3 or 4 aliquots. Preparations are available for intravenous and intramuscular use. Adverse reactions mainly affect the gastrointestinal tract. Chlortetracycline often stimulates vomiting which is too severe to permit its continuation. Oxytetracycline and tetracycline may initiate acute diarrhea which is usually mild and unlikely to interfere with the completion of a short course of treatment. In infants the cessation of therapy may be followed by an annoying continuance of mild diarrhea which rarely has important consequences.

Other Antibiotics

A complete listing and evaluation of the antibiotics currently available is beyond the scope of this text. New preparations are continually being discovered and added to the armamentarium. Similar to the broad-spectrum antibiotics are preparations such as erythromycin, Magnamycin, oleandomycin, and streptonivicin. Bacitracin, polymyxin and neomycin are powerful agents whose usefulness is hampered by their toxicity when absorbed into the

body. They are used topically or in otherwise desperate situations where a calculated risk must be taken. Neomycin is poorly absorbed from the intestinal tract and is useful in the treatment of certain types of infantile diarrhea.

ACTH AND CORTISONE

Physiology and Nursing Care

In health the pituitary gland produces small amounts of a substance called adrenocorticotrophic hormone (ACTH) which enters the blood stream, circulates through the body and eventually reaches its target organ, the adrenal cortex. There ACTH stimulates the production of steroid hormones among which are cortisone (compound E) and hydrocortisone (compound F). These substances enter the blood stream from the adrenal cortex and exert a remarkably widespread and varied influence upon the internal workings of the body. Many of these effects are as yet incompletely understood. Information comes from a number of types of study. Deficient production of the steroid hormones can be observed in persons with Addison's disease in which the adrenal cortex is destroyed by disease, or in persons who have had their adrenals removed for the control of advanced cancer. A rare disorder known as Cushing's syndrome affords opportunity to observe the effects of excessive production of ACTH by the pituitary gland with consequent increased production of cortisone by the adrenal cortices.

Since 1949 first ACTH and then cortisone has become available for clinical use, and their effects upon the body in both health and disease have been studied widely. In most respects they have the same sort of action. It must be remembered that ACTH cannot influence an individual whose adrenal cortices are unable to respond.

The nurse who cares for a child under treatment with these substances will have the responsibility for observing the favorable effects that reverse the course of the disease, but in addition she should be alert to the appearance of undesirable effects from the therapy itself. The nature of the favorable effects will depend upon the disease under treatment. Some of the undesirable effects are described below.

Increase in Weight. Daily weights of the children receiving these substances are necessary because prolonged administration of large doses of these substances may produce side effects which decrease their therapeutic usefulness. Increase in weight is a side effect which is due to several factors. The steroid hormones produce a retention of salt, sodium in particular, within the body which holds water in the tissues. In addition, the child deposits fat, usually in a peculiar distribution which is more obvious about the face, the shoulders and the hips. A round moonlike face and hunched shoulders are characteristic. At the same time the child's appetite usually increases, often becoming voracious. The changes in the body and the facial contours are not often of critical significance, but in certain diseases the retention of salt and fluids may be dangerous. In rheumatic fever, for instance, excessive increase in blood volume must be prevented because of the danger of heart failure.

Increased Excretion of Potassium. The retention of sodium in the tissues may be accompanied by an increased excretion of potassium. The substances produced by the adrenal cortex increase the renal tubular resorption of sodium and the excretion of potassium in the urine. Increased excretion of potassium also results because some of the excess sodium passes into the cells to replace the potassium that has been lost. Cellular potassium deficits, hypopotassemia, hypochloremia and alkalosis may result. The effects of potassium loss are not immediately visible to the nurse and can be determined only by chemical analysis of the blood or by periodic electrocardiograms, which are sensitive indicators of potassium deficiency in the myocardium. If tissue depletion of potassium proceeds too far, very serious muscular and circulatory weakness appear quite suddenly. Intake and output of urine must be recorded carefully. In some instances 24-hour urine collections will be indicated.

Hypertension, Convulsions or Psychotic Behavior and Increased Susceptibility to Infection. These other undesirable effects may result from prolonged or high-dosage administration of cortical steroids or ACTH. Daily blood pressure readings must be taken in order to discover changes in the blood pressure level. Rise in blood pressure, the appearance of convulsions or manifestations of psychotic behavior demands cessation of treatment for they may be very difficult to control. Fortunately, these symptoms rarely occur.

Children who are receiving these substances have an *increased susceptibility to infection* and sometimes display very poor resistance to even the most trivial childhood diseases. Therefore, these children must be protected from exposure to contagious diseases and to the common communicable diseases such as colds, sore throats and bronchitis. When patients under hormone therapy are placed among other children it is common practice to give them some type of antibiotics as protection even before they show any evidence of infections.

Hirsutism, Acne, Glycosuria and Wound Healing. Other effects which may be attributed to treatment with ACTH or cortisone are hirsutism, the increased growth of hair on the face and the body, acne and glycosuria. Wound healing may be delayed.

Technic of Administration

Unlike other drugs, there is little difference in the amounts of these substances which are administered to children of different sizes. Usually the initial daily dose is fairly large (50 to 200 mg.) in order to obtain an initial response. As symptoms are brought under control the dose is decreased to a point at which it will just control the undesirable features of the disease. The determination of appropriate dosage is an individual matter which must be varied according to the child and the nature of his disease.

ACTH must be given by injection. The intramuscular route is used ordinarily, but the substance may also be given intravenously. It disappears rapidly from the circulation, so that the total daily dose is usually given in 4 aliquots about 6 hours apart. Slowly released ACTH is also available in the form of gels which need to be given only once a day.

Cortisone (and hydrocortisone) is ordinarily given in pill form by mouth. Depending upon the total dose administered, 2, 3 or 4 portions may be spaced through the 24-hour period.

Meticortin and Meticortalone (which are also known as prednisone and prednisolone) are chemical modifications of cortisone and hydrocortisone, respectively. They are about 4 times as powerful in suppressing inflammation yet retain salt to a lesser degree. Dosage is usually about one fourth of that of cortisone. The dangers of hypertension are not completely avoided by these compounds.

Diseases That Respond to ACTH and Cortisone

These substances have been found to exert an ameliorating influence upon an amazingly large and diverse number of disorders. In many instances their effect seems to be one of suppressing the symptoms of the disease rather than that of producing a permanent cure. When the drugs are stopped the disease usually returns to its expected state after a variable interval. Thus their greatest usefulness lies in tiding children over the severe symptoms of an illness which is ordinarily self-limited. In addition, they prolong life and ameliorate discomfort for those whose difficulties are inevitably progressive.

No complete list of the conditions which are favorably affected is possible because the substances are not yet completely tested. The group of collagen diseases which includes rheumatoid arthritis, rheumatic fever and some rarer disturbances, is influenced favorably. Many allergic disorders such as hay fever, asthma and drug sensitivities, are also responsive. Some of the inflammations of the eye and the skin, ulcerative colitis, nephrosis, leukemia, purpura and hemolytic anemia are also benefited temporarily or permanently. Further discussion will be found under the consideration of the individual disease states.

SITUATIONS FOR FURTHER STUDY

1. What understanding does the nurse need when nursing a child who requires intravenous therapy?

2. What observational skills does the nurse require when nursing a child requiring intravenous therapy to replace fluids, calories and electrolytes lost during the acute stages of diarrhea?

3. What are the symptoms of dehydration? Why is dehydration serious for an infant?

4. Describe the ways in which you

helped a child to co-operate with you in meeting his oral fluid requirements?

5. Observe an infant of from 1 to 2 years of age and describe his reaction to restraint.

6. How do you imagine a 1-year-old child feels when he is completely immobilized and having fluid administered via a scalp vein? Describe a child for whom you are caring who is receiving fluids via the scalp vein. What substitute satisfactions were you able to provide

for him? What was his response to you, his doctor, his mother and the treatments he was receiving?

7. What are the nurse's responsibilities in administering medications?

8. Describe a situation in which you helped a child to co-operate in the process of taking his medicine. What were the factors that helped you to be successful? How did the child respond to his ability to co-operate with you?

9. How is the therapeutic usefulness of ACTH increased? How can the nurse help to minimize or prevent the nontherapeutic effects of the hormone?

10. Describe a child receiving ACTH therapy. What was his reaction to the drug? How did he respond to the nursing care which he required during the time he was receiving ACTH therapy?

BIBLIOGRAPHY

Greenman, Lawrence: Sodium restriction during ACTH therapy, Am. J. Nursing 53:444, 1953.

Wallinger, E. M.: Intramuscular injections for children, Am. J. Nursing 48:112, 1948.

Wilkins, Gladys: The patient, the nurse, and the low sodium diet, Am. J. Nursing 53:445, 1953.

Wilson, L. D.: ACTH and cortisone in clinical practice, Am. J. Nursing 50:649, 1950.

Infant Nursing

CHAPTER TEN

Care of the Newborn

To his parents the newborn infant is the culmination of plans, hopes and fears experienced during the long period of gestation. Understandably, parents are likely to be in a state of emotional instability and suppressed excitement during the early days of the infant's life. Parents of first-born children are apt to find that their relief over the successful conclusion of labor and delivery is soon followed by concern over the normality of their child and over their ability to give him the proper care. Every aspect of his physique and behavior will be subjected to their anxious scrutiny. It is important that those who are assisting with the early care of the infant be able to help parents become comfortable in the care of their child and to discriminate between aberrations that are of temporary or trivial significance and those that may have far-reaching consequences to the infant. In the discussion below, the more or less normal peculiarities of the newborn infant are separated from the important diseases and abnormalities that may affect him.

IMMEDIATE CARE OF THE NEWBORN

After the cord is cut, the baby should be received into a warm blanket and placed immediately upon a table or in a crib where resuscitative measures can be carried out if needed. Mucus should be aspirated gently from the pharynx. If respiration is not initiated spontaneously within a minute or two, resuscitative measures should be commenced. These are described later in this chapter under Asphyxia.

Whenever the circumstances of delivery will permit, ligation of the cord is delayed until it has stopped pulsating so that the infant will receive as much of the blood contained in the placenta as possible. Permanent ligation or clamping should be secure, and the cord stump should be covered with a sterile dressing.

Most states have laws requiring the instillation of silver nitrate into the conjunctival sacs at birth in order to prevent gonorrheal ophthalmia. The eyelids are cleansed gently with cotton, then separated, and a few drops of a 1 per cent solution of silver nitrate are instilled. After a minute or two the lids should be separated again and the silver nitrate flushed out with normal saline solution. Some states now permit the use of penicillin in place of silver nitrate, since it is equally effective and much less irritating. A solution of penicillin containing 2,500 units per cc. is instilled daily for 4 days.

Before the baby leaves the delivery room, some means of identification should be provided. This may be in the form of a necklace or a bracelet of lettered beads, a tape with a number, or a military type of "dog tag" fastened around the wrist. Many hospitals also make simultaneous records of the prints of the infant's foot and palm and of the mother's fingerprints in order to have conclusive proof of identity.

The preliminary appraisal of the infant should include observation of the color of his skin and mucous membranes and of the character of his respirations. The general behavior and degree of activity should be noted, and a cursory examination for the presence of abnormalities should be made. The length and the weight should be recorded; preferably, the head and the chest circumferences should be measured as well.

When the infant is born in a hospital, usually the foregoing procedures will be the responsibility of the delivery-room staff. They should be completed with minimum exposure of the infant before he is sent to the nursery.

EARLY ADJUSTMENT TO LIFE OUTSIDE THE UTERUS

At birth suddenly the newborn infant is required to take over a number of important functions which his mother previously performed for him, i.e., carrying oxygen to his tissues through the activity of heart and lungs, ingesting his food, regulating his body temperature, defending himself against infection, and eliminating his wastes through his kidneys and bowels. In addition, he must attract attention to his wants and discomfitures through the medium of his cry. Several of these functions depend upon the integrity of his brain and central nervous system. The persons in attendance upon the newborn must assist him to carry out many of these vital activities. Even with minimal aid, more than 90 per cent of newborns make a rapid and satisfactory adjustment. The small fraction who have difficulty in so adapting require special attention, particularly during the first day or two of life. From the tables in Chapter 5, it can be seen that of all infants who fail to survive the first year, well over half of them die in the first month of life, and nearly a third die during the first day. Careful observation of *all* infants during the early days will speed the recognition of those who are going to have difficulty.

GENERAL ASPECTS OF ADJUSTMENT

Activity

This varies a great deal among newborns. For a period of a few hours to 2 or 3 days, many will be quite sleepy and inactive, due presumably to the effects of maternal medication during labor or to the compression of the brain during its passage through the birth canal. Such inactivity need occasion no alarm if the respirations and the color are normal, if the infant arouses at least momentarily on mild stimulation, and if the cry and the sucking response are present. After the period of somnolence is over, the newborn still sleeps much of the day, but in a tentative sort of way with spontaneous movements of the extremities, fitful turning and prompt awakening after mild stimulation. In small or slender infants, rapid and vigorous response to mild disturbances may appear during the first few days.

Tissue Oxygenation

This is gauged by the color of the skin and by the type of respiratory behavior. Normal skin color ranges from a delicate pink to a ruddy red. It is most constant on the trunk and the face. The hands, the feet and the upper lip are not always reliable indicators, since they may have a dusky hue during repose but become pink when the sluggish circulation is stimulated by crying or increased activity. Infants who are having difficulty in oxygenating their tissues respond instead with an increase in the depth and the extent of cyanosis during crying. In deeply pigmented infants observation of the skin coloration is more difficult. Reliance must be placed upon the appearance of the mucous membranes.

The newborn breathes with shallow, rapid respirations. The rate varies from 30 to 80 per minute, and the rhythm may be irregular. The abdomen usually moves more than the chest, bulging with inspiration and falling with expiration. The excursions of the chest are effortless when the infant is resting; during crying they become slower and deeper. Rapid, labored or grunting respirations indicate imperfect aeration of the lungs, particularly if they are accompanied by retraction of the chest wall during inspiration and by cyanosis of the skin or the mucous membranes. Miller has emphasized that resting respiratory rates which are persistently above 40 per minute indicate abnormal ventilation.

The pulse rate is not easily determined in the newborn. By auscultation of the chest the rate in a healthy infant is found to be from 120 to 160 per minute.

Body Temperature

The body temperature of the newborn falls immediately after birth to around 96° F. in spite of efforts to maintain warmth. During the first half day it climbs slowly to a range of 98°

to 99° F. where it stabilizes in the full-term infant. Deviations beyond this range may indicate improper environmental temperature, insufficient fluid intake or early illness.

Ingestion of Fluids and Food

This can be commenced very soon after birth. The healthy newborn is able to suck and swallow as soon as he has recovered from the immediate effects of delivery. Early feedings must be given cautiously to forestall overloading of his stomach, vomiting, and aspiration into the trachea. Usually it takes about a week before he is able to consume the requisite amount of food and fluid for his body needs. A fuller discussion of feeding is given in the following chapters. Persistent nausea, vomiting or choking during feeding should serve as a warning that there may be an anomaly of the upper gastro-intestinal tract.

Weight Loss

A loss of from 5 to 10 per cent of the initial weight is common during the first 10 days of life. The newborn's weight curve is bound to dip during the first few days because of his inability to consume his full complement of food. Some infants who have an excess quantity of tissue fluid at birth lose weight rapidly during the first 48 hours of life, as the kidneys excrete large amounts of urine. Obviously, such infants cannot be expected to regain their birth weights as rapidly as the average.

Elimination of Urine and Stool

Often elimination takes place at the time of delivery. During the first 2 or 3 days, urine production may be scanty, and the urine highly concentrated. A record should be made of the time of the first voiding. It may not appear for 12 to 24 hours after delivery, occasionally even later. The first stools passed are composed of meconium, a tarry green substance which is replaced after

2 or 3 days by transitional stools. Failure to pass meconium during the first day may indicate an intestinal abnormality, particularly if there is associated abdominal distention or vomiting. The first passage of stool should be recorded as well as the frequency and the type of stool passage thereafter. The number of stools passed per day varies considerably from one infant to another. The consistency of the stool is determined in part by the type of feeding, a subject which is discussed more fully later on.

Susceptibility to Infection

This condition exists during the early months of the infant's life. He comes suddenly from a completely sterile environment into a world teeming with bacteria. Eventually, he will be able to defend himself against most of these organisms.

Until the infant has built up his own defenses against infection, measures must be taken at home and by the hospital to minimize the opportunities for harmful bacteria to enter his food or the air that he breathes, or to infect his skin. In the home, his contacts should be reduced by excluding unnecessary visitors. His formulas should be prepared with sterile technic. His skin, clothing, bedding, and the hands which attend him always should be clean. Members of the household who harbor infections should be kept at a distance. The same sort of precautions should be exercised in the hospital with even greater strictness because the number of persons involved in his care is much greater, and many babies are being cared for in one unit. In the hospital, individual equipment and meticulous aseptic technic are essential to protect him from infection.

Crying

The infant's cry has meaning and needs to be heeded because it is his only way of communicating discomfort from hunger, distention, loneliness, an uncomfortable position, chilliness, excess warmth, functional insufficiency or disease. The newborn infant is a helpless creature who is completely dependent upon those in his environment for the satisfaction of his needs. A crying baby is in need of care. Discovering his need and fulfilling it is important emotionally as well as physically.

NORMAL ASPECTS OF THE NEWBORN

POSTURE

Before birth the infant's body is packed into the egg-shaped confines of the uterus. During pregnancy the mother or the obstetrician will often note changes in the baby's position. But after birth many newborns show the effects of habitual intra-uterine postures. With a little gentle manipulation the infant can be restored to such a position, and, even though it be a bizarre one, he generally prefers it. Thus, babies delivered by cephalic presentation usually keep their knees doubled up on the abdomen, and indeed it may be impossible to extend their legs fully. Often the lower legs bow outward, and the soles of the feet turn toward each other as a consequence of the squatting position in utero. In contrast, a breech-delivered baby has legs that are fully extended and is more likely to be knock-kneed than bowlegged. Infants delivered from brow or face presentations prefer to lie with heads extended backward rather than in the more universally acceptable position of flexion upon the chest. These postural peculiarities gradually correct themselves as muscles and ligaments lengthen and the curvature of bones is slowly corrected during growth. Treatment is seldom required unless there has been interference with the growth of bone or marked displacement of bony structures, such as occurs in clubbed feet.

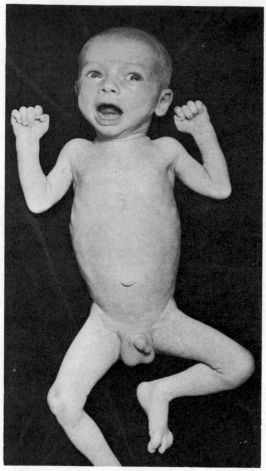

Fig. 26. Cutis marmorata, showing the pattern of congested capillaries on the trunk and the extremities.

Tonic Neck Reflex

Two postural reflexes are peculiar to the first few weeks of life. The tonic neck reflex may be observed in the sleeping position of the newborn—head turned to one side with the arm and the leg on that side extended and the arm and the leg on the opposite side drawn up. At times the position of the extremities can be seen to reverse if the head is turned to the opposite side, either actively or passively.

Moro Reflex

The Moro reflex or startle response is elicited when the infant is awakened suddenly or is caused to fall a short distance onto a bed or a table. It consists of an embracing motion of the arms and general tensing of musculature, usually with an accompanying cry. Both these reflexes are evolutionary heirlooms that have no importance to the modern infant.

Skin

The skin of the newborn varies considerably from one baby to another in respect to its color, texture and general toughness. Many have skin that is poorly supplied with natural oils, making it easily irritated and prone to infection.

Hospital routines for initial care differ. Some leave most of the vernix caseosa on at birth to act as a temporary protective vanishing cream. Others bathe the infant completely and then anoint him thoroughly with a bland oil or an ointment with antibacterial properties. Soaps containing hexachlorophene are particularly effective in eliminating skin bacteria. For some infants, water acts as an irritant if applied too frequently. Those whose skin is dry, or parchmentlike, or peeling, or those who have cracks and fissures or deep folds which cannot be kept dry, profit from liberal applications of oil and a minimum use of water.

Mongolian Spots

These irregular areas of greenish-blue pigmentation are concentrated over the lower back. They are present universally in infants of Asian extraction, are frequent among Negroes and the Mediterranean races, and are rarely found on Caucasian infants. They disappear by school age. They have no relation to mongolian idiocy.

Pigmented Nevi

Pigmented nevi, or moles, either brown or black in color, may be found at birth. The larger ones may be cosmetically undesirable, but otherwise they have no significance. Large, flat areas of brown pigment are called *café au lait* spots.

Cutis Marmorata (Fig. 26)

This term describes a faint purple marblelike pattern of the skin capillaries in small infants visible during periods of inactivity or chilling. It is a normal phenomenon which is abolished by an increase in the circulation through the skin. The coldness and the occasional blueness of the normal infant's hands and feet has been described already.

Telangiectasia

Telangiectasia or widening of the skin capillaries is extremely common at the nape of the neck, less common over the forehead, the eyelids and along the midline of the scalp and the trunk. These flat, dark-red or purple areas of skin have sharp but irregular borders. Sometimes they are called "stork bites." They fade out but do not disappear entirely as the infant's skin becomes thicker during normal growth. Occasionally, a similar area of skin will precede the development of a strawberry hemangioma. This is a raised, bright-red collection of small blood vessels which is seldom present at birth but appears during the second or third week of life. Such tumors almost invariably break up and disappear spontaneously before the fourth year of life. No treatment is required.

Forceps Marks

These marks may be identified over the face at the time of birth but invariably disappear within a day or two.

Bruises

After difficult deliveries sometimes bruises are present on the face and the scalp. They are common about the buttocks and the external genitalia of breech-delivered infants. Even large bruises clear up within a few days, leaving no scar.

Milia

Milia are small white lumps about the size of a pinhead, seen usually on the face. They are small collections of the secretions of sebaceous glands trapped beneath the surface of the skin. They eventually establish an opening to the surface and disappear.

Blebs

Sometimes a similar collection of material is found in larger blebs in the skin folds of the neck, the axilla or the groin. They too disappear rapidly once the superficial skin is broken.

Hives

Occasionally, hives are seen on the second or the third day of life. They are

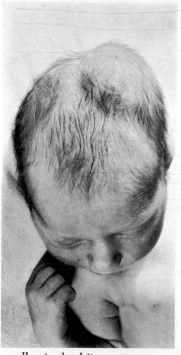

Fig. 27. Cephalhematoma of left parietal bone. (Davis, M., and Sheckler, C.: DeLee's Obstetrics for Nurses, Philadelphia, Saunders)

small raised white spots surrounded by an area of erythema. They look much like small insect bites. Although they probably are due to some allergic response derived from the mother, they have no known relation to allergy in later life.

HEAD AND NECK

Pressure applied to the head before and during labor may produce a number of temporary changes which disappear shortly after birth without affecting the infant's welfare.

Molding of the Skull

Molding of the skull with overriding of the bones along the suture lines results when the head is pushed through a tight birth canal. The skulls of most infants delivered by cephalic presentation show some such overlapping of the bones with elongation of the occipital portion of the skull. These irregularities disappear during the early weeks of life.

Breech-delivered infants usually have heads that are flattened in the occipital region. Cesarean-delivered infants, of course, have symmetrically round or slightly square heads.

Caput Succedaneum

This is a poorly defined area of edema of the scalp which indicates the first portion of the head to pass through the uterine cervix. A caput usually is gone by the third day.

Craniotabes

This term is used to describe areas of softening of the flat cranial bones. It is most common along the suture edges but sometimes is present in the center of the bone. The condition results from a combination of intra-uterine pressure and minor disturbances of the mother's calcium metabolism. The areas calcify rapidly after birth and seldom can be identified after 2 months.

Fig. 28. Facial paralysis in a newborn baby, in this instance resulting from a spontaneous delivery.

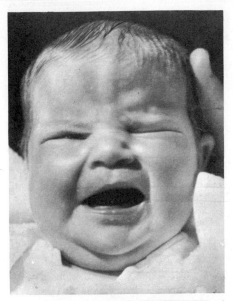

Cephalhematoma

This is a collection of blood beneath the fibrous investment of one of the flat cranial bones, usually the parietal (Fig. 27). It is most common in first-born infants whose heads have been subjected to prolonged compression during labor. Often inconspicuous at first, the swelling enlarges rapidly during the first 2 or 3 days, producing a smooth, fluctuant, prominent mass, the margins of which are limited by the edges of the cranial bone involved. Some of the smaller hematomas absorb rapidly. The larger ones usually calcify gradually, beginning at the base and eventually converting the swelling into a firm bony lump which remains until it is gradually engulfed by the increased size of the skull. Cephalhematomas produce no outward pressure on the brain and are innocuous except for their peculiar appearance. Aspiration of the contents of the swelling is unwise because of the danger of infection.

Petechiae

Petechiae are tiny hemorrhages into the skin which are sometimes seen sprinkled over the face, the scalp and the neck. They result from the sudden compression of the chest and the abdomen during delivery. They clear up within a few days.

Subconjunctival Hemorrhage

This flame-shaped collection of blood on the white portion of the eyeball results from the same mechanism. It usually takes a week or slightly longer to disappear.

Facial Paralysis (Fig. 28)

This may result from intra-uterine pressure upon the facial nerve as it runs through the cheek. When the infant cries, the paralyzed side of the mouth fails to retract backward and upward as it should. The nerve usually recovers its function during the first 6 to 8 weeks of life. Infrequently, the paralysis is permanent.

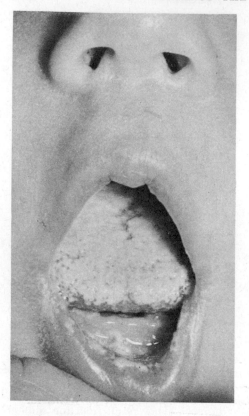

Fig. 29. Thrush. (Potter, E. L.: Pathology of the Fetus and the Newborn, Chicago, Yr. Bk. Pub.)

Hematoma of the Sternocleidomastoid Muscle

This is a small firm lump in the belly of the muscle which results from tearing of muscle fibers when traction is exerted upon the head (or shoulders in a breech delivery). The lump disappears slowly, and unless excessive fibrosis takes place during healing, it does not interfere with the function of the muscle.

EYES

Chemical Conjunctivitis

Irritation by the silver nitrate instilled into the eyes at birth may result in a chemical conjunctivitis. On the second day of life the eyes are red, swollen shut, with pus exuding from between the lids. If there is any suspicion that the process might be infectious, the pus should be examined for the presence of bacteria. The eyes should be cleansed gently or irrigated with warm saline solution. In spite of the initial severity, the inflammation subsides within a few days, leaving no harmful effects upon the eyes.

Obstruction of the Nasolacrimal Duct

This condition may be recognized toward the end of the newborn period by excessive tearing and the accumulation of small amounts of pus in the eye without inflammation of the globe itself. In most instances the duct opens up spontaneously during the first few months of life, requiring no special treatment.

MOUTH

Several features of the normal newborn's mouth may occasion unnecessary concern. Frequently, the gums are rough, almost serrated. The frenulum of the upper lip may extend down, partially cleaving the upper gums. Posteriorly, the gums are usually very white. On either side of the mid-line of the hard palate a raised white plaque, called an epithelial pearl, may be seen. Concern over tongue-tie is usually unjustified. The newborn's tongue is normally short and broad with the frenulum extending out to the tip. It cannot be protruded much beyond the gum margin until its shape is changed by elongating growth in later months.

Thrush

Thrush (Fig. 29) is a trivial infection of the mouth, caused by a fungus which usually is derived from the mother's vaginal secretions during birth. The tongue and the mucous membranes are diffusely red and speckled with closely adherent white patches. The infection is easily cured by a few applications of aqueous gentian violet solution or 1:1,000 Merthiolate solution.

UMBILICUS

Granuloma

After the cord separates, healing usually takes place promptly at the navel. Occasionally, a small piece of granulation tissue remains uncovered by epithelium and grows to form a granuloma; the weeping surface produces a chronic discharge. The granulations may be cauterized with a silver nitrate stick which terminates the discharge by drying up the weeping surface.

Umbilical Hernia

This is the result of a defect in the anterior abdominal wall through which a loop of intestine may bulge out under the skin when the infant cries or strains. Although unsightly and often worrisome to the mother, such hernias produce no important symptoms. All but the larger ones close over spontaneously by the second or the third year as the abdominal muscles strengthen when the child begins to stand. Application of abdominal binders or adhesive strapping have little effect in hastening the closure of the defect.

MALE GENITALIA

Hydroceles

The testes are normally descended at birth but may be placed high in the inguinal canal. Frequently, they are surrounded by small collections of fluid called hydroceles. These latter absorb during the early months.

Circumcision

The prepuce is usually long and tightly adherent to the glans. Since there are no significant medical reasons for or against circumcision, the choice should be left to the parents. If the operation is to be done, it should be completed during the newborn period. If it is not done, the mother should be instructed in gradual stretching of the prepuce to permit its retraction behind the glans for proper cleansing. She should be warned that a tight prepuce must be restored promptly to its original position lest it become trapped behind the coronal ridge, swell progressively and lead to a paraphimosis which may have to be relieved surgically.

HORMONAL EFFECTS

During the latter part of pregnancy, hormones are transmitted from the mother to the infant. Both male and female infants may show enlargement of the breasts with secretion of "witches milk" which may persist for a period of 4 to 6 weeks. In addition, female infants commonly have marked enlargement and swelling of the external genitalia. Occasionally, there is a small discharge of blood simulating menstruation. No treatment is indicated except ordinary cleanliness.

SIGNIFICANT DISORDERS OF THE NEWBORN

Congenital Malformations

About 2 to 3 per cent of all newborns have significant malformations discovered at birth. Some are easily and immediately recognized; others are concealed. Details are given in Chapter 16.

Disorders That Depend Upon the Mother's Condition During Pregnancy

Syphilis

Syphilis may be transmitted from the mother to her unborn child (Chap. 25). Other infectious diseases are rarely passed from mother to child before birth.

Diabetes

Diabetes in the mother increases the hazard to her infant, especially if the disease is of long duration or poorly controlled. Infants of diabetic mothers usually are oversized for the gestational age, edematous, and bothered by excessive secretions of mucus from the pharynx and the stomach. Repeated aspiration and careful observation are necessary to prevent interference with the respiratory exchange. Symptoms of low blood sugar, such as irritability or convulsions, are seen occasionally on the first or the second day of life. Some of these babies require temporary care in an incubator to supply additional warmth and oxygen. Infants of diabetic mothers who are delivered by cesarean section run a greater risk of resorption atelectasis than do normal infants delivered by the same route. They also run an increased risk of being born with a congenital abnormality.

Anoxia

Anoxia occurs when the infant's vital organs, the brain in particular, have their oxygen supply seriously reduced. It may occur before birth if the mother suffers from some severe illness, such as extreme anemia, heart failure, shock or pneumonia which prevents her circulation from supplying the placenta with adequate amounts of oxygenated blood. It may occur also from compression of the umbilical cord within the uterus, or from premature separation of the placenta from the inner wall of the uterus (abruptio placentae). Anoxia is a serious circumstance to the infant, and when it is recognized, usually steps are taken to deliver him rapidly. At birth the infant is usually limp and unresponsive, and measures to support him are of vital importance. He has difficulty establishing his respirations and maintaining his body temperature. External warmth, oxygen and the resuscitative measures described under Asphyxia (p. 233) usually are required. Infants may recover quickly and completely from brief periods of anoxia; but after prolonged oxygen lack, the brain is damaged to such an extent that respiration either cannot be established at all or can be maintained for a few hours only after birth. It is believed that some of the central nervous system disturbances that appear in later life (cerebral palsy, for instance) may be the aftermath of nonfatal periods of anoxia experienced during or just prior to birth.

Erythroblastosis Fetalis

This is an acute hemolytic anemia occurring at birth in an infant whose mother has become sensitized to his red blood cells. Most often the disease depends upon sensitization to the Rh factor; infrequently, it may concern the A and B substances of the blood cells or other antigens. Only Rh-negative women, i.e., those who lack the Rh factor in their red blood cells, are capable of becoming sensitized to it. About 15 per cent of all Caucasian women are Rh-negative. (Only a very small percentage of Negro and Asian women lack the Rh substance.) If an Rh-negative woman marries an Rh-positive man, some or all of the infants of such a marriage will be Rh-positive. During such a pregnancy, blood from the Rh-positive fetus may find its way back across the placental circulation into the mother's blood stream where it can stimulate the mother's body to form antibodies against the Rh factor. These antibodies are capable of clumping and destroying Rh-positive cells. If they pass back through the placenta into the infant's blood in sufficient quantity, the symptoms of erythroblastosis result. Actually, the disease never appears in the first Rh-positive child of an Rh-negative woman. It seems as though additional stimulation of antibody formation by a second Rh-positive child is required before the mother can form antibodies in sufficient amount to damage the child. Also, it should be emphasized that most Rh-negative women never become sensitized, even though they bear several Rh-positive children. The popular misconception that every Rh-negative woman is threatened with erythroblastotic babies is far from true. However, once a given mother has borne an infant with the disease, there is a very strong probability that future Rh-positive infants will be affected similarly.

The cardinal symptoms of erythroblastosis are jaundice and anemia, which are present at birth or appear during the first 36 hours. *Any infant who is found to be jaundiced on the first or the second day of life should be brought to the doctor's attention because he requires thorough investigation.* In severe cases the mother delivers a stillborn fetus or one suffering from *hydrops fetalis*, which is characterized by extensive edema, marked anemia, jaundice, and enlargement of the liver and the spleen. Similar findings of lesser intensity are present in infants afflicted with milder forms of the disease. If no treatment is given, both the anemia and the jaundice are likely to increase in severity during the first few days of life.

Sometimes hemorrhages into the skin are present, and occasionally a fatal pulmonary hemorrhage occurs on the fourth day.

Infants who are severely jaundiced run the risk of serious damage to the brain (kernicterus). The symptoms of this complication appear from the third day on and consist of vomiting, spasticity, convulsions and inability to feed. Kernicterus is often fatal shortly after its appearance. Survivors suffer from severe forms of mental retardation with spastic paralysis.

Mild forms of erythroblastosis produce no symptoms except slight jaundice and anemia—indeed, cases may be overlooked entirely unless special laboratory tests are performed. The effect of the antibodies obtained from the mother is temporary. If the infant survives the tenth day of life without evidence of complications, his outlook is good. Except for anemia which is corrected easily by transfusion, erythroblastotic infants suffer no additional consequences of the disease after this time.

The treatment of erythroblastosis consists in the transfusion of Rh-negative blood to combat the anemia. The Rh-negative cells will persist in the infant's circulation, since they are unaffected by the antibodies received from the mother. While repeated simple transfusions are often effective, the more elaborate technic of exchange transfusion is to be preferred. Through a catheter inserted into the umbilical or some other large vein, small amounts of the infant's blood are withdrawn, and an equal amount of the Rh-negative donor's blood is injected. The procedure is continued until most of the circulating blood of the infant has been replaced. This technic not only provides new red cells, but also removes the harmful maternal antibodies and the products of the destruction of the infant's red cells which produce jaundice. Even moribund infants are sometimes salvaged by the prompt application of this treatment.

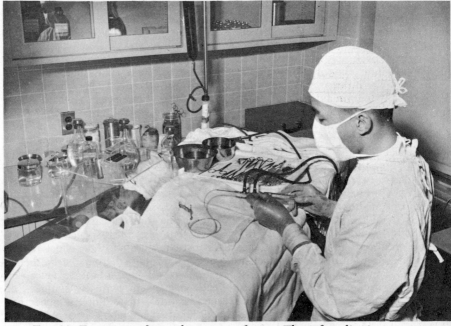

Fig. 30. Equipment for exchange transfusion. The infant lies in an oxygen hood with long umbilical cord protruding onto the sterile field. The plastic catheter is inserted into the umbilical vein of the cord. The operator removes blood into the syringe, ejects it through one tube, refills the syringe from the reservoir of Rh-negative blood and injects it into the infant. This sequence is repeated until approximately 500 ml. of blood has been withdrawn and replaced.

Exchange transfusion (Fig. 30) requires considerable preparation and is frequently an emergency procedure. Hence, it is desirable that the birth of an erythroblastotic infant be anticipated so that preparations may be made in advance. This can be done if all pregnant women are Rh-typed, and if Rh antibodies are sought periodically during pregnancy in the blood of those who might be expected to produce an erythroblastotic baby.

The nursing care of an infant with erythroblastosis consists of careful observations and supportive measures which provide protection during the period when he is receiving medical treatment. Babies born with erythroblastosis frequently require measures to combat shock. When the birth of an infant with erythroblastosis is anticipated, an incubator and oxygen should be in readiness to maintain the infant's temperature and to combat cyanosis. These babies are lethargic, due to generalized weakness and anemia. Frequent change in position prevents atelectasis and intercurrent infections.

Usually, the infant's strength to suckle is greatly reduced, indicating a need for a method of feeding that will conserve his energy. A nipple with enlarged holes or a medicine dropper may be required for feeding a weakened infant. With all methods of feeding, patience in feeding the infant slowly enough to prevent aspiration is necessary.

In caring for an infant with erythroblastosis, the nurse must be constantly on the alert to detect untoward symptoms. The nurse must not only assist with the replacement transfusion but also she must observe the infant's response during the procedure and in the period after it is completed. Untoward symptoms that need to be brought to the attention of the doctor include increasing weakness and jaundice, edema, pigmentation of the urine, increased respirations, cyanosis of the face or the nailbeds, and convulsions that result when the basal nuclei of the brain become damaged.

Hemorrhagic Disease of the Newborn

This is a condition in which spontaneous bleeding occurs during the first week of life. Hemorrhages may occur into the skin, from the orifices of the body, or from the umbilicus. Blood passed in the stool is called *melena*. Large hemorrhages or very numerous small ones occasionally threaten life from the loss of blood.

The disturbance is due to a failure of the blood to clot properly, which in turn is caused by an insufficient production of prothrombin, one of the main activators of the clotting mechanism. The body requires vitamin K in order to manufacture prothrombin. Before birth the infant obtains vitamin K from his mother; after birth it comes from his food or from the synthetic activity of the bacteria which invade his intestinal tract shortly after his birth. All infants have relatively low levels of prothrombin in the blood during the first few days of life. Premature infants and full-term infants whose mothers have not provided them with adequate amounts of vitamin K may suffer decreases of prothrombin to such low levels that hemorrhage occurs.

Treatment consists in supplying vitamin K by intramuscular injection, following which the infant begins to produce prothrombin at an adequate rate within an hour or two. In severe cases

where significant blood loss has occurred, transfusion is desirable to supply red blood cells and to correct the prothrombin deficiency at once. Prevention of hemorrhagic disease is advocated by some. Routine vitamin K injections are given either to the mothers a few hours before delivery or to the infants immediately after birth.

DISORDERS DUE TO TRAUMA AT BIRTH

Intracranial Injury

This is the most common and serious form of birth trauma. Since the head is the largest portion of the infant body which must traverse the birth canal, it is most likely to be damaged when delivery is difficult. Sudden, violent alterations in the shape of the skull, such as occur with precipitate delivery or difficult forceps or breech extractions, are more likely to result in injury than is the gradual molding of a slowly progressing labor. Temporary or permanent damage is suffered by various portions of the brain if their blood supply is compromised by edema or hemorrhage from large blood vessels that have torn or have burst in response to the unusual stresses. Large hemorrhages occur most commonly from the veins coursing in the membrane that separates the two halves of the brain (falx cerebri) or in the membrane that divides the cerebellum from the cerebrum (tentorium cerebelli). In premature infants the delicate vessels of the choroid plexus may burst, resulting in a hemorrhage into the ventricular system of the brain.

Following intracranial injury, the infant is abnormally sleepy, difficult to arouse, does not demonstrate the Moro reflex and may be unable to suck or to swallow. If intracranial pressure is high, his respirations are slow, irregular and periodic; his heart beats slowly; his fontanel bulges; and his eyes turn inward. There may be generalized spasticity of the muscles with backward arching of the head and the neck and extension of the legs. Evidence of irritation of the cerebral cortex may be present in the form of generalized convulsions or convulsive twitchings of muscle groups. The body temperature may be elevated or may hover at subnormal levels. In mild cases the symptoms are limited to general listlessness, poor appetite and occasional vomiting.

The prognosis following intracranial injury varies considerably, depending upon the extent and the location of the damage. When large or vital areas of the brain are affected, the immediate mortality is high, and infants who survive are likely to show spastic paralysis or mental retardation in later years. When the brain damage is less extensive, recovery may ensue with reasonably normal mental development. Neurologic complications, such as hemiplegia, convergent squint or convulsive attacks may appear later. In some cases recovery is complete without any residua.

Treatment is unsatisfactory, for there is seldom any opportunity to stop the bleeding or control the increased pressure within the skull. While waiting hopefully for the symptoms to subside spontaneously, general supportive measures are used. If there are convulsions, phenobarbital is indicated. Vitamin K usually is given in order to minimize bleeding. Unresponsive infants are not fed or handled any more than necessary, and measures to supply warmth or decrease elevated temperature are instituted. Sometimes it is possible to relieve intracranial pressure by withdrawing bloody fluid from the spinal canal or from the surface of the brain by tapping the dura at the lateral angle of the fontanel. The latter procedure may be repeated effectively if the bleeding has become localized to a walled-off area over the surface of the brain (subdural hematoma). The best management of intracranial injury is to prevent it through judicious obstetric management of the mother. Under ideal circumstances it is possible to reduce the infant deaths from this cause to less than 1 per thousand live-born babies.

Fractures

Sometimes fractures occur during birth. The clavicle suffers most frequently. It is broken by direct pressure of the finger during extraction of the shoulder. No special management is required, for this bone heals rapidly with the formation of a callus but without producing much pain or disability. Occasionally, linear fractures of the skull are discovered in infants whose birth has not been unusually difficult. Unless there is associated intracranial hemorrhage, such cracks are of trivial importance and heal quickly. Rarely, the humerus is broken during efforts to sweep the arm down over the face during breech delivery; or the femur may be fractured during version and extraction. Breaks of an extremity are usually apparent from the abnormal angulation that they produce. They heal well when immobilized in corrected position.

Brachial Palsy

This is a partial paralysis of one arm which results from excessive stretching of the nerve fibers that run from the neck through the shoulder and toward the arm. The trauma is produced by the forcible pulling of the shoulder away from the head during obstetric maneuvers. The most common type of paralysis involves the muscles of the upper arm and spares those of the hand and the fingers. The arm is held at the side with the elbow extended and the hand rotated inward. In mild cases when the injury is the result of stretching of nerve fibers that have not broken, recovery is rapid and may be complete within 3 weeks. More commonly, the fibers are stretched to such an extent that they break within their sheaths. Recovery from paralysis then depends upon the regeneration of nerves which are guided back to the appropriate muscles by the intact sheaths. Regeneration usually takes from 2 to 3 months. During the waiting period, the muscles of the shoulder should be manipulated gently and given massage to prevent contractures from forming. When recovery fails to take place within 3 months it probably indicates that the nerve roots have been torn loose from their connections with the spinal cord and that recovery will not occur unless the pathways can be restored surgically—a very difficult feat.

Asphyxia or Respiratory Failure

Initiation of Respiration in the Normal Infant

Once the newborn infant is separated from his mother he takes over the responsibility for oxygenating his blood through the activity of his own lungs. Under optimal circumstances the baby is born with a small amount of thin fluid in his respiratory passages. Perhaps even before his body is delivered, the stimulus of chilling or of manipulation, or the chemical changes taking place in his blood as the flow from the placenta is diminished, will activate the respiratory center in his brain. Thus a series of reflex muscular activities is set in motion, and they cause him to gasp and emit a cry—a most welcome sound in the delivery room! During the first few cries, most of the amniotic fluid in his lungs is expelled, and the air sacs become distended with air. Thus, oxygen is brought in contact with the lung capillaries. Adjustments are made in the fetal blood circulation which throw a larger proportion of blood through the lungs. The respiratory center in the brain gives periodic signals that remind him to breathe, and within a few seconds the infant is ready to oxygenate his own tissues and participate in his own survival.

Causes of Asphyxia

Taking over the responsibility for oxygenating his own blood through the activity of his own lungs is a critical step for the newborn infant, for if he fails to discharge this duty within a matter of a few minutes, he will either die or suffer irreparable damage. Infants who have difficulty in making this transition are said to suffer from asphyxia. The term is admittedly a broad one which encompasses respiratory failure from a number of causes. The asphyxiated infant presents an emergency which must be dealt with before there is time for more than a cursory examination. Frequently, the exact reason for this difficulty is not immediately apparent.

The normal sequence of events cited above may be impeded if (1) the respiratory movements are adequate but the air passages are obstructed, (2) the respiratory center fails to emit the proper signals to the muscles that move the chest and the diaphragm, (3) the respiratory movements and the airways are adequate but intrinsic factors in the lungs or the chest interfere with proper expansion of the lungs, or (4) respiratory movements, airway, lungs and chest are all normal but oxygenation of the blood is incomplete because of an abnormality of the heart or its major vessels.

Obstruction of the Air Passages. In actual practice attention is first directed to the infant's *airway*. Even before the first breath is taken, the secretions of the mouth and the nose should be sucked out gently to prevent them from being drawn back into the lungs. Thick mucus may block branches of the bronchial tree and prevent full expansion of the lungs. Inhaled meconium is an even worse offender, since it is very irritating and difficult to remove. During suction of the mouth the infant should be held inverted to promote drainage from the trachea. If these measures are deemed insufficient to clear the airway, an operator skilled in the use of the tracheal catheter or the infant bronchoscope should be called to deal with the secretions below the larynx. On rare occasions the airway may be blocked by congenital abnormalities of the larynx or by compression of the trachea by an anomalous structure within the chest.

Inactivity of the Respiratory Center. This condition is the most hazardous aspect of asphyxia. Under normal conditions, a fall in the oxygen content of the blood triggers the center to send out its signals. But the center will fail to respond if the oxygen concentration falls too low or if it is already damaged by prenatal anoxia, by intracranial injury, or by the injudicious administration of sedatives or anesthetics to the mother during the course of delivery.

If the infant has made no effort to breathe during the first minute after birth, resuscitative measures are begun. Frequently, a torpid respiratory center can be aroused by physical stimulation of the infant's skin through rubbing, slapping, or blowing upon it. Usually, oxygen is administered so that the maximum benefit will be derived from any respiratory effort, no matter how feeble. If a tracheal catheter is in place, oxygen can be carried directly into the lungs. Caution is needed in regulating the pressure so that the delicate lungs are not damaged by overdistention. Similar care must be exercised if any of the methods of artificial insufflation are used, i.e., mouth-to-mouth breathing, inflation of the lungs through a catheter, mechanical respirators or other devices. There is considerable difference of opinion about the actual effectiveness of these methods.

Drugs are sometimes but not dependably effective in stimulating respiration. Caffeine is the most dependable; epinephrine, Coramine, alpha-lobeline and Metrazol are also used. Recently, an antagonist for the morphine group of drugs (Nalline Hydrochloride) has appeared which seems to be effective in infants who are narcotized by overdosage of the mother.

Intrinsic Disorders of the Lung. ATELECTASIS. Chief among the intrinsic disorders of the lung which produce asphyxia is atelectasis. This term indicates that areas of the lung are collapsed without air in the alveoli (air sacs) and consequently are useless for respiratory exchange. At birth the lungs are normally collapsed and devoid of air, but with the first breath many air sacs inflate, and with each succeeding breath more areas are opened until expansion is complete. Atelectasis may be due to the initial failure of the air sacs to open up. This in turn may depend upon incomplete development of the lung, or feeble respiratory movements, or blockage by mucus in the small ducts leading to the air sacs. The anterior and superior portions of the lung open most easily so that atelectatic areas usually are found posteriorly at the base of the lung.

The symptoms depend upon the extent of the collapse. Small areas of atelectasis are often discovered accidentally when a chest roentgenogram is taken for some other purpose. No discernible symptoms may be present. Moderate degrees of atelectasis produce mild cyanosis but little distress. When extensive portions of the lung are involved there is cyanosis, labored or grunting respirations, weakness and ultimately exhaustion. Treatment consists of continuous administration of oxygen and saturation of the inspired air with water vapor. Oxygen is given so that those areas of lung that are open will have the maximum effect in oxygenating the blood passing through. The moist atmosphere is desirable in order to liquefy secretions and make it easier for the infant to cough them up. Frequent changes of position offer the best opportunity for the collapsed areas to open. Since there is danger that the inactive portions of lung will become infected secondarily, often some type of antibiotic is administered.

RESORPTION ATELECTASIS. A peculiar type of atelectasis is seen in some premature and some cesarean-delivered infants. It is called resorption atelectasis because the lungs seem to expand fairly well at first and then collapse again in spite of vigorous respiratory efforts on the part of the infant. This disorder often ends fatally within the first 48 hours. The lungs examined after birth reveal a peculiar hyaline membrane lining the walls of some of the alveoli. The origin of the membrane is not known.

The course of atelectasis depends upon the infant's general condition and the extent of the collapse. Vigorous infants with mild or moderate degrees of collapse usually improve slowly but progressively and seldom have symptoms that extend into the second week. They suffer no permanent damage to the lung. Feeble, weak, or anoxic infants have a poorer chance of survival. Among premature infants the outlook depends in part upon the birth weight—the smaller the infant the poorer his prognosis. Infants of 1,000 Gm. birth weight or less usually succumb because their lungs have not yet reached a stage of development that will support extrauterine life.

MALFORMATIONS, INTERSTITIAL EMPHYSEMA AND PNEUMOTHORAX. Other varieties of intrinsic disease of the chest or the lung include malformations, interstitial emphysema and pneumothorax. The lung may be completely absent on one side; or the diaphragm may be defective, permitting the intestines to invade the chest; or one or both lungs may be seeded with cysts containing air. Interstitial emphysema results when air is admitted into the space between the air sacs from a tear in the lining of one of them. If a large amount of air becomes trapped in this way, there will be insufficient room within the chest to permit expansion of the alveoli. Pneumothorax in the newborn is an extension of the process just mentioned. Air passes into the pleural space and collapses the lung, rendering it temporarily useless.

Congenital Malformations of the Heart and the Great Vessels. These abnormalities are considered in Chapter 18.

Nursing Care

Because the incidence of respiratory distress due to anoxia, asphyxia and resorption atelectasis is more frequent in babies who are born prematurely, postmaturely, by cesarean section and to mothers with complications of pregnancy, careful observation of these babies is imperative to prevent death. Their breathing is rapid with retraction of a moderate or severe degree and an expiratory grunt. Flaring of the nostrils, mottled skin, cyanosis, limpness and symptoms of shock are other associated symptoms. Symptoms develop rapidly, leaving the baby weak, apprehensive and close to the point of exhaustion. Therefore, early recognition of respiratory distress which enables the doctor to order supportive measures immediately is a lifesaving measure.

The baby with respiratory distress needs a nurse who can institute supportive measures immediately and watch him with undivided attention. Aspiration of gastric contents to prevent their inhalation and suctioning to keep the airway free of secretions are emergency measures. Oxygen, humidity and warmth must be provided constantly during the period of distress and be kept at a *constant level.* Feeding or administration of fluids is often deferred for the first few days, since by the end of that time either death or definite improvement is likely to occur. Infants who continue to have respiratory difficulty after this period need to be fed by gavage. Handling should be gentle and reduced to a minimum to avoid stimulation they cannot tolerate. Preventing distention is important, for it impedes normal expansion of the lung. Observing the infant's response to change in position helps the nurse to discover the position which gives him the most comfort. Prevention of infection is an important part of the nursing care for the addition of otherwise trivial disease may prove to be fatal to an infant who is already desperately ill.

Postnatal Infections

During the latter portion of the pregnancy the mother transmits to her infant antibodies against some of the infectious diseases to which she has become immune. Passive immunity of this sort protects the infant for a variable time after birth—about 6 months in the case of measles, probably less than 3 months for chickenpox, and not at all for whooping cough. Unfortunately, such a protective mechanism exists for only a few diseases. To most of the infectious ills of man, the newborn is highly susceptible. In fact, he may even become infected by those bacteria that normally dwell in his intestines (colon bacilli) or on his skin (staphylococci). The special measures which are designed to shield him from infection have been discussed earlier in this chapter. When these safeguards fail, the character of the ensuing infection has special implications for the newborn.

Sepsis

Sepsis occurs when bacteria gain access to and multiply in the blood stream. Thus, organisms are transported to all parts of the body and may set up secondary areas of infection almost anywhere. The portal of invasion is not always apparent. Sometimes the route passes from an infected umbilicus through the umbilical vessels to the liver and thence to the general circulation. At other times invasion appears to take place through normal skin or through the mucous membrane of the intestinal or respiratory tract.

The symptoms of sepsis are not uniform. In some cases there is a dramatic rise in temperature, rapid weight loss, convulsions, jaundice and hemorrhagic phenomena. Abscesses appear in the skin, or pus is coughed up from the lungs. To an experienced eye, the nature of the disease is obvious at once. In other cases the onset is more insidious. The temperature may remain normal or fall to subnormal levels. Sudden weight loss in spite of a reasonable food intake may be the only warning of trouble. Usually those caring for the infant sense that something is amiss, but the true state of affairs may not be uncovered until a systematic search for infection is made by taking cultures of the blood, the spinal fluid and the secretions of the nose and the throat.

In all cases cultures are most important, for treatment rests mainly upon the use of antibiotics, the rational use of which depends upon isolating the invading bacterium and determining its sensitivity to the drugs that are available. In addition to specific antibacterial therapy, transfusions and oxygen are commonly needed.

The prognosis of sepsis depends to a great extent upon the speed of recognition of the disease and the accuracy of antibiotic administration. Even with good care the mortality is high. If meningitis occurs, complications such as hydrocephalus, convulsions or mental retardation must be feared as sequels, even when a bacteriologic cure is obtained.

Pneumonia

Pneumonia in the newborn is always a serious disease. The added burden of infection is frequently more than the lungs can tolerate, for even in the healthy newborn they are tenuously prepared for their new function of respiration. Furthermore, the bacteria responsible for pneumonia of the newborn are less likely to respond to the common antibiotics. Instead of pneumococci and streptococci, the infant is more likely to be infected by staphylococci, colon bacilli, or other varieties of intestinal organisms. Pneumonia occasionally begins before birth when there is premature rupture of the membranes with infection of the amniotic fluid. When present at birth it is difficult to differentiate from atelectasis.

Epidemic Diarrhea

Epidemic diarrhea of the newborn is, as the name implies, a highly contagious disease which sweeps rapidly through nurseries into which it is introduced. The course is usually severe, and the mortality may run as high as 25 to 50 per cent of those affected. A single causative agent has not been clearly identified. However, several epidemics have now been traced to particularly virulent strains of colon bacilli—organisms which can be distinguished from normal intestinal bacteria only by special laboratory methods. The disease is presumed to gain access to the nursery either by breaks in technic during formula preparation or by spread from infected mothers or personnel who do not recognize disease in themselves.

The management of epidemic diarrhea is similar to that described for diarrhea in the older infants (Chap. 13). Rigid isolation technic must be used to limit the spread of the epidemic. Neomycin given orally is usually effective against the enteropathic strains of colon bacilli. Admission of infants to the nursery is discontinued, and unaffected infants and their mothers are dispersed to their homes as rapidly as possible. Personnel responsible for the care of infants outside the area should not be permitted to enter it.

Impetigo and Furunculosis

Impetigo and furunculosis of the skin occur more easily in the newborn than in the older child, because the resistance to skin bacteria is lower. These disorders are described in Chapter 15. The reputation of impetigo as a scourge of newborn nurseries probably is unwarranted today when the disease can be controlled rapidly with antibiotics.

Tetanus

Tetanus of the newborn is practically unknown in the United States but still occurs in countries where hygienic care of the umbilicus is so poor that tetanus spores may gain access to and grow in its recesses. The disease is described in Chapter 25.

Gonorrheal Conjunctivitis

Gonorrheal conjunctivitis (ophthalmia neonatorum) is losing its importance as a cause of congenital blindness, due in part to the impact of state laws that require prophylactic treatment of all infants at birth and in part to the advent of penicillin which provides an effective cure of the infection in both the mother and the child. The disease is acquired during birth by contamination of the infant's eyes with the infected secretions of the mother's vagina. The symptoms are similar to those of chemical conjunctivitis of the newborn but become evident on the second or the third day of life rather than in the first 12 to 24 hours. Prompt differentiation is important, for a delay in the treatment of gonorrheal conjunctivitis may permit ulceration and scarring of the cornea to occur. False security sometimes arises from the knowledge that silver nitrate presumably has been instilled in the birth-room. The technic of instillation of the drops into the eyes of a newborn infant is sufficiently difficult, however, that drops sometimes fail to get into the sacs. When the disease is suspected, smears and cultures of the pus should be made, but treatment usually is initiated before the laboratory results are known. Penicillin given by injections and by direct instillation into the conjunctival sacs at frequent intervals results in prompt healing.

Tuberculosis

Tuberculosis is practically unknown during the newborn period, but it must be kept in mind as a disease to which the small infant is highly susceptible. It is hazardous for him to go home into an environment in which he will come in contact with someone harboring an active form of tuberculosis. Special efforts should be made to see that not only his mother but all other members of his family as well are free from the disease. When this is impossible vaccination with BCG should be considered.

PREMATURITY

DEFINITION

A premature infant is one who is born before the conclusion of the normal period of gestation. Ideally, the determination of prematurity should be based upon the length of time that elapses between conception and birth. Methods for estimating the date of conception are so notoriously inaccurate that a less-debatable standard of classification—the birth weight—has been adopted universally. By international agreement a premature infant is now defined as one which weighs less than 2,500 grams (5½ lbs.) at birth. In setting this standard it is admitted that some infants who are actually premature by gestational age (less than 37 weeks) will be classified erroneously as mature; and, conversely, that some infants who are small for reasons other than short gestation periods will be labeled wrongly as premature.

CAUSES

A physiologic reason for prematurity is apparent in only about half the cases. Abnormal conditions in the mother are the most frequent explanation—toxemia of pregnancy, uterine bleeding, early rupture of the membranes, chronic heart, kidney or thyroid disease, diabetes, syphilis, tuberculosis, acute infections, accidents, or abdominal operations. When there is more than one fetus in the uterus, the excessive size sets off premature labor approximately 3 times out of 10. Some varieties of severe malformation of the fetus are responsible for premature labor.

Research to discover other causes of prematurity is urgently needed, for the majority of premature infants are born to women who show no symptoms of physical illness. Studies that have been done already disclose the fact that good prenatal care which included an adequate protein intake decreases the incidence of toxemia and prematurity.

INCIDENCE

Accepting the definition of prematurity stated above, most obstetric services find that from 5 to 8 per cent of their liveborn babies arrive prematurely. Because certain races normally have small infants, the incidence of prematurity is higher in population groups that have a large proportion of Negro or Asiatic mothers.

PREVENTION

The medical profession is attempting to prevent prematurity through improved services to all expectant mothers. Care that protects the infant as well as the mother is being provided for expectant mothers with placenta praevia and premature rupture of the membranes. Mothers with placenta praevia are hospitalized where bed rest and transfusions can be provided. Instead of inducing labor when membranes rupture spontaneously, some obstetricians are prescribing antibiotics, bed rest and careful perineal care. With special care which includes support to help the woman to adjust to her pregnancy, obstetricians are finding that the pregnancy continues for days and in some instances to term.

HANDICAPS

It is to be expected that an infant born before he has completed the biologic steps desirable for extra-uterine life will have a more difficult time making the adjustment than will the infant who is appropriately mature. This hypothesis is confirmed by mortality figures which show that the premature s chances of failing to survive are 10 to 15 times as great as the risk run by a full-term child. Of all the infant deaths occurring in the first month of life, more than half are in babies who were born prematurely. The handicaps that the premature must surmount in order to survive differ in kind, number and severity, depending upon the degree of his immaturity. The smaller the infant is at birth, the more arduous his struggle for survival. After a general survey of the problems that all prematures face and the care that these handicaps necessitate, the characteristics, the prognosis and the additional nursing care for infants with different degrees of immaturity will be considered in more detail.

Prenatal Disturbance

The same prenatal disturbance that produced the premature birth may constitute a serious handicap. An infant hastily delivered because of his mother's toxemia of pregnancy may be ill from the effects of the maternal disease; one who was extracted because of maternal bleeding may have suffered anoxic damage to the brain as described previously. Syphilis in the mother may mean both premature birth and an infection for the infant. Erythroblastosis or severe anomalies may pose insuperable handicaps for the premature infant.

Difficulty in Establishing Respiration

There are many reasons why difficulty in establishing respiration is by all odds the most common single cause of death among premature infants. In the very immature infant the fault lies within the lungs themselves, for important structural changes take place during the second half of pregnancy which enlarge the potential air sacs and bring them into closer approximation to the lung capillaries. Failure of this change to proceed to a critical point in the development of the lung accounts for most of the deaths attributed to "previability." In addition, the small premature is handicapped by weakness of the muscles that move his chest wall and by the plasticity of the bony framework which permits it to retract during inspiration, cutting down the effective expansion of the lungs within. Frequently, the stimulation of the respiratory center in the brain is irregular. An added hazard of the first few days is resorption atelectasis, a peculiar variety of lung disorder which has been mentioned above and is primarily a disease of premature infants.

Even when the respiratory apparatus permits survival, symptoms of respiratory difficulty are apparent. The small premature infant is likely to show irregular, periodic breathing interspersed with long moments of apnea. Mild cyanosis is intermittently present.

The administration of oxygen relieves cyanosis and increases the rate and the regularity of respiration in the premature infant. However, its use must be tempered by the realization that oxygen in high concentration in the inspired air is the main cause of retrolental fibroplasia in the premature infant. The former practice of placing all prematures routinely in oxygen until respiratory sufficiency was proved has now given way to the cautious administration only when need is clearly demonstrated by the infant's condition. Since it has been shown that the danger from oxygen mounts rapidly when the concentration rises above 40 to 50 per cent in the inspired air, most premature nurseries require periodic testing of the concentrations in incubators, or use a supply which cannot yield more than 40 per cent. Use of higher concentrations cannot be categorically forbidden but should be regarded as an emergency procedure.

The water content of the atmosphere in the incubator should be kept as high as possible, for if the secretions within

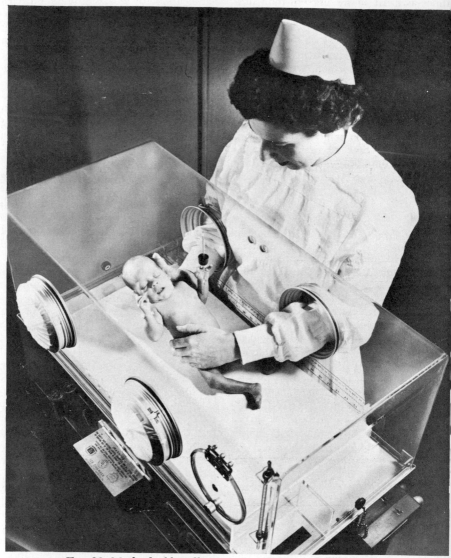

Fig. 31. Method of handling a premature baby in an Isolette.
(Air Shields, Inc., Hatboro, Pa.)

he bronchial tree are allowed to dry out, they will block the exchange of air and produce additional areas of atelectasis. In many nurseries devices are now used to create a mist or fog within the incubator in which the smaller infants are housed.

The question of respiratory adequacy usually is settled within the first 2 or 3 days of life. If the infant survives this period he may still have some unexpanded areas of lung, but unless he is handicapped further by infection, the areas of atelectasis will be of decreasing importance to him. As with most other handicaps, the frequency and the severity of atelectasis are greater the less mature the infant is at birth.

Body Temperature

The premature infant has difficulty in regulating his body temperature, for it responds rather promptly to changes in the temperature of the surrounding environment. When placed in cold or drafty surroundings he has trouble conserving his body heat. As a result, his temperature may fall to subnormal levels. The factors that interfere with his efforts to hold or produce body heat are the relatively large surface area in proportion to his body size, the lack of an insulating layer of fat beneath his skin, poor reflex control of his skin capillaries, and the smallness and the inactivity of his muscles—the main source from which body heat is obtained. When the premature is placed in a hot environment, poor control over his skin capillaries and the lack of an adequate sweating mechanism prevent him from losing heat, and his body temperature rises accordingly.

Some type of mechanical incubator is highly desirable if not essential to the small premature infant in order to keep him at a stable temperature and to supply adequately humidified air (Fig. 31). Now it is recognized that environmental temperature should be adjusted so that his body temperature ranges between 35.5° and 36.5° C. (96° to 98° F.) rather than attempting to push it up to the accepted normal range for older infants. At such lower levels stability is obtained more easily. The premature nursery should be kept warm (80° F.) and free of drafts. In hot climates and seasons, air conditioning is desirable. The humidity of the air should be kept between 55 and 65 per cent. Premature infants dehydrate easily. In humidified nurseries it has been found that initial loss of weight is less, the regaining of birth weight is more rapid, body temperature stabilizes more easily, and the incidence of respiratory infections and gastro-intestinal disturbances is lower.

Poor Resistance to Infection

The premature infant's resistance to infection is notoriously poor. He receives less than the usual quantity of protective substances from his mother's blood and is denied the benefits of her early milk (colostrum). In addition, his ability to manufacture his own body proteins, including antibodies, is below par.

Protective measures to prevent infection are imperative because even trivial infections may be devastating to him. The organization of the nursery facilities should be such that prematures are kept in a unit separated from other children and even from the nursery for full-term newborn infants. None but a minimum number of essential personnel should be permitted within the unit. Isolation and aseptic precautions should be observed. The mere suggestion of an infection in one of the personnel should be considered as an adequate reason for excluding that individual from the unit until recovery is complete. Prematures born outside of the hospital and those who develop infections should be kept in a separate area. Modern incubators provide additional safeguards within the nursery. Some are so designed that the infant's complete care can be carried out without removing him from the enclosed space of the incubator. It is desirable to sterilize the clothing that comes in direct contact with the infant's skin and also the cotton and the oil that are used for cleansing. The nurse needs to be constantly alert to observe symptoms which might indicate the onset of any type of skin, respiratory or gastro-intestinal infection. In some nurseries it is standard practice to administer antibiotics to all small prematures until they have made a promising start and whenever any suspicion of infection arises.

Biochemical Handicaps

A large number of biochemical handicaps of the premature infant can be enumerated. These arise in part from his extremely rapid growth rate, in part from the immaturity of organs such as the liver and the kidneys, and in part from his failure to linger within the uterus long enough to acquire his full complement of certain essential materials.

The premature infant grows more rapidly than the full-term infant and requires a relatively large amount of food to supply building materials and energy. No other human being grows as rapidly as the premature infant. It is not uncommon for him to double his initial birth weight in the brief span of 2 months! In order to do this, if calculated in terms of calories per unit of weight, his requirements are from 30 to 50 per cent greater than those of the full-term infant.

The immaturity of the premature infant's digestive and nervous systems complicates the technic of meeting his food requirements. The limited capacity of his stomach must not be exceeded, for vomiting and aspiration of food into his lungs are to be avoided at all costs. The mere ability to suck and to swallow is sometimes lacking or too exhausting for him to perform frequently. Special methods must be used to convey food into his stomach. The ability of his intestinal tract to digest the food brought

to it is also limited, particularly in respect to fat which he tolerates poorly. Care must be taken to see that too much is not forced upon him, for if his tolerance for digestion is exceeded diarrhea may result.

Immaturity of the liver accounts in part for the premature's poor resistance to infection (he forms antibody protein poorly); for his tendency to bleed (he forms prothrombin poorly); for his tendency to become edematous (his total serum protein concentration is low); and for his susceptibility to jaundice (his liver cannot adequately clear the blood of the pigments which result from the normal postnatal destruction of circulating red blood cells). Immaturity of the kidneys contributes to his limited tolerance for salt, to his tendency to become edematous and to the mild state of acidosis in which the premature normally lives.

The premature infant is born before he has fortified himself with his full quota of Vitamins A, C, D and K and of the minerals phosphorus, calcium and iron, yet the rapidity of his immediate postnatal growth demands an unusual supply of these substances. During the last 2 months of pregnancy the full-term infant draws upon his mother for stores of vitamins and minerals and therefore is protected temporarily from the vitamin-deficiency diseases such as rickets, scurvy and hemorrhagic disease of the newborn. Prophylactic quantities of the corresponding vitamins usually are given to the premature in double the dosage recommended for the full-term infant.* Calcium and phosphorus are present in milk in abundance to satisfy the needs of prematures. Iron is not supplied in adequate amounts by most feedings. Even when the diet is supplemented with medicinal iron, absorption is poor during the first 6 to 8 weeks of life. However, it is commonly

* Liberal use of Vitamin K prophylactically is now suspected as a cause of kernicterus in prematures. Dosage of menadione should not exceed 1 to 2 mg.

added in the hope of preventing as far as possible the anemia that regularly develops in the growing premature.

Retrolental Fibroplasia

Since 1940 a disease peculiar to premature infants has been recognized. In its fully developed form retrolental fibroplasia involves both eyes and produces complete or nearly complete blindness due to separation and fibrosis of the retina. It now constitutes the chief cause of neonatal blindness and is the object of intensive study by many institutions that care for prematures.

The main peculiarities of the disease are that it apparently did not exist before 1935; that it attacks the most immature infants more frequently than the larger prematures; that its incidence is extremely variable among different populations of prematures; and that its effects are not immediately apparent but are discovered only after weeks or months have elapsed. If the eyes of all premature infants are examined at regular intervals with the aid of an ophthalmoscope, the early pathologic changes may be observed some time before the infant reaches a weight of 1,500 to 1,800 Gm. These consist of dilation of retinal veins, hemorrhage and exudate into the retina and areas of separation of the retina from the inner surface of the eyeball. In some infants these changes regress, but in others there is progressive detachment of the retina until it is brought forward into an irregular, useless fibrotic mass retaining perhaps some light perception but no useful vision. The matted retina can be seen through the pupil as a greenish opacity. Unless routine ophthalmoscopic examination of eyes is made, loss of vision may be easily overlooked in small infants until they are 3 to 4 months of age.

Experimental and clinical study has demonstrated that the main factor in the causation of retrolental fibroplasia is oxygen poisoning. The premature's delicate retinal vessels are unusually susceptible to high concentrations of oxygen and go into spasm which in turn leads to leakage of blood or serum through their walls. Extensive clinical study has shown that retrolental fibroplasia can be virtually eliminated from premature populations if oxygen is restricted to emergency use and if concentrations are never allowed to exceed 40 per cent. Most nurseries now monitor concentrations in incubators by periodic testing and adjustment of the flow of oxygen, or by valves in incubators which presumably limit the concentrations attainable, or by using a mixture of oxygen and nitrogen which makes it impossible to exceed 40 per cent concentration of oxygen. Careless and unnecessary use of oxygen is to be condemned, yet occasions arise when it cannot be withheld if the infant's life is to be saved. Other factors such as excessive salt intake and overtransfusion may play a role in the causation of retrolental fibroplasia.

NURSING CARE OF THE PREMATURE

In spite of the many hazards that beset prematurely born infants, from 75 to 85 per cent of them will survive if given reasonably adequate care. Better obstetric practices, new medical discoveries and improved mechanical aids are all contributing to better care for these infants. But the benefits of such advances are easily erased if the daily nursing care of the infant is slighted. Many a prematurely born child owes his life in a very real sense to the devotion, the skill and the judgment of the nurses who ministered to his early needs. The requirements of care differ with the initial size of the premature and will be considered separately for each of the main subdivisions by weight.

Prematures of 400 to 1,000 Gm.
(14 oz. to 2 lbs. 3 oz.)

With good luck and meticulous care about 10 per cent of these infants can be reared. Fetuses of less than 400 Gm. are classified as abortions. They never develop effective respirations and die

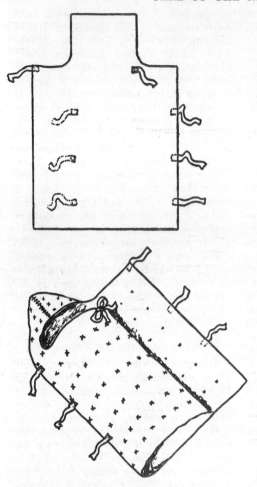

FIG. 32. Illustrating method of making jacket for a premature infant.

within a short time after birth. Infants of birth weights between 400 and 1,000 Gm. are called previable and generally are not expected to survive but some show unusual strength and survive despite their initial handicaps. Infants of such small size are infrequent. They comprise about 0.5 per cent of all live births and about 7 per cent of premature births.

Many external evidences of immaturity are present in this group of premature infants whose gestation period ranges from 20 to 28 weeks and length measures from 28 to 35 cm. (11 to 14 in.). The head is proportionately quite large, with high forehead and small facial features. The eyes are tiny, scarcely visible; the ears are soft and poorly developed; the chin recedes. The extremities are spindly, with tiny muscles and soft rudimentary nails on the fingers and the toes. The skin may be covered with lanugo hair. The subcutaneous tissues are usually full, giving the appearance of plumpness. But if the infant survives a few days the skin hangs loosely on his body, demonstrating that the original appearance was due to edema rather than subcutaneous fat.

Nipples and genitalia are small, and in male infants the testes are often undescended. Activity of the infant is limited to the respiratory efforts, which may be weak and unpredictable. The soft chest wall retracts excessively during inspiration, and the mouth often opens in a gulping fashion. The sucking, swallowing and gag reflexes are usually absent in these very immature infants. They seldom cry. Cyanosis may be present constantly or during periods of prolonged apnea.

If he can weather the first 48 hours of life, the previable infant has a chance of ultimate survival. Deaths are usually due to failure to establish respirations, and less commonly to intracranial hemorrhage.

The first objectives of nursing care are to maintain a stable, appropriate body temperature, to conserve body heat and muscular energy, and to support the respiratory effort by the administration of humidified air and oxygen supplemented by stimulation as indicated. The infant should be placed at once in an incubator, preferably one that has been preheated to 90° to 95° F. Oxygen in a concentration of 40 per cent should be available. The highest concentration of water vapor that can be obtained with the available apparatus should be maintained. Then the infant should be disturbed only for necessary suction aspiration of secretions from the mouth and the nose and for the injection of vitamin K and antibiotics as prescribed. Stimulants or periodic brief inhalations of a 5 per cent carbon dioxide in oxygen mixture may be required if the respiratory effort fails.

Constant nursing care during the first 24 hours after birth is essential. Respirations, color, activity, temperature, cry, condition of the skin and the cord, the bladder and bowel function should be observed. A bulb syringe or a suction set consisting of a mouthpiece, 4 inches of rubber tubing, a Murphy drip bulb and a No. 8 or 10 catheter should be in readiness in the infant's unit. When cyanosis and difficult breathing occur the nurse should pass the catheter through the mouth and into the back of the throat to remove by suction the mucus obstruction. This should be done *before* carbon dioxide 5 per cent in oxygen is administered. Carbon dioxide stimulates respiration. If it is given before mucus is withdrawn by suction, the infant may aspirate as he inhales.

When mechanical incubators are not available for the care of a small premature, other means of supplying external heat must be provided. Stabilization of body temperature may be attempted by wrapping the infant in a close-fitting parka made of outing flannel or of alternate layers of cotton and gauze (Fig. 32). A bed constructed within a box or a large basket and heated by hot-water bottles or electric lamp may serve to keep the immediate environmental temperature suitable. A thermometer placed between the blankets and the infant and bottles of water at a temperature of from 100° to 105° F. can be used as aids in controlling the temperature. When the water is changed, it should be done at the bedside to avoid a prolonged drop in environmental temperature. The room should be kept at a temperature of 85° to 90° F. The infant's temperature will stabilize more readily when environmental temperature is elevated than when he is heavily clothed and covered with additional blankets. His temperature should be taken every 2 to 3 hours until stabilization is acquired; thereafter, twice daily is sufficient. Administration of oxygen through a mask is serviceable but gives poor humidification and variable control of concentration.

Administration of food or fluid to these delicate infants usually is deferred for a day or two until they have had a chance to establish their respirations and to lose the edema fluid with which they were born. Since early feedings must be small in volume, additional fluid may be given by subcutaneous injection. Glucose solutions are generally preferred to salt-containing fluids which may result in a return of edema.

In the absence of the normal sucking and swallowing reflexes, the first food must be administered by gavage. This process of tube feeding is also least tiring to the infant. The technic is as follows:

Equipment for gavage (Fig. 33) consists of a sterile catheter (No. 8 or 10F), a medicine glass containing sterile water, a glass syringe barrel, and the prescribed food. The infant is placed on his back for the treatment. The distance from the tip of the nose to the ensiform process should be marked on the catheter with an indelible pencil before preparation of the equipment. This distance corresponds to that from the lips to the lower part of the esophagus immediately above the cardiac orifice. This site for the end of the catheter is

preferable in order to avoid vomiting. The catheter should be connected to the syringe barrel, lubricated with sterile water and passed into the esophagus through the mouth. When the marked portion of the catheter reaches the lips, the mouth of the syringe barrel is placed in the medicine glass of water to test the position of the catheter. The tube is not likely to enter the larynx and the trachea, but if it should, air will bubble through the water in the glass on expiration by the baby. In addition, the baby would become cyanotic, and if he were sufficiently vigorous he would have a spasm of coughing at the time the tube was inserted. After the tube has been passed properly, the syringe barrel is held stable in one hand, and the food is poured into the barrel with the other. After the food is poured, the barrel may be elevated sufficiently to allow the food to run slowly into the stomach. After the food has run in, the tube should be removed, *first having*

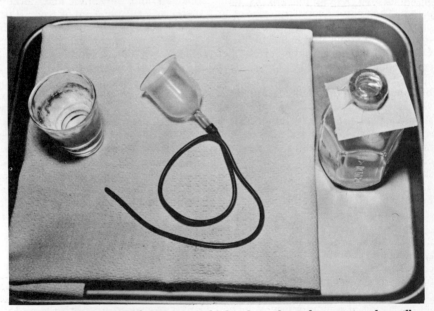

Fig. 33. Equipment for gavage. The bottle to the right contains the milk mixture. The medicine glass contains sterile water for catheter lubrication and testing for anatomic position.

been tightly pinched or bent onto itself.
Because the infant tends to gasp as the
tube is removed, every precaution must
be taken to prevent aspiration of milk
that may have remained in the tube. At
the end of the feeding, the infant should
be turned on his right side to lessen
stomach-emptying time. If a tendency
to regurgitation exists, the infant's head
and thorax should be elevated slightly.

The type of food, the amount, the
frequency and the method of feeding
are prescribed in accordance with the
infant's weight, physical response to
ingestion of food and to his ability to
suckle. Although breast milk is used
sometimes as a feeding for small prematures, artificial formulas consisting of
half-skimmed milk with added salt-free
carbohydrate are generally preferred.
The quantity of feeding must be restricted to a few cubic centimeters at a
time until the infant's capacity is
learned. Overloading his stomach must
be avoided at all costs, for a single
episode of vomiting and aspiration may
prove to be fatal. Not only is regurgitation to be avoided but also abdominal
distention. Distention is a cause of
cyanotic attacks because it interferes
with respiration, which is chiefly dia-
phragmatic. Gavage feedings may be
given as often as every 2 hours. The
amounts given are increased gradually
until the food intake reaches 120 to 140
calories per kilogram (55 to 65 calories
per pound) of body weight. Water-
miscible preparations of vitamins A, B,
C and D which may be added to the
gavage feedings are available. When the
infant begins to suck on the gavage
tube, cautious trials may be made with
feedings from a dropper.

Carefully given medicine-dropper
feedings protect the premature infant
and increase his pleasure in the feeding
experience. A medicine glass containing the prescribed feeding should be
kept warm throughout the procedure.
After the infant's diaper has been
changed and the nurse's hands thor-

oughly washed, the nurse should support his head and shoulders with one
hand and open his mouth by applying
gentle pressure to the chin. Milk is
dropped from a medicine dropper,
sheathed in rubber tubing, well back
onto the tongue, a drop at a time until
the infant's ability to swallow has been
ascertained. The feeding should not be
hurried or forced. Gentle pressure on
the back of the tongue may be used to
stimulate swallowing. Food should not
be left in the mouth at the conclusion of
the feeding. The infant may be supported partially erect for a while in
order to permit bubbling. Then he
should be placed on his right side with
head slightly elevated to facilitate
gastric emptying.

During the initial medicine-dropper
feedings, the nurse should observe him
for signs of fatigue. If the feeding experience leads to cyanosis and increased
lassitude instead of pleasure, resumption of gavage feedings is indicated until
he demonstrates increased capacity to
participate with comfort.

The necessary early caution in feeding, combined with the loss of edema
fluid, results in a rather sizable loss of
weight during the first 2 weeks. Ordinarily, it takes from 3 to 5 weeks at
least for the previable infant to regain
his initial weight and make a steady
daily increment. Three months or more
may elapse before such an infant reaches
the premature graduation weight of
2,500 grams.

The prognosis of the previable infant
is difficult to estimate. Too few of those
who survive are observed in follow-up
studies, and as a result any accurate
estimate of the long-range prognosis is
impossible. Previable infants who survive generally have rather large heads
with narrow faces and slender body
habitus. Their early growth and development is likely to be at least 3 months
retarded for their chronologic age. Most
of them catch up gradually, and some
at least reach adult life with perfectly

normal mental competence. The risk of retrolental fibroplasia is a significant one in these small infants. Medicinal iron usually is given at 4 to 6 weeks of age. Administration must be started cautiously in order to avoid vomiting or diarrhea.

Prematures of 1,000 to 1,500 Gm. (2 lbs. 3 oz. to 3 lbs. 5 oz.)

Since most of these infants have reached a stage of pulmonary maturity that can support life, the anticipated survival rate is distinctly better—from 40 to 50 per cent. Most of the deaths will occur in the first 48 hours of life from resorption atelectasis, pulmonary hemorrhage, or the effects of anoxia or intracranial injury. The number of infants born with weights in this range is slightly greater than the number of previable infants—a little over 0.5 per cent of total live births and about 10 per cent of all premature births. The gestational age ranges from 28 to 32 weeks, and the infants measure from 35 to 40 cm. (14 to 16 in.) in length.

The physical features are similar to those of the previable infant but less extreme in their divergence from the normal term infant. Periodic and ineffectual respiratory effort is common but not universal. Temperature regulation is poor. The sucking, swallowing and gag reflexes may be present at birth, but gavage feeding is still required as an introductory measure.

The early nursing care is identical with that of the previable infant but is required for a shorter period of time. Many infants in this group will be able to dispense with gavage feedings and the mechanical incubator within the first weeks of life. Initial weight losses are usually marked, but the food intake can be increased at a more rapid pace, and the birth weight is often regained by 3 to 4 weeks of age, and steady weight progress is made thereafter.

Prematures in this group can tolerate more handling after their initial adjust-ment to extra-uterine life has been made. The exposure incident to a daily soap-and-water bath should be avoided in most instances, at least for the first week or two. Warmed oil baths may be given every other day until the infant reaches the weight of 5½ pounds. On alternate days care should be given to the head and the genitalia as the entire body and behavior are observed to appraise the general condition. During the period of adjustment daily weighing may be eliminated. When the infant is weighed, exposure should be prevented. The scale should be balanced with a diaper or paper that completely covers the scale pan, and with whatever clothing is to be used. The infant should be covered with a blanket while being carried to the scales. Before the infant is weighed, he should be dressed in the clothing provided. This method prevents undue exposure and lessens the amount of handling.

These infants, too, will bear the marks of their prematurity for many months after birth—large, narrow heads, important degrees of anemia, retardation of growth and development by at least 2 months. Their chances for eventually having normal mentality and size are good. The risk of developing retrolental fibroplasia is still significant if oxygen is used heedlessly.

Prematures of 1,500 to 2,000 Gm. (3 lbs. 5 oz. to 4 lbs. 6 oz.)

The added maturity greatly improves the rate of survival in this group of infants, so that 75 to 80 per cent may be expected to live. The gestational ages approximate 32 to 35 weeks, and the length at birth varies from 40 to 43 cm. (15½ to 16½ in.). About twice as many infants are born with weights in this range as in the preceding group—somewhat over 1 per cent of total live births and about 20 per cent of all prematures.

The physical characteristics of extreme prematurity are less marked. Heads are not as large relatively, edema is less common, and some of the infants show a modest amount of subcutaneous fat. Although initial respiratory difficulty will create a problem for some of them, routine use of high humidity is no longer necessary. The ability to stabilize body temperature is much better, so that most of these infants can be transferred rapidly to a heated crib or an ordinary crib in an evenly warmed room. The sucking, gag and swallowing reflexes are regularly present unless the infant is abnormal in some manner apart from his prematurity. Feeding by gavage is generally unnecessary.

Medicine-dropper feedings may be necessary temporarily for some of these babies, but the majority of them soon indicate their ability and eagerness for sucking activity. The more vigorous infants in this group may be fed from a bottle with a soft-rubber nipple after the initial dropper feeding. The nipple should be chosen with care. It should not have holes that are too large or too small. When the nipple holes are too small, the infant becomes unduly fatigued; when they are too large the baby is forced beyond his capacity and he is deprived of the pleasure and the exercise that sucking supplies.

As soon as the infant's physical condition permits, he should be fed according to his manifest hunger needs and held throughout the feedings. Like the full-term infant, he, too, needs freedom from frustration, as well as cuddling associated with his feedings. From the moment of birth the nurse should be sensitive to the discomforts and the hazards that the prematurely born infant is experiencing, both physically and emotionally. Nursing measures that preserve life and provide gratification should be carried out. He needs a soothing, warm and tranquil environment; he requires interest in him as an individual and care that takes into account his emotional as well as his physical needs. It is possible to gratify an infant when he signals his distress,

be it from insufficient sucking, hunger or sheer loneliness and a need for closeness, without exposing him to infection, overfeeding, or fatigue.

Within this group steady weight gains are generally established by 2 to 3 weeks of age, and growth and development proceed at a rate that is about 1 to 2 months behind the average for the chronologic age. The risk of retrolental fibroplasia is greatly diminished but not entirely absent.

Prematures of 2,000 to 2,500 Gm. (4 lbs. 6 oz. to 5 lbs. 8 oz.)

The degree of prematurity is mild in this group of infants, and a proportional reduction in the handicaps permits from 90 to 95 per cent or even more of them to survive. The bulk of the premature infants fall within this weight range—about 4 per cent of the total births and from 60 to 65 per cent of all the premature births. The gestational ages approximate 35 to 38 weeks, and the infants measure from 43 to 47 cm. (16½ to 18 in.) in length.

Apart from smallness, the physical characteristics and care differ little from those of full-term infants. Slenderness and hyperactivity are common. Mechanical apparatus for the regulation of body temperatures or for the administration of oxygen and humidified air is seldom required. Bottle feeding may be commenced at once, and the infants can be picked up and held during feeding. Some of the larger and more vigorous members of this group can be cared for in the regular nursery or may visit their mothers. Most of them will begin to gain weight steadily after 10 days to 2 weeks. Few of them will have to remain within the confines of the premature nursery for more than a month. Immediate direct breast-feeding is feasible for some of the larger infants; eventual nursing can be carried out for most of them. Mothers should be encouraged to keep their supplies of breast milk flowing by regular emptying of the breast with manual expression or by the use of a breast pump. The main reason for segregating these large prematures from the full-term infants is to shield them from infection and to give them the benefit of skilled assistance in their early feedings.

Growth and development proceed at a pace that is only temporarily behind that of other infants of the same age. Nearly all of them will catch up within the first 6 months of life. Retrolental fibroplasia is seldom found in infants of this degree of maturity.

MATERNAL PREPARATION

Preparing the mother for the care of her prematurely born infant should begin in the immediate postpartum period and continue until she has developed confidence in her ability to understand and meet his needs. To alleviate the mother's anxiety the nurse must be able to understand the emotional problems common to those who give birth to prematurely born infants. Also, she must satisfy the mother's need to learn about her infant and offer reassurance which will help her to assume the responsibilities entailed in his care after he leaves the hospital. The necessity for frequent, cautious feeding, for the administration of vitamins, for avoidance of infection and for periodic medical examination can be emphasized in a way that not only ensures protective care of the infant but also conveys the nurse's confidence in the mother's ability to meet his needs as well. A practical demonstration with opportunity to practice various aspects of the infant's care and to share her feelings concerning him and his care must be offered to the mother before she takes him home.

Many mothers of prematurely born infants also need the help of the visiting nurse during the period when they are becoming adjusted to their maternal role. Ideally, the nurse should visit the home before the infant leaves the hos-

pital. In such a visit the nurse can center her interest in the mother in an attempt to understand her problems as she anticipates taking over the care of her baby. Also, she can appraise the physical surroundings, the available equipment, and the mother's readiness to give her infant care. She will need to discover the supportive supervision that the mother will require in the period when she begins to take over the responsibility of his care. She will need to return later after the baby has been discharged to render assistance in accordance with her individual requirements.

The mother of a premature infant often requires extended counseling and support to alleviate anxiety and to help her to understand his changing needs. Her attitude toward the infant is easily distorted by the anxieties that assail her at various stages of his early life. At first she is concerned about whether or not he will survive. Then she worries about his prospects for achieving ultimate normal development. At the time of departure from the hospital she is likely to be anxious about the special precautions and requirements of his care and perhaps be dubious about her ability to carry them out as expertly as the nurse. She often believes that he will need the same protective care that he required when he was smaller and one among many in a hospital nursery. The infant's early behavior at home is not always reassuring, for often he is emotionally unstable, requires frequent, self-regulated feedings and much more attention and holding than the average full-term infant who has just emerged from the hospital. This is especially true if he has been in a busy nursery and subjected to rigid schedules which have prevented him from acquiring a degree of trust. In so far as she can honestly do so, the nurse should offer reassurance and encouragement rather than criticism and hints at additional topics for concern.

After the mother has weathered the

first months at home, she will need help to direct her attention to the infant's needs to become gradually prepared for the socialization process. She may need help in recognizing her infant's developing powers and signs of readiness to explore, to begin learning to tolerate small amounts of frustration and to develop increasing amounts of independence. Like any other child, he must learn to deal with disappointment and frustration and gradually learn to adjust himself to social living. If his mother shields him from such experiences for too long a period he is likely to be an unhappy child, poorly prepared for neighborhood and school life.

Certain personality characteristics have been observed in infants born prematurely. Investigators who have studied children who were born prematurely found that they showed a tendency to prolonged thumb-sucking, maternal overdependence, negativism, emotional instability, difficulty in establishing bowel and bladder control and in mastering speech.

Investigators have ascribed the premature behavior syndrome to certain physical and environmental factors. The prematurely born infant's nervous system is less mature than is that of the full-term infant. He is exposed to extra-uterine existence before he is ready to adapt himself to it. As a result he experiences more frustration and untimely stimulation than the full-term infant. In addition, he must begin life with the care of many people rather than with the care of one mother who can provide

warm, consistent care. Early in life he requires extra protection and solicitude. Many mothers have difficulty in accepting the fact that the original delicate condition which required special protective measures was a temporary phenomenon. They overprotect and infantilize their children after they have approached the status normal for their age. Simultaneously, however, in their eagerness for them to stand well with other children of their age, they expect performance that is beyond their capacity to achieve. Under such circumstances disturbances in the mother-child relationship are inevitable.

Assisting mothers in observing their infants' individual readiness for experiences which help them to adjust to the social customs of their society can help to prevent the premature behavior syndrome that Shirley describes. The behavior expected should conform to the infant's biologic age rather than to his extra-uterine chronologic age. Over-expectancy produces tension within the child; therefore, learning becomes more difficult. Permitting the infant the gratification that comes when his signal of need is met early in life and observing clues that indicate his preparedness for less dependent care and more self-directed activity is the kind of guidance that any young child requires, be he premature, physically handicapped or normal. Both infantilization and unreasonable expectations which demand more than the child can accomplish with comfort and satisfaction prevent healthy ego growth.

SITUATIONS FOR FURTHER STUDY

1. What are some of the characteristic fears of the new mother? How can the nurse help to alleviate them?

2. What adjustments must the newborn infant make to extra-uterine life?

3. What are the physical and emotional needs of the infant during the neonatal period?

4. What are the dangers of anoxia? How can the nurse function to prevent it?

5. Select a newborn infant in the pediatric ward, observe him and describe the way his physical condition frustrates his emotional needs. How could you lessen his frustration? De-

scribe the nursing care that you think he needs.

6. From observation of a prematurely born infant of from 800 to 1,000 Gm. in weight, list the characteristics that differentiate him from a full-term infant. As a result of these physiologic characteristics, what are his nursing needs? How would his nursing care differ from that required by a premature infant of 2,000 Gm. in weight?

7. Study mortality-rate statistics of infants born prematurely. At what period of life do most deaths occur? By what measures could this rate be reduced?

8. How do you think a mother would feel giving birth to a premature infant? Observe her behavior as you help her learn to take care of her baby before she takes him home. Provide her with an opportunity to talk about her feelings and write a report of the understanding you acquired during the experience.

BIBLIOGRAPHY

Adams, Margaret: Appraisal of a newborn infant, Am. J. Nursing 55:1336, 1955.

Blake, F. G.: Nursing care during the adjustment period (birth to 3 months): its influence on the child's feelings about the world in The Child, His Parents and the Nurse, chap. 3, p. 53, Philadelphia, Lippincott, 1954.

Drorbaugh, James E., and Fogg, Marguerite F.: Respiratory distress in the newborn infant, Am. J. Nursing 56: 1559, 1956.

Dunham, E. C.: Premature Infants; A Manual for Physicians, ed. 2, New York, Harper, 1955.

Grayson, Robert, and Cranch, Gene S.: Care of the foreskin, Am. J. Nursing 56:75, 1956.

Greene, D. M.: Caring for the premature baby, Am. J. Nursing 50:458, 1950.

Lundeen, Evelyn, and Kunstadter,
Ralph: Care of the Premature Infant, Philadelphia, Lippincott, 1958.

Miller, H. F., and Conklin, E. V.: Clinical evaluation of respiratory insufficiency in newborn infants, Pediatrics 16:427, 1955.

Parmelee, A. H.: Management of the Newborn, Chicago, Year Book Pub., 1952.

Patz, A.: The role of oxygen in retrolental fibroplasia, Pediatrics 19:504, 1957.

Potter, Edith: Pathology of the Fetus and the Newborn, Chicago, Year Book Pub., 1952.

Prugh, D. G.: Emotional problems of the premature infant's parents, Nursing Outlook 1:461, 1953.

Shirley, Mary: A behavior syndrome characterizing prematurely-born children, Child Develop. 10:115, 1939.

Vaughn, V. C.: Treatment of erythroblastosis fetalis, Am. J. Nursing 52: 320, 1952.

CHAPTER ELEVEN

Breast Feeding

IMPORTANCE

Human milk remains the ideal food for the young infant despite all advances in the knowledge of artificial feeding. Infants fed human milk have fewer illnesses and have better chances of survival than those artificially fed. When well supervised, artificial feeding has a high degree of success, but breast feeding is likely to be successful with little or no supervision. Human milk contains no harmful bacteria, whereas cow's milk must be guarded carefully in this respect. Human milk requires no modification. It contains all the nutritional essentials in adequate, even though minimum, amounts, with the exception of vitamin D and iron. From a strictly medical point of view it is doubtful whether breast feeding is superior to artificial feeding in survival value for the infant in areas where standards of medical care are high and

where the infant mortality rate is correspondingly low. However, in communities where infantile disease is still rife, and educational opportunities are primitive, human milk is far safer than artificial food.

Successful breast feeding has significant advantages in the construction of a happy mother-child relationship. To the infant it is the natural mode of feeding which automatically satisfies his desires for food, sucking, warmth and closeness to his mother. To the mother it can be a rewarding symbol of the transmission of the love she feels for her child as well as a satisfying contribution to his physical needs. Unfortunately, not all mothers are physiologically and psychologically attuned to capitalize upon this form of gratification. Some of the reasons will be considered below.

253

CONTRAINDICATIONS

On the Mother's Part

Tuberculosis

If the mother has active open tuberculosis, not only should the infant be kept from her breast, but also he should be completely isolated from her because of the communicability of the infection. If the maternal tuberculosis is active but not transmissible (closed), nursing is generally not advised because of the physical strain on the mother. When tuberculosis is latent or presumably healed, there is no contraindication to breast feeding.

Chronic Disease

A mother who is ill from a serious chronic disease usually cannot be subjected to the strain of nursing her child. Some chronic illnesses such as psychosis, frequent convulsions or uncontrolled insulin reactions may make breast feeding inadvisable because of hazard to the infant.

Acute Disturbances

Severe acute illnesses on the part of the mother and major surgical operations constitute valid reasons for temporary weaning. During the period of temporary weaning, effort should be made to maintain the milk secretion by periodic emptying of the breasts.

Menstruation, should it occur during lactation, is not an indication for weaning, even though during the first day or two the baby may be somewhat disturbed. The occurrence of pregnancy is not an indication for sudden weaning. Although weaning is desirable because of the strain on the mother, it should be accomplished gradually. Medication of the mother is not usually a contraindication to breast feeding. It is probable that no commonly used drug given mothers in customary amounts is secreted in the milk in sufficient quantity to affect the infant deleteriously.

Mastitis

In the event of the mother's developing mastitis, use of the affected breast should be discontinued. If both breasts become inflamed, complete weaning is necessary. Lesser degrees of nipple disorders require management, as discussed later in this chapter. Inverted, cracked, fissured or painful nipples often can be restored to service by proper attention.

Psychological Aversion

Attempts to persuade mothers who have an aversion toward breast feeding to nurse their infants are usually futile within a brief period. Occasionally, the mother will have an intellectual desire to use the natural method because she accepts its advantages, but if this is not accompanied by emotional comfort, the attempt may disturb her excessively.

On the Infant's Part

Local Deformity

An infant with a cleft lip and palate is usually unable to suckle at the breast. Sometimes when the deformity involves the lip only an early surgical repair will permit nursing if the mother's supply has been maintained. Obstruction of the nose or marked hypoplasia of the mandible often make it mechanically impossible for an infant to nurse successfully.

Prematurity

Whether or not a premature infant can nurse at the breast depends largely upon his initial size. Larger prematures will be strong enough to nurse almost at once or will be released from the special nursery after a brief period so that the problem of maintaining the mother's supply is not arduous. When graduation from the premature nursery is delayed beyond 3 to 4 weeks the likelihood of keeping the mother's breasts flowing is diminished.

Illness

Any condition which debilitates the infant interferes with nursing. Acute illnesses may require only a few days of bottle feeding, and then a return to the breast is possible. Longer illness or congenital malformations such as cardiac disorders may weaken the infant so as to make nursing too exhausting for him to attempt.

PREPARATION OF THE MOTHER

PSYCHOLOGICAL

The mother's conscious and subconscious attitudes toward breast feeding have a very important bearing upon her ability to produce milk. Several trends in modern American culture contribute subtle influences which are making it more difficult for women to accept and enjoy the process of natural feeding. Factors such as advanced education, professional training, out-of-the-home employment and the hectic, highly organized pace of life in our large cities frequently interfere with the mother's ability to relax and they make her impatient over the inefficiencies and the uncertainties of breast feeding. Delivery of milk to the infant will be impeded by maternal worry over the adequacy of her supply or by the necessity for haste in the completion of the feeding so that she can get on to something else.* In addition, some women have a distinct aversion to nursing which is rooted in unwholesome or prudish attitudes toward sex and the maternal role. These attitudes are the product of their own upbringing; they are not easily

* An important connection between nervous tension and the delivery of milk from the breast is embodied in the "let-down" reflex which has been demonstrated in lactating animals and women. Stroking of the nipple or the presence of the infant produces reflex contracture of the alveoli of the mammary gland, pushing milk down into the ducts which discharge at the nipple. Fear, excitement, anger and embarrassment may inhibit this reflex and prevent milk present deep in the gland from coming down to the nipple.

modified but generally must be accepted as valid reasons for giving up breast feeding after a preliminary exploration.

During the prenatal period much can be done by those who attend and advise the mother in creating a wholesome attitude toward breast feeding. In communities where artificial feeding is manifestly risky it can be assumed and urged that the mother will nurse her infant. But in areas with low infant mortality rates the degree to which a mother should be "sold" on its advantages requires some individualized judgment. Nursing cannot honestly be regarded as a medical necessity for such infants but it can be advised as a procedure which will yield dividends in emotional satisfaction and easy adjustment for both mother and baby, provided that the mother can relax and allay her fears and doubts. Prenatal advisors can do much to reassure and solve practical problems in advance which may lead some hesitant mothers to give nursing a reasonable trial. The danger of "overselling" lies in the creation of a sense of guilt, defeat or frustration in the mother who does her conscious best to provide milk but still fails.

DIET AND HEALTH

Unfortunately, mother's milk is not adequate in all instances. Dairymen realize that the health and the food of the cow influence the quality and the quantity of the milk, and these same factors influence the milk of the human mother. Mothers cannot secrete into their milk vitamins which they do not ingest in sufficient amount. Mothers in poor health or with nutritional deficiencies cannot be expected to secrete either an abundance of milk or a milk of good quality. Appropriate attention to the health and the diet of the mother is conducive to and often essential for successful breast feeding.

The diet of the lactating mother need differ qualitatively in no way from that which is suitable for her at other times. No food will have an ill effect on the milk if it does not cause a disturbance in the mother. For example, the prejudice against "acid" foods is unfounded.

A mother who is secreting from a pint to a quart of milk daily, with an energy

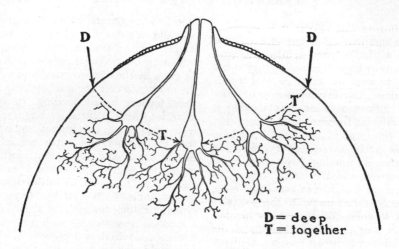

Fig. 34. Schematic representation of the breast. (Moore: Nutrition of Mother and Child)

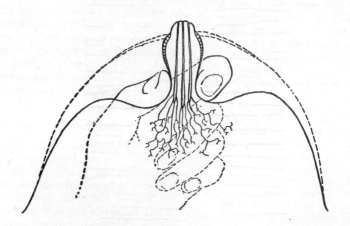

Fig. 35. Schematic representation of the manual expression of milk from the breast. (Moore: Nutrition of Mother and Child)

value of from 300 to 700 calories and with the accompanying protein, minerals and vitamins, must eat at least that many more calories than her customary allowance in order to supply a good quality of milk without depleting her own body supplies. Some mothers who are ingesting a restricted diet and secreting little milk secrete more when the diet is improved. Too often the diet is incomplete irrespective of lactation, and during this period it is especially important that all of the essential food materials be included in adequate quantities. Although the milk may contain calcium from the body stores (bones), it cannot contain vitamins unless they are ingested regularly by the mother. Allowances recommended for the mother during lactation are as follows: 3,000 calories, 100 Gm. of protein, 2 Gm. of calcium, 8,000 units of vitamin A, 1.5 mg. of thiamine, 150 mg. of ascorbic acid, 3 mg. of riboflavin, 15 mg. of niacin and 400 units of vitamin D. In order to obtain these amounts of nutrients, it is necessary to include in the diet at least 1 quart of milk, preferably more. The daily diet also should contain 1 or 2 eggs, 1 serving of meat and an abundance of fruits and vegetables.

CARE OF THE NIPPLES

Fissuring, cracking and infection of the nipples is one of the commonest causes of failure early in breast feeding. During pregnancy the breasts should be inspected for adequate protrusion of the nipples. If the nipples are retracted or adherent so that they fail to protrude when pressure is applied to the base, attempts to bring them out should be made by massage, the use of a breast pump, or by wearing plastic nipple shields with a central hole underneath a brassiere. Some insurance against blocked alveolar ducts may be obtained by having the mother manually express breast secretions twice a day during the latter weeks of pregnancy. Procedures for toughening nipples have doubtful value.

EMPTYING THE BREAST

Manual Expression

For one who has mastered the technic, the most effective method of emptying the breast is by manual expression.

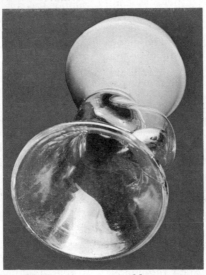

FIG. 36. Common type of breast pump.

The principle of this method is indicated in Figures 34 and 35. The thumb and the finger are placed on the opposite sides of and about 1 inch from the nipple; then while in this position they are pressed deeply into the breast. Then the thumb and the finger are brought toward each other with sufficient pressure to empty the underlying milk sacs. Sometimes better success is attained when the bringing together of the thumb and the finger is followed by a forward motion. This series of motions is repeated with a frequency found most efficient in the individual case. There should be no movement of the fingers on the skin; the skin and the fingers should move together. The milk should flow from the nipple in streams, not drops, during the period of pressure.

Breast Pump

The cheapest, simplest and most commonly used type of breast pump is that shown in Figure 36. A negative pressure is obtained by applying the pump with the bulb compressed and then allowing the bulb to expand. The nipple and the areola are drawn into the conical glass with resultant compression of the milk sacs and a consequent flow of milk. The negative pressure must be released by pressure on the bulb to allow the milk sacs to refill and then be reapplied. This process is repeated over and over until the breast is empty. This method is slow and not highly efficient. A similar but more efficient method uses this same principle of intermittent negative pressure, but the suction is produced by an electrically operated machine pump.

CHARACTERISTICS OF HUMAN MILK

The milk that is secreted during the first few days after the birth of the baby is small in amount and differs much from that secreted after lactation is established. This early milk is known as colostrum. It is of a lemon-yellow color and consequently looks "rich" as compared with later milk. It has a relatively high protein content, and much of the protein consists of globulin. The globulin is considered to have a biologic and immunologic importance for the infant.

On about the third or the fourth day the amount of secretion increases greatly. The breasts become distended and often tender. A gradual transition takes place in the appearance and the composition of the milk. Most of the transition occurs within a week or two, and by the end of the first month it has been completed. After lactation is established, the milk contains approximately from 3.5 to 4 per cent fat, 7.5 per cent sugar, 1.25 per cent protein and 0.2 per cent mineral salts. It has an energy value of 20 calories to the ounce. The composition remains practically constant throughout the period of lactation. At any one withdrawal the first milk that comes from the breast is low in fat, and the last milk relatively rich in fat. Thus any sample taken for analysis should be an entire breast content. Milk analysis usually gives little information of value in determining the difficulty when a breast-fed baby is not thriving. No validity can be given to the common statement that the milk is weak or watery because of its bluish appearance. This is the normal appearance of human milk because the fat is white in color rather than yellow like cow's milk.

Details of the differences between cow's milk and human milk are given in the next chapter. It should be emphasized that the protein and the fat of human milk are more readily digested by the infant and that consequently the bulk of his stools is frequently smaller. Some healthy infants fed at the breast alone will go 3 or more days without passing a stool. In other infants the breast milk has a highly laxative quality so that stool passage is rather frequent, and the color of the movements is green instead of the usual golden yellow. Stools of the breast-fed infant are acid in reaction and have a buttermilk odor due to the fact that a type of bacteria normally grows in them which is different from that present in the stools of artificially fed infants.

Breast milk can be stored from wet nurses or from lactating mothers who have an excess. It is usually pasteurized and frozen or canned for future use. Some communities have established breast-milk centers or banks for the collection of surplus milk which can then be made available for premature infants or those with special nutritional problems whose mothers cannot supply enough for their needs.

TECHNIC OF BREAST FEEDING

The time at which a newborn infant is first placed at the breast varies in different hospitals. In some the babies are put to breast as soon as the mother and the baby indicate a readiness to be together; in others, babies are not put to breast until 6 to 12 hours after birth. During the first few days, the infant gets very little from the breast. To supply fluids and a few calories, 5-per-cent sugar solution is offered approximately every 3 or 4 hours.

The object of placing the baby at the breast is to stimulate the flow of milk and to establish a mutually enjoyed experience for the mother and the baby. For this reason, it is important that the mother be prepared for the experience, that the baby be awake and ready to participate in finding his source of supply of milk and that the nurse remain to help make feeding time a pleasant and comfortable experience for both of them (Fig. 37).

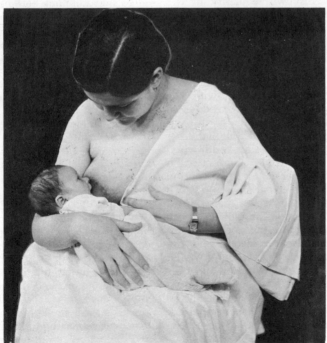

Fig. 37. A suitable position of a baby at the breast. The head is supported, and the nose is free from the breast.

Mothers should be aware of the "rooting" reflex which makes the infant turn instinctively toward the warmth of the breast when it is applied to his cheek. He cannot distinguish this from the warmth of a palm which is mistakenly used to try to guide his mouth to the nipple by turning his head. Instead he appears to refuse the breast by turning away from it and toward the warm palm.

SCHEDULE

Regularity in following a feeding schedule seems to be necessary in some nurseries for the newborn. In others, more flexibility exists, and the babies are taken to their mothers whenever they show a need for closeness or food. At home or under the rooming-in type of hospital care, the feeding schedules can be governed by the infant's spontaneous demands for food. By observing the infant, his own regularity in the need for food will become apparent. As he grows and matures his shifting requirements will be signaled promptly to his mother. It is possible to plan a schedule which maintains flexibility in accordance with the individual infant's demands without interfering with the mother's plan of work or freedom to carry on desired activities.

Establishing irregular eating habits or "spoiling" the baby does not result when a schedule has evolved from observation of his needs; rather, it aids in prevention of poor food habits and anxiety by supplying food when he really feels a need for it. When an infant is allowed to cry with hunger because the clock does not indicate the time for feeding, he becomes emotionally overwrought. When food finally is given, he relaxes and falls asleep from fatigue without his nutritional needs being satisfied or he eats so hastily that digestion becomes impaired.

Many infants, who are fed on a self-regulatory schedule, will select schedules that closely follow the traditional 4-hour intervals. Some of the smaller ones or those who are tense or insecure or are attempting to make rapid increments in size may require feedings at 3-hour or even 2-hour intervals for a time. During the third to the seventh day of life a period of constant demand for food is quite common. In most instances, once the mother recovers from her own excitement and begins to understand her infant's needs, a regular feeding pattern emerges. The intervals between nursing periods may not be exactly equal—often the period of satisfaction in the late afternoon and the early evening is relatively shorter. During the 24-hour period, few infants will require less than 5 feedings; most of them desire 6, 7 or 8. In some cases even more frequent feeding is desirable for brief periods. When the latter behavior persists over protracted periods it may be necessary to inquire into the adequacy of the mother's milk supply.

To substitute one bottle feeding for a breast feeding each 24 hours is frequently of great advantage. Such a plan serves several useful purposes. It allows the mother greater freedom, without which in certain cases she would find nursing too great an obstacle to her social routine. It also keeps the infant accustomed to the bottle, so that if weaning suddenly should become necessary or when the normal time comes for weaning, the infant will accept the new method of feeding without serious objection.

In most instances, the supply of milk is abundant enough so that the infant may obtain sufficient from a single breast, and it is desirable to offer alternate breasts, one at one nursing and the other at the next. By satisfying the infant at one breast, that breast is emptied more thoroughly, and the production of milk is encouraged. When both breasts are given at a single nursing the infant may overfeed, and intestinal disturbance and discomfort result. In some instances when a 4-hour schedule is selected, the baby may be put to both breasts in order to get sufficient milk. When this is done, the breasts should be alternated in being offered first.

LENGTH OF TIME AT BREAST

The average time for an infant to remain at the breast is about 15 minutes. The time depends on the sucking need and the strength of the infant, the amount of milk available and whether or not the breasts are difficult to empty. Some infants will obtain sufficient and be satisfied in 10 minutes or less. When there is little milk, in a very few minutes the infant may give up the attempt to obtain it. The only method of determining with certainty whether the infant has obtained a sufficient amount is to weigh him before and after feedings. In general it is unwise to recommend this procedure to the mother, for the information obtained may be inaccurate and it is more likely to stimulate anxiety than to reassure. The flow of milk is much more rapid at the beginning of a feeding than later; about half or more of the total quantity is taken by the infant in the first 5 minutes, more than a quarter during the next 5 minutes, and very little after this time. Many infants who remain at the breast for long periods swallow air in considerable amounts and

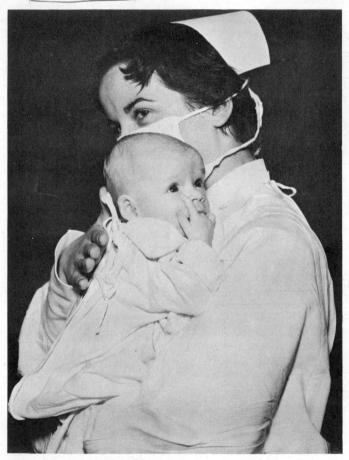

FIG. 38. Holding an infant for "bubbling."

this may lead to vomiting, colic and fretfulness.

Every infant swallows some air during feeding, and for this reason it should be the custom to hold an infant upright and pat him on the back until the air is belched (Fig. 38). The infant always should be so held after each feeding and many infants before feeding as well. Occasionally, for young infants it is desirable to allow opportunity for eructation during the course of the feeding.

DIFFICULTIES ENCOUNTERED IN BREAST FEEDING

The difficulties encountered in breast feeding are to be explained chiefly by either overfeeding or underfeeding, and the diagnosis of the difficulty is made largely by the application of common sense.

OVERFEEDING

Overfeeding of breast milk is a rather uncommon source of difficulty. Occasionally, a mother may produce so much milk that the infant easily takes more than he can digest properly. Vomiting, distention and restlessness may result. Ordinarily, the milk supply adjusts itself within a few days, and the symptoms subside. All-night feeding with the baby sleeping in the mother's bed should be discouraged because of the risks of overfeeding, mutual disturbance of rest and the danger of the mother's rolling onto the infant during sleep.

UNDERFEEDING

The intensity of the signs and the symptoms of underfeeding depends on the degree of deficiency of the diet. There may be a slow gain, no gain or a loss in weight. The stools may remain yellow, may be varying shades of brown or, with complete starvation, will be dark green. The stools are more commonly infrequent but they may be loose and green, similar to stools of overfeeding. There may or may not be excessive crying; if there is, it is due to hunger rather than to colic. If the underfeeding is marked, there is usually disturbance of sleep. There may be some difficulty in differentiating the colic of overfeeding from the hunger of underfeeding, especially in the presence of loose green stools. Parenteral disease may be the cause of weight loss when the milk supply is normal.

The investigation in a case of suspected underfeeding can begin properly with the determination of the amount of milk received by the infant, and this is accomplished best by weighing the baby before and after feeding. Since the amount of milk obtained at different feedings may vary, it is well to take the average of several feedings or, better, to determine the actual amount taken over a 24-hour period. If the infant has received an inadequate amount of milk, the fault may be with the mother or the baby. The next logical step is to determine how much milk remains in the breast. If little or none can be obtained, then the supply is inadequate. If the supply is adequate, the difficulty may be that the nipples are inverted or small or it may be that the infant is unable to suckle properly. Inverted nipples may be drawn out sufficiently by manipulation or by the suction of a pump. Nipples too small or too much inverted for successful breast feeding seldom are encountered. Feeding the baby by means of a nipple shield may be successful, although there is a tendency for the milk to diminish gradually with this procedure. The infant may be too feeble to suckle. He may suckle for a short time and then fall asleep exhausted. A baby with an occluded nose cannot obtain his food satisfactorily; he will grasp the nipple as if hungry, suckle for a brief time and then cry. Many new mothers do not know how to hold the infant in a comfortable position for feeding, or the breast may be allowed to occlude the infant's nares.

The treatment of these various causes of underfeeding is obvious once the cause is determined. A baby should not be weaned from the breast merely because of insufficient milk but should be given milk from a bottle in addition to that obtained from the breast. Often sufficient milk may be obtained by giving both breasts at each feeding. At the same time, measures which have been mentioned previously—improving the diet of the mother, helping her to see her need for rest and shortening the feeding interval—should be undertaken to increase the supply of milk. Occasionally, because of such measures the supplementary feedings may be discontinued.

INANITION OR DEHYDRATION FEVER

It is appropriate to consider in connection with starvation a condition known as inanition fever. This name is given to a febrile illness occurring in the first 5 days after birth. The temperature usually does not rise above 102° F., and no evidence of local disease is present. The condition is associated with loss in weight, often rapid, and a persistence of the meconium nature of the stools. The degree of prostration is directly proportionate to the duration of the illness, and its general nature is that of progressive weakness. In the milder forms, there is much crying and restlessness; in the more severe forms, the infant is limp and apathetic, with perhaps a feeble whine. The condition always is associated with dry or nearly dry breasts and always is relieved within a few hours by the administration of food or even an abundance of fluid. The symptoms are due to dehydration. The treatment is to supply fluid primarily and food secondarily, the effect being rapid disappearance of the fever and prostration and recovery of the lost weight.

MIXED FEEDING

Mixed feeding means that an infant is fed in part at the breast and in part artificially. Such a method of feeding may be used from necessity because of inadequate supply of milk or it may be used as a convenience to the mother in order that she may have liberty for social engagements or be relieved of night nursing. When started early it also gets the infant accustomed to the bottle, so weaning from the breast will be accomplished with fewer difficulties. An older infant who has been fed only at the breast frequently will starve himself seriously rather than take his milk in any other manner than that to which he is accustomed. If the infant is gradually accustomed to the bottle early, it is possible to avoid this difficulty.

When artificial feeding is chosen only for the convenience of the mother, usually a bottle feeding is given in place of a single feeding at the breast. When it is employed from necessity, the same plan may be used to a limited extent. However, it is to be remembered that if an infant is fed less than a certain minimum at the breast—usually 5 feedings—the supply of milk tends to decrease. If it becomes necessary to give considerable amounts of supplemental food, the mother's milk supply is conserved best by having the baby feed regularly at the breast and by giving the necessary amounts of supplemental food immediately after each breast feeding.

ADDITIONS TO THE DIET OF THE BREAST-FED INFANT

Certain supplements to the milk diet of the infant are required whether he is fed artificially or at the breast. These supplements are discussed more fully in the chapter on artificial feeding. The only noteworthy difference between the requirements of the breast-fed baby and the one artificially fed is in the need for additional ascorbic acid. When the mother is ingesting appropriate amounts of ascorbic acid, her milk contains a supply of this vitamin adequate for her infant. Although orange juice or other food containing ascorbic acid is unnec-essary for the breast-fed infant, the giv-ing of such foods serves a useful pur-pose. An adequate supply of ascorbic acid is made more certain, and the in-fant has desirable early experience with variety in his diet. Other food needs of the breast-fed baby are the same as those of the baby who is fed artificially.

WEANING

There are many reasons why weaning is indicated during the first year of life. The more important reasons for wean-ing on account of disease or abnormality in the mother or the infant have been discussed. Even when the mother is well and the baby is thriving, a time comes when breast feeding is no longer ad-vantageous. It is pointed out elsewhere that milk is deficient in certain essen-tials. When these deficiencies are pro-vided by proper food additions and when total food is ingested, infants may be fed successfully at the breast well into the second year. However, the in-fant begins to indicate readiness for a change in method of feeding before the end of the first year. In the latter part of the first year, also, the infant's ability to digest foods more complex than milk is increased greatly.

From observation of infants and from practical experience, it seems to be a wise rule that all infants, with certain exceptions to be noted, be weaned from the breast at from 6 to 10 months of age, and that cow's milk be substituted. If the infant must be weaned before 6 months of age, bottle feeding is the usual substitute; if late in the first year, feeding from a cup is to be recom-mended. Babies accustomed to a for-mula usually can take undiluted milk at from 6 to 8 months of age. However, if they have not been accustomed to whole milk, a sudden change to un-diluted milk may cause a digestive dis-turbance. In these instances, diluted milk should be presented. When wean-ing at any age, the formula at first should be weaker than is customary for the age. The dilution need not be con-tinued for more than a few days. Prep-aration for weaning, signs of readiness for learning new ways of drinking and a method of weaning are discussed in Chapter 4.

If a breast-fed baby comes under ob-servation because of acute illness at an age when normally he should be weaned, weaning usually is not advis-able until the infant is well. If the illness is due to food, it is more likely to be caused by improper food other than the milk.

More than at present, summer for-merly brought many serious digestive disturbances to babies. With excellent reason, weaning in the summer was avoided, and the second summer was feared. When heat is retained by an in-fant through mismanagement of his hygiene in regard to bathing, clothing and ventilation, digestion and absorp-tion of food are impaired, and gastro-intestinal disturbances develop. Im-proper food or food contaminated with bacteria aggravates these disturbances or becomes a primary cause. With the application of our present knowledge of the proper choice and preparation of foods, with present methods of steriliza-tion and refrigeration and with good hygiene, the average infant has no more difficulty if weaned in the summer than at any other time. If circumstances are such that these various conditions are not likely to be satisfactory, weaning may well be deferred.

SITUATIONS FOR FURTHER STUDY

1. What advantages and disadvantages do you see in breast feeding?

2. If an expectant mother showed interest in discussing methods of feeding her baby with you, what would you do?

3. Observe a mother who has a newborn baby on breast feeding in the pediatric unit and describe the interaction between the mother and the baby and the mother and yourself. How would you interpret your role in this situation?

4. What is the "let-down" reflex? How might the mother-nurse relationship influence the functioning of this reflex?

5. What advantages and disadvantages do you see in self-regulatory schedules during the early months of an infant's life? Can you see disadvantages in a rigid 4-hour schedule? What might be the outcome of the method of feeding? What signs would indicate a baby's need for food? What influences a mother's choice of method of feeding her baby?

6. Observe a normal infant of from 2 to 3 months of age to determine times when he indicates a need for food. How does he express it? How can you differentiate between behavior that indicates hunger and behavior that indicates a need for affection or social stimulation? Keep a chart showing periods when food is demanded. Is the time between periods regular?

7. If a 7-month-old baby, who had been breast fed up until the time he was brought to the hospital, showed difficulty in adjustment to your nursing care, how would you interpret the behavior?

8. If when her baby was 6 months of age a mother asked you how to prepare her infant for weaning from the breast, what suggestions would you give her?

9. How can the nurse function to make breast feeding an enjoyable experience for both the infant and the mother? What are your attitudes toward breast feeding? What attitudes toward breast feeding have you encountered in mothers?

BIBLIOGRAPHY

Barnes, G. R., Jr., Lethin, A. N., Jr., and Jackson, E. B.: Management of breast feeding, J.A.M.A. 151:192, 1953.

Bartram, J. B.: In Nelson, Textbook of Pediatrics, ed. 6, Philadelphia, Saunders, 1954.

Meyer, H. F.: Essentials of Infant Feeding for Physicians, Springfield, Ill., Thomas, 1952.

Wright, F. H.: Infant Feeding, Journal-Lancet 77:65, 1957.

CHAPTER TWELVE

Artificial Feeding

When human milk is not available to the infant, a substitute source is required. Because of its commercial availability cow's milk is far and away the most common basis of infant formulas. Occasionally, the milk of the goat is used, and rarely mare's and ass's milk has been employed. In recent years it has also been found possible to rear an infant without any milk at all by substituting preparations made from vegetable sources. However, well over 90 per cent of artificially fed infants receive some modification of cow's milk. The milk from different breeds and herds of cows varies only in its fat content. In the United States this difference disappears in the processing of milks, since dairies usually reduce the fat content to the minimum required by law. Thus, milk from all sources is essentially of the same composition.

Artificial feeding with cow's (or any other animal's) milk must be undertaken with the realization that three automatic safety factors of breast milk have been lost: (1) sterility, (2) maximum digestibility and (3) nearly complete vitamin coverage. Any scheme of artificial feeding must be designed in such a way as to control these deficiencies insofar as possible. It will be impossible here to consider in detail all of the ways in which these objectives can be met. Only the general principles as they apply to the common modifications of cow's milk will be presented. The reader is referred to the references, particularly the handbook by Meyer, for details and additional varieties of infant foods.

CONTROL OF BACTERIA

As he grows up the infant will eventually have to learn how to defend himself against the bacteria which surround him. In the early months of life his immunologic defenses are notoriously poor; hence it is prudent to shield him against sudden exposure to infectious agents in large numbers or wide variety. A more

266

compelling reason for care in formula preparation is that milk is an ideal medium for the transmission of disease. Pathogens introduced accidentally into a supply may disseminate disease to large numbers of infants or children in a community or in a hospital if proper care is not exercised. The educational value of careful formula instruction to parents should not be overlooked. If properly schooled in this aspect of care, they may extend the principles to other aspects of the infant's hygiene. The age at which sterilizing measures may be relaxed is a matter of varying opinion among physicians and will have to be determined in part by medical and social circumstances. Some insist upon careful technic throughout the first year of life or even longer; others are willing under good hygienic circumstances to shift infants to pasteurized milk around 5 to 6 months of age.

Milk taken by the infant from the human breast is sterile except for a trivial number of bacteria from the skin and the surrounding environment. A comparable degree of sterility could be achieved by having the infant nurse directly from the cleansed udder of the cow—a cumbersome procedure which was actually tried around the turn of the century in a frantic attempt to find a safer form of artificial feeding. As obtained from the cow under the cleanest conditions, milk contains from 100 to 1,000 bacteria per cubic centimeter. Since it is an excellent food for bacteria as well as for infants, these organisms multiply rapidly during any period required for processing and transportation. By the time clean milk reaches the consumer the bacteria have usually increased to between 10,000 and 50,000 per cubic centimeter. Milk which is not carefully collected or preserved may have several million bacteria per cubic centimeter. Depending upon the kind of bacteria such milk contains, it may or may not taste sour or be capable of transmitting disease to the infant. How-

ever, it should be considered unfit for infant feeding. The grading of market milk into Grades A, B, etc., is determined by local regulations of production and handling. Only Grade A milk should be used for infants, and even then its bacterial content must be reduced by methods described below.

PARTIAL BACTERIAL CONTROL

Certified Milk

In this form of control the milk is produced under conditions of rigid supervision by public authorities. The health of the cows, the methods of milking and storage, and the bacterial content of the milk must meet high standards. Since it is an expensive form of bacterial control which is not always entirely reliable, certification of milk is seldom used today.

Pasteurization

Shortly after it is obtained from the cow the milk is heated to a temperature of 150° F. for 30 minutes, or by the "flash" method, to a higher temperature for a shorter time. The conditions are sufficient to kill most pathogenic bacteria but do not render the milk completely sterile. They do not alter the taste of the milk or interfere with cream formation. Following pasteurization the milk must be kept refrigerated in order to hold down growth of the surviving bacteria. Most health departments now require pasteurization of all milk for general sale, but local farms and dairies do not always treat their milk in this fashion. In general, fresh pasteurized milk is deemed suitable for the older infant or child, but it must be sterilized by heat when used in formula preparation.

METHODS OF STERILIZING MILK

Boiling

In the home the simplest method of sterilizing milk is to bring it to a boil for at least 3 minutes. Bacteria may also be killed by exposure to steam or by autoclaving the milk at appropriate combinations of temperature, pressure and time.

Evaporated Milk

The milk is first reduced to about half its original volume, then sealed in airtight containers and sterilized by heat. Evaporated milk needs no refrigeration and remains sterile until the can is opened. It is very popular in infant feeding because of its foolproof safety, low cost and ease of storage and shipment. It is possible to skim the milk partially before evaporation, to homogenize it or to add vitamin D.

Dried Milk

The raw milk is sprayed into a warm low-pressure chamber or onto hot rollers. Thus, nearly all of the water is extracted, and the powder is collected and sealed in air-tight tins. The milk is usually pasteurized before being dried. It may be skimmed or may have carbohydrate added to it before processing. Like evaporated milk, it is sterile and easily kept and packaged.

Proprietary Milks

A great many commercial varieties of sterile canned milk are available either as evaporated liquids or dried powders. These are produced by the processes enumerated above but in addition have been subjected to various chemical modifications to increase digestibility or restore lost vitamins.

Condensed Milk

This is essentially evaporated milk to which has been added a heavy concentration of carbohydrate. It is no longer used in infant feeding and is mentioned merely to distinguish it from evaporated milk with which the laity sometimes confuses it.

FORMULA PREPARATION IN THE HOME

The exact method used to prepare formula in the home will depend upon the ingredients to be used and upon the intellectual and economic status of the parents. Instructions must be precise but tailored to individual circumstances. Whatever the method employed, its objective is to provide a day's supply of formula which is sterile at the conclusion of its preparation and will remain so under refrigeration until each individual bottle is ready for use. The desirability of cleanliness of the mother's person, the kitchen and the utensils is obvious. Even though bottles and nipples are going to be sterilized they should be thoroughly cleansed and well rinsed before use. Detergent soaps in particular must be carefully removed since some of them are poisonous if ingested in any significant amount. Once items have been sterilized they should be handled in such a way as to avoid subsequent contamination even from presumably clean hands. Sterilized nipples can be housed in sterile screw-top jars or may be left on the bottles with protective tops or inverted into those which are so designed.

The "terminal method" of sterilization is most likely to result in sterile formula. The ingredients are measured into each of the clean bottles, and then the units with their nipples or caps are given a final sterilization in steam. The method has some disadvantages which limit its usefulness. It cannot be applied to formulas made from acidified or cultured milks. Certain of the proprietary formulas which contain added vitamins will suffer a reduction in the concentration of some of these vitamins if terminally sterilized. Under some conditions of temperature and local water supply, a scum may form within the bottles which clogs the nipple holes and interferes with feedings. A simple modification of terminal sterilization avoids these difficulties and makes it applicable to all formulas prepared from liquid proprietary or evaporated milks. The water (with added carbohydrate if ordered) is measured into each bottle, and the units with their nipples, caps and accessory equipment, such as a funnel, forceps and can-opener, are steam sterilized and cooled. Then the milk is added directly from the can through the sterile funnel and the bottles are capped and refrigerated at once.

HOSPITAL FORMULAS

In maternity and children's hospitals the responsibility for formula preparation usually is vested in a dietitian or a graduate nurse who has had appropriate training. Scrupulous care is required lest the milk room serve as a focus for the dissemination of disease to all the infants within the institution. Clean quarters separated from the infected areas of the hospital, and a staff free from the responsibility for sick patients are desirable. The terminal method of sterilization as described above is gaining increasing favor as a safeguard. In large hospital units formula can be prepared rapidly and in large batches if suitable autoclaves are available. The milk room must also guard against mistakes and later contamination of formulas by careful planning of the labeling, the distribution, the local storage and the final preparation of the bottles. Periodic bacterial cultures of the formulas produced affords a check upon the adequacy of the technic.

CHEMICAL MODIFICATION OF MILK

The major chemical differences between cow's milk and human milk are summarized in Table 7. Both are dilute fluids composed of about 90 per cent water and 10 per cent solid constituents. Their energy values are the same (20 calories per ounce) since the lower content of carbohydrate in cow's milk is

TABLE 7. APPROXIMATE COMPOSITION OF HUMAN AND COW'S MILK

	HUMAN	COW'S
Water—per cent	88	88
Energy—calories per ounce	20	20
Protein—grams per cent	1.5	3.4
(Casein)	(0.4)	(2.8)
(Lactalbumin)	(0.8)	(0.4)
Fat—grams per cent	3.8	3.8
Carbohydrate—grams per cent	7.0	4.8
Minerals—milligrams per cent	0.20	0.72
(Ca)	(0.04)	(0.15)
(P)	(0.02)	(0.15)
(Na)	(0.015)	(0.055)
(K)	(0.055)	(0.150)
(Fe)	(0.0001)	(0.00004)
Vitamin A—International Units per quart	2,000	2,000
Vitamin D—International Units per quart	50–100	3–5
Vitamin C—milligrams per quart	45	20 (raw)
Nicotinic Acid—milligrams per quart	1.7	0.85
Riboflavin—milligrams per quart	0.47	1.6
Thiamine—milligrams per quart	0.05	0.25

Data from several sources, chiefly Macy, I. G., Kelley, H., and Sloan, R., The Composition of Milks, National Council Bulletin 119, 1950.

exactly compensated by an increase in protein. The minerals are 2 to 3 times as plentiful in cow's milk on the average. The natural content of both vitamin C and D is low, and the former is usually decreased further by procedures used to sterilize cow's milk.

Historically, the goal in formula preparation has been to achieve a product which simulates breast milk as closely as possible. It is now recognized that infants have a wide range of digestive tolerance, and that exact compliance with this goal is unnecessary for most of them. The theoretic basis for some of the modifications of cow's milk is considered below.

PROTEIN

As seen in the table, the total concentration of protein in cow's milk is more than twice that in breast milk. However, the quality of the protein differs by virtue of its higher content (85%) of casein and lower content (15%) of lactalbumin. Complete digestion of the protein yields an ample supply of the essential amino acids (those which the body is unable to synthesize from other materials).

A major consideration in the modification of cow's milk is the quality of curd formed in the stomach. When milk meets the gastric juice the casein portion is coagulated into a curd while the lactalbumin remains in solution. Digestion of the curd depends upon its physical qualities of particle size—large curds being tough and difficult for the digestive juices to manage; small, flocculent curds yielding more readily. The high concentration of casein in cow's milk favors formation of large curd coagulums and slows digestion, gastric emptying time and later absorption. It is thus imperative to modify the casein by partial digestion (or denaturation) before it is admitted to the stomach. Historically, this was achieved by diluting the milk and by boiling. Modern methods which accomplish a similar result are the procedures of evaporation and drying of milk. Thus the same methods which sterilize are also effective in changing casein so that it will form smaller curds. Additional methods of predigestion are by treating the milk with acid or alkali or with a proteolytic enzyme. Homogenization which is primarily directed at breaking the fat up into small particle size also has a modest effect upon the character of the resulting curd. Pasteurization is too mild a process to influence the protein significantly. One or more of these processes of protein alteration is invariably used in the construction of infant formulas, whether in the home or during the processing of the milk before sale.

Preparations are available which increase the protein content of formulas. Essentially, these consist in milks to which has been added casein which has been pretreated with a proteolytic enzyme (protein milk), or of supplements which consist of casein completely reduced by hydrolysis to its constituent amino acids.

FAT

Although the total content of fat in cow's and human milk is approximately the same, there are differences in the types of fatty acids contained within the fat which render cow's milk somewhat more irritating and less readily digestible. Premature babies in general and individual full-term infants may require reduction or alteration in the fat of the formula offered. The process of homogenization, which by forcing milk through a small aperture under high pressure results in dispersion of the fat into very fine globules which remain uniformly suspended in the milk, aids digestion by providing a larger surface area upon which the lipases of the intestinal tract can act. Dilution and partial or complete removal of the fat are also used in the modification of formulas.

When the fat content of milk is reduced by partial or complete skimming, its energy value is significantly reduced, since fat supplies 9 calories per gram as contrasted with only 4 for proteins and carbohydrates. Thus the formula must be given in larger volume to meet the energy requirements, or it will have to be fortified by the addition of calories in another form, usually as carbohydrate.

Some commercial preparations remove the fat from cow's milk completely and replace it with another, more digestible type such as olive oil.

Most full-term infants are able to accept the fat of cow's milk in its original concentration. When intolerance of a formula is manifested or during disease, particularly diarrhea, it is common practice to reduce the intake of fat in the infant's formula.

CARBOHYDRATE

The same form of carbohydrate is present in both milks (lactose), but its concentration is higher in breast milk. Traditionally, it has been the practice to add carbohydrate to formulas of cow's milk in order to reach the same concentration. If dilution or skimming is employed in the formula construction, carbohydrate addition is desirable in order to increase the energy value and avoid the necessity of feeding unusually large volumes. Some physicians now believe that the addition of carbohydrate to whole or evaporated milk formulas is unnecessary and that infants profit by receiving a higher proportion of their calories in the form of protein.

A great many types of carbohydrate have been used as supplements in the construction of formulas. In addition to simple sugars such as dextrose, levulose and lactose, various residues of starch digestion are employed. Control of intestinal fermentation and of the laxative effect of the formula is imputed to the proper selection of carbohydrate. The importance of this aspect of infant feeding has been overemphasized.

MINERALS

In ordinary formula construction no attempt is made to reduce the concentration of minerals, which is two or three times as high in cow's milk as in human milk. Commercially, it is possible to produce milk which is very low in its content of sodium and other minerals. Occasionally, the high mineral content of cow's milk must be considered in feeding prematures or infants with cardiac or renal diseases. The high concentration of phosphorus renders the artificially fed infant somewhat more susceptible to tetany of the newborn. Both human and cow's milk are deficient in iron which must be obtained from other foods or from therapeutic administration.

FORMULA CONSTRUCTION

The tasks of prescribing and preparing artificial formulas for infants have been greatly simplified by modern technics of food packaging and by a change in the philosophy of infant feeding. Old-fashioned complicated recipes for home use are becoming obsolete, for it has been amply demonstrated that most infants thrive on simple milk modifications, and for the few who do not there is now available a multiplicity of canned prepared mixtures. In the past it was deemed necessary for the physician to calculate an infant's nutritional dosage exactly and for the parents to follow his directions precisely. But today it is generally recognized that such an approach is impractical because of wide individual differences in the food requirements of infants. The supervisor of infant feeding usually selects a formula and instructs the parents about the probable limits of intake which will be required, on the one hand to support growth, and on the other to avoid digestive disturbances from overeating. The parents are then encouraged to allow the infant to indicate his individual desire in respect to amounts and frequency of feeding within these broad limits. Periodic evaluation by the supervisor is required to judge whether or not the result is satisfactory.

The selection of a formula by a hospital, a clinic or an individual physician is based upon past experience and upon the economic circumstances of the clientele. Formulas based on evaporated and dried milks are the most economical. Proprietary preparations are more convenient but also more expensive. Some of the commonly used formulas are discussed below.

EVAPORATED MILK FORMULAS

Evaporated milk is popular as a base for formulas because of its low cost, general availability, sterility, and convenience in storage and handling. In the United States, government supervision keeps the more than 400 different brands equivalent in composition so that they may be used interchangeably. For newborn infants evaporated milk is usually diluted with water in a ratio of 1:2 or 2:3. For older infants it is reconstituted to the strength of whole milk by adding an equal volume of water. Although the addition of carbohydrate is traditional, it may be omitted. When sugar is added the concentrations used ordinarily range from 5 to 8 per cent.

Nearly all brands of evaporated milk are now fortified by the addition of 400 international units to the 13-oz. can. Thus an infant whose daily formula intake includes the contents of a can of evaporated milk will simultaneously receive his quota of vitamin D.

The caloric value of evaporated milk formula depends upon its degree of dilution and the amount of carbohydrate added. The weakest dilution ordinarily used (1 part evaporated milk to 2 parts of water) yields about 14 calories per ounce. A dilution of equal parts of evaporated milk and water has about the

same energy value as whole milk—21 calories per ounce. Each 1 per cent of added carbohydrate increases the energy value by 1.2 calories per ounce.

FRESH-MILK FORMULAS

When pasteurized or certified milk is used as the basis of a formula it must be boiled in order to modify the curd and to complete sterilization. Soft curd and enzyme-treated liquid milks require no additional modification of the protein but must be boiled if sterility is desired. For older infants these various fresh milks may be used as they come. Ordinarily, water in amounts not exceeding one third of the volume of milk is added as diluent for younger infants. Carbohydrate additions may be made in the customary 5 to 8 per cent strengths. Many fresh milks are fortified by the addition of vitamin D.

Formulas of this type have no particular advantage over evaporated milk. They are more expensive and more cumbersome in preparation. In addition, they require continually fresh supplies of milk and refrigerated storage.

The caloric value of formula prepared from fresh milk is 20 calories per ounce when the original milk is not modified. Dilution reduces the caloric value proportionally; the addition of carbohydrate increases it as noted above.

DRIED MILK FORMULAS

Dried powdered milk is available in canned and sterilized form and can be reconstituted to its original strength by the addition of boiled water. Like the fresh milks it may be diluted or sweetened as desired. Some dried milks are partially skimmed, and others completely skimmed, so that on reconstitution they yield lower caloric values. Dried milk has the advantages of low cost and convenient storage in bulk and is more commonly used as a formula base by institutions than in the home. Vitamin D is not usually added to the powdered milks and hence must be given as a supplement.

PROPRIETARY FORMULAS

A variety of commercially prepared formulas are packaged as powders or as liquids which upon proper dilution with boiled water provide a "complete" dietary for the infant, even including an adequate intake of the several vitamins required. These preparations are generally quite satisfactory and convenient in all respects but suffer the disadvantage of somewhat increased cost. Special attention is usually given to making the reconstituted mixture resemble breast milk as closely as possible. The details of composition and caloric and vitamin contents must be obtained from the labels or the literature concerning the individual product.

FORMULAS FOR PREMATURES

Because of the premature's relative inability to digest and absorb the fat of cow's milk, the most generally used formulas are based upon skimmed or partially skimmed milk. The energy value lost by the removal of fat is more than compensated by the addition of carbohydrate, since it is desirable to meet the energy needs of these small infants without having to feed excessive volume. Modifications of the formula originally proposed by Powers consist of half-skimmed milk to which from 7 to 10 per cent carbohydrate is added. Another approach is to use evaporated milk in more than the usual dilution and add carbohydrate in similar high percentage. Proprietary milks with low fat content are also used, frequently with addition of carbohydrate. The exact caloric value of such mixtures varies but it is usually above 20 calories per ounce and may run as high as 27 calories per ounce. Vitamin supplementation is particularly necessary for the premature infant.

HYPOALLERGIC FORMULAS

For the infant who is allergic to cow's milk it is necessary to alter or to avoid the protein fraction. When sensitivity is mild, the degree of protein alteration accomplished by evaporation, by drying or by boiling may be sufficient to avoid trouble. More drastic alteration of protein can be accomplished by prolonged heating of cow's milk which is the basis for some hypoallergic milks. Avoidance of cow's milk proteins is achieved by using milk from another species of animal such as goat's milk (or human milk when it is available), or through substitution of one of the artificial milks prepared from vegetable proteins such as soybeans or almonds, or a milk which contains protein only in the form of its constituent amino acids. Goat's milk is quite similar to cow's milk and can be obtained in certified, dried, or evaporated form and used similarly. It is notorious in its ability to produce anemia and must be supplemented with appropriate hematinics. The milks of vegetable origin have the disadvantages of unpalatable taste and somewhat lower nutritional value but can be used as exclusive sources of protein over long periods of time.

VITAMIN SUPPLEMENTATION

When the type of basic feeding for the infant has been determined it is necessary to take stock of the vitamins it contains in order to be sure that daily requirements will be met. Only under unusual circumstances will vitamin A be lacking, since both breast and cow's milks contain an adequate concentration. However, when milk is skimmed much of the vitamin A is removed with the fat component, and unless it is restored or obtained from other foods, the intake may fall below the required 1,500 units per day. Vitamin A in good concentration is present in the fish liver oils which are used to supply vitamin D.

It may also be given as carotene, which is a precursor of vitamin A.

A deficiency of members of the B-complex group of vitamins is likewise unlikely, since both breast and cow's milk contain adequate concentrations. However, the optimal intake of many of these substances is not fully determined for infants, and many physicians believe that supplements are desirable if not essential. The individual members of the group may be added as synthetic chemicals or as mixtures in wheat germ or yeast preparations or they may be obtained through the early addition of other foods to the infant's diet.

Care must always be taken to be sure that the minimum of 25 mg. of vitamin C is being consumed. The breast-fed infant will receive most of his allotment if his mother is ingesting a diet well supplied with the vitamin. But the infant whose main food is heated cow's milk will receive little or no vitamin C from this source. Orange and other citrous fruit juices have been the time-honored media for supplying ascorbic acid. One ounce of fresh orange juice or 2 ounces of constituted frozen orange juice per day will usually cover the infant's needs. Because infants sometimes dislike or vomit orange juice it has become the more common practice to administer synthetic ascorbic acid in pill or liquid form or as part of a multiple vitamin concentrate. Overdosage with vitamin C is harmless.

Since most of the fresh and evaporated milk and nearly all of the proprietary formulas contain 400 units of vitamin D per quart, it has become a debated point as to whether or not additional supplements are wise. Because small infants do not take a full quart of formula daily, and because there is no harm in giving 2 or 3 times the minimum required dose, it is a widespread practice to "make certain." Breast-fed infants and those raised upon skimmed milk formulas surely must be given extra vitamin D. Cod-liver oil has given place to concentrates made from the livers of percomorph fishes. Prematures require higher dosage than full-term infants.

Multiple vitamin concentrates containing at least A, C and D and sometimes B-complex offer an easy way of making certain that the infant's vitamin needs are covered. Undoubtedly, there is some economic waste in prescribing these mixtures for all infants no matter what the nature of their formulas, but within reasonable limits, no harm results. Misunderstanding of the function of vitamins occasionally leads to excessive dosage, particularly of vitamin D, in which case appetite and even growth may be hampered by the toxic effects of prolonged overdosage.

TECHNIC OF FEEDING

In addition to determining the type of mixture to be used for the artificially fed infant, the physician or the nurse must initiate the procedure by making a tentative estimate of the daily quantity which will be required to meet nutritional needs and to satisfy hunger. Most newborn nurseries start during the first few days of life by offering full-term infants 1½ to 2 ounces about every 4 hours. (The feeding of prematures is considered in a previous section.) Even by the time he is ready to leave the new-born nursery, some intimation of the individual infant's appetite and feeding frequency may be obtained. Intelligent and stable parents can be encouraged to permit him some freedom in determining the rate at which he will take the chosen formula. For them it is desirable to set maximum and minimum daily limits within which framework feeding behavior can be considered as normal. After the initial period of adjustment, perhaps by the end of a week or 10 days of life, infants will not gain satisfactorily unless they are taking at least 80 calories per kilogram of body weight. From the infant's weight and the known caloric value of his formula the minimal desired intake can thus be readily calculated. Few normal infants will be peacefully satisfied with less than this minimum. At the other extreme are to be found those infants who are very active, fussy, or ravenous, due to an unusually strong growth impulse. Parents of such a child will need to know how rapidly and to what lengths they may safely go in making increases in formula in an attempt to appease the child's appetite.

With most of the formulas in common use it is permissible to make gradual increases up to 150 calories per kilogram of body weight or even a little more. Infants who consistently demand higher levels of food intake should be watched carefully for evidence of intolerance or should be studied for the possibility of abnormality.

The reasons for individualized or "demand" feeding schedules for small infants have been considered in the preceding chapter on breast feeding. Not all physicians subscribe to this approach; some exercise varying degrees

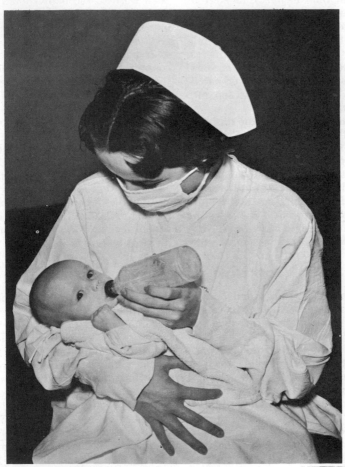

Fig. 39. Position of a baby for feeding.

of tighter control over the times and the amounts of feeding. When dealing with parents of limited intelligence or those who are ritualistic by nature or too upset by anxiety, it is sometimes necessary to issue more didactic instructions. In the authors experience the prompt accession to the small infant's legitimate demands for food is a most important cornerstone upon which to construct a wholesome mother-child relationship not only in respect to feeding but also as a foundation for mutual confidence and pleasure in other aspects of their future life together.

At feeding time the milk is taken from the refrigerator and warmed to body temperature by placing the bottle in a container of warm water. If a sweet-milk formula is overheated in this process, it can be cooled, and no harm is done. However, if acidified milk is overheated, the curd is likely to clump and separate from the whey.

After warming the milk, the nipple is placed on the bottle without contamination of the tip, the temperature is tested by sprinkling a few drops on the inner aspect of the wrist, and the speed of flow is observed. When the bottle is turned up, the milk should drop out rapidly but not run in a stream. If the holes are too small, they can be made larger with a hot needle.

The size of the nipple holes must be geared to the type of formula that is being fed and to the needs of the individual infant. Acidified milk is thicker than sweet milk and requires slightly larger nipple holes. Sick infants with lowered vitality require a nipple with comparatively large holes. The hungry infant who sucks vigorously should be given a nipple with small holes to prevent him from getting his food too rapidly and to provide ample opportunity for sucking.

After the infant's diapers have been changed and the nurse's hands have been washed, the baby should be held during his feeding (Fig. 39). The infant's need for emotional warmth at feeding time has been cited in Chapter 4. If holding the baby for feedings is contraindicated medically, the bottle should be held throughout the feeding unless the infant is desirous of holding it himself.

After feeding, the young baby should be "bubbled," cuddled until he is ready for sleep and placed in bed. If he does not seem to be comfortable after being put down to rest, he should be "bubbled" again. Some babies need to be "bubbled" before, during and after feeding. It takes time to discover the way of feeding which best meets the individual infant's requirements.

ADDITION OF OTHER FOODS

Although milk is the foundation of the infant's diet and the main source of his nutritional intake during the early months, by itself it will not be adequate indefinitely. The age and the sequence of introduction of the "solid" foods is governed by custom, fads, whims and personal prejudices more than by the logic of nutritional need. Old-fashioned custom left solids out of the diet at least until the second half of the first year; modern enthusiasm witnesses the consumption of meat and cereal in the premature nursery. It seems clear that, contrary to older ideas, very young infants can accept and utilize fruit, cereal, vegetable, meat and eggs at the very beginning of extra-uterine life if these substances are converted into finely divided semiliquid mixtures. Whether or not there is any advantage in rushing them into the infant dietary is a moot question.

Most pediatricians now initiate solid foods sometime between 1 and 3 months of age. Cereal is a traditional first choice because of its bland taste and the ease with which it can be made into a gruel by dilution with milk. The infant's initial difficulty is mainly mechanical—he mouths the food as he would the nipple and appears to be pushing it out of his mouth, whereas in reality he is trying to sweep it backward along the roof of his mouth and over the top of his tongue so that it will gravitate into his pharynx. His efforts are helped if the early feedings are fluid and if the feeder aids him by guiding the mixture well back in his mouth. After a little practice he learns how to accept thicker material and to transport it backward with little help. After his initiation on cereal, puréed fruits and vegetables and well-strained meat and liver may be added in order. Eggs can be given raw, poached or soft-boiled. Since the yolk holds the most important items (iron, riboflavin and protein), ordinarily it is given first. Nutritionally, the infant is most in need of vitamin B and iron to supplement his milk and vitamin concentrate. Thus it would be most logical to offer eggs, meat and vegetables as the first nonmilk foods. Commonly, however, these are reserved until last, and the more acceptable cereal and fruit are used for an introduction.

In addition to the value of specific nutrients, early feeding of solid foods offers an opportunity to cultivate a cosmopolitan appetite before the infant's tastes are too firmly fixed. Most infants are relatively agreeable about trying new foods up until the age of 5 or 6 months, at which time they begin to show resistance to innovations. Therefore, it is desirable to have a wide selection of foods in their habitual diet before this age is reached. The manner in which foods are offered has some bearing upon the final result. If the feeder urges or forces a food which the infant dislikes, he may not only acquire a permanent aversion to this item, but the recurring struggle may condition him adversely to the whole process of eating so that it becomes a time to fight rather than a period of relaxation and enjoyment. If the feeder, on the other hand, is too tentative and shies away from further efforts when the infant shows his first evidence of displeasure, the particular item usually does not have a sufficient trial. Often it is possible to tide a small baby over his dislike of a food by mixing it with fruit or some other item which he relishes and then gradually shifting the proportions of the mix until he is ready to accept the new food in unadulterated form. Persistent rejection or vomiting of an item of food should be taken as an indication to omit the offending substance at least for a few weeks. Sometimes a later trial will be met with quiet acceptance.

Home preparation of foods for the infant's use is being supplanted by the inexpensive and conveniently packaged prepared foods now available in any grocery store. Cereals are precooked and reduced to a powder which can then be made into a paste or a liquid by the addition of formula or water. Fruits, vegetables, fish and meats are puréed or finely ground, sieved, sterilized and put up in small jars or cans which after opening can safely be kept in the refrigerator for 2 or 3 days before being discarded. Egg yolk is also available in canned form. Coarser grades of foods are prepared in the same manner, known as "chopped" or "junior" foods to be used during the transition period from strained to table foods. If foods are prepared at home for the small infant, they should be thoroughly and simply cooked, finely subdivided, and then strained.

TRANSITION TO ADULT FOODS AND METHODS

By the age of 5 or 6 months infants can be started on cup-feeding and finger-feeding in preparation for the time when they will be able to take over the process and eat without assistance. The period of transition varies considerably from one infant to another. The introduction of more advanced technics does not mean that the infantile methods should be discarded at once, for many infants like to explore their own abilities for a time and then revert to the comforts of previously learned dependence upon adult help or upon the bottle. Emphasis should be placed upon teaching and encouraging the use of new methods rather than upon forbidding the old. Although most infants will have completed the transition early in the second year of life, many will want to retain a bottle at bedtime until the third year in spite of advanced behavior in other respects.

Introduction of the cup is best made at a time when the bottle is not in use or even in sight. Many infants will accept water or orange juice readily from the cup but balk at taking milk from such an unaccustomed receptacle. Independent use of a cup will not be achieved until the infant is able to sit up well in a high chair or at a table. Mothers must be prepared for the inevitable period of experimentation when he discovers the joys of pouring his milk out on the tray or directly on the floor. The mess can be minimized if he is offered repeated small quantities rather than a full cup or glass.

Finger-feeding is usually initiated with some firm, readily dissolvable food such as zweibach or dry thin toast which the infant 5 to 6 months old can carry to his mouth and safely chew upon. As his interest increases and he becomes more facile in the use of his hands, other soft lumpy items such as dices of well-cooked vegetable, crisp bacon, crackers, bread, peas and even nonsplintering bones can be proffered for independent use. By 8 to 9 months of age he will be able to hold and mess with a spoon, but efficient use of this utensil usually is not achieved much before 12 to 14 months. Prior to this time the infant may learn to scoop up his food but he usually inverts the spoon on the way to his mouth and spills most of its contents down his bib. Mothers and nurses must be willing to tolerate his inefficiency, for without trial there can be no learning.

SITUATIONS FOR FURTHER STUDY

1. What safety factors of breast milk have been lost when a baby is fed a formula? How is safety of the milk supply ensured?

2. Compare the composition of human and cow's milk. How is cow's milk modified to simulate human milk?

3. How must a premature infant's formula differ from that prepared for the full-term infant? What characteristics of the premature make this difference necessary?

4. What principles of feeding an infant do you deem to be essential?

5. What principles of introducing solid foods do you use in caring for a baby under 1 year of age? Why do you feel that these principles are important? How do you react when an infant will not take the food you offer? What reasons can you discover for his disinterest in feeding? Describe a situation in which you discovered the cause of disinterest, redesigned your plan of care for him and observed the results.

6. How do you react when a baby tries to learn the properties of foods through manual experimentation? Describe a situation in which you were able to modify your attitudes and permit a baby to have this kind of learning experience.

BIBLIOGRAPHY

Lanman, J. T.: Modern Trends in Infant Nutrition and Feeding, Scientific Report Series No. 14, New York, Sugar Research Foundation, 1952.

Meyer, H. F.: Essentials of Infant Feeding for Physicians, Springfield, Ill., Thomas, 1952.

Wishik, S. M.: Feeding Your Child, Garden City, New York, Doubleday, 1955.

CHAPTER THIRTEEN

Digestive Disorders of Infancy

DIGESTION IN INFANCY

The digestive equipment of the infant is adequate for its task, but only when the food is appropriately chosen, prepared and administered. The expected rate of growth of the infant is far in excess of that which occurs at any later time. Consequently, in proportion to his size, an infant requires several times as much food as does an adult. Because of the immaturity of the digestive functions, the infant's food must differ from that of the older person in quality as well as in relative quantity. Even with the simple diet that babies customarily receive, the amount of food necessary approaches closely the digestive capacity. Digestive capacity is decreased by illness, particularly by certain common infections, with the result that digestive disturbances are much more common in infancy than at any other age period. Such disturbances, when they occur, are more serious for the infant than for the older person. By them he is deprived of much or all of his food through vomiting,

diarrhea and food refusal. When deprived of food, the infant uses his body stores at a much greater rate than an older person, and serious consequences are more quickly evident. In order to prevent or to manage the digestive and nutritional disturbances of infancy, more detailed knowledge and attention are required than for feeding older children or adults.

SALIVARY DIGESTION

Salivary digestion is concerned only with the digestion of starch. Even when starch is fed as part of a young infant's diet, the extent to which it is digested by saliva is small. Whatever importance salivary digestion may have is attained at a later age.

GASTRIC DIGESTION

The important factors in gastric digestion are hydrochloric acid and the two enzymes—pepsin and rennin. The pepsin enzyme acts on protein, breaking it down to simpler products, which are

279

further digested later by other enzymes in the intestine. No digestion of sugar or starch occurs in the stomach, and little if any of fat. Hydrochloric acid serves several useful purposes. When in sufficient concentration, it inhibits bacterial growth, activates the enzyme, pepsin, and to some extent influences the pyloric reflexes. The amount of acid present at birth is small, but it increases progressively. It is decreased by any illness and by severe malnutrition. When human milk is fed, the gastric acidity finally reached is optimum for peptic digestion. Although cow's milk is neither acid nor alkaline, it has the property of binding small amounts of acid without changing its reaction. To bring about the same degree of acidity it is necessary to add 3 times as much acid to cow's milk as to human milk. Modifications of cow's milk which have proved to be more or less uniformly successful in infant feeding have the common property requiring relatively small amounts of acid to bring the acidity to a point optimum for peptic digestion. They also have in common the production of a fine curd in the stomach.

Soon after the ingestion of milk the casein is precipitated by the enzyme rennin. Because of the small amount of casein in human milk, the precipitate is divided finely. Unmodified cow's milk, because of the larger amount of casein, gives rise to a large rubbery curd which may resist complete breaking up, and parts of it may be passed eventually in the stool as tough lima-beanlike masses. Cow's milk that has been boiled or has been subjected to heat incident to evaporation or drying gives rise to a curd resembling that of human milk, although usually somewhat coarser. When cow's milk is fed to an infant, less difficulty is encountered if the milk has been heat-treated than if it has not been modified in any way. Milk to which acid has been added in such a manner and quantity as to make a fine curd is better tolerated than either plain boiled or raw milk. The fineness of the curd undoubtedly contributes to the ease of digestion, and it is probable that this factor is of greater importance than the degree of acidity reached in gastric digestion.

Practically no absorption takes place from the stomach. The stomach may be expected to be empty in from 2 to 3 hours when human milk is fed, and in from 2½ to 3½ hours with customary modifications of cow's milk. Emptying of the stomach is delayed by a high proportion of fat in the food and by illness of the infant.

DIGESTION IN DUODENUM AND SMALL INTESTINE

Although much has been said in the preceding discussion concerning gastric digestion, it is in the duodenum and the small intestine that the greater part of digestion is accomplished. Protein that escapes gastric digestion is acted on by the pancreatic secretion, and the resultant products are further broken down into amino acids by an enzyme secreted by the mucous membrane of the intestine. The amino acids are absorbed and either converted to body protein or burned. Fats are changed into soaps and glycerin by pancreatic secretion and bile. These are absorbed from the small intestine to be reconstructed into body fat or burned. Another enzyme of the pancreatic secretion converts starch into sugar. Complex sugars are changed to monosaccharides (dextrose, levulose and galactose) by the secretions of the small intestine before absorption. The ability to digest starch is relatively feeble at birth, but it increases rapidly. If starch is fed in the very early months of life, a portion of it is likely to pass through the intestinal tract unchanged. Usually this does no harm, and only occasionally are fermentative processes set up.

CHIEF FUNCTION OF LARGE INTESTINE

The chief function of the large intestine is to absorb water. Though it is capable of absorbing amino acids, salts and simple sugars, it is seldom called on for this purpose. Before reaching the large intestine, practically all the protein and its products will have been digested and absorbed. Sugars reaching the large intestine are fermented quickly by the bacteria present in enormous number. Some soaps remaining from fat digestion pass into the colon, though little or no digestion or absorption takes place.

The period required for food to pass through the gastro-intestinal tract varies from 8 to 36 hours, depending largely on the degree to which different food substances stimulate peristalsis.

Bacteria are not present in the intestinal tract at birth but gain entrance soon thereafter. They are not present in important numbers until food is given. In the presence of food they multiply greatly. The prevailing type of bacteria present depends on the type of food that the baby receives. With human-milk feeding the bacteria are pre-dominantly gram-positive; with customary formulas of cow's milk they are gram-negative. That one of these two types is more beneficial to the baby than the other has not been shown. The gram-positive types are associated with the slightly acid stools of low protein-high sugar feeding; the gram-negative types, with the alkaline stools of relatively high protein feeding. Certain bacteria which grow in an alkaline medium are the cause of ammoniacal excoriations of the skin of the diaper region, a condition which may occur in an otherwise normal baby; it is discussed under Ammonia Dermatitis. Only under abnormal conditions do acid excoriations of the buttocks occur. Their cause is discussed under Diarrhea. Bacteria are unevenly distributed in the intestinal tract. Under normal conditions few are found in the stomach, the duodenum and the upper jejunum. The number increases progressively down the tract, the greatest number being in the colon. Their abnormal presence in the duodenum is discussed under Diarrhea.

STOOLS

Meconium

Meconium is the term applied to the first stools passed after birth. Meconium consists of partially dried intestinal secretions which have gradually accumulated in the lower tract. It is dark brownish-green in color, semiformed, and is usually passed from 4 to 6 times daily. The stools continue so until food is ingested. About the third day, with the ingestion of food the stools begin to change, and by the fourth or the fifth day they have assumed the characteristics that persist for the subsequent months.

Character of Stools

The character of the stools is determined by the type of food. Normal stools of infants fed on milk are composed of approximately 20 per cent solids, chiefly soaps, and 80 per cent water.

Human Milk

When human milk is fed, the stools may be passed only once or twice a day or may occur after every feeding. Characteristically, such stools are unformed but not watery; the color is bright or golden yellow or occasionally light green; the odor is unobjectionably aromatic; the reaction is acid. After the initial adjustment to breast feeding some infants will have soft stools that are passed very infrequently, e.g., only every third or fourth day.

Cow's Milk

When cow's milk is fed in customary formulas, the stools are firmer than those from human milk and are passed less frequently, usually from 1 to 3 times daily. Although yellow, they seldom have the bright yellow color of the stool from human milk. The reaction is neutral or slightly alkaline, and the odor is more or less foul. The differences between the stools from human and from cow's milk are due to the differences in the composition of the food. A high-sugar, low-protein diet (human milk) tends to cause more frequent stools, which are acid in reaction. A low-sugar, high-protein diet tends to cause the reverse condition.

COLOR OF STOOL

The color of stools when milk is the principal food is influenced chiefly by the rate at which the food passes through the intestinal tract. A diarrheal stool usually is green; a soft stool, yellowish; and a firm pasty stool, light yellow or almost white. These variations are due to the fact that the bile pigment in the upper intestine is green, but after it has remained for some time in the intestinal tract chemical action occurs which changes the green to yellow, and after further stay in the tract the yellow pigment is changed to a colorless pigment. When diarrhea occurs, the green bile coloring passes through the intestine so rapidly that it is not changed. A yellow stool, if exposed to the air for some time, often turns green on the surface, due to a process of oxidation. This change of color is of no significance. The feeding of cereals, malt preparations or skimmed milk may lead to stools which are less yellow or even of brownish color. Certain drugs, such as bismuth and iron, may color the stools black. With atresia of the bile ducts the stools are gray or clay-colored because of the absence of bile (acholic stools). (See Plate 1.)

MUCUS, PUS AND BLOOD

A slight amount of glairy mucus may be seen normally in the stools, especially those from breast-fed infants. A larger amount of mucus in the stools of either breast-fed or artificially fed babies is an indication of irritation of the intestinal tract and is often seen when diarrhea is present. Pus does not normally occur in stools. When it is found, it indicates an inflammation of the intestinal wall (ileocolitis or dysentery). When severe inflammation of the wall of the intestine occurs, blood as well as pus may appear in the stools. The blood may be bright, or, if its source is higher in the intestine, it may be altered to a brownish or black color. It is mixed in streaks in the stool, or the whole stool may be bloody. Bloody stools also occur in association with intussusception. Small streaks of blood occurring on the outside of constipated stools usually mean nothing more than a slight crack or fissure at the anus.

CURDS

Curds occurring in stools are of three varieties: soap, casein and mucus. Soap curds are most frequent. They are small and soft and are easily mashed with a spatula. They occur normally in the stools of breast-fed infants and are seen also in loose stools of artificially fed babies. The presence of soap curds indicates that peristalsis has been rapid, and that there has not been sufficient time for the absorption of water and the compression of curds into firmer masses. The occurrence of soap curds does not necessarily indicate that too much fat is being fed. They occur in the stools no matter what causes the increased looseness.

Casein curds are seen in the stools only of infants fed raw or pasteurized cow's milk. They are hard, tough, usually yellowish, and about the size and the shape of a small lima bean. Mucus in the stool in excess may become dry and rolled up in the form of small balls or stringy curds. Parents sometimes mistake the mucous strings for intestinal worms.

COLIC

Infants in the first few months of life who have frequent fits of sudden crying are commonly regarded as suffering from colic. There are many theories about the nature of colic which govern the type of treatment. It is entirely possible that several factors may be responsible and that the behavior observed is merely the response of an immature infant to any of a number of types of discomfort.

Infants who suffer from colic are generally small at birth (5 to 7 lbs.). They tend to be lean with tense muscles and a nervous system which easily is triggered into a maximum response by the slightest of stimuli. During much of their day such infants are either asleep or violently protesting their discomfort. They do not remain long in the middle ground of quiet, satisfied wakefulness. The symptoms tend to be worse in the early evening and the nighttime hours than they are during the day. The persistence of this type of behavior is variable. In many instances it ceases rather abruptly—often without any particular change in regimen. Such a welcome cessation may come at from 3 to 4 weeks or as late as from 3 to 4 months. The colloquial designation "3-month colic" suggests the average duration and enforces the suspicion that it is predetermined and not related to treatment.

The behavior of an infant with colic usually is suggestive of paroxysmal abdominal pain due to excessive accumulation of gas in the intestine or the stomach. Crying starts abruptly with loud screams, clenched fists and legs that are drawn up on the abdomen. During the general muscular contraction, gas may be expelled from the anus or may be belched up from the stomach. The traditional efforts to explain and treat colic center around control of the gas production within the intestinal tract.

Excessive air-swallowing often is considered as an important factor. Too-rapid feeding during which the infant gulps down air is blamed sometimes. Small nipple holes or a breast that yields little milk can result in vigorous sucking and swallowing efforts which also carry an excessive amount of air into the stomach. Depending upon the individual situation, the feeding procedure may need to be altered. Frequent burping of the baby during and after feeding usually is advised. The use of carminatives such as peppermint water and fennel tea to aid in relaxation of the cardiac sphincter of the stomach is a household remedy that is not generally very effective. Enemas, suppositories and rectal tubes to relieve distention of the lower bowel are advised sometimes, but the same result usually can be achieved by turning the infant on his abdomen.

The accumulation of gas in the intestine is attributed by some to intestinal indigestion from overfeeding or from excessive use of carbohydrate, which fosters intestinal fermentation and produces gas within the lumen of the bowel. On this basis, various modifications of the amount and the type of formula are made.

Another approach is the attempt to reduce the vigor of intestinal movements by the use of drugs such as atropine and its derivatives, phenobarbital and banthine. The local application of heat by the use of a hot-water bottle also is advocated by some.

Yet another theory holds that colic is largely emotionally conditioned. The fact that many colicky infants are relieved of their distress merely by being held or permitted to suck on a pacifier is cited as evidence that the disturbance may be due to insufficient emotional satisfaction. Mothers are encouraged to give their infants additional cuddling and closeness as a temporary measure.

Whatever the importance of these various factors, at the present time it cannot be said that colic has a single etiology or appropriate treatment. The measures that are important for relief of the individual infant (and its mother) must be worked out by trial and error in each instance.

CONSTIPATION

Constipation exists when the bowels move infrequently or with difficulty or both. Usually it produces no symptoms, although there may be local pain from the passage of a large hard fecal mass. Occasionally in infancy streaks of blood are found on the outside of the stool, the blood having come from a fissure at the anus. Only rarely and only in infancy does constipation cause prolapse of the anus or the rectum. General symptoms from constipation either do not exist or are too vague to be identified.

Constipation results when the stimulus to peristalsis is insufficient or when the intestine fails to respond to a normal stimulus. Since the normal stimulus to peristalsis is food, insufficient food results in constipation. Intestinal irritability varies in different infants and children and from time to time in the same infant or child. Constipation results also when the intestinal content is of such consistency from absorption of water in the lower bowel that it is difficult for it to move onward even though peristalsis is active.

Certain anomalies of the intestinal tract lead to constipation. Constipation from such causes is uncommon as compared with those due to causes associated with food. The constipation accompanying pyloric stenosis in infancy is due to the dearth of food passing the pylorus. The constipation of megacolon is caused by mechanical interference in the lower part of the colon.

In infancy, underfeeding or persistent vomiting may cause constipation. Usually with insufficient food the stools are small and infrequent, although occasionally as a result of underfeeding the stools may be as numerous as from 8 to 10 a day. Constipation in a breast-fed baby is most frequently due to underfeeding. However, in some instances the stools are infrequent when the amount of food seems to be adequate.

When constipation is present in either a breast-fed or an artificially fed baby and the food seems to be adequate and the infant is thriving, the addition of fruits and vegetables to the diet, or an increase in the amount of these if they already are being fed, often serves to give the little increase in stimulus that is necessary. Strained orange juice usually is not laxative because the dextrose is absorbed so quickly. Prune juice is somewhat laxative.

Drugs preferably should not be used in the management of constipation. If laxatives seem to be necessary in the beginning of treatment they should be given regularly and not occasionally as apparently needed. The amount should be decreased gradually until none is being taken. For infants, magnesia magma (milk of magnesia) is effective and relatively mild.

Enemas may be necessary at times to relieve difficult situations but they are too likely to lead to habitual need of increased stimulation to be useful as a regular means of relief. In addition, they may evoke rebellious feelings in the child and make him feel attacked, punished or robbed. Suppositories also may lead to habitual need and are contraindicated, both for physical and psychological reasons. Suitable massage of the abdomen often is recommended and at times may be of benefit.

VOMITING

Vomiting is a much more common symptom during infancy than in childhood or later life. Much of it is due to trivial or temporary causes, but it can betoken serious illness which should be recognized promptly so that appropriate treatment can be instituted. The symptoms must always be evaluated in the setting of other indications of the state of the infant's health.

COMMON CAUSES
Gastric Distention

Gastric distention from any cause results in vomiting in infancy. When the stomach is overfilled with food, it reacts by expelling the excess. Expulsion of food from this cause may be no more than a little regurgitation of a small or moderate amount of partly altered milk, which pours out of the mouth with no expulsive effort. This safety-valve action of the stomach in rejecting excessive amounts of food tends to protect the infant from the more serious consequences of overfeeding. A few infants have a small gastric capacity and are unable, without vomiting, to take all the food needed when it is offered in the usual dilutions. In such cases it is necessary to use a more concentrated food. When food is given at such short intervals that the stomach is not empty before the next feeding, vomiting often results from overfilling the stomach. When food is taken too rapidly, insufficient food leaves the stomach during the feeding, with distention and vomiting as a result. Some of these difficulties are avoided when the infant's appetite is allowed to determine the amounts and the times of feeding.

A common cause of overdistention of the stomach is the gas that it contains in addition to food. The gas is chiefly swallowed air and may be present in large amounts. All babies swallow some air. The amount swallowed is increased when they are hungry or when the food intake is insufficient or when the milk is obtained from the nipple with difficulty. When the infant is lying on his back, the air cannot escape without first forcing out part of the fluid. Abdominal bands or clothes that are too tight have the same effect as gastric distention in producing vomiting.

Gastric Irritation

Newborn babies often vomit from the irritation produced by the presence of mucus in the stomach. In the older infant, reflex vomiting may result from the ingestion of unusual foods, foods which are highly spiced, or foods to which the infant is allergic. An excess of fat in the feeding or the presence of disease will often slow down the discharge of food from the stomach, permitting fermentation by the bacteria present and leading to an accumulation of irritating products of partial or abnormal digestion.

Acute Infections

Both vomiting and diarrhea may be the initial symptom of infections outside of the gastro-intestinal tract, most commonly in the pharynx or the ears. It is usually a feature of the initial stages of the disease and abates rapidly as spontaneous or therapeutic improvement takes place.

Voluntary Vomiting and Rumination

Some infants and young children are able to bring up food from the stomach at will. Others initiate vomiting by putting a hand into the mouth. When voluntary vomiting becomes a regular habit without known provocation, it is spoken of as rumination. Rumination usually occurs only in infancy. In certain instances, voluntary vomiting is a reaction of the infant or the child to unusual foods or foods that he does not like. Occasionally, vomiting develops as a result of the infant's or the child's re-action to his environment and manage-ment, such as the forcing of food. Vomiting from these latter causes is amenable to proper management, al-though often the environment must be changed completely to accomplish the desired result.

Nursing Care of Infants Who Vomit

When an infant shows a tendency to vomit, unusual care in feeding is neces-sary. In each case the infant's tolerance should be noted. The nursing care should be planned to eliminate unnecessary movement of the infant after feed-ing. Too much handling and tossing about of an infant often leads to vomit-ing. Treatments leading to emotional strain should neither precede nor follow feeding. The food should be kept warm and given slowly. Care in "bubbling" the baby is especially important. He should be held up after each feeding and should be patted gently on the back until the air is expelled. Holding the infant in an erect position allows the air bubble to lodge at the cardiac orifice, from which location it may escape easily without causing vomiting. Some infants have to be held up in this manner before and during feeding, as well as after-ward. Placing the infant on his side and elevating the head of the bed after feed-ing tends to prevent vomiting and aspiration; in this position gas is ex-pelled from the stomach more freely.

In the case of very weak babies, such as those prematurely born, vomiting is to be guarded against by every means possible. In these instances the vomitus is likely to be aspirated. The resultant pneumonia is serious and often fatal.

When vomiting occurs, skin irritation will be prevented by care of the skin of the face, behind the ears and in the folds of the neck. Charting is important. Not only is it necessary to chart the estimated amount of vomitus and the relation to feeding, but the type, the nature, the color, the consistency and the odor and the presence or the absence of nausea also may aid in diagnosis. Differentiation should be made between regurgitation, projectile vomiting and the vomiting that occurs at the time that air is expelled.

Infants who ruminate must be ob-served closely and provided with substi-tute satisfactions. Ruminator caps have been devised. These fit firmly over the chin and the throat and prevent move-ment of the tongue and the throat muscles which bring the food back into the mouth. At the time of feeding, the cap is loosened. Immediately after feeding the cap should be readjusted, and an effort should be made to divert the infant's attention to something that is interesting and pleasurable to him. Constant attention until the infant falls asleep or until the food has left the stomach is necessary. Such a method provides a substitute wholesome satis-faction for one that is essentially de-priving.

Occasionally, arm restraints are ordered to prevent the infant from in-itiating vomiting with his hands. How-ever, restraints without play materials and a close personal relationship often are not only ineffectual but also suffi-ciently frustrating to create additional emotional tension which tends to fix rather than eliminate the habit.

VOMITING ASSOCIATED WITH DISEASE OF OTHER ORGANS

Abnormalities of the central nervous system, particularly those which lead to an increase in intracranial pressure, us-ually are accompanied by vomiting which is automatic in character and not associated with feeding. Congenital hy-drocephalus, subarachnoid or subdural hemorrhage and acute meningitis and encephalitis are some of the infantile disorders in which it may be a prom-inent symptom. Severe or chronic coughing, such as that associated with pertussis or acute bronchitis or broncho-pneumonia, may precipitate vomiting during the coughing paroxysms. Adrenal insufficiency is accompanied by persistent vomiting. Severe renal disorders, such as hydronephrosis or congenital cystic kidneys, may produce uremia with its associated emesis.

OBSTRUCTION OF THE GASTRO-INTESTINAL TRACT

Congenital Malformations

Vomiting of bile-containing fluid during the newborn period should raise the suspicion of an abnormality of the intestinal tract which interferes with the patency of its lumen. These conditions are considered in more detail in Chapter 16. Some types of malformation permit a delay in the appearance of symptoms until later in infancy. Strangulation of inguinal hernias may be included in this category.

Pyloric Stenosis

Congenital hypertrophic pyloric stenosis is commonly classified as a congenital abnormality of the intestinal tract. It is considered here because its late onset places it outside the newborn period and makes it a constant topic of concern whenever an infant's early ad-

justment is marred by chronic vomiting.

Symptoms. Vomiting is the outstanding symptom. It seldom begins earlier than 2 or 3 weeks or later than 2 months of age; it progresses gradually in frequency and force until most of the ingested food is expelled, often in a projectile manner which carries it over the side of the bed. The vomitus is never bile-stained but may contain mucus or streaks of blood. The stools usually decrease in size and number. Chronic loss of food results in a decline in the infant's rate of gain in weight until progress ceases and then reverses. The infants are uniformly hungry and chronically so, being willing to eat immediately after vomiting. Dehydration follows the weight loss and may reach life-threatening proportions. Unlike most other types of dehydration, it is associated with alkalosis of the body fluids rather than acidosis. The infants have no fever except during dehydration or intercurrent infection. Pain is not obvious apart from the discomfort of chronic hunger. An observant attendant will often notice upper abdominal distention after feeding within which peristaltic waves can be seen to sweep across the abdomen from left to right, reversing

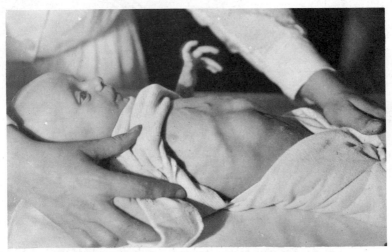

FIG. 40. Showing peristaltic waves of pyloric stenosis.

themselves just prior to or during vomiting (Fig. 40).

Pyloric stenosis is about 3 times as common in male infants as it is in females. It appears to involve first-born children primarily and has some tendency to recur within certain families, suggesting a hereditary background. Its incidence among Caucasian infants has been reported as high as 1 in 150 liveborn males. It is uncommon in Negroes.

Mechanism. The symptoms are readily understood from the findings at operation or at autopsy. The pyloric canal —the channel through the distal, muscular end of the stomach which conducts food into the duodenum (Fig. 41)—is greatly narrowed by a combination of muscular hypertrophy, muscular spasm and edema of the mucous membrane within the canal. Behind the obstructed channel the wall of the stomach is thickened, due to hypertrophy in response to its efforts to force material through the narrowed channel. This hypertrophy accounts for the visible abdominal waves and for the ability of the stomach to propel vomitus out of the mouth with some force.

The inability of food to pass readily through the pylorus into the duodenum accounts for the decline in weight and the decrease in volume of stool. Little or no food absorption occurs from the stomach, but some water may be taken up before passage into the duodenum. Thus the malnutrition of these infants is usually more severe than the dehydration. The fluid being lost from the body in the vomitus is primarily acid in character because of the hydrochloric acid in gastric juice. The deficit of acid ions can be compensated by the kidneys and the lungs for a time, but beyond a certain point the reaction of the blood plasma shifts into the alkaline range.

Diagnosis. The diagnosis can be suspected from the history which is usually typical in respect to the age of onset, the character of the vomiting and its progressive course. In addition, the infants have a characteristic hungry, pinched, anxious facies which experienced nurses soon learn to identify. Observation of peristaltic abdominal waves is possible in advanced cases, and a skilled clinician can frequently feel the hypertrophied pyloric muscle

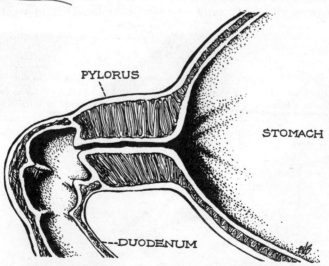

Fig. 41. Showing hypertrophied circular muscle of the pylorus in pyloric stenosis.

through the abdominal wall. Changes in the chemical anatomy of the blood will often demonstrate the loss of chloride and help to indicate the severity of the disturbance. Final proof of the diagnosis may be obtained by roentgen examination with barium. Enlargement of the stomach, delay in passage of the barium into the duodenum, a narrowed, elongated and curved pyloric canal, and bulging of the hypertrophied pyloric muscle into the antrum of the stomach are findings which support the clinical impression. In early or mild cases the roentgen findings may not support the clinical diagnosis, and it is presumed that the chief obstructing mechanism is spasm rather than hypertrophy of the pyloric muscle. Infants whose troubles simulate pyloric stenosis but are not regarded as having the fully developed disorder are often said to have *pylorospasm*, an entity of somewhat vague definition which occupies the middle ground between normality and true pyloric stenosis.

Treatment varies with the severity of the disease and the concept of its pathogenesis. Medical management can be tried where the diagnosis is uncertain or the symptoms relatively mild. In Europe there is greater enthusiasm for medical management of the severely affected infants than in the United States, where the prompt termination of symptoms and excellent prognosis from skillful surgical correction wield greater influence in the decision. Medical management, even when successful, is likely to be a prolonged and inconvenient process. It is not usually undertaken in successfully breast-fed infants or in those whose disease has carried them into obvious dehydration, chemical imbalance or significant malnutrition. In the latter case the hazard of temporizing with medical management may convert the infant into an increasingly poorer operative risk.

The symptoms of pyloric stenosis tend to decrease after the age of 3 or 4 months. If an infant has been treated with more or less success up to this age, usually medical treatment is continued. As time passes, little diminution of hypertrophy occurs, but the lumen enlarges with growth.

Medical Treatment. This includes several or all of the following procedures: gastric lavage, refeeding after vomiting, thickening the formula with cereal, administration of atropine derivatives or sedatives or both.

Atropine is given to abolish the spasm of the pyloric sphincter. A 1:1,000 solution of atropine sulfate (½ gr. to the ounce) is used. The solution should not be kept longer than 2 weeks. The dose is given in a small amount of water 20 minutes before each feeding. The dose at the start is one drop of the solution. The amount is increased rapidly until flushing of the skin occurs, and then this amount, or an amount slightly smaller, is given before each feeding. Doses above 3 or 4 drops usually are to be avoided. Eumydrine, an atropine derivative with less marked side effects, is used in an initial dose of 0.05 mg. once a day, increasing to a maximum of 0.5 mg. per day. Phenobarbital may be used in individual doses of 15 mg. 2 or 3 times daily.

If thickened feedings are to be used, the formula should be one suitable for the age of the infant, but thickened with cereal. Food thus thickened is not vomited as easily as customary formulas. In those instances in which it may seem desirable not to use a thickened feeding, the formula should be one that produces very fine curds in the stomach.

Refeeding is often of value. If a portion of the food is vomited within an hour after feeding, approximately this same amount of additional food may be given. The entire feeding may be retained under these conditions.

Surgical Treatment. The surgical treatment of choice for pyloric stenosis is known as the Rammstedt or Fredet-Rammstedt operation. It consists of an incision through the hypertrophied circular muscle down to, but not through, the mucosa and parallel with the pyloric lumen. This procedure allows the pylorus to expand so that food will pass. The operation is over quickly, and the baby is little disturbed by it.

Preoperatively, the infant should be brought into the best condition of hydration and electrolyte balance which can be achieved within a period of 2 or 3 days. Fluids are restored by intravenous or subcutaneous saline which simultaneously helps to correct the chloride deficit. Potassium-containing solutions are usually advisable after renal function has been established, since any significant degree of cellular dehydration is associated with a loss of potassium. In severely affected infants plasma or blood may be required to correct anemia or to bolster plasma proteins. Feeding is usually continued up until the time of operation in the hope that some of the nutriment will pass through the pylorus. Immediately prior to operation the stomach should be emptied in order to prevent vomiting and also to simplify the surgical procedure by deflating the stomach. Often the tube is left in place during the operation.

Parenterally administered thiamine and ascorbic acid are sometimes given to promote rapid healing of the wound.

Following operation, the parenteral administration of fluids is continued until oral intake is sufficient to meet the infant's fluid needs. Feedings by mouth are usually begun in 12 to 24 hours with glucose solution in small amounts and the volume and the strength of the formula increased according to a prearranged scheme which is designed to forestall vomiting. Barring the unusual complications of poor healing of the abdominal incision or persistence of vomiting due to incomplete division of the pyloric muscle or to accidental perforation of the duodenum, recovery is usually rapid enough to

permit a full intake of food within a week.

Preoperative Nursing Care. Gastric lavage in a baby is carried out in the same manner as in an adult, with a few minor differences. The infant may be recumbent or held in the lap of an assistant. In either case, restraint by means of wrapping in a sheet usually is necessary. A catheter (size 10 or 12 French) connected to a funnel by 2 feet of rubber tubing is moistened in sterile water and passed rapidly into the stomach. Passage into the larynx is practically impossible. If by chance the catheter should go into the larynx or the trachea, breathing would stop, and cyanosis from suspended respiration would develop rapidly. As evidence that the tube is in the stomach, the infant is able to breathe (not through the tube), and usually gastric contents will appear in the funnel. In infants, when the tube has been inserted 9 inches from the gums or the teeth it reaches well into the stomach. Coughing, gagging and redness of the face caused by passage of the tube cease quickly if the tube is held without motion. After siphoning off the stomach contents, an amount of fluid somewhat less than the gastric capacity is allowed to run in. An initial failure to flow, due to a column of air in the tube, can be corrected by "milking" the tube gently.

The stomach is emptied by lowering the funnel and the tube below the level of the child. The process is repeated until the water returns clear. Usually from 1 pint to 1 quart of fluid is required. Suitable amounts for each washing are: 1 week, 1 ounce; 1 month, 2 ounces; 6 months or more, 4 to 6 ounces. For removal, the tube is pinched tightly in order that fluid may not leak into the pharynx and cause choking. Gastric lavage is seldom required more than twice daily. The fluid commonly used for lavage is either sterile water or normal saline.

Atropine is a toxic drug when given

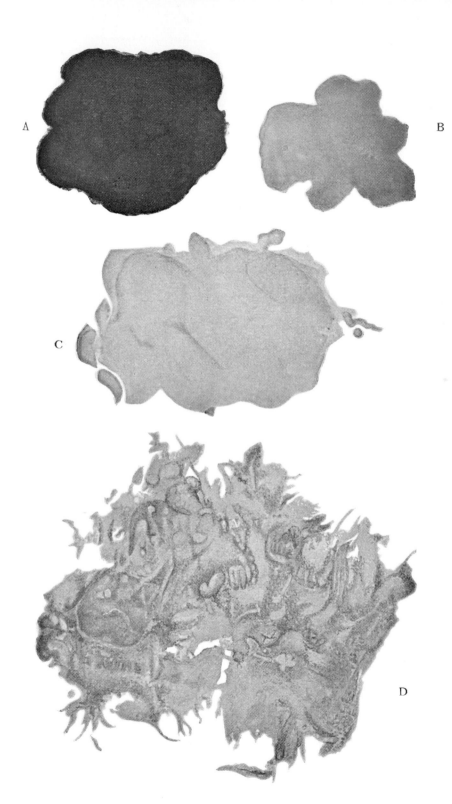

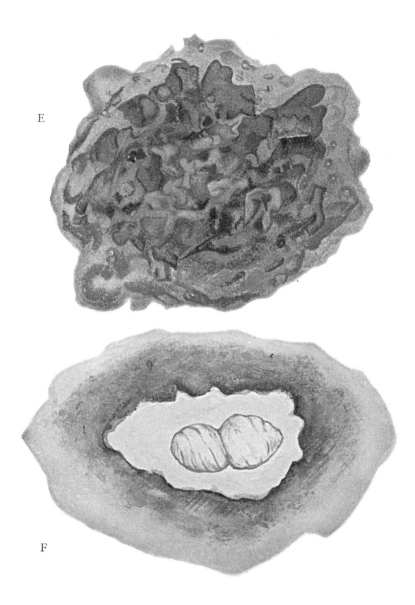

E

F

PLATE 1

Infants' stools as observed in the diaper by which any fluid portion has been absorbed. (A) Meconium stool of the newborn infant. (B) Stool of the breast-fed infant. (C) Stool of the artificially fed infant. (D) Stool of the infant with diarrhea. (E) Stool of the infant with dysentery. (F) Acholic stool of the infant with atresia of the bile ducts.

in overdosage. It should be diluted with water and given with a medicine dropper. When the dosage has been increased cautiously until flushing occurs, the flushing appears soon after the drug has been given and disappears after a short time. The effect is transitory and harmless. The flushing is the most obvious sign that the tolerance without harmful effect has been reached. In some instances, atropine in a flushing dose causes moderate fever. High fever should be reported.

A thickened feeding should be so thick that it will not drop from an inverted spoon. A baby may be fed with a spoon, or the food may be placed in a large "Hygeia" nipple, the tip of which has been cut off so as to leave a large hole. The nipple is placed in the infant's mouth, and the food is pressed into the end of the nipple by a spoon or a spatula.

When unthickened feedings are ordered, the formula should be given with such care that the likelihood of vomiting is decreased. Infants with pyloric stenosis tend to suck their hands and get a great deal of air into the stomach. Bubbling before the infant begins to eat is often necessary. Because he is hungry he tends to eat his food rapidly, and the food must be given slowly if vomiting is to be prevented.

Charting accurately the approximate amount vomited, the type and the color, and its relation to feeding aids in diagnosis. Refeeding the infant an equivalent of the amount vomited should be done when it is directed.

Impairment of nutrition causes lowered resistance to infection, and every means possible should be used to prevent the infant from developing intercurrent infection. Technic to protect the baby from infections should be carried out. Position should be changed frequently. If the infant has a lowered body temperature, extra warmth should be added to keep his temperature stable and in a normal range. Lamps attached to a bed cradle can be placed over the infant to give this additional warmth. Supportive treatment, such as blood transfusions and fluids parenterally, is given the infant to supplement his food and fluid intake. Urine output should be noted, and accurate charting of the stools is important.

Postoperative Nursing Care. When the infant returns from the operating room, he should be placed on his side to prevent aspiration of vomitus. Additional warmth will be needed to prevent shock. The quality of the pulse, the type of respiration, and the color of the infant's skin should be noted frequently. If shock does occur, the foot of the bed should be elevated, and additional warmth should be supplied. Position must be changed, but it should be done gently to prevent vomiting.

Customs differ as to when the first feedings are given after operation. If the pyloric mucosa has not been punctured at operation, no strong contraindication exists to feeding small amounts soon after operation when a local anesthetic has been used or as soon as recovery occurs from general anesthesia. However, peristalsis is impaired by the operation, and some vomiting is usual when food is given early. Because of impaired peristalsis and resultant vomiting, it is customary in some hospitals to leave a nasal tube in the stomach for about 24 hours and to defer feeding for the same length of time, maintaining body fluids by parenteral administration. While the nasal tube is in place, the infant's arms should be restrained to prevent removal of the tube. When feedings are resumed, they are ordered in small amounts. Hunger is observed soon after operation, and to prevent vomiting from hurried feedings, the food should be given by medicine dropper. During the early period if vomiting is frequent, it is best to feed the baby in bed with his head slightly elevated. When the feedings are increased and tolerance is noted, they may be given by

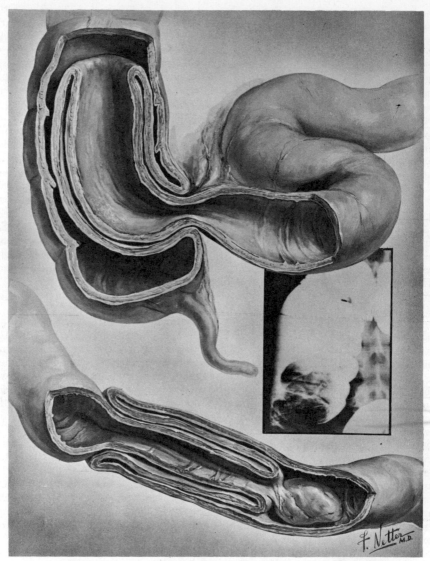

FIG. 42. Intussusception. (*Top*) Ileocolic variety. (*Insert*)
Roentgen appearance. (*Bottom*) Ileoileal variety. (Ciba
Collection of Medical Illustrations)

nipple and bottle, with the infant in the
nurse's lap where he can be cuddled
and bubbled more effectively. The
amount of food is increased as the
infant shows greater tolerance for it.
His behavior before and after feeding

is a guide to his tolerance and food
needs.

If the infant received breast feedings
prior to operation, the feeding of human
milk should be resumed subsequent to
operation. At first, he can be fed ex-

pressed milk in order to regulate the quantity, but within 2 or 3 days he can be placed directly at the breast and allowed to suckle for the usual length of time. During the period when the milk is being expressed, the breasts should be emptied completely in order to maintain the supply.

Until the stitches have been removed, protection of the dressing will help to prevent wound infection. Applying the diaper low, below the dressing, prevents wound contamination.

Intussusception

Intussusception is the invagination of a portion of the bowel into the portion immediately distal to it. This telescoping effect is illustrated in Figure 42. It probably is caused by hyperactive peristalsis in the proximal portion of the bowel with relative inactivity of the distal segment. Although it may occur at any level of the small or the large intestine, nearly always it is discovered at the junction of the ileum and the colon. As the bowel invaginates it carries along its mesentery. Thus the blood supply is cut off, and if the condition continues, the bowel will become gangrenous. Death may result if the condition is not recognized and corrected. Most of those who develop intussusception are infants, and usually they are robust boys who have been thriving.

Symptoms. The disease may begin suddenly with a shriek of pain and rapidly appearing symptoms of intestinal obstruction—vomiting, constipation, abdominal pain and eventually prostration and shock. At times the origin of symptoms is more insidious, with indefinite discomfort, poor appetite and unexplained vomiting. Despite the constipation characteristic of obstruction, small bloody stools containing mucus and little or no fecal matter may be passed. The tumor mass that results from intussusception may be palpated through the abdominal wall or may be detected with the finger on rectal examination if it has progressed far enough down the colon.

Treatment. Intussusception requires immediate relief, for the mortality rises sharply with increasing duration of symptoms. In rare instances the intussusception will reduce spontaneously, but this is not an outcome that can be awaited with safety. In some instances the barium enema given to confirm the diagnosis will exert enough retrograde pressure to reduce the telescoped bowel, and the fluoroscopic examination or films will demonstrate that complete relief has been achieved. Usually, however, prompt surgical exploration is indicated in order to reduce the intussusception before irreversible gangrene of the bowel has occurred. In the latter instance, resection of bowel is necessary—a procedure which is poorly tolerated by a seriously ill infant.

Nursing Care. The postoperative symptomatic care of the infant is not unlike that given after other types of abdominal operation. If simple reduction of the bowel is accomplished, feedings may be started shortly after peristaltic activity is audible in the abdomen. If resection of gangrenous bowel is necesssary, constant gastric suction and parenteral administration of fluids are required for several days. During this period an infant may find some measure of solace in being permitted to suck on a pacifier or a nipple, and in being held.

DIARRHEA

Diarrhea is a common symptom among infants which has particular import because of fluid loss which threatens the relatively unstable water balance of the human young. Like vomiting, it has multiple causes. In a small minority of instances the reason for diarrhea is obvious or can be inferred from other events taking place around or within the infant. Usually its exact basis is unknown. It either remains obscure or is not clarified by laboratory study until after the crucial period of illness has passed. Thus the practical management of diarrhea is a symptomatic approach which attempts to correct the physiologic changes from moment to moment, while keeping a wary eye open for specific etiologic agents which may require appropriate antibiotic attack.

ETIOLOGY AND PREVENTION

Diarrhea results from an increase in the rate of peristalsis which carries the intestinal contents along so rapidly that they are expelled before the large intestine has had time to reabsorb water in the usual way. A change in the color of the stools also depends upon rapid passage of material through the tract. Bile pigment which enters high up in the duodenum is ordinarily changed by the chemical action of the intestinal contents from green through yellow to brown. If passage through the intestinal canal is too rapid, this reaction is not completed by the time the stool emerges.

Minor degrees of diarrhea are sometimes ascribed to noninfectious factors such as the mechanical and chemical irritation resulting from bulky or undigested food; or from antibiotics or drugs; or from allergic response to specific items of diet; or from increased irritability due to nervous tension; or as a nonspecific effect of any illness which depresses the tolerance for food. This variety of diarrhea can be prevented only through a knowledge of the individual infant's idiosyncrasies and avoidance of foods and drugs known to upset him.

Practically all of the serious diarrhea and much of the milder afflictions are associated with or directly due to infec-

tion. Past experience has demonstrated the urgency of handling infants with diarrhea as though they had a disease which could be readily transmitted to others either by direct contact or by contamination from their stools. Some of the bacterial agents responsible for diarrhea are well-known and can be isolated by culture of the stools. These include the dysentery group of organisms (Shiga, Flexner, Sonne and other types), the typhoid bacillus and the salmonella group of related bacteria. In recent years certain antigenic types of colon bacilli (enteropathic *E. coli*) have been added to this list as a definite cause of epidemic diarrhea, particularly among newborn infants. Other bacteria such as staphylococci, pseudomonas and proteus organisms have often been suspected as specific causes of infantile diarrhea, but their guilt has been more difficult to fix with certainty. The epidemiologic characteristics of old-fashioned "summer diarrhea" from which incriminating bacteria could not be cultivated have for a long time placed it under the suspicion of being a virus infection. Proof of this etiology has been obtained on infrequent occasions. Diarrhea has also been attributed to "toxic effects." Some theories have regarded it as being analogous to food-poisoning and due to the action of soluble toxins from bacterial growth accumulating in contaminated and poorly refrigerated formula. Other theories have blamed changes which take place within the infant's body during the course of infections of the nose, the throat and particularly the ears and the mastoids. It is quite likely that each of these theories offers the correct explanation for some cases of diarrhea.

The prevention of diarrhea which is due to a communicable infection is achieved through careful formula preparation, through isolation of sick infants and through general public health improvements in safeguarding milk, water supplies, sewage, and the control of

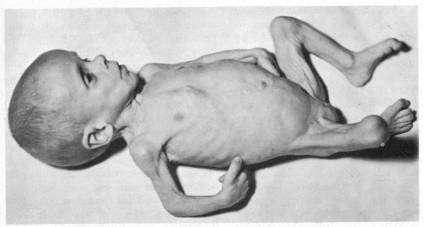

FIG. 43. Dehydration, showing loose skin and sunken eyes.

insects. Where these measures and standards of personal hygiene are of dubious quality it becomes increasingly important to encourage breast feeding of small infants, for the incidence and the severity of diarrhea is much lower among those receiving mother's milk.

MILD DIARRHEA

Diarrhea which is not severe enough to produce significant dehydration or acidosis may be classified as mild. The distinction is admittedly arbitrary, and all gradations will be found in practice between that which is described here as mild, and that which is considered later on as severe. In mild diarrhea the infant may appear quite well except for an increase in the frequency and the fluidity of his stools. Sometimes there is irritability, loss of appetite or disturbance of sleep. Infrequent vomiting and lesser degrees of fever may also occur. Treatment consists of a decrease in food intake, particularly with reduction of the carbohydrate and fat in the formula, and of an increase in water intake to compensate for fluid loss. Unsweetened boiled milk or boiled skimmed milk or even brief starvation for 12 to 24 hours are usually employed. If there is no vomiting, water or a balanced salt solution is given by mouth in amounts to meet the normal fluid requirements plus the estimated loss in the stools. Mild diarrhea usually responds to such changes within 2 to 3 days so that the usual schedule can be gradually resumed. Occasionally, a mild diarrhea is associated with prolonged intolerance for fat and the infant must be kept on a low fat formula for several weeks in order to prevent recurrence of symptoms. Kaolin products and pectin or scraped apple have been used to speed the resumption of normal stools in mild diarrheas, but the wisdom of their usage is debatable. Diarrhea which remains mild is a nuisance but not a serious disease.

SEVERE DIARRHEA

Symptoms

Diarrhea may progress from a mild to a severe illness within a matter of hours or over the course of several days. As the frequency and the volume of stools increases the infant becomes more restless and fretful. Stool passage may become painful, partly due to griping and partly due to the tenderness of the skin in the diaper area which rapidly becomes inflamed or even ulcerated from the irritation of constant moisture and the acid stools.

In dysentery the stools may become bloody or have gross pus in them. In any type of diarrhea there may be mucus present. Vomiting may interfere with attempts to assuage the infant's thirst.

Between the lack of food and the loss of fluid the infant begins to lose weight progressively. The mucous membranes of the mouth become dry and cracked. The skin dries and loses its normal elasticity so that it does not snap back into place when pinched up into a fold and then released. The fontanel and the eyes become sunken, and the face adopts a pinched and anxious look at first followed later by impassivity with eyes half-closed (Fig. 43). The urine becomes scanty in amount and dark in color. Fever may appear if it has not already been present as part of an infection. These are the main signs and symptoms of dehydration.

With significant degrees of dehydration there may be changes in the respirations which betoken acidosis. These consist of an increase in depth of respiration with a sighing quality often present. The rate may be slowed or accelerated. Grayish color of the skin and cold extremities in spite of an elevated body temperature indicate sluggishness of the peripheral circulation due to decreased plasma volume.

Severe diarrhea sometimes begins quite abruptly with high fever, listlessness, extreme toxicity and convulsions or coma. The onset may be so sudden that little warning of the disease is available for liquid stool may accumulate within the intestinal tract and not be expelled until after the toxic symptoms begin. The prognosis in diarrhea with this type of onset is particularly serious, and such infants constitute a therapeutic emergency.

Physiologic Alterations

The principles of water and electrolyte balance and fluid administration are presented in Chapter 9. During severe diarrhea the loss in weight is due primarily to loss of water from the body, which in turn is chiefly intercellular water (interstitial fluid). This compartment of the body fluids is used up first, and its loss accounts for the symptoms of sunken fontanel and eyes and loss of skin elasticity. The body is not able to maintain the plasma volume indefinitely, and when water loss becomes severe there is also shrinkage in plasma volume which accounts for hemoconcentration, for poor peripheral circulation and for the small volume of urine. The water of the body cells themselves (intracellular water) is also lost, but the changes are more subtle and less easily recognized clinically. Loss of vigor and dulling of the sensorium are probably external manifestations of the loss of intracellular water.

The losses sustained are not merely losses of water, however, for the electrolytes of the body fluids invariably accompany them. Restoration of water to the body must be combined with a restoration of the lost electrolytes as well. Usually in diarrhea a number of factors conspire to produce acidosis. The liquid stools carry off a disproportionate amount of basic electrolytes. The normal products of metabolism are acid, and when starvation and fever are present the quantities produced are increased. When the blood flow to the kidney is decreased by shrinking plasma volume, the excretion of these products is hampered. For a time the kidney is able to select an excess of acid radicles for excretion and thus tends to correct the acid-base balance in the blood. Similarly, the lungs, by hyperventilation, blow off more carbon dioxide than usual in an attempt to increase the excretion of carbonic acid. But eventually these measures become insufficient, and the pH of the blood begins to change from its normal range of 7.35 to 7.45 downward toward 7.0, the level which is barely compatible with survival.

When dehydration has progressed to the point where intracellular water is being lost, the body loses potassium from within the cells. Unless special care is taken to replace potassium during treatment, the function of cells such as those of the myocardium and other muscles may be impaired by falling concentrations of this important element. Excessive potassium administration must also be feared, since high blood levels are equally dangerous.

The losses of both water and the individual chemical substances do not always follow the same pattern. Recently it has been discovered that a few infants lose more water than electrolytes during diarrhea and have inordinately high levels of sodium and other ions in the blood. Such infants are likely to show evidence of central nervous system impairment, such as coma or convulsions, and suffer an unusually high mortality rate.

Treatment

Acidosis and Dehydration. In diarrhea of any severity the most urgent aspect of treatment is relief of acidosis and dehydration. Ideally, these procedures should be guided by repeated determinations of blood components such as the hemoglobin, hematocrit, carbon dioxide content (or combining power), pH, sodium, chloride, potassium and nonprotein nitrogen. The technics for obtaining blood for such determinations have been described in Chapter 9. If the recent weights of the infant before he became ill are known, the present figure provides an important measure of the quantity of water lost. The other measurements assist in computing the relative losses of water and electrolytes and in judging the level of kidney function.

Infants who appear moribund at the time of admission are often given a sizable injection of physiologic saline or Ringer's solution into the peritoneal cavity in order to initiate rehydration rapidly. Continuous intravenous infusion is always advisable when severe diarrhea is present, for the poor condition of the circulation makes absorption from the subcutaneous spaces slow and unreliable. The mechanical problem in establishing a continuous infusion in a small infant in circulatory collapse is often great. When success has been attained the flow through this lifeline must be regarded as precious, for its failure endangers the infant's survival. The physician must determine the desired type of solution and rate of dosage; but the nurse has an important part in policing the flow to make sure that it is running at the predetermined rate and to keep accurate track of the amounts infused.

Many schemes are used for estimating fluid and electrolyte losses and for restoring deficits. Isotonic solutions of glucose, sodium chloride and the more complicated salt mixtures are generally used as the main basis for restoring water. If plasma volume can be bolstered to the point where kidney function improves progressively, the natural mechanisms for correcting acidosis begin to operate again. More rapid correction of acidosis is often accomplished by injecting calculated amounts of sodium bicarbonate or ⅙ molar sodium lactate solution. After urine flow is established, solutions containing potassium, such as Darrow's solution, are usually added in order to permit this substance to re-enter the cells which are undergoing hydration. In anemic or starved infants plasma or transfusions are used as supportive measures. Once the major electrolyte defects have been corrected and vomiting has ceased, the intake of water and salt can be gradually shifted over from the intravenous or subcutaneous route to the oral one.

Management of Feeding. In addition to correcting the deficits already suffered, it is imperative to prevent additional ones from being incurred through the persistence of diarrhea or vomiting. A preliminary period of starvation is always advisable in severe diarrhea. The length of this period must be determined by changes in the clinical condition and the extent of the diarrhea. Usually at least 24 to 48 hours rest must be given to the intestinal tract and in severe instances the starvation may be prolonged to as long as a week. When feedings are resumed, water, glucose or balanced salt solution are offered first to test the irritability of the tract. If these are tolerated, small amounts of dilute skimmed milk, lactic acid milk or breast milk are tried; and the amounts and the strength of the feedings is increased at a rate which is judged to be slow enough to prevent recurrence of the symptoms. During prolonged periods of starvation the intake may be augmented by the use of parenteral vitamin solutions, by plasma, transfusions, or intravenous amino acid mixtures.

Other Aspects of Treatment. If high fever is present it should be controlled by sponging in order to forestall convulsions. Sedatives are usually avoided in these desperately ill infants because they may be dangerous and may confuse the clinical indications of progress. In the presence of upper respiratory infection, antibiotics should be given to bring the associated disease under control as rapidly as possible. Direct attack upon the etiologic agent causing the diarrhea will have to depend upon the results of laboratory studies of the stools. Where specific infection with dysentery or salmonella organisms is suspected, the use of sulfonamides or chloramphenicol is rational. Neomycin given orally is generally effective against pathogenic strains of *E. coli* and some of the other agents implicated in infantile diarrhea. It is too toxic for parenteral administration.

Nursing Care. In addition to her important responsibilities in monitoring the parenteral fluids, the nurse has several challenges in caring for the infant with severe diarrhea. Strict isolation technic must be maintained in order to protect other infants in the ward. Hands should be washed carefully, and stools and diapers disposed of in appropriate containers. Charting the number and the description of the stools and the frequency of urination must be accurate. At the beginning of the disease, nursing maneuvers are often obstructed by the necessity for maintaining a particular position of the infant in order to keep his intravenous fluids running. While changes of position and protection of his diaper area are desirable, sometimes they must yield to the necessity of keeping him quiet.

In the endeavor to prevent redness and excoriation of the buttocks, the diapers should be changed frequently, and the buttocks and the genitalia cleansed with oil on cotton. If redness or excoriation should appear, a further protection against the acid stool is afforded by a bland ointment or paste.

Often it may be desirable to avoid contact of the skin with the stool to a greater degree and to have the affected skin exposed to warm air and light to promote healing. Keeping the infant on his abdomen gives the greatest exposure, but care must be taken to prevent irritation of the skin of the knees, the toes and the chin and, above all, suffocation. The equipment to be used for exposure to light depends on what is available and to some extent on the season of the year. A bed cradle with a lamp attached in the dome serves well, or the lamp may be attached to the side of the crib with tape. The lamp should be equipped with a 25-watt bulb, protected by a shade or a wire cage and adjusted 12 inches from the infant's body. The precautions are to prevent overheating and burns. After cleansing the buttocks and the genitalia, the infant should be placed comfortably on his abdomen or on his side.

With or without a bed cradle, a tent which leaves the infant's head in the open may be made. A sheet may be used to form the tent, covering the lower portion of the bed, and a folded diaper to form the front.

Judicious use of mothering procedures, such as the pacifier, stroking and holding the infant, are important elements of nursing during the period of recovery.

EPIDEMIC DIARRHEA OF THE NEWBORN

A highly communicable type of diarrhea occurring in newborn nurseries has been recognized with increasing frequency. Originally, the etiology was obscure. Various types of bacteria were implicated, and a virus origin was suspected. More precise methods of investigation have disclosed that many of these epidemics are due to particular strains of the common inhabitants of the intestinal tract—E. coli. These pathogenic strains are presumably carried by healthy adults who handle the newborn infant. Unfortunately, it is very difficult to identify such individuals by stool culture methods and thus to prevent their contact with small infants. Scrupulous technic in the nursery and prompt recognition of the epidemic form of the disease followed by rigorous isolation and dispersal of exposed infants are the only preventive measures that can be used. Fortunately, most strains of pathogenic E. coli have been found to yield promptly to neomycin given by mouth. With this treatment, the previously high rates of mortality among these infants have been reduced considerably. The clinical picture is that of a rapidly advancing toxemia without fever or symptoms other than watery, explosive stools and progressive weight loss. General management is the same as that described above.

CYSTIC FIBROSIS OF THE PANCREAS—MUCOVISCIDOSIS

Although this disorder is a generalized affliction of several portions of the body, it is considered here because its onset is usually recognized during infancy through its effects upon the digestive tract. Historically, attention focused upon the pathologic changes of the pancreas and upon the lack of pancreatic secretions which determined the nutritional defect. Later investigations have emphasized the hereditary nature of the disease and its widespread effects upon secretions of glands in the intestine, the bronchial mucosa and the skin.

ETIOLOGY AND PATHOGENESIS

The condition is inherited and is transmitted as a recessive trait. This implies that each of the parents must be a healthy carrier of a defective gene which appears in one-fourth of their offspring in double dosage and results in the full-blown disease. Recently, it has become possible to recognize the recessive carrier state by analysis of the sweat of parents and siblings of affected children.

Practically all children with the genetic defect have abnormally high concentrations of sodium, potassium and chloride in the secretions produced by their sweat glands. This portion of the disorder is of minor consequence except in hot weather when they may suffer excessive salt depletion. Of greater clinical significance are the changes produced in the excretions of the pancreas, the intestinal glands and the bronchial mucus-secreting glands. The degree of involvement of these different structures varies somewhat, so that individuals with the general disease may be affected in different ways and with different degrees of severity. Thus meconium ileus may be present at birth when the viscosity of the secretions of the intestinal tract is so

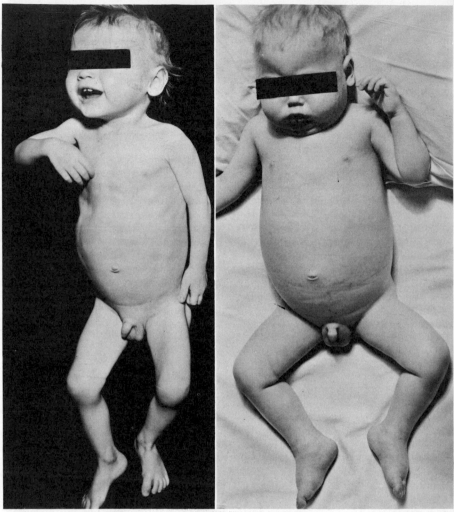

Fig. 44. (*Left*) Infant of 1 year, snowing moderate malnutrition from cystic fibrosis of the pancreas.

Fig. 45. (*Right*) The same infant at 2 years of age, showing congestive heart failure as a result of pulmonary fibrosis.

marked that the gummy intestinal contents cannot pass through. Obstruction of the ducts of the pancreas by thick secretions blocks the egress of important digestive enzymes produced within the gland and leads to abnormality of stools and nutritional failure. Most important of all is the effect of abnormally thick bronchial mucus within the lungs in blocking off small segments of lung and encouraging chronic infection and fibrotic changes. Symptoms of this complication may appear in early infancy or may be delayed until later childhood. Treatment of the digestive aspects of cystic fibrosis is effective, but methods available for controlling the pulmonary complications are likely to be temporary. Progressive changes in the lungs lead to fibrosis, which in turn may interfere with circulation of blood through the lungs and result in heart failure. Children who die of cystic fibrosis of the pancreas usually succumb to the immediate or remote effects of pulmonary disease.

SYMPTOMS

The symptoms of meconium ileus appear within hours or a few days after birth and consist of vomiting, abdominal distention and failure to pass meconium. Often the exact cause of the obstruction cannot be determined before surgical exploration of the abdomen. The treatment consists of irrigation of the obstructed lower ileum and usually resection of the portion containing the mass of inspissated meconium. A double opening is then left to provide one channel for the discharge of intestinal contents and a second opening through which the lower segment of the intestines can be opened up gradually by postoperative irrigation with solutions containing proteolytic enzymes. The immediate mortality from meconium ileus is high, and even when recovery takes place the child must face the other aspects of his basic disease.

Symptoms which indicate insufficiency of pancreatic enzymes are more insidious in their onset but usually are discovered before the age of 6 months. The stools tend to be large in volume, mushy but not usually watery. They have an offensive odor, and when the diet contains much fat some of it comes through undigested. The infant's appetite is usually good, if not ravenous, yet in spite of a normal food intake his weight increases at an abnormally slow rate (Fig. 44).

Pulmonary symptoms may arise spontaneously or after an acute respiratory infection. They consist of a chronic cough and obstructive bronchitis. Infants may escape this complication but

are prone to show during later childhood evidence of increasing emphysema by chest roentgenogram and chronic or recurring bronchitis on physical examination. In the later stages of pulmonary disease clubbing of the fingers and chronic cyanosis appear, and when fibrosis of the lungs is taking place the heart enlarges, and the child becomes dyspneic and edematous (Fig. 45).

DIAGNOSIS

The diagnosis is usually suspected in infancy from the clinical picture of low-grade diarrhea, good appetite, failure to gain weight and cough. It may be confirmed by demonstrating the absence of normal concentrations of trypsin in the secretions obtained by drainage of the duodenum. Measurement of the concentration of sodium and chloride in the sweat now offers an additional means of supporting the diagnosis. The following procedure is used for *duodenal aspiration:* Equipment: radiopaque catheter No. 10 to 12 French, medicine glass of water, 20-ml. syringe, an indicator, test tubes, adhesive tape and elbow restraints. After the restraints have been applied to prevent removal of the tube, the catheter is lubricated with water and passed through the nose and the stomach and into the duodenum. Fluid is aspirated through the tube, and its reaction is tested: gastric secretion is acid, and duodenal content is alkaline. If the fluid is definitely alkaline (pH above 7), the infant is examined fluoroscopically to verify the position of the catheter. If the fluid has a pH of less than 7 by indicator, the head of the bed is elevated, the infant is restrained on his right side, the catheter is inserted an inch or two further, and the upper end is made secure to the infant's face with adhesive tape. Fluid is withdrawn, and its reaction is tested at intervals until an alkaline reaction indicates that the end of the catheter has passed into the duodenum. After fluoroscopic verification of the position, fluid is withdrawn. The material obtained from the duodenum in cases of cystic fibrosis is very viscid and sticks to glass. The finding of such material is pathognomonic of cystic fibrosis. The fluid is tested for tryptic activity. Successive dilutions are made, usually up to 1:100. These are tested with gelatin. A simple procedure is to apply a large drop of the fluid of the various dilutions to the gelatin surface of a photographic film and incubate for 1 hour. In the presence of tryptic activity, the treated portion of the gelatin digests and leaves a clear spot on the film. The test for tryptic activity in the stool is carried out in the same manner as with duodenal secretion. Early in cystic fibrosis, tryptic activity may still be present and disappear later.

TREATMENT

The management of cystic fibrosis of the pancreas consists of diet regulation and protection against pulmonary infection. The diet should be low in fat and starch but high in calories and vitamins. High protein foods such as skimmed milk, protein milk, cottage cheese, casein hydrolysates and lean meats should be offered in amounts which will supply 1½ to 2 times the usual quantity of protein. Fruits and vegetables are well tolerated except for those with a high starch content. Bananas

have particular virtue because of the high content of easily digested carbohydrate. In actual practice the individual child's tolerance for fat and starch differs somewhat, so that his mother learns by experience what he can and cannot take without suffering adverse results as revealed by the character of his stools. Vitamins should be presented in water-soluble form because of the difficulty in fat absorption. The level of intake of most of the vitamins is kept at 2 to 3 times the normal. Usually the absent digestive enzymes are replaced with pancreatic preparations which can be mixed with the child's food. They are given in the form of granules or powder. Older children can take the preparation in capsules or tablets at mealtime.

Respiratory infections, even when the child has no symptoms, should be studiously avoided. Prophylactic administration of sulfonamides or broad-spectrum antibiotics is customary in order to abort them when unwitting contact has occurred. Treatment of fully developed respiratory disease should be guided by careful bacteriologic investigation of the organisms present and of their susceptibility to the various antibiotics available. The latter are frequently given by inhalation in the hope of carrying them directly to the seat of bacterial action.

SITUATIONS FOR FURTHER STUDY

1. How would you help a mother who described symptoms of colic to you? Symptoms of constipation?

2. What would you do if you were a visiting nurse and a mother told you that her baby vomited?

3. What knowledge must the nurse have to teach mothers ways of preventing infantile diarrhea?

4. Observe an infant with severe diarrhea. Describe his appearance, symptoms, treatment and behavior. Observe the baby's response to you from day to

day and record the changes which occur. How do you account for these changes?

5. A normal infant 6 months old is being cared for in an underprivileged home. On visiting this home during the early summer months, what parent counseling would aid in the prevention of diarrhea?

6. A child 2 years old is being discharged from the hospital after a dysentery infection. If you visit this home prior to his discharge, what observation

would you make, and what would you help the parents to learn about his care at home?

7. Observe an infant with cystic fibrosis of the pancreas. How do his symptoms affect him physically and emotionally? Describe your relationship with him and show how you used it in providing nursing care during the period he was being subjected to diagnostic study.

BIBLIOGRAPHY

d'Sant Agnese, P. A.: Fibrocystic disease of the pancreas, Pediatrics **15**: 683, 1955.

Gibbs, G. E., and Smith, Kathryn: Cystic fibrosis of the pancreas, Am. J. Nursing 49:783, 1949.

Gross, R. E.: Congenital hypertrophic pyloric stenosis and intussusception *in* The Surgery of Infancy and Childhood, Philadelphia, Saunders, 1953.

Herweg, J. C., Middelkamp, J. N., and

Thornton, H. K.: Escherichia coli diarrhea, J. Pediat. 49:629, 1956.

Levine, M. I., and Bell, Anita I.: The treatment of "colic" in infancy by use of the pacifier, J. Pediat. 37:750, 1950.

Schwachman, Harry: Pancreatic Fibrosis (pamphlet), Boston, The Children's Medical Centre, 1954.

Stevenson, Stuart, and Bonine, Gladys: Mucoviscidosis, Am. J. Nursing **56**: 866, 1956.

CHAPTER FOURTEEN

Nutritional and Vitamin Deficiencies

GENERAL DISCUSSION

The nutritional deficiencies are considered in the section on infant nursing because most of them have their greatest incidence during the early months when growth is very rapid and specific needs must be amply satisfied. In addition, it is desirable to understand what sort of illness is being avoided when careful supervision of the infant's diet is invoked.

In countries which have ample food supply and a high general level of education and hygiene, vitamin deficiency diseases are rare. However, even in the United States occasional infants suffer from neglect, poverty or ignorance of dietary requirements. None of the disorders which are to be described arises suddenly, for the infant has a store of nutrients within his body which must be exhausted before disease appears. (A notable exception is vitamin K deficiency which appears shortly after birth.) Most of the concern over vitamin deficiency in well-fed families is the product of advertising campaigns which have led the public to use vitamin preparations in wasteful amounts.

Deficiencies may be single in their occurrence or may be combined with other defects in diet. Some of the conditions are due to a generalized failure to ingest enough food. Others are due to an isolated lack of single chemical items. Infants can also suffer the symptoms of vitamin and food deficiency when they have abnormalities of absorption or of metabolism which prevent proper utilization.

SPECIFIC VITAMIN DEFICIENCIES

VITAMIN A

Since vitamin A is widely distributed in the fat of animal meats and milks and in the carotene component of vegetables, deficiency occurs only under the unusual circumstances of a very limited diet or of imperfect absorption. Infants fed upon skimmed milk products, or older children receiving little except starchy foods are potential victims. Diseases such as the celiac syndrome in which fat absorption is impaired may also be accompanied by clinical evidence of avitaminosis.

Lack of vitamin A results in changes in the character of the epithelium of the skin, the conjunctiva and the cornea, of the bronchial mucous membrane and of the urinary tract. In addition, it interferes with the metabolism of the visual purple of the retina so that accommodation to dim light is slow or imperfect. Clinically, the disease is usually discovered by noting changes in the eye. Dryness of the conjunctiva leads to infection and ulceration which, if not checked promptly, can result in scarring of the cornea and permanently defective vision. The skin becomes thickened and dry with prominence of the hair follicles. Changes in the bronchial epithelium court infection so that chronic bronchitis, atelectasis and emphysema may complicate the illness. The loss of dim light perception or night-blindness is difficult to discover in infants or young children. Treatment of this deficiency with 10 times the usual daily requirements (20,000 units) can be expected to yield clinical improvement within a few days.

Vitamin B Complex

Thiamine

Beriberi results from deficiency of thiamine (vitamin B_1). The disease is common in parts of the world where polished rice constitutes a large part of the diet. It is not common in this country, occurring less often from low intake of thiamine than from failure of absorption, as in chronic diarrhea.

Beriberi usually is insidious in its onset, being the result of a long-continued partial deficiency of thiamine. Except in the acute (wet) form described below, it is not seen in infants. Only after a period of vague and indefinite symptoms does the disease become fully manifest. During the prodromal period, the complaints made are referable to many systems, but most prominently to the nervous system. The mental symptoms are such as to lead to a diagnosis of neurosis in the older child. Undue anxiety is shown, along with lassitude, general weakness, easy fatigue and lack of interest in normal activities and personal care. Irritability and inattentiveness may be present.

After beriberi is fully developed, the symptoms are referable chiefly to the peripheral nerves, the heart and the alimentary tract. The gastro-intestinal tract shows altered motility, with constipation more often than diarrhea. Anorexia is constant, and nausea and vomiting may be present. The signs of peripheral neuritis appear, preceded and accompanied by burning, tingling and numbness of the hands and the feet. Tenderness is present over the nerve trunks and the calves. Muscle weakness may be marked. The muscle of the heart also becomes weakened, the symptoms being the same as those of myocarditis from other causes and may include rapid heart rate, dyspnea, pain over the heart and thready pulse.

Sometimes generalized edema is present. Then the disease is known as wet beriberi in contradistinction to the dry beriberi unassociated with edema. No doubt the myocardial changes contribute to the production of edema, but it is not clear that these are the sole cause. Wet beriberi is likely to be a more acute disease than dry beriberi, with rapid onset of the acute symptoms and sometimes with sudden death.

Beriberi responds dramatically to thiamine. For those severely ill, parenteral administration may be desirable; otherwise, the oral route is satisfactory. For infants, 10 mg. daily in divided doses is ample, and for older children, twice this amount. Half the amounts stated are adequate when the disease is mild. After the symptoms have disappeared, the normal daily allowance is all that is required, except when the disease is dependent on chronic diarrhea which persists. It is seldom that deficiency of any component of the vitamin B complex exists alone; consequently, the treatment with thiamine should be supplemented by administration of the complex or food materials containing it, such as yeast. Complete rest in bed is necessary, at least until full recovery from the myocardial disease.

Riboflavin

Riboflavin deficiency is almost always associated with deficiency of other members of the B complex. Its chief features are inflammation of the eye and about the mouth. In the eye there is dilatation of blood vessels, tearing, sensitivity to light, burning and dimness of vision. About the mouth a low-grade inflammatory reaction at the corners occurs which is also known as cheilitis and perlèche. The tongue becomes smooth, and there may be a greasy inflammation along the side of the nose. The symptoms seldom progress to a point where they threaten loss of function. They can be reversed by administration of 3 to 10 mg. of riboflavin daily.

Nicotinic Acid

Pellagra is caused by dietary deficiency of niacin (nicotinic acid), a member of the vitamin B complex. It is endemic in the southeastern United States, southern Europe and a few other regions. Where it is endemic, it exists at least in a latent form throughout the year. It becomes manifest notably in the spring, the symptoms increase in frequency and severity until early summer and then recede to the winter low level. Deficiency of niacin usually is partial rather than absolute. The effects of partial deficiency appear to be cumulative. With each successive year of deficiency the recurring manifestations are more apparent and more severe. In the first 2 years of life, gross lesions are uncommon. They increase in frequency with the age in pellagrous families. The

severe disease of many adults has its beginning in childhood.

The occurrence of pellagra is dependent on dietary habits. A typical diet of a pellagrous family in the southeastern United States is greatly restricted in variety and includes chiefly salt fat pork, corn bread and syrup. It is lacking in vegetables, fruit, lean meat, milk and eggs. It is deficient in almost all nutritional essentials. Whole cornmeal contains a moderate amount of thiamine and other members of the vitamin B complex but contains little niacin. Also corn protein is deficient in tryptophan, an amino acid that decreases to some extent the need for niacin. As a rule, babies of pellagrous mothers must be weaned early because of lack of milk. The subsequent diet usually is unsatisfactory. The children take over the dietary habits of the family. Once these habits are established, they are difficult to change, regardless of availability of better foods.

In this country the death rate, and presumably the incidence, of pellagra reached a peak about 1928. The decline since that time has been attributed largely to extensive use of dried yeast.

The symptoms of niacin deficiency in its earliest stages are vague and ill-defined, but with continued deficiency the manifestations characteristic of pellagra make their appearance.

Lesions of the mucous membranes of the alimentary tract are usually the first to appear. The changes are those of inflammation, and the most characteristic visible changes occur in the tongue. A subjective sensation of burning precedes and accompanies an intense glossitis. The tongue becomes very red, swollen and smooth. Inflammation of the mouth and the gums usually is present also. The gums become red and ulcerated, much of the ulceration being caused by Vincent's organisms (see Vincent's Angina). Similar inflammatory lesions may be present in the pharynx and the stomach, and more or less throughout the alimentary tract. Anorexia and abdominal pain develop early. Enteritis and proctitis cause diarrhea with foul watery stools. Abdominal pain becomes severe, and distention is marked. Intensity of inflammation necessary to produce diarrhea is not as common in children as in adults. Many children have only soreness of the tongue and the lips and abdominal pain. Often they are constipated, with only occasional attacks of diarrhea during the spring and the summer. There have been instances of babies in whom only diarrhea was present. Exacerbations of the alimentary symptoms of pellagra and the appearance of the characteristic dermatitis occur concurrently.

The mucous membranes of the genitourinary tract also may become affected, and the lesions may become manifest as urethritis or vaginitis. In association with these lesions, as in the case of those in the mouth, Vincent's organisms grow profusely.

The skin lesions of pellagra are due to an inflammation similar to that produced by sunburn. They are initiated by exposure to the sun, and they tend to heal gradually if sunshine is excluded. Because exposure to sunshine usually is symmetrical, the dermatitis also is symmetrical. It occurs in its characteristic form on exposed parts, especially the back of the hands and the neck. On the arms it extends up to the line of the sleeve. Coincident with the appearance of lesions on parts exposed to the sun, or subsequently, a somewhat different type of dermatitis may appear on unexposed parts subject to irritation. The parts commonly affected are the elbows, the knees and the ankles, where the affected skin remains dry, and the axillae and the perineum, where a moist type of dermatitis appears. The characteristic lesions on exposed parts pass through the same stages as do those of sunburn, though the course is slower and more chronic. The initial redness deepens, and pigment is deposited gradually. The older the lesion the greater the brownish pigmentation. The skin becomes thickened, rough and scaly. In some instances, seldom in childhood, the initial inflammation is sufficiently severe to produce large blisters. In practically all instances, the edges of the area of inflammation are sharply demarcated. A sensation of burning is present in the early stages.

The nervous and mental symptoms of pellagra increase in number and severity with continuation through years of niacin deficiency and recurring attacks of manifest pellagra. The more severe varieties of mental disturbances, such as mental confusion, delirium, mania and dementia, observed in adults, are not commonly present in the child. The milder nervous symptoms shown by the child may be due as much to chronic illness as to more specific effect on the nervous system, if not more. The children become tired and apathetic and lacking in normal childhood interest. Because of their physical status and consequent inability to concentrate, they do poorly in school. They become irritable, fretful and apprehensive; they sleep restlessly.

The general nutritional status of pellagrous children is poor. Because of inadequate diet and poor health with anorexia, the children are undernourished in both stature and weight.

The prognosis in children with treatment is excellent, much better than in adults. Response to treatment is prompt, often dramatic. With or without treatment, and with continued dietary deficiency, the recurrences become increasingly severe and eventually lead to death.

The treatment consists primarily of giving niacin or preparations containing it. Either niacin or its amide is given in a dosage of from 50 to 300 mg. daily, depending on the size of the child and the severity of symptoms. It should be given in divided doses, 10 mg. at a time for the small child and 20 mg. for the older child, in order to obtain better absorption and to avoid unpleasant subjective sensations which may occur with larger doses.

Dried brewers' yeast also is effective. An appropriate amount for a child up to 6 or 7 years is 45 Gm. daily, for an older child 60 Gm. The yeast may be mixed with milk. It is given in divided doses.

Niacin deficiency seldom exists alone. Consequently, attention must be paid to the entire diet. Deficiency manifestations most commonly associated with pellagra are those caused by lack of other members of the vitamin B complex, particularly thiamine. Symptomatic treatment, such as parenterally administered fluids for dehydration and transfusion for anemia and severe malnutrition, is to be given as indicated.

Other Members of the B Complex

A number of other substances are recognized as members of the vitamin B complex. Isolated deficiency of pyridoxine (B_6) has been identified as a cause of convulsions in small infants receiving a proprietary formula which was lacking in this metabolite. Folic acid or pteroylglutamic acid is discussed under diseases of the blood in Chapter 23. Vitamin B_{12}, the pernicious anemia factor, is important to adults but seems to have little significance for infants and children. It has been offered as a means of stimulating growth in children, but the evidence is controversial. Other substances which belong in the complex and have important metabolic functions yet are not recognized clinically by symptoms of deficiency are choline, biotin, pantothenic acid and inositol.

VITAMIN C—SCURVY

Scurvy is caused by deficiency of ascorbic acid (vitamin C) in the diet.

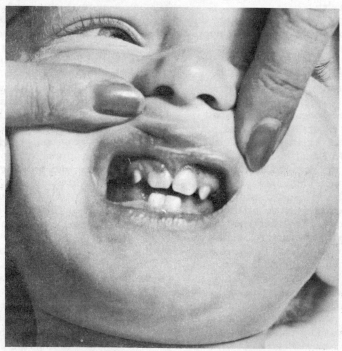

FIG. 46. The characteristic gum changes of scurvy.

Scurvy occurs only in those whose diet is abnormally restricted. For this reason, scurvy is rare in children and adults. In infancy, the diet is much more limited, and it is chiefly at this period that scurvy occurs. At present, scurvy is uncommon even in infancy as compared with former years. Most mothers now know that the artificially fed baby should have orange juice or some equivalent source of ascorbic acid. Even without a special source of ascorbic acid, the diet usually is not completely devoid of this material. A partial deficiency causes scurvy to appear somewhat later than if the deficiency were absolute. Scurvy is rare in the first 6 months and has its highest incidence in the second 6 months. It disappears as soon as foods containing vitamin C are included in the diet.

In its early stages, preceding the clinical signs by which it may be recognized, scurvy is characterized by indisposition, fretfulness, pallor, diminished appetite and failing nutrition. Pulse and respiration rates are increased. These symptoms continue through the manifest phases of the disease. The important manifestations are a tendency to hemorrhage and changes in the bones.

The hemorrhages of scurvy occur through the capillaries because of loss of cement substance between the cells of the capillary walls and because of arrested growth of connective tissue and its collagen-supporting structure. They are not caused by any change in the blood. Hemorrhage may occur in many places. Blood may appear in the urine or the stool. Small hemorrhages may appear within the skin, the appearance often resembling the effect of a bruise. Hemorrhage occurs in the gums and is usually limited to the site of erupted teeth. The gums become dark and swollen and bleed easily. Their appearance is strikingly suggestive, almost diagnostic, of scurvy (Fig. 46).

The bone changes are dependent in part on hemorrhage, but the important diagnostic changes as shown by roentgenograms are produced by impaired growth of osteoblasts and capillaries, especially at the points of growth of the bones. No difficulty exists in the deposit of mineral in the newly formed bone, but the newly calcified bone is not converted to trabeculated bone in a normal manner. As a result, there is present an abnormally heavy line of calcification immediately beyond a zone of rarefaction caused by impaired osteoblastic activity. For the same reasons, the trabeculae of the bones become thinner and less well defined in roentgenograms. Bone-marrow cells may largely disappear, a factor in addition to hemorrhage in producing anemia. In advanced scurvy, epiphyseal separation may occur from slight trauma.

The characteristic hemorrhages are in the long bones and are subperiosteal. They start at the growing end of the bone and strip off the periosteum, producing subperiosteal hematomas.

One of the characteristics of scurvy is pain and tenderness of the extremities, especially of the legs. The baby resents handling, the legs are not moved voluntarily, paralysis is simulated, and the thighs and the legs are held flexed with outward rotation of the hips (Fig. 47).

Moderate anemia is constantly present in scurvy, and severe anemia may develop. Slight fever is often present, and the temperature may be as high as from 102° to 103° F. when the disease is acute.

The diagnosis of frank scurvy is seldom difficult. Scurvy with pseudoparalysis is easily differentiated from diseases causing true paralysis by careful observation. Most hemorrhagic diseases other than scurvy which occur in infancy have characteristic blood changes. Roentgenograms show definitely diagnostic changes in the bones.

Scurvy responds quickly to ascorbic acid, whether given in crystalline form

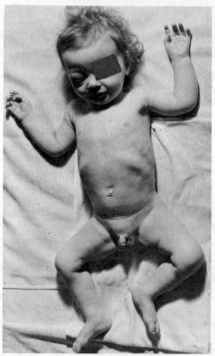

FIG. 47. Illustrating the characteristic posture of an infant with scurvy and periorbital hemorrhage.

or as foods naturally containing this material. The pain and acute symptoms are relieved within a few days. A longer period is required to recover from anemia and nutritional and bone changes. For the first few days of treatment, from 100 to 200 mg. of ascorbic acid may be given daily in divided doses. Subsequently, the normal allowance is sufficient.

Nursing Care

All procedures are associated with pain when the infant first comes under care. Nearing his bed often produces reactions of fear. Gentleness in handling is important. If taking up the infant for feeding is accompanied by excessive pain and poor acceptance of food, it is reasonable to feed him in bed with his head elevated. As soon as the acute symptoms subside, holding the infant for feeding should be resumed. Because of pain on motion, the infant tends to lie in one position, a symptom which

must be kept in mind in attempts to prevent intercurrent infection. As much of the needed care as possible should be given at one time; avoidable handling should be eliminated. When upper bedclothing is used, the weight should be reduced by the use of a bed cradle.

VITAMIN D—RICKETS

Infantile Rickets

Rickets can occur only when growth is active. The counterpart of rickets in those fully grown is osteomalacia. The more rapid the growth the more likely is rickets to develop. The most rapid growth occurs in infancy, and it is almost exclusively among infants that rickets occurs as a deficiency disease.

Rickets is more common in artificially fed than in breast-fed babies. It occurs chiefly in the temperate zones, where babies may have long periods without sunshine. It is more common in dark-skinned races because some of the ultraviolet rays are filtered out by the pigment. Rickets is not common in the tropics, even in dark-skinned races with the poorest of diets. Rickets is seasonal. It begins to be active when babies are more closely housed for the winter. Its activity is at its height in the northern hemisphere in March and subsides as babies are allowed sunshine again in the spring.

The disturbance of calcium and phosphorus metabolism is evidenced by poor retention of these materials by the body, by abnormal blood levels of calcium, phosphorus and phosphatase, and by faulty mineralization of bones. Normally, the blood of an infant contains from 10 to 12 mg. of calcium and from 5 to 7 mg. of phosphorus for each 100 cc. of serum. When rickets is present and active, the blood calcium may be expected to be from 9 to 10 mg., and the phosphorus less than 4 mg. for each

100 cc. When the product of the calcium and the phosphorus values is less than 30, rickets is present and active. The occasional finding of very low calcium and normal or high phosphorus is explained subsequently under Tetany. Phosphatase is an enzyme which increases in the blood in proportion to the severity of the rickets.

The growth in length of the long bones takes place in the shaft at its junction with the epiphysis. This area of growth change is the metaphysis. The normal process of increase is by growth of cartilage cells (osteoid tissue) and mineralization of these cells at such a rate that only a thin layer of osteoid tissue is present. In rickets, the deposit of calcium and phosphate in the newly grown cartilage is deficient. The roentgenogram shows a raggedly calcified bone end. The osteoid tissue continues to grow, producing enlargement of the

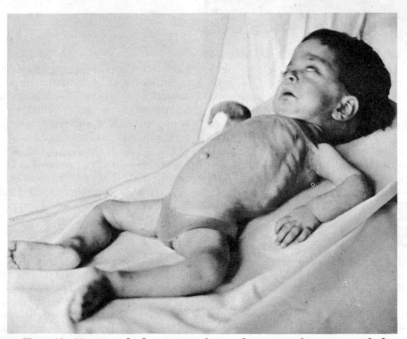

Fig. 48. Very marked active rickets, showing enlargement of the head from "bossing," a marked "rosary," enlarged epiphyses and inability to stand or sit.

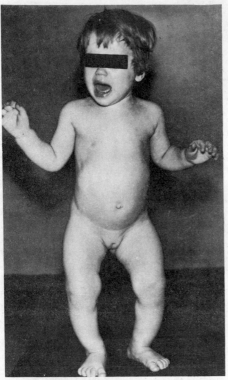

Fig. 49. This 18-month-old child shows the effects of rickets: bowed legs, large wrists and large skull with prominent bosses.

end of the bone by overgrowth or a mushrooming effect of pressure on soft tissue. Enlargement of the bone end becomes apparent on inspection and palpation. This same process produces small knobs at the junction of the ribs with the cartilage near the sternum. Because of their distribution, these enlargements have been designated collectively a rachitic rosary (Fig. 48).

The shafts of the long bones eventually become soft from lack of mineral, and they may bend according to the direction in which stress is put on them (Fig. 49). The pull of the diaphragm on the softened ribs, particularly when combined with nasal obstruction, causes deformities of the chest, the most common of which is depression of the ribs at the line of attachment of the diaphragm (Harrison's groove). Softening of the spine may result in scoliosis or kyphosis. The bones of the skull sometimes become sufficiently soft to permit

indentation by the finger as though they were made of stiff parchment. This condition is known as craniotabes and occurs chiefly in the occipital bones of young infants. Sometimes overgrowth occurs on the parietal and frontal bones of the skull, producing bosses and giving to the skull a somewhat square shape. Rickets causes delay in eruption of teeth and in closing of the fontanel. Whatever the bone changes may be as a result of rickets, they tend to occur similarly and equally on the two sides of the body.

Muscles as well as bones suffer in rickets. As rickets advances, the muscles show a general weakness and loss of tone. Because of these changes, sitting, standing and walking are delayed, or the baby may retrogress in these acts if they were already established. The abdominal wall is relaxed, and the abdomen protrudes when the child is erect. Constipation may result from loss of muscle strength. Ligaments about joints may become lax and permit unusual mobility. Sometimes the spleen is enlarged by simple hyperplasia, and the liver may be increased in size.

The diagnosis of active rickets is made by finding the characteristic changes in roentgenograms of bones or abnormal blood levels of calcium and phosphorus, or both. Also, blood phosphatase is increased above the normal. Rachitic changes are found roentgenographically at the wrist when they are evident in any other bones.

Rickets is not a direct cause of death, though it may be a contributing factor by predisposing to other diseases. With rare exceptions, rickets subsides, even without treatment, by the time the period of infancy has passed, because growth is not so rapid, and the child can get more sunshine under his own power. The deformities of rickets may persist. There is considerable tendency for moderate deformities to disappear in the period from 2 to 5 years of age. Severe deformities remain unless corrected by operative or mechanical means. Some deformities, such as those of the chest, are not easily amenable to corrective procedures.

The treatment of rickets consists primarily of the administration of vitamin D. The larger the dosage the more quickly the healing process begins. Since the baby is not ill, and no emergency exists, moderate rather than massive dosage is preferable. Vitamin D in the amount of from 1,500 to 3,000 units daily may be expected to produce evidence of recovery in the blood in about a week, and in the bones in approximately 2 weeks (Fig. 50). Some of the high-potency cod-liver oils contain 900 units to the teaspoonful. Of these, from 2 to 3 teaspoonfuls daily suffice. Concentrated preparations may be preferred to low-potency oils because of the bulk of oil required for the larger doses. In any case, a large dosage serves

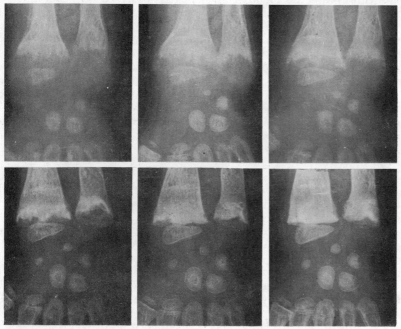

FIG. 50. Showing various stages in the healing of active rickets. The increase of calcification as observed from time to time is evident.

a useful purpose only until the healing process has well begun; thereafter a maintenance dose of from 300 to 400 units daily is adequate. Except for correction of existing dietary faults, no other treatment is necessary in most instances.

In a few instances, corrective appliances may be desirable during the healing stage of rickets and subsequently. These appliances would be for the correction of deformity such as bowlegs or knock knees. Operative correction of deformity, if necessary, is deferred until the rickets has healed completely.

Rickets in Childhood (Late Rickets)

Older children sometimes show bone changes similar to those observed in infantile rickets. The similarity exists in the nature of the bone deformities, in the roentgenographic evidence of rickets and in the amounts of calcium, phosphorus and phosphatase in the blood. By all these criteria the condition is rickets. However, in this country clinically recognizable rickets is infrequently caused by dietary deficiency.

Severe dietary deficiency was the cause of rickets reported in children of central Europe after World War I. For normal bone mineralization not only must vitamin D be present, but also there must also be appropriate amounts of calcium and phosphorus. Rickets has been reported in India among high-caste girls who were kept closely housed under the system of purdah during late childhood and adolescence.

Late rickets is uncommon in this country. When it does occur, it is nearly always due to some metabolic disturbance which is unrelated to the intake of minerals and vitamin D and makes normal retention of calcium and phosphorus impossible. Several varieties of such disturbances have been recognized. Infantile rickets usually does not last long enough to produce permanent stunting of growth, whereas late rickets dependent on a metabolic disorder is a

chronic disease, and stunted growth is a common occurrence.

In some instances of late rickets, the difficulty seems to lie in a defect in the mechanism by which vitamin D promotes the utilization of calcium and phosphorus. In this variety which is also known as "resistant rickets," response is observed when the intake of vitamin D is greatly increased. The necessary increase may be so great that only a small margin exists between the therapeutic and the toxic dose. Children under treatment must be observed frequently and carefully. Dosage may range as high as several hundred thousand units per day.

Chronic acidosis from any cause is likely to produce rickets. In this condition, calcium is used to help neutralize the excessive amounts of acid. In most of these instances, improvement or recovery occurs with the continued administration of alkali.

Renal rickets is a term applied to rickets observed in association with chronic nephritis. Usually some acidosis is present, causing increased excretion of calcium, but an equally important factor is the failure to excrete phosphates. The increased concentration of phosphate in the body affects adversely the deposition of calcium in bone. Since the underlying renal defect is not usually correctible, the treatment of renal rickets is unsatisfactory.

Rachitic Tetany

Tetany is a condition of increased excitability of nerves and muscles which is associated with a decrease in the portion of the blood calcium which is free, that is, not bound to the blood proteins. Reduction of this free or un-ionized calcium may occur when the total blood calcium level falls to 7.5 mg. per cent or below (certain instances of rickets, celiac disease, hypoparathyroidism) or when the acid-base balance of the blood is shifted toward the alkaline side as a result of hyperventilation, prolonged

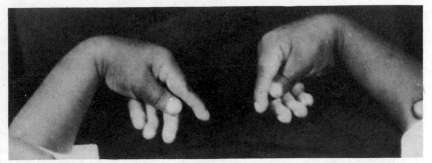

FIG. 51. Showing the characteristic position of the hands in the carpal spasm of tetany.

vomiting or excessive intake of sodium bicarbonate. Tetany will be referred to in the discussion of some of these conditions. Rickets is not the only disease in which it is a manifestation, but it is the most common cause among infants. Tetany must be distinguished from tetanus, which is a totally different entity.

Tetany due to vitamin D insufficiency has the same seasonal and age incidence as rickets since the basic cause is identical. Regular administration of vitamin D to a rachitic infant will produce a brief and transient fall in blood calcium. But when the vitamin D dosage is irregular and small, the calcium level may remain low, and the symptoms of tetany appear. The general irritability of nerves and muscles declares itself in three distinctive ways—convulsions, laryngospasm and carpopedal spasm. A given child usually does not display all of these symptoms. The convulsions are not different from those of other origin, and unless tetany is suspected, the true reason may be overlooked. Laryngospasm is due to brief spasm of the adductor muscles of the larynx which pull the vocal cords together, creating a high-pitched inspiration as the infant draws his breath through a narrowed glottic passageway. Although the attacks produce alarming interference with respiration, they almost invariably subside spontaneously before asphyxia takes place.

Carpopedal spasm is the most common symptom of tetany. It consists of a painless flexion of the wrists and the proximal metacarpal joints with extension of the thumb and the fingers into a characteristic position shown in Figure 51. A similar but less obvious combination of muscle contractions may take place in the feet. The position is assumed from time to time when the ionized blood calcium remains low. Incipient tetany may be disclosed by Trousseau's sign, which consists in producing carpal spasm by temporarily cutting off blood circulation to the arm with a tourniquet. Latent tetany may also be disclosed by tapping certain nerves which run close to the surface. In tetany the facial muscles will contract when the facial nerve is tapped (Chvostek's sign). The peroneal sign is a similar brief contraction of the muscles which evert the foot when the peroneal nerve is tapped as it runs around the head of the fibula. Confirmation of the clinical suspicion of tetany must always be sought in a determination of the blood calcium level.

Treatment of the associated rickets is usually sufficient to abolish tetany. However, rapid alleviation of laryngospasm or convulsions is usually desired. This can be achieved by oral administration of calcium, preferably in the form of an acid-producing salt such as calcium chloride. Approximately 1 Gm.

a day in divided doses is used for infants. Even more rapid alleviation of symptoms may be achieved by the cautious administration of calcium or magnesium salts intravenously.

VITAMIN K

Vitamin K is necessary for the liver to use in its manufacture of prothrombin, which in turn is essential to the blood-clotting mechanism. Vitamin K is sometimes deficient in the newborn infant or the premature. Symptoms are those of spontaneous bleeding, and control is achieved by administering certain synthetic quinones which provide the basic material necessary for the synthesis of prothrombin. Intestinal bacteria and a wide variety of foods provide sufficient vitamin K in later infancy and childhood so that the disorder is encountered only under peculiar circumstances. Liver disease may render the body unable to synthesize prothrombin; then replacement therapy is required via transfusions. On occasion, heavy antibiotic dosage may sterilize the intestinal tract to a point where vitamin K-producing bacteria are no longer present. Salicylate therapy over long periods of time may interfere with the synthesis of vitamin K. In the newborn period from 1 to 2 mg. of a synthetic preparation such as Synkavite, Hykinone or menadione is sufficient to correct hemorrhagic disease. For older children, from 5 to 10 mg. per day should be given as long as the conditions which interfere with prothrombin formation persist.

PROTEIN DEFICIENCY—NUTRITIONAL EDEMA

The body is compelled to burn its own tissues when the energy intake is less than the requirement. Eventually, the body reservoirs of fat disappear, and some of the body protein is broken down for energy production. If the amount of protein in the diet is low at the same time, some of the protein tissues of the body must be broken down to provide the necessary amino acids for renewal of more essential protein tissues. In severe or long-continued depletion, the body protein destroyed includes that of the blood plasma. When the blood protein, particularly the albumin fraction, becomes low, edema results. When edema occurs as a result of protein depletion, it is designated nutritional edema. During World War I it was known also as war edema, having been the result of the famine of war conditions.

Nutritional edema is insidious in its onset, usually being the result of many months of deficiency. The edema may be local or general, depending on the degree of deficiency. Edema from low blood protein may result also from wasting diseases of various types in which the intake and the absorption of energy and protein do not equal the need; it is the type of edema that occurs in nephrosis. This type is to be distinguished from that resulting from cardiovascular disease, as in glomerular nephritis and in heart disease with decompensation.

The only treatment required for starvation edema is the giving of a good diet. In other instances, the underlying disease, such as chronic diarrhea or celiac disease, requires appropriate management.

GENERAL MALNUTRITION—STARVATION

Extreme malnutrition in infancy has been known by the terms marasmus, infantile atrophy, decomposition and athrepsia. Of these terms, athrepsia, meaning lack of food, best fits the condition, which is essentially a starvation.

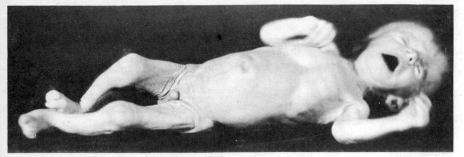

FIG. 52. A malnourished infant.

Extreme malnutrition may be the result of prolonged underfeeding. It also may be the result of emotional deprivation which interferes with food intake. In other instances, malnutrition results from loss of food through vomiting or diarrhea, and perhaps through associated therapeutic underfeeding. In still other instances it is found in association with chronic infections. Infections decrease available food by decreasing appetite and lowering powers of digestion and by increasing the combustion of food within the body, thus causing a disproportion between the food available and that required.

In all conditions stated, the amount of food absorbed from the intestinal tract is inadequate to meet the needs of the infant. Since the infant must continue to burn food, such foods as are available in the body are used. Thus the fat deposits disappear, and emaciation becomes apparent. Probably every organ in the body suffers by loss of material for combustion. The volume of the blood is diminished because part of its protein has been burned. Because of depletion and poor circulation the digestive glands have decreased capacity. As a consequence, less food can be ingested without the production of a gastro-intestinal disturbance. With continued disproportion between absorption and combustion, there comes a time when the infant is able to digest and absorb successfully only a portion of the amount of food

actually required. When food is given within the limits of digestive ability, the stools are normal in character. Diarrhea is induced easily, either by increase in food in an attempt to cause gain in weight or by intercurrent infections.

An athreptic infant has decreased resistance to infections and is subject to infections of all kinds, notably pyelitis, bronchitis, upper respiratory infections and furunculosis. Infection thus becomes a part of a cycle in the production of increasing degrees of malnutrition. Continued combustion of essential body tissues must be fatal eventually.

The appearance of an extremely malnourished infant is striking. Emaciation is the prominent feature. The eyes are sunken, but alert; the cheek bones are prominent; the facial appearance is that of an aged person (Fig. 52). The fat at the center of each cheek disappears late because its composition differs from that of other fat deposits. These "sucking pads" are present in all but the most severely malnourished. The bony skeleton becomes more prominent over the entire body. The hands and the feet become clawlike; the skin is often of paper thinness, hanging in folds. The skin at first is pale and later a characteristic grayish white. The head appears too big for the body, because the brain continues to grow even though certain other parts of the body waste.

Other characteristics also may be

prominent. Hunger may be great in the beginning and difficult to satisfy. As emaciation continues, hunger may disappear. In extreme cases the cry is feeble, the heart rate is slow, the heart sounds are weak, and the body temperature becomes subnormal. As emaciation increases, activity of the baby decreases, and the basal metabolic rate becomes lower. Growth in body length (skeletal growth) continues at a retarded rate long after growth in weight has ceased, but even growth in length eventually ceases and after it has stopped it does not start again until growth in weight has continued for weeks.

The most obvious features of marasmus are those caused by deficiency in calories. However, other deficiencies may become evident. Nutritional anemia is relatively common. Nutritional edema occurs occasionally as a result of protein deficiency. Rigidity of the muscles, especially those of the legs and the neck, which is observed occasionally, has been attributed to niacin deficiency. Xerophthalmia from vitamin A deficiency has been observed. Rickets rarely occurs because of the slowness of bone growth.

As activity of the baby decreases, the possibility of development of bedsores increases. These are most likely to appear on the head but may occur at any pressure point. Thrush is relatively common. Severely athreptic infants sometimes are subject to periods of collapse or syncope, in which they may die. The syncope is accompanied by large and sudden weight (water) loss, lowered body temperature, low heart rate and increased impairment of circulation. Such syncopal attacks frequently are associated with unsuspected hidden infections such as mastoiditis.

The measures for prevention of malnutrition in infancy are much the same as those stated for the prevention of diarrhea. Breast feeding should be encouraged, especially in unfavored groups. The baby should be under competent supervision as to growth progress, diet, emotional and physical hygiene. Infections should have prompt and appropriate treatment.

If an athreptic infant is to recover, it is essential that the amount of food ingested be increased to a point at which the infant will gain. At the same time it is necessary to keep the food within the limits of digestive capacity. Satisfaction of both these therapeutic indications is sometimes most difficult. The food requirement is high. As much as from 200 to 250 calories for each kilogram of body weight (100 to 120 calories to the pound) daily may be necessary. The digestive capacity is low, and food in excess of the capacity is a potent cause of diarrhea and consequent further weight loss. In meeting this therapeutic problem, considerable care must be taken in the choice of food, and such measures should be employed as tend to increase the ability of the infant to utilize the food successfully.

In the selection of food a type should be chosen that is easily digestible, one that offers a medium relatively unfavorable to bacterial growth. It is desirable also to use a concentrated food, since vomiting is very likely to occur if the large amount of food needed is offered in customary dilution. Two types of food meet these requirements fairly well. When human milk is available, it may be fortified by the addition of dried milk and further modified to advantage by partial acidification. When only cow's milk is available, a good preparation is undiluted acidified whole milk with added carbohydrate. When a tendency to diarrhea exists, somewhat less sugar and fat than customary should be given, or the added sugar may be changed to a type quickly absorbable, such as dextrose. At times it is desirable to increase the food value of the cow's milk formula by the addition of dried skimmed milk. Too much attention should not be given to moderately increased frequency of the stools if the baby is making good gains in weight and the condition is satisfactory otherwise.

Malnutrition is often accompanied by specific vitamin deficiencies. A liberal intake of all vitamins is needed to correct prior deficits and to support the rapid growth which follows recovery. Vitamins B and C may be given parenterally.

Moderate dehydration is common in athrepsia even in the absence of diarrhea. Loss of interstitial fluid is characteristically a part of the loss of body weight in malnutrition. Replacement of this fluid and its maintenance in interstitial tissues are two of the first essentials in recovery. Parenteral administration of fluid from time to time as indicated is helpful in hastening recovery.

The ability of the infant to utilize food may be increased by restoring the blood volume by means of transfusions. Transfusions hasten recovery and often permit survival in an otherwise hopeless case. A suitable amount of blood to give at one time is 20 ml. for each kilogram of body weight. In extreme malnutrition, transfusions at intervals of several days to a week are indicated.

Nursing Care

The body temperature of athreptic infants must be guarded much as in the case of prematurely born infants, although seldom is an incubator necessary. If additional clothing fails to supply the necessary warmth, a lamp-heated bed (see under Diarrhea) is useful. Preventing infections, careful feeding and close observation for signs of collapse comprise the specific physical care.

The baby with marasmus must have abundant emotional warmth given with each feeding. He needs extra cuddling, sucking, interest and care which helps him to feel that those in the world are giving and responsive to his needs. Every effort should be made to supply him with continuity of maternal care.

KWASHIORKOR

From various parts of the world syndromes of complex nutritional deficiencies in children have been reported. Though very infrequently discovered in the United States, these disturbances have importance because of the numbers of children affected elsewhere on the globe. Kwashiorkor, the variety found in Africa, is probably the best studied. It affects children at the age of weaning from the breast when an automatically complete diet is forsaken for the limited native fare which is mainly carbohydrates and a few vegetables with little or no milk or animal protein. The result is retardation of growth, nutritional edema, depigmentation and various kinds of eruption of the skin, peculiar changes in hair color which may make it appear reddish or gray, and enlargement and fatty infiltration of the liver. The latter, when well advanced, makes it extremely difficult to reverse the nutritional defect. Mortality rates are high among those with the well-developed syndrome. Treatment follows the principles outlined above for general malnutrition.

MINERAL DEFICIENCIES

Insufficient intake or utilization of some of the minerals results in certain specific diseases. These are discussed elsewhere. Defects in calcium and phosphorus metabolism have been discussed in association with lack of vitamin D. Anemia due to iron starvation is considered in the chapter on diseases of the blood. Iodine deficiency affects the thyroid gland primarily and is considered in the chapter which deals with endocrine disorders. The possible relation of fluoride lack to dental caries is discussed in Chapter 20.

SITUATIONS FOR FURTHER STUDY

1. In teaching a mother methods of giving vitamin concentrates and orange juice to a young infant, what points would you include?

2. By what methods can nutritional anemia be prevented?

3. By what process does tetany develop in a child with healing rickets?

4. Give care to a baby with marasmus and record his behavior at feeding time each day and your response to it. Write a summary showing the trend which took place in the nurse-child relationship.

BIBLIOGRAPHY

Elliott, M. M., and Park, E. A.: Rickets *in* Brenneman's Practice of Pediatrics, vol. 1, chap. 36, Hagerstown, Md., Prior, 1948.

Jelliffe, D. B.: Social culture and nutrition, Pediatrics 20:128, 1957.

McIntosh, R.: Infantile scurvy *in* Brenneman's Practice of Pediatrics, vol. 1, chap. 35, Hagerstown, Md., Prior, 1948.

CHAPTER FIFTEEN

Infantile Skin Disorders

CONGENITAL AND HEREDITARY DISORDERS

Disorders of the skin that have a congenital or hereditary basis are numerous and diverse in characteristics. In Chapter 10 some of the more common aberrations seen in the newborn infant are described, and the significance to the child is indicated. Individual variations in the pigmentation, the texture, the reactivity to stimuli and the degree of oiliness of the skin are so great as to defy comprehensive description. The more serious congenital disturbances are too rare to warrant inclusion in a short text, and the reader should consult one of the treatises on dermatology for a full description and illustrations.

INFECTIONS

BACTERIAL INFECTION

Impetigo Contagiosa

Impetigo contagiosa is a skin disease caused by an infection that invades the superficial layers of the skin. The infection tends to spread from one area to another on the affected person. It is transferred easily to other persons by direct or indirect contact. Both streptococci and staphylococci are causative agents.

The individual lesion varies in size from 3 mm. to 3 cm. or more. It appears first as a vesicle located superficially in the skin, with a loose and often wrinkled, rather than a tense and distended, top. Soon purulent material can be seen through the skin covering. The skin immediately surrounding the lesions shows no change from the normal. The pustule ruptures easily, and the exudate over the lesion tends to dry and form a crust. The crust eventually falls off, leaving an area slightly reddened. Soon all trace of the presence of the lesion disappears. The individual lesion runs its course in a week or two, but the disease has no uniform duration. Because of continued auto-inoculation, it may persist for many weeks.

The number of lesions on the body varies greatly, the total number depending on the amount of reinoculation from earlier lesions. Exposed parts (hands and face) are chiefly affected,

321

but the lesions may be in any location, especially in babies. No symptoms of consequence are associated with the disease, and rarely are complications or sequelae encountered. In a few cases of severe impetigo, acute hemorrhagic nephritis has occurred as a complication. When the infection occurs in the newborn, the lesions usually are large blisters, and often the condition is designated as pemphigus neonatorum.

The treatment consists of removal of the crusts and the tops of bullous lesions and the application of some germicide. The crusts may be removed by washing gently with warm saline solution. Perhaps the germicide most extensively used is an ointment containing 3 per cent ammoniated mercury. The ointment should be applied at least twice daily to areas where it cannot be protected by dressings from being rubbed off. Often other types of germicide are preferred, such as a 3 per cent aqueous solution of gentian violet or silver nitrate in concentrations up to 5 per cent. These solutions are painted on and not used as wet dressings. Antibiotic ointments are usually quite effective. Preparations containing bacitracin, polymyxin, chlortetracycline, erythromycin and neomycin are employed commonly. Ointments containing sulfonamides and penicillin are generally less effective and are more likely to result in sensitization of the child.

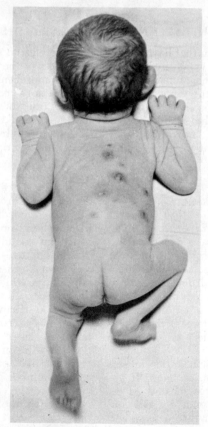

Fig. 53. Furunculosis or pyoderma.

When local therapy is not effective within a few days, it may be necessary to give an appropriate antibiotic systemically. If the impetigo is superimposed upon scabies or pediculosis, the underlying condition also should be treated.

Furunculosis

Furunculosis is a condition in which multiple small abscesses or boils are present in the skin. While a furuncle may occur at any age, multiple lesions, constituting furunculosis, occur chiefly in infants and especially in infants who are malnourished. The furuncles are caused by pyogenic bacteria, chiefly staphylococci, which gain entrance to the skin by way of the hair follicles. They are most common about the head but may occur in any location and may be generalized (Fig. 53).

Symptoms of furunculosis in a baby are few or lacking. Little or no fever is present in most instances. No doubt, furunculosis produces some constitutional effects, but such effects are vague and usually undetectable.

In the management of the skin disease, meticulous cleanliness is important. The hair should be shaved around any lesions on the scalp, and that area should be cleansed with green-soap solution several times daily. Incision is indicated only after the furuncle has pointed. In some instances, it may be desirable to hasten maturation of the lesions by the use of hot compresses. Draining furuncles should be covered in order to prevent spread of the infection. The dressing should be changed frequently enough to keep the drainage from the surrounding area. Elbow restraints may be necessary to prevent the infant from removing the dressing and transplanting the infection to other areas of the skin. Application of an antibiotic ointment may assist in destroying the infecting organisms as they emerge in the contents of the boil. Systemic treatment is often desirable. The selection of the antibiotic to be used can be made best by isolation of the infecting organism from the pus expressed from within the furuncle and determination of the sensitivities of the particular agent recovered. Stayphlococci in particular have become resistant to many of the commonly used antibiotics.

Modification of the diet to exclude as much carbohydrate as possible seems to aid in healing the lesions. Yeast or other preparations containing vitamin B complex are also useful.

INFECTION WITH OTHER AGENTS

Skin disorders may also be due to virus infection (warts, herpes), to fungous infections (ringworm) or to infestation with lice or mites. These afflictions are more commonly observed among children and are treated under the chapters dealing with the etiologic class of agents.

DISORDERS DUE TO PHYSICAL AND CHEMICAL AGENTS

REACTIONS TO BODY EXCRETIONS

Miliaria

Miliaria (miliaria rubra, "prickly heat") is the result of inflammation about the sweat glands in association with sweating from any cause, whether summer heat, excessive clothing or febrile illness. It is more common in babies than in those older. It is manifest by a bright-red papular rash. Some of the lesions may be topped by a small vesicle; others may become pustular. The rash tends to be most prominent about the neck and the body folds.

Treatment includes management of the hygiene to avoid sweating. Frequent bathing without soap is useful. Some simple dusting powder should be applied to the affected areas. The occasional use of calamine lotion is helpful, especially if itching is present.

Intertrigo

This inflammation of the skin occurs in body folds where moisture accumulates and two moist surfaces remain in contact. It is more common in obese infants. The infant's skin reacts more easily to irritation than does the skin of the older person. In infants, intertrigo may occur in the axilla, between the upper parts of the thighs, in the folds of the groin and the neck and in any other location where two skin surfaces come together. The affected skin is red and sometimes more or less raw from the loss of the outermost layer of skin. Intertrigo may be both prevented and treated by keeping the skin dry and clean in the body folds. Exposure of the affected areas to permit complete evaporation of moisture is desirable whenever possible. Clothing should be light and porous, and any material such as plastic or rubber diaper coverings which holds in moisture must be avoided until the lesions heal. In some cases the intertrigo becomes infected secondarily by skin bacteria or fungi. Application of mild antiseptics, antibiotics or fungicides may be necessary.

Diaper Rashes

In infancy, irritation or excoriation of the skin beneath the diapers is a common annoyance. In addition to the irritant effect of moisture from sweat and urine, there may be the burning erythema produced by organic acids in the stool or by ammonia which results from bacterial decomposition of the urine.

Diarrheal stools contain large amounts of organic acids which may result in a chemical burn of the skin if allowed to remain in contact with it for any appreciable length of time. The lesions produced have a characteristic distribution which conforms to the area of soiling by the stool. Dermatitis from this cause clears up when the diarrhea is brought under control. Prompt cleansing of the skin, preferably with a bland

oil, helps to prevent this form of diaper rash. Mechanical protection against the next stool may be given by smearing a layer of protective ointment over the affected area. A number of proprietary preparations are available for this purpose.

Diaper irritation from urine generally is due to the formation of ammonia by bacterial action on the urea normally present as a constituent of urine. The bacillus responsible is a common inhabitant of the intestinal tract, particularly of the artificially fed infant. Since it readily contaminates the perineum and the buttocks of the infant, it has easy access to urine in the wet diaper unless this is replaced rapidly by a dry one. The distribution of ammonia dermatitis corresponds to the spread of urine—mainly over the buttocks in an infant who habitually sleeps on his back, mainly over the anterior abdominal wall in an infant who sleeps face down.

Ulceration of the Urinary Meatus. This is a common disorder of circumcised male infants which probably depends upon the same general mechanism. It may occur even in the absence of any associated diaper rash. A small ulcer is produced at or just within the opening of the urinary meatus at the tip of the penis. A small crust forms over this ulcer, which is washed away easily by the stream of urine, producing pain and the appearance of a small drop of blood on the diaper. If the crust remains firmly attached, the urinary stream may be diverted to one side, or occasionally the opening will be blocked temporarily.

Treatment of ammonia dermatitis consists in thorough drying of the affected parts by persistent exposure to the air and by application of bland oils and protective ointments. Prevention may be achieved by measures designed to interfere with the growth of the bacteria which produce ammonia. Diapers may be given a final rinse in 1:5,000

G. 54. Weeping and crusted
ezcema of face, arms and legs.

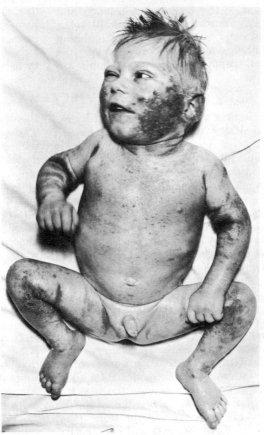

mercuric chloride solution or one of the proprietary antiseptics prepared for this purpose. Whichever substance is used, the diaper should be hung up wet so that the antiseptic can remain in the diaper in good concentration.

Seborrheic Dermatitis

In the common form of this disorder, surface lipids, scales, serum and dirt accumulate into yellowish crusts on the scalp in infants which, if neglected, may become thick, irritated or secondarily infected. Periodic removal of the crusts and the scales with a soap-and-water shampoo or the application of a bland oil is sufficient for mild accumulations. Ointments containing salicylic acid. or sulfur are useful in removing heavy scales. The tendency toward seborrheic dermatitis of the scalp usually decreases when the infant reaches a year of age. Occasionally other parts of the body are affected.

EXOGENOUS IRRITANTS

A very large number of substances are capable of stimulating a sensitivity reaction after repeated contact with the skin. Infants and young children are generally more likely to acquire such sensitization because of their relatively thin skins. In its mild form this contact dermatitis or allergic dermatitis appears as an area of redness with mild itching. In a more severe form it may result in swelling or even blistering. The main problem in treatment is to discover the offending substance and prevent further contact with it. Bleaches and detergent soaps used in laundering clothing or diapers are perhaps the most common sources of trouble to-day. Occasionally, such items as rubber pants or sheeting, plastic substances, cosmetics, adhesive gum, nail polish, iodine, or dyes from clothing are found to be responsible.

ECZEMA

Eczema is a dermatitis caused by internal or external irritants and having distinctive characteristics which make it differ from the dermatitis of bacterial inflammation. It tends to run a chronic course with periods of remission and exacerbation. Eczema occurs at all ages but it is considerably more frequent in infancy than at any time later. In the majority of cases, the eczema appears before 6 months of age, though seldom in the first month.

MANIFESTATIONS

Eczema of infancy differs from that occurring later in its greater severity and in the distribution and the general nature of the lesions. The common type of infantile eczema occurs most often in fat or well-nourished babies. The lesions are most severe on the face but they may appear also on the scalp, the forearms, the legs and the trunk (Fig. 54). In the early stages and in exacerbations, the superficial epithelium is lost, and the skin surface is raw and oozing. The exudate tends to dry, forming crusts. The skin is not thickened.

A less-common type, more frequent in malnourished babies, is characterized by a reddened, thickened, scaly skin. The lesions of this type may appear anywhere on the body. This latter type is the most common in older children, except that it is more likely to be limited in the body folds, especially at the elbows and the knees.

Infantile eczema is accompanied by considerable itching or burning, and as a consequence the baby, if permitted, will rub or scratch most of the time, thus aggravating the condition markedly. Remissions and exacerbations of the eczema occur at irregular intervals. The eczema usually is much worse in winter and better in summer, often disappearing entirely in the warm months only to recur in the fall. In the majority of instances, the skin heals between 1 and 2 years of age, and the eczema does not recur. In some infants the lesions change gradually into those of neurodermatitis (Chap. 26) which continues into later childhood.

ETIOLOGY

The cause of infantile eczema cannot be stated with the definiteness and the accuracy that one desires. That allergy is a large factor in many instances is an acceptable belief, but any claim that it is the cause in all cases is not supportable by the evidence at hand. Approximately three fourths of the older babies with eczema have positive reactions to various proteins when applied to the skin by customary testing methods. Babies in the first half year, especially those under 4 months, seldom present good evidence of skin sensitivity to test proteins, even though the eczema may be caused by these proteins. The food proteins to which infants most commonly are found sensitive are egg white; various cereals, especially wheat; cow's milk; fruit, especially apple and orange; and potato.

Even though a considerable proportion of babies with eczema have positive skin reactions to test proteins, only about one third or fewer of them will obtain relief from their eczema when removal of the supposedly offending protein from the diet is the only therapeutic measure employed. Factors other than allergy seem to play an important role. The skin of the infant is more sensitive and delicate than that of the child and reacts to milder stimuli. A large factor in the increased sensitivity of the infant is the large water content of the body, in which the skin shares. The extracellular or the interstitial water of the body of the infant is fully twice that of the adult, and the skin normally contains as much water as that of an edematous adult. Thus it is that many infants can have eczema without allergy and that treatment other than removal of the responsible allergen is necessary. This also explains why eczema is aggravated by the trauma of rubbing and scratching, by local infections which are acquired so easily in the affected areas of skin, and by sudden marked changes in temperature such as those to which the baby is exposed when taken outdoors in winter.

There are those who believe that eczema is caused or aggravated by dietary factors apparently unrelated to allergy, such as an excess of fat, an excess of sugar or an excess of total food. It is difficult to state the exact degree of truth in such a belief. In general, it may be stated that the eczema of well-nourished babies decreases when the babies lose weight, and that weight loss may result when the diet is restricted sufficiently in any of the ways stated. In ordinary circumstances this should not be considered as a good method of management. Any success it may have probably is dependent on loss of water from the body and therefore from the skin. Interstitial water never exists alone but always has in solution definite quantities of certain salts, chiefly sodium chloride. Therefore, any type of diet that tends to increase salt retention also would increase the water content of the skin and aggravate the eczema. The converse likewise would be true.

Babies with eczema have been found to have a low unsaturated fatty acid content of the blood, and the feeding of fats high in unsaturated fatty acid content has been suggested in treatment. Such therapy has not met with much clinical success. However, a diet relatively high in fat and low in carbohydrate (ketogenic type) has a dehydrating effect and could be beneficial in eczema.

Infants with eczema are prone to infections both of the skin itself and of the respiratory tract. Hospitalization carries a certain risk to the infant by placing him close to others who are infected. Isolation procedures are thus desirable for protection, though often undesirable for psychological reasons. *The eczematous infant must be kept away from children who have recently been vaccinated against smallpox and must not be vaccinated himself,* for the vaccina virus can diffusely infect his weeping skin and produce serious or fatal disease (Chap. 24). Individuals with herpes virus infections or streptococcal or pneumococcal infections are also a potential hazard. The debilitated eczematous infant does not fare well with severe respiratory disease, particularly pneumonia.

NURSING CARE

Ideally, the infant with eczema should be restrained as little as is absolutely necessary to prevent scratching and infection. It has been observed that these infants cry less than other babies. When they are frustrated, angry and unhappy they scratch instead of crying. If a nurse is in constant attendance, she can follow the baby's cues and give him affection or food or help him find a satisfying activity according to his specific need at the moment. The baby with eczema improves physically and psychologically when he has a continuous warm relationship with a nurse who recognizes his need to express his feelings overtly and to use his powers in independent, learning activities.

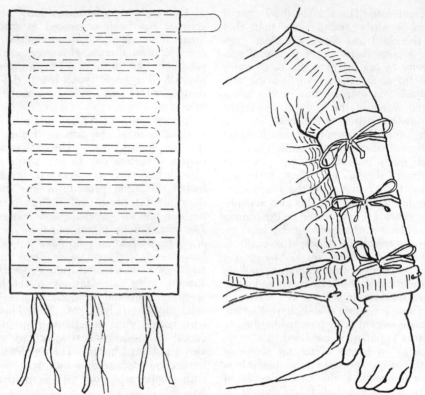

Fig. 55. Elbow cuff restraint. (*Left*) Elbow cuff for use in treatment of eczema. (*Right*) Elbow cuff applied.

Restraint

When constant attendance is not possible, it is necessary to employ some means that will prevent scratching or rubbing. Elbow cuffs that prevent flexion at the elbows are of assistance, but usually the arms must be held with additional restraint to prevent rubbing of the face with the upper arms. Restraints must be applied securely and in a kind fashion. They must be adjusted securely because the baby's discomfort and desire for activity drive him to find methods of freeing himself. A few minutes without restraint may undo the nursing of the past weeks and produce open lesions that become infected easily. They must be applied in a kind

fashion to minimize feelings of anger at being restrained.

A good type of elbow cuff is one splinted with tongue blades (Fig. 55). It is more comfortable for young infants to have the tongue blades cut to about 4 inches in length. In order to retain the cuff securely, the shirt sleeves should be folded over the lower end of the cuff and pinned to it. Ankle restraints are necessary if eczema is present in the legs. When the weather is warm or when the infant tends to perspire profusely, it is advisable to eliminate the use of the shirt. To keep the cuff restraints in position, a 4-inch strip of old linen can be brought across the shoulders and down the arms and then pinned back over the cuff.

Fingernails and toenails must be cut short. If necessary, gloves or stockings can be put on the hands and pinned to the cuffs to minimize scratching.

Protection by Pliofilm

When an infant tends to rub his face on his shoulders, a bib of Pliofilm prevents excoriations. Such a bib may be made of an 8-inch square of Pliofilm with tabs of adhesive and tape at the corners for pinning it into position. In some institutions, Pliofilm covers over the head of the mattress have been used with excellent results. When the Pliofilm bib and mattress covers are used, the infant can be turned from side to side and on his abdomen without danger of increasing the severity of the lesions. Changes in position are important in the prevention of respiratory infections, a complication to which the infant with eczema is very susceptible.

Local Applications

The selection of appropriate dermatologic remedies and their meticulous application are useful in all cases of eczema and, in addition to other general measures discussed, are sufficient in many instances to bring about recovery without recourse to radical dietary changes. If the skin is moderately infected when the baby comes under care, an antibiotic ointment, such as bacitracin or neomycin, may be used until the infection has disappeared. Systemic use of antibiotics may be necessary to control severe infection. In instances of more severe infection, wet packs of normal salt solution serve better than an ointment. If the skin is not infected or if the infection has been treated effectively, a protective or soothing ointment is indicated. Such an ointment may be 2 per cent ichthyol or Lassar's paste. If satisfactory improvement is not obtained with the soothing ointment, a stimulating ointment, such as 6 per cent tar ointment or carbonis detergens cream, is indi-

cated, but only after the protective ointment has failed. When tar ointment is used, exposure to the sun should be avoided because the ointment contains a photosensitizing fraction that produces skin irritation as a result of exposure to sunshine.

Ointments containing hydrocortisone or related adrenal steroids are useful in controlling the inflammatory reaction. General use of these hormones is to be avoided.

Ointments should be applied liberally and bandaged in place with 2-inch elastic bandage. Applying the ointment with long strokes has been found to produce a more soothing effect.

In order to ensure satisfactory retention of ointments or wet dressings applied to the face, it may be necessary to use a mask. A mask is prepared by cutting holes in a piece of old linen or cotton stocking, the holes corresponding in shape and location to the eyes, the nose and the mouth. The mask should be large enough to go around the head and should be held in position with attached tapes. Binding and friction must be avoided when adjusting the mask.

Cleansing the Skin

Oil applied by means of cotton, or water to which sodium bicarbonate and starch have been added is used for cleansing. The use of soap is not advisable. When ointments are being used, it is customary to cleanse the skin once daily or less frequently. Cleansing should be done gently without rubbing. If itching is intense and restraint is being used, only one extremity at a time can be released for cleansing.

Sometimes a colloidal bath is desired. In preparation, an infant-sized tub is filled with water at 95° F., and ¼ cup each of soluble starch and sodium bicarbonate is mixed in thoroughly. Floating toys should be at hand to divert the infant's attention and prevent scratching during the procedure. A diaper should be placed in the bottom of the tub to prevent the baby from slipping, and a firm hold is necessary to prevent the child from feeling insecure in the tub. During the time the infant is in the tub (15 to 20 minutes), the washcloth should be used to pour water over the infant's head and body. Rubbing the skin may produce a paroxysm of itching.

Diet

Usually it is not possible at the first examination to determine whether or not infantile eczema is on an allergic basis. Whether or not special dietary measures are instituted at the beginning of treatment, they may be employed if response to local treatment is not definite and prompt. More than half the babies with eczema will respond to local treatment without dietary change. If the eczema is dependent on allergy to foods, the offending foods should be omitted from the diet, while at the same time the diet should be kept "complete."

One good method of management is to use what is known as an elimination diet. This is accomplished by starting with a simple basic diet which is hypoallergenic to the extent that improvement in the eczema is permitted and then adding one food at a time to determine the infant's reaction to each food. In such a scheme, new foods should be introduced in small amounts. The diet and the skin changes should be charted in full in order to determine the foods to which the baby is sensitive.

The chief article of the basic diet should be some form of milk or milk substitute. Prolonged or high heating of protein alters its character in such a way that it is less allergenic, often sufficiently so that babies who are sensitive to the raw protein can take the cooked protein without disturbance. It is the alteration produced by heat that gives to evaporated and dried milk a considerable degree of usefulness in the management of babies with allergic eczema. Babies sensitive to cow's milk often are able to take goat's milk. Synthetic "milks" are commercially available. Some of these are prepared from soybeans. One is prepared from hydrolyzed casein. Regardless of which of these various foods may be chosen, the formula must be supplemented by vitamins C and D and perhaps other essentials, depending on the food chosen. In the dietary management of babies with eczema, foods are to be avoided on the basis of actual demonstration by feeding, not on the basis of skin tests.

Psychological Aspects

Eczema is rarely dependent completely upon sensitivity to foods but often is aggravated by either internal or external environmental irritants. Feathers, wool, kapok and certain dusts may irritate the child. The common factors among these materials should be eliminated. Stuffed toys may contain allergenic factors. Emotional factors also may play a part in producing eczema. Many investigators who have studied children with eczema have found emotional disturbances in the mother-child relationship. Dunbar concluded that a climate with "smother love" was the characteristic emotional climate to which the child with eczema was subjected. She felt that many of these children experienced conflict between their desire for affection and their fear lest they be hurt if they sought it. Other investigators found these children overprotected and recipients of domineering love. Some believed that a frustrated need for love was one of the dynamic factors operating to produce the condition.

A baby with eczema should be held for feedings the same as one does in the case of a healthy child. Such holding gives him a change in position and the affection that he needs for normal emotional growth. Time of feeding should be gauged by his need for food. Awakening a baby with eczema robs him of necessary sleep and increases his need to scratch. Often excellent results are obtained by giving the baby increased opportunity to suck. It reduces tension and brings relaxation. A pacifier has been found to be effective in giving the baby increased comfort. However, other sources of pleasure also must be provided. He needs both stimulation from a satisfying, non-smothering type of relationship with a parent figure and sufficient opportunity to meet his need for sucking.

In preventing scratching, the nurse must not lose sight of the fact that her patient is a human being who needs the same satisfactions and opportunities for learning as does the healthy infant. He needs freedom for self-directed play and opportunities to develop his powers. Restraints should be removed each time the infant is fed, and his arms and legs should be exercised. If he is old enough to be interested in self-feeding, his interest in learning should be encouraged. As soon as the skin lesions show sufficient improvement, the outer restraints should be removed and the infant allowed to move about and play freely under close supervision. Toys suited to his individual needs should be introduced. Diversion prevents scratching and gives the infant needed experience with play materials.

When caring for a child with eczema, the nurse must also direct her interest to the needs of the mother. The nurse not only needs to reflect upon her feelings toward the child with eczema but also she should reflect upon her reactions to his mother. Mothers of babies with eczema are often unusually fearful and agitated and see the baby's condition as evidence of their failure to fulfill the mother role. Some tend to handle the baby less than do mothers of normal infants, and the manner of handling is usually less gentle. Others overstimulate the baby with excessive handling. Some hesitate to restrain and to restrict the baby's diet because it frustrates their deep need to overprotect. Many mothers fear that their infants are afflicted with a chronic disease that may produce scars and prevent normal development.

The mothers of babies with eczema need much help before they assume complete charge of the infants. Providing the mother with an opportunity to talk about her feelings toward her child and the amount of care he requires not only meets her need to share her burden with another person but also gives the nurse increased understanding of her as a person. If the nurse knows of what the mother is fearful, she can help her gain increased mastery of the feeling. Detailed instructions and demonstrations of care are important but they are not enough to ensure continuity of nursing care for the baby. Experience can verify this statement. It is not unusual to see recurrences very soon after the baby has been discharged from the hospital. Recurrences can be minimized if the mother has opportunities to take care of her baby in the presence of an understanding nurse. During such experiences, the nurse should direct her interest to the mother. Supporting her through experiences which are fear-provoking builds up her self-confidence, increases her feelings of self-esteem and frees energy for the building of a warmer relationship with her child. The nurse can help the mother find ways to restrict scratching which minimizes her feelings of guilt and provides her child with opportunities to use his extremities in play. She can increase her hope, clarify any misconceptions she is harboring and help her feel more comfortable with her baby.

Nervous mannerisms are seen frequently in children with eczema. The long periods of restriction with constant frustrations tend to produce emotional instability, insecurity, aggression, extroversion, restlessness and an unusual drive to dominate. Parental anxiety often is reflected in their behavior. When frustrated in play, these children not uncommonly revert to scratching, even though their skin shows little or no irritation. Some studies have indicated superior mental ability in these children. If this is true, it is not to be wondered at that they are eager to investigate their environment when once freed from the restraints that have limited and angered them. To prevent these nervous mannerisms, it is necessary that the nurse understand the problems of the mother and help her to feel the need to give her child more opportunities to develop his independence in play and in learning to do things for himself.

ACRODYNIA (ERYTHREDEMA, PINK DISEASE)

Acrodynia is a peculiar disorder which is seen sporadically in infants during the first 2 years of life. It is characterized by a prolonged course during which there is swelling, itching and peeling of the fingers, combined with general irritability and evidence of irritation of the sympathetic nervous system.

ETIOLOGY

Until recently the cause of acrodynia was obscure. The finding of mercury in the urine of nearly all infants who suffer from the disease and the successful treatment with BAL, which is an effective agent in some heavy metal poisonings, has demonstrated that mercury poisoning is an important aspect of the disease. Since a child who has contact with mercury appears only rarely to suffer from acrodynia, it is presumed that an individual sensitivity to mercury is necessary or that some additional factor which has not yet been recognized must be involved.

Fortunately this unhappy affliction of infants is disappearing from most areas of the United States. The declining use of mercurial teething lotions and pow-

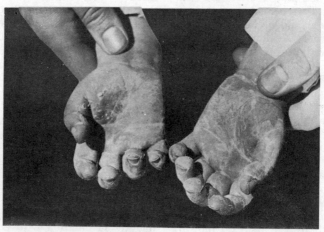

FIG. 56. The hands in acrodynia.

ders, anthelmintics and local ointments may be responsible.

Symptoms

Usually the onset is insidious, and it is often difficult to determine from the history the relative time of onset of the various symptoms. When the disease has developed sufficiently for identification the symptoms are numerous. Perhaps the one pathognomonic feature and the one without which the diagnosis is uncertain consists of the changes that take place in the hands and the feet (Fig. 56). In the outspoken disease, the palms and the soles are bluish red and slightly swollen. Associated with this change is an annoying or painful itching or stinging which causes frequent or nearly constant rubbing and scratching. As the disease becomes older, the thickened skin of the palms and the soles begins to desquamate. The redness of the hands fades gradually at the wrist into the normal color of the arm, and there is no sharp line of demarcation such as is found in pellagra.

One finds that the disposition and the behavior of the child have changed. Early in the disease there is hyperesthesia of the skin and the muscles, which results in resentment at being handled and contributes to fretfulness and irritability, which are usually present. As the disease advances, the deep reflexes diminish, and a progressive muscular weakness becomes apparent. The result is decrease of such activity or effort as is represented by sitting, standing or walking. The most characteristic attitude is to lie in a knee-chest position, usually on the front, sometimes on the side, with the face buried in the pillow or the bedclothes. Covering of the face is to be accounted for by photophobia, which is present in the majority of cases. Insomnia is often a conspicuous feature. Partial or complete loss of appetite is usual.

In the early stage, an acute exanthem often is to be noted. The rash is a diffuse erythema and more often than not is associated with profuse perspiration, in which case the rash is chiefly miliaria. Acute upper respiratory infection is common. At least a moderate amount of fever usually is present. Tachycardia and elevation of the blood pressure are common. The white blood count may be normal or increased considerably.

As the disease progresses, weight loss becomes increasingly apparent, with a resultant poor nutritional state. Perspiration frequently becomes excessive. Salivation may be conspicuous. In many of the more severe illnesses stomatitis develops, with swollen tender gums and loosening or even loss of teeth. In a few cases, a patchy alopecia is to be observed. In some cases, a profuse nasal discharge persists throughout most of the course of the illness.

In severe illnesses the course is slow, and in a few instances the disease has persisted for as long as a year. The duration of the milder illnesses may be as short as 6 weeks. Despite the severity and the persistence of this disease, the mortality is low, and death, when it occurs, usually is due to some intercurrent infection such as pneumonia.

Treatment

Intramuscular injection of BAL every 4 hours during the acute stage of the illness and then at decreasing intervals as the symptoms subside is reported to to be effective in acrodynia. Symptomatic treatment includes control of respiratory infections which are often present, sedation and general nursing care.

Nursing Care

The child with acrodynia presents a picture of abject misery. He rarely smiles, is irritable, negative, temperamental and prone to exaggerated emotional responses. However, at times he is apathetic and withdrawn. At other times he is hyperactive; he may chew on his fingers and pull out his hair. He perspires profusely and shows symptoms of excessive thirst because of fluid loss through the skin.

The child with this disease is difficult yet challenging to nurse because results are slow and discouraging, and his responses to thoughtful, kindly given care are different from those of the usual child. He is so miserable that he can give little in return for all that he gets. Expert nursing care assists him in adjusting to a disease that deprives him of normal satisfactions. It does not bring rapid and dramatic results but it lessens the severity of his discomfort. Symptoms of nervous instability can be minimized with poise, insight and kindness. If the nurse does not understand him, he will feel unloved as well as physically uncomfortable. Although the child may seem to be uninterested in everything and everyone within his environment, efforts to relieve his anxiety and physical discomfort must never cease.

Physical nursing care consists of protective measures, good skin and mouth care and the provision of thoughtful, patient feeding experiences. Padded cribsides are frequently necessary to protect the child from injury. Elbow restraints to prevent finger chewing and hair pulling are indicated in periods when the child cannot have the constant attention of his nurse. Baths twice daily are necessary to keep the skin clean and free from pyogenic infection. If sponge baths bring discomfort, tub baths should be given. The child should be lifted carefully and held securely to prevent his slipping in the tub.

When the illness is severe, teeth drop out or become loosened, and the gums are swollen, red and spongy. In cleansing the mouth, care must be taken to prevent traumatization of the delicate buccal mucosa. Protection from bright lights should be provided. If sun treatments are ordered, the child should be provided with goggles.

Attention to nutrition might be considered as one of the major factors leading to recovery. The child with acrodynia presents many problems in relation to food intake. Because he loses much fluid through the skin, he needs high-vitamin, high-caloric fluid drinks at frequent intervals. Since the child with acrodynia has little or no appetite, patience and ingenuity are needed to encourage an adequate intake of food. Often he cannot handle feeding utensils because his hands are painful, his muscles are hypnotic, and he fatigues easily. He requires feeding and kind firmness to help him to understand that he is expected to take the small amounts of food that are offered at short intervals. Gavage feedings may be necessary. Many times gavage feedings are preferable to forced feedings because invariably the resistance they evoke causes hyperirritability and vomiting.

Sedatives are often necessary for wakefulness, which may last for long periods of time. Often the child falls asleep from sheer exhaustion. When he does, he should be covered lightly to prevent chilling. He has poor resistance, low vitality and is unusually susceptible to respiratory infections. Every possible precaution must be taken to protect him from cross-infection.

SITUATIONS FOR FURTHER STUDY

1. How would you help a mother who was troubled by her infant's diaper rash?

2. Observe an infant with eczema and describe his behavior when he shows signs of frustration. How might frustration be prevented? Plan his care to prevent it and record your observation of change in behavior and in the appearance of the infant's skin.

3. Observe the mother of an infant with eczema. What did she talk about?

What were her chief concerns? How were they reflected in her behavior with her baby? Describe the way in which you helped her to feel more competent and comfortable with her baby.

BIBLIOGRAPHY

Andrews, G. C.: Diseases of the Skin, ed. 4, Philadelphia, Saunders, 1954.

Becker, S. W., and Obermayer, M. E.: Modern Dermatology and Syphilology, ed. 2, Philadelphia, Lippincott, 1947.

Bilderback, J. B.: Acrodynia in Nelson, Textbook of Pediatrics, ed. 6, Philadelphia, Saunders, 1954.

Bivings, L.: Acrodynia, a summary of BAL therapy reports, J. Pediat. 34: 322, 1949.

Deutsch, F., and Nadell, R.: Psychosomatic aspects of dermatology with special consideration of allergic phenomena, Nerv. Child 5:339, 1946.

Dunbar, H. F.: Mind and Body: Psychosomatic Medicine, p. 190, New York, Random, 1947.

Hill, L. W.: Eczema and Poison Ivy (pamphlet), Boston, The Children's Medical Centre, 1954.

Lofthouse, E. M.: Infantile eczema, Am. J. Nursing 49:500, 1949.

Miller, M. L.: A psychological study of a case of eczema and a case of neurodermatitis, Psychosom. Med. 4:82, 1942.

Stone, H. M.: Psychological factors in infantile eczema, Am. J. Nursing 53: 449, 1953.

Warkany, J., and Hubbard, D. M.: Adverse mercurial reactions in the form of acrodynia and related conditions, Am. J. Dis. Child. 81:335, 1951.

CHAPTER SIXTEEN

Congenital Malformations

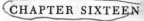

The care of a congenitally malformed child presents the nurse with several challenges. The physical aspects of nursing care may be complex and demanding and frequently are frustrating and discouraging. The emotional aspects of nursing care are trying, until the nurse faces her feelings and learns to handle them constructively. Initial experiences with malformed infants and their parents are bound to create tension and conflictful feelings. Talking these feelings over with a helpful instructor or head nurse will help the inexperienced nurse to keep them within her awareness where they can be handled with increasing comfort. In addition, the nurse must confront the disappointed parents whose attitudes toward the malformed child commonly need to be converted from hopeless despair to a constructive, realistic plan for salvaging his assets. To face the latter challenge the nurse should have knowledge about the ultimate prognosis of the particular deformity, the degree to which it can be modified by modern treatment, and the steps which will be necessary either to eliminate the defect or to help the parents and the child toward an optimum disposition of his life. This chapter will consider only defects which are apparent at birth or soon afterward. It cannot hope to cover the infinite variety of known deformities but will present the peculiar problems of some of the commoner abnormalities. In the chapters on diseases of the various organ systems will be found additional information about malformations which evade discovery until later infancy or childhood.

INCIDENCE

Anomalies cover such a wide range of severity from the fatal to the trivial that an exact statement of incidence depends upon what changes are included within the definition. At one extreme it is possible to say that almost every infant has some anomaly such as a pigmented mole, facial asymmetry, or slight webbing of the toes. At the other extreme the definition may be limited to those defects which seriously interfere with function of the body; roughly 1 per cent of newborns will be found to be thus afflicted. More exact are the figures for malformations which result in death during the first year of life. As detailed in Chapter 5, approximately 1 out of 7 or 8 of the deaths which go to make up the infant mortality rate can be attributed to anomalous development. Over the years this incidence has not changed much because measures for preventing malformations are not very effective. In contrast, the surgical technics for correcting or ameliorating those anomalies which are compatible with life have been greatly improved in recent years so that this aspect of pediatric care is assuming more and more importance.

ETIOLOGY

The construction of the human body begins at conception with the division of the fertilized ovum, first into 2 cells, then into 4, 8, and so on until the process has been repeated an estimated 44 times by the conclusion of the 40-week period of gestation. Along the way the dividing cells differentiate into the many types found in the completed body, and group themselves into masses and layers which form the organ systems. These latter undergo a predetermined sequence of changes in shape through the development of curves, bulges, ridges, tubes, projections and tunnels as they progress toward their final anatomic form. Simultaneously, the whole growing mass of protoplasm migrates into the fallopian tube, traverses it rapidly and fixes itself to the wall of the uterus. Here it develops a placenta through which it eventually acquires nourishment by way of the maternal circulation. During later growth the fetus distends the uterus so that it occupies a large fraction of the maternal abdominal cavity. Malformations arise when the expected changes in this complicated assembly-line fail to take place in proper sequence or to the proper extent. Interferences at any stage may affect the final form of a portion or even of the whole of the body. It is small wonder that malformations occur; it is the miracle of reproduction that the intricate changes follow the blueprint exactly in more than 9 out of 10 gestations.

Some malformations are determined even before fertilization of the ovum takes place. The genetic material of the ovum itself or of the sperm which fertilizes it may be such that it will direct the growth of the new individual along aberrant lines. The science of genetics studies the way in which traits, both normal and abnormal, are passed along from parent to child through the activities of the genes. Some of the anomalies of man are known to follow the same rules of transmission as those which have been established for animals by research and experimentation. Such hereditary or genetically transmitted malformations are identified by their occurrence in other members of the child's family. Those which are passed along by a dominant type of inheritance are relatively easy to identify, but those with a recessive mode of transmission may appear too infrequently to permit adequate study. The reader is referred to treatises on genetics for further elaboration of the methods of transmittal of traits. It should be noted that a given abnormality such as cleft palate can at times be the result of genetic factors and at other times be due to influences upon the fetus developing in utero which have no hereditary basis.

The first 12 weeks of fetal development are a crucial period in which the major organ systems of the body complete the transformation into their final shapes, albeit not their final sizes. Any interference with growth during this "organogenetic" period may result in permanent deformity of the organ or part involved. In experimental work with animals it has been shown that various types of disturbance of the mother during the corresponding period of gestation can be used to produce anomalies in the young. Deprivation of oxygen or of certain vitamins, administration of hormones, poisons, antimetabolites and cortisone or exposure to irradiation from radium or roentgen rays are among the methods used to interfere with the normal development of animal fetuses. In man it has been suspected that similar influences upon the pregnant woman might be responsible for anomalies, but only a few such examples have been definitely established. Exposure to radium, roentgen rays and the atomic bomb have resulted in the delivery of infants with abnormalities of the brain. Maternal infection with rubella is generally accepted as being responsible for a combination of defects of the eye, the heart and the brain. Infants who are subjected to the hormonal disturbances of a mother who has diabetes during pregnancy suffer a distinctly greater incidence of congenital malformations.

In the latter two thirds of pregnancy the adverse effects upon the fetus are better understood. Disease of the mother may be transferred to him (syphilis, toxoplasmosis, and rarely other infections). Antithyroid drugs given to the mother may result in her child having a goiter at birth. Erythroblastosis is the effect of abnormal antibodies in the mother upon the red blood cells of the child. In fact, the mechanisms of many of these defects is now so well understood that we no longer regard them as congenital malformations. During the last few months of pregnancy some infants appear to remain in one position and to suffer in consequence pressure effects from the uterus or from bony prominences of the maternal skeleton. Positional anomalies of the feet, the legs, the jaw and the face are explained in this fashion. The reason why certain infants fail to change position is not understood.

Prevention of malformations is largely an unrealized hope. Careful supervision of maternal diets in pregnancy, exact regulation of diabetes, and shielding of mothers insofar as possible from infectious disease and from radiant energy probably prevents some malformations, but it must be admitted that our understanding of the mechanism of malformation is too inexact as yet to permit the prevention of more than a small percentage.

HEREDITARY IN-BORN ERRORS OF METABOLISM

Although in-born errors of metabolism do not produce symptoms which are apparent at birth, they have such importance to our understanding of the origin of congenital abnormalities that they deserve brief discussion here. Some are relatively common disorders (sicklemia for example), but most are rare conditions (galactosemia, Gaucher's disease, phenylketonuria) in which an enzyme necessary for the completion of a biochemical reaction within the body is congenitally missing. A rapidly increasing number of such disorders is

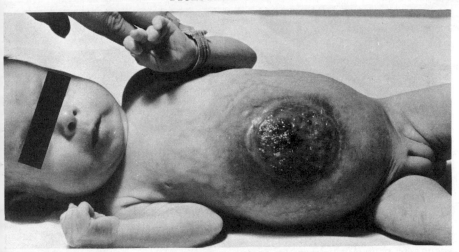

FIG. 57. Omphalocele.

being discovered, most of which are found to have a recessive mode of inheritance. This means that to be affected by the disease, a child must receive a pair of abnormal genes—one from his father and the other from his mother. The parents who themselves carry the abnormal gene in single dosage are not affected with the disease. However, their union makes it possible for them to bear children with 1 chance in 4 of receiving the double dose of the gene and manifesting the disease. Sickle cell anemia is a good illustration. About 10 per cent of American Negroes have an abnormal gene which causes them to manufacture chemically abnormal S-hemoglobin in their red blood cells. When present in single dosage the gene does them no harm, for only a relatively small fraction of their hemoglobin is S-hemoglobin. Its presence can be recognized by electrophoretic tests upon hemoglobin obtained from

their red cells or by a simpler test of the red cells themselves for the sickling trait. However, when two individuals who have the asymptomatic sickle trait produce children, about one fourth of the offspring will receive two abnormal genes and in consequence will produce such a large proportion of S-hemoglobin that the symptoms of sickle cell anemia will result. While 10 per cent of Negroes carry the abnormal gene, only about 0.25 per cent have it in double dosage and suffer from sickle cell anemia. It can be understood that abnormal genes which are less frequent in the population as a whole will produce disease with corresponding rarity. The rarity itself makes study difficult. It is quite possible that many disorders whose origin we do not now understand will eventually be found to depend upon the conjunction of two rare recessive genes.

DIGESTIVE TRACT

OMPHALOCELE

Omphalocele is a rare but important anomaly in which the contents of the abdominal cavity protrude into the root of the umbilical cord or through a defect in the skin of the anterior abdominal wall (Fig. 57). The protruding mass may be small in size or large

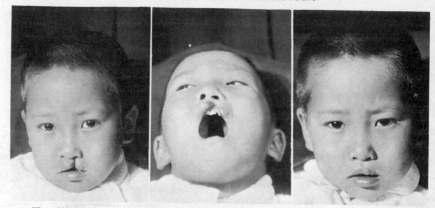

FIG. 58. (*Left*) Incomplete cleft lip. (*Center*) Complete cleft palate. (*Right*) Cleft lip repaired.

enough to contain much of the intestines and the liver. It is covered with a delicate membrane rather than skin. Immediate surgical repair is necessary before the sac ruptures and infection is introduced into the abdominal cavity. In about half of the instances of omphalocele, other congenital defects are present. Surgical repair is made difficult by the small size of the abdominal cavity which may make it almost impossible to mobilize enough skin to cover over the defect. This problem and the presence of other anomalies lead to a high postoperative mortality.

CLEFT LIP AND PALATE

The deformity of cleft lip (harelip) or cleft palate or both combined (Fig. 58) results from failure of growth and union of the bony and soft tissue structures on one or both sides of the midline of the palate and the upper jaw. The failure in union may be on one or both sides of the lip alone, or it may extend backward into the upper jaw and even through into the nasal cavity. The defect of the palate posteriorly is a failure of mid-line closure which may occur alone or in conjunction with clefts in the lip or the anterior palate. These anomalies are fairly common, occurring in between 1:500 and 1:1000 newborns. In some families there is a clear hereditary transmission. In other instances no etiologic basis is known. Sometimes isolated defects of the palate are associated with very marked hypoplasia of the lower jaw (Pierre Robin syndrome), suggesting that the palate has been prevented from closing by backward pressure of the tongue and the jaw due to intra-uterine anteflexion of the head upon the chest.

Plan of Treatment

The general plan of treatment and the prospective outcome depend upon the extent and the combination of the deformities. Surgical repair of the lip and the upper maxilla usually is performed within the first few weeks of life. Where only the lip is involved, the result of early operation may be final and quite satisfactory. Involvement of the maxilla usually foreshadows irregularities in later dentition and perhaps some abnormality of growth. Defects of the palate are more difficult to handle, and their correction usually is deferred until at least the second year and often later in order to take advantage of changes which occur with growth. Cleft palates usually foreshadow speech difficulties and may be attended by recurrent infections of the upper respiratory tract and the middle ear. When it is deemed advisable to postpone surgical repair of the palate, prosthetic speech appliances are fitted so that speech development can approximate the normal. Prostheses are used after the deciduous teeth have become fully erupted and the child has developed emotionally to the point where he can accept the use of the speech appliance. Prostheses have been used for children as early as 2½ years. Sometimes speech proceeds normally without the benefit of formal speech training. In most instances, however, speech therapy is imperative. Sometimes prostheses are used as interim devices before the palate is repaired or when the palate is repaired in two or more stages. In instances when the deformity is too severe for adequate plastic repair, prosthetic speech appliances are used as a permanent means of speech rehabilitation. As the child grows, the appliance must be modified accordingly.

An important aspect of the initial management is the problem of dealing with the disappointment and the anxieties of the parents. Considerable justified reassurance can be given when the defect is confined to the lip. If the palate is also involved, parents usually can be assured that much improvement is to be expected but that it will take time, skillful judgment and care, and patience on their parts to help the child adjust to his deformity and to assume a relatively normal place in the community.

The optimum management of a child with a cleft palate requires coordinated efforts of the pediatrician, the plastic surgeon, the dentist, the speech therapist, the social worker and the nurse. In large metropolitan areas and in state Crippled Children's programs there is an increasing tendency to provide cleft palate clinics where the several specialists can work jointly with easy consultation among themselves. When such facilities are available to an infant with cleft palate, early referral even within the first few weeks of life is desirable so that changes taking place with growth can be observed and appropriate plans for ultimate corrective measures can be made accordingly.

Nursing Care of Cleft Lip

The artificial feeding of infants who cannot feed at the breast may be successful when carried out in the usual manner, if the hole in the nipple is larger than customary and the nipple is soft. A "lamb's nipple" often serves better than those in common use; they are longer and softer. Otherwise, feeding may be by means of a medicine dropper, a bulb or a spoon. When an infant with a cleft lip sucks, he is likely to swallow excessive amounts of air; more frequent bubbling is necessary to prevent regurgitation.

To accustom the infant to the postoperative method of feeding, he should be fed with a rubber-tipped medicine dropper a day or two before operation. Insertion of the dropper into the corner of his mouth will prevent interference with the suture line and will prevent much suction on the repaired lip. Feedings should be given slowly and at a rate suitable to the capacity of the individual infant, the milk mixture being kept warm continually throughout the procedure.

The nurse should observe the infant for signs of respiratory or gastro-intestinal disease during the preoperative period, for it is imperative that surgery be performed when the infant is in the best possible physical condition. Protective isolation precautions are helpful in preventing cross-infection. Arm restraint immediately after the operation is necesary, and the effect is less distressing to the infant if he has become accustomed to it before. If the infant is old enough to turn himself onto his abdomen and face, a jacket restraint to keep him on his side or back will also be necessary.

After operative repair of the lip, the infant needs observation and meticulous care. Water may be given as soon as he is awake and able to swallow. Milk feedings are resumed within 3 to 4 hours postoperatively. The infant with a cleft lip repair requires slow, careful feeding and adequate bubbling to prevent regurgitation. After feeding he should be placed on his side to prevent aspiration of any regurgitated milk or mucus that may accumulate. Support with a rolled bed pad will be necessary to keep him in this position. A sterile bulb syringe should be in readiness to aspirate mucus from the mouth. Arm and body restraints should be in readiness for application immediately after his return to the ward. Tongue-depressor arm restraints will prevent the infant from getting his hands to his mouth but will not prevent him from rubbing his face with his upper arms. For this reason, the cuffs should be pinned securely to the shirt. Periodically, he should be given relief from his restraint. His arms should be massaged and exercised one at a time. Restraints should not be removed for weighing, nor should both be removed at one time during the morning bath. The infant's position should be changed frequently to prevent both hypostatic pneumonia and discomfort. Crying causes tension on the suture line. His need for emotional satisfactions are no different from the normal infant. The infant who has had a surgical repair of the lip cannot suckle; therefore, he needs extra cuddling to keep him free from anxiety and tension.

A tray containing sterile swabs, hydrogen peroxide or saline, forceps in alcohol, and a paper bag should be in readiness when the infant returns from the operating room. Careful and frequent cleansing of the entire suture line to promote healing is a major responsibility of the nurse. Should there be sloughing of the sutures, the vermilion border of the lip becomes uneven, and additional repair makes a good cosmetic effect impossible. Cleansing of the suture line should be done after feeding and as often as serum collects. When a crust forms, scar formation is more prominent. Tightly twisted toothpick swabs moistened in hydrogen peroxide or saline are used to remove serum and milk. Cleansing should be done gently to avoid injury, and excess solution should be removed with dry swabs. All sutures need care, including those on the inner surface of the lip.

During the first 48 hours after operation, difficulty in breathing may be encountered. When bilateral clefts have been repaired, the infant must become accustomed to nasal breathing, a type not required before. In some instances a sterile airway made of a small piece of ¼-inch rubber tubing is sutured to the corner of the infant's mouth before he leaves the operating room. If no airway has been inserted and difficult breathing is observed, downward pressure on the chin to open the mouth will bring relief. If a Logan bar has been applied to prevent suture tension, care should be taken to keep the adhesive strapping dry and clean. Moisture loosens it, and then its effectiveness is negligible.

After sutures have been removed and the wound is entirely healed (2 to 3 weeks), bottle or breast feedings may be resumed. If the mother still has breast milk, she should be encouraged to maintain her supply during the period in which the infant is having surgical repair. The use of pumped milk during the postoperative period is an added advantage to the infant.

When a cleft lip has been repaired successfully in a baby who has an associated cleft palate, the improved appearance usually has a remarkable psychological effect on the parents. It gives them hope and helps the mother to face the future care that the infant with cleft palate requires. Before the infant leaves the hospital, the mother should be assisted in learning how to feed her baby effectively and how to prevent respiratory infections. Many infants with cleft palates can learn to suckle from a bottle if the nipple bulb is soft and long, and if the holes are large enough. If the usual method of feeding can be used, the mother is less inclined to feel that her child is abnormal. These babies require slow feeding to prevent excessive air swallowing and regurgitation. Holding them in a sitting position helps to prevent the food from going into their nostrils.

ATRESIA OF THE INTESTINAL TRACT

Atresia of the Esophagus

Failure of the embryonic development of the esophagus to result in a continuous tube connecting the pharynx with the stomach is a serious but rather uncommon congenital malformation. Several variations of this condition are known. The most common one consists of a blindly ending pouch at the upper end of the esophagus and an errant lower segment which runs upward from the stomach and opens through a fistula into the trachea near its bifurcation. At the time of birth, air enters the stomach by way of the trachea, the fistula and the lower segment of the esophagus. Attempts to swallow liquids or even the normal secretions of the mouth result in rapid filling of the blind pouch and overflow of liquid into the larynx and the trachea. The infant chokes, coughs and turns blue whenever attempts are made to feed him. Unless the situation is corrected quickly, he will contract bronchitis or pneumonia from the repeated aspiration of food and secretions. Rarely, the esophagus is fully open but communicates with the trachea by an abnormal fistula. The same sort of symptoms result, and the treatment is identical.

Diagnosis of atresia is made by stoppage of a catheter at the site of atresia or by a roentgenogram with iodized oil in the esophagus; barium never should be used for this purpose because of the danger of pneumonia from its aspiration.

Treatment and Nursing Care. Only prompt surgical treatment offers any hope of correcting the defect and saving life. Surgical treatment consists of ligation of the fistula and end-to-end anastomosis of the upper and the lower segments of the esophagus. This procedure is successful in some instances. Occasionally, a stricture develops subsequently at the site of anastomosis; the stricture usually is overcome satisfactorily by dilatation. In a few instances anastomosis is not possible at the primary operation because of shortness of the lower segment or the wide separation of the two segments. In such cases the fistula is ligated, the upper segment of the esophagus is brought to the surface, and gastrostomy is done. Subsequent feeding is by way of the gastrostomy.

If the esophagus has been brought to the surface, the exposed portion should be protected by a sterilized gauze dressing held securely in place by a knit binder of the type used as an abdominal binder. After the first few months, when salivary glands become more active, frequent change of dressing is necessary. Saline solution should be used to cleanse the area, and the surrounding skin should be kept scrupulously clean. Frequent change of position is desirable to help prevent respiratory infection.

If gastrostomy has been done, feedings are begun several hours postoperatively. A tray is required, containing the warmed formula, a funnel and an empty feeding bottle and a nipple. Before compression of the gastrostomy tube is released, the funnel should be attached and partially filled with the formula. Further to prevent air from entering the stomach, the funnel always must contain fluid. Elevation of the funnel should be sufficient to allow the food to run in slowly. When the milk is at the level of the end of the funnel, the tube should be folded onto itself and compressed with a rubber band or a clamp. While the milk is running into the stomach, the infant should be given an empty bottle with a nipple to suck. The nipple provides normal sucking activity, exercises the muscles of the jaw and relaxes the musculature. When opportunity for sucking is not provided, the infant will suck his fists to satisfy his needs. It has been observed that unless the infant is comfortable and happy, the formula fails to run into the stomach. When the feeding is completed, the infant should be picked up for a period of attention. Normal babies have pleasure associated with their feedings. Babies with gastrostomies usually require long periods of hospitalization, and unless attention is paid to their psychological needs, they do not thrive.

The skin around the gastrostomy tube should be kept clean and protected with zinc oxide or aluminum paste. The adhesive strips that hold the tube in place should not adhere to the gauze dressings that encircle the tube. Reinforcing the inner side with an additional piece of adhesive makes the necessary dressing change possible without removing the adhesive tape. Such removal frequently displaces the tube.

Atresia of the Duodenum

Strictly speaking, this term should be applied to the failure of the duodenum to open into a continuous tube, connecting the stomach with the upper small intestine. Also, it is used to describe obstruction in the duodenum due to valves or diaphragms within the lumen or from bands, kinks and abnormal pressure from without. The symptoms of all these conditions begin immediately after birth and consist of persistent nausea with vomiting of bile-stained fluid. Diagnosis may be confirmed by x-ray examination, which will show that neither air nor barium passes out of the duodenum. Treatment is by surgical relief through release of the obstructing

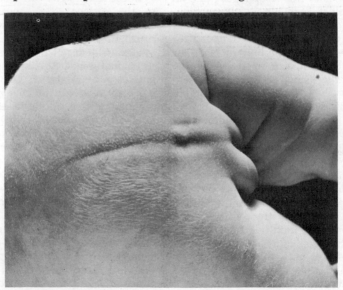

Fig. 59. Imperforate anus. (Potter, E. L.: Pathology of the Fetus and the Newborn, Chicago, Yr. Bk. Pub.)

mechanism or by an anastomosis which bypasses the area of atresia.

Atresia of the Small Intestine

Single or multiple regions of the small intestine which have failed to canalize properly in their development are not very uncommon. The symptoms and the treatment are like those of duodenal atresia. The lower they are along the course of the intestinal tract, the later the symptoms will occur and the greater the accompanying degree of abdominal distention.

Atresia of the Rectum and the Anus

Abnormal development of the lower intestinal tract may be apparent on inspection of the infant if no anal opening is found (Fig. 59) or if the initial attempt to take the baby's temperature reveals a shallow blind pouch instead of a normal anus. At other times the failure of the infant to produce meconium and the progressive distention of his abdomen lead to the discovery of an incomplete canalization of the rectum in spite of an externally normal anus.

In the normal embryologic development of the lower bowel, a blind pouch within the abdomen descends toward the perineum and meets another pouch which is invaginating the skin in the region of the anus. The ends of the two pouches fuse, and the septum between them breaks through to form a continuous passageway. The mildest form of atresia is that in which the development is complete, except for the disappearance of the membrane between the two pouches. This situation is relieved easily by splitting the membrane with a small knife introduced into the anus. Even if the two pouches have not quite met, the surgeon may be able to join them from below and make a proper anastomosis at once. The opening must be dilated periodically for several months afterward to prevent its constriction during scar-tissue formation. More serious abnormalities result when the internal blind pouch lies at some distance

from the skin of the perineum or aberrantly joins the vagina, the urethra or a fistulous opening into the perineum. Often primary union cannot be undertaken in these circumstances, and a temporary colostomy is necessary until a later, more extensive operation can be performed.

Volvulus

Early in fetal life a large portion of the intestinal tract lies in the umbilical sac outside the abdomen and in a position reversed from that which is normal later; that is, the ascending colon is on the left. With continued fetal development the intestine gradually is withdrawn into the abdomen with concurrent rotation to the newly and permanently normal position. After withdrawal and rotation, the mesentery attaches to the posterior wall of the abdomen, and the transverse colon becomes attached to the stomach by the gastrocolic ligament.

In a few instances, rotation of the bowel is faulty, in that it is incomplete or absent. In such circumstances, the mesentery cannot attach in the normal places or in the normal manner. The abnormal attachment may give rise to peritoneal bands which may cause obstruction subsequently by pressure on the bowel at some point or by entangling a loop of bowel. A bowel with incomplete mesenteric attachment is not well anchored and at any time may become twisted in such a manner as to cause obstruction and to cut off the blood supply to a portion of itself. Volvulus is the term applied when obstruction occurs from twisting of the intestine. Volvulus from abnormal rotation may occur at any time in the first few years but is much more common in early infancy. The only treatment is prompt surgical attention, with cutting of constricting bands or with the untwisting of a twisted intestinal loop. Often some anchoring of unattached bowel is indicated.

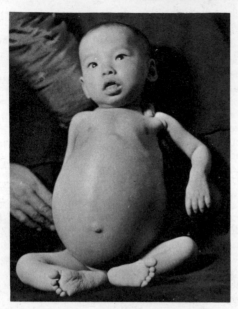

FIG. 60. A baby with Hirschsprung's disease.

MEGACOLON

Megacolon is most commonly a primary congenital abnormality (Hirschsprung's disease). The essential lesion is partial obstruction in the distal portion of the colon, which causes obstinate constipation, enlargement of the abdomen and dilatation and hypertrophy of the colon. When the bowel is examined at operation or at autopsy no gross explanation for the obstruction can be found. The fault appears to lie in an abnormality of the innervation of the intrinsic musculature of the bowel wall, which under normal circumstances, produces the co-ordinated peristaltic movements that propel feces and gas downward toward the anus. In Hirschsprung's disease one or more segments of the colon do not participate properly in co-ordinated peristaltic activity, either because the essential ganglion cells are absent from the muscles or because there is a disturbance of the balance between the activities of the sympathetic and the parasympathetic nerve fibers. Stool reaching such an area is not passed along normally, and the bowel proximal to it eventually hypertrophies in its attempt to force the accumulating mass through the malfunctioning segment of bowel. Often such an area can be identified by a small barium enema and careful study of the activity of the area between the rectum and the sigmoid colon.

Megacolon may also occur as a disorder secondary to anatomic (rectal stricture or rectovaginal fistula with a small opening) and psychogenic obstruction. Of course, in these instances successful treatment will depend upon the ability to provide an adequate channel by surgical measures or to correct the emotional disturbance that leads to spastic withholding of stool.

Symptoms

The symptoms of megacolon are manifest early in infancy. Constipation that persists in spite of treatment, and progressive enlargement of the abdomen are the first symptoms (Fig. 60). Periodically, the distention may be so great as to cause discomfort, vomiting and interference with respirations. The absorption of toxic materials retained in the bowel may produce nausea, lethargy or even collapse when the obstipation has been prolonged. Unless close attention is given to bowel evacuation, the accumulation of dry fecal masses may lead to inflammation or even ulceration of the bowel so that once the obstruction is relieved, diarrhea ensues. The effort of the colon to pass the fecal mass along is often apparent by peristaltic activity which is visible through the abdominal wall. Malnutrition may be present as a consequence of vomiting or food refusal. In some of the milder cases spontaneous recovery may take place. Children who continue with the disorder unrelieved may have a serious social problem because of inability to control the escape of gas under pressure. An occasional child who reaches adolescence will learn how to evacuate his bowel successfully by the use of his abdominal muscles.

Diagnosis

Diagnosis is seldom difficult. The combination of gross enlargement of the abdomen, visible peristalsis and obstinate constipation with passage of stools of excessive size is regularly present in all cases. A roentgen study of the colon is indicated in order to confirm the diagnosis and to identify, if possible, the main area of disturbed peristalsis. This procedure should be undertaken cautiously in instances where the obstruction can be identified as anatomic or functional in the lower rectum, for the addition of barium to the retained fecal mass above such an obstruction may turn a partial intestinal obstruction into a complete one.

Treatment and Nursing Care

These may be considered under three general headings—emergency relief of fecal impaction, long-term medical management and surgical treatment.

Intestinal obstruction from fecal impaction requires prompt relief. Various types of enemas are used to soften the impacted mass and increase the effectiveness of bowel contractions. Because of the large size of the colon, the enemas are only partially returned. It is possible to produce water intoxication in these patients if excessive amounts are run in without being recovered. Normal saline solution is probably safer to use than plain water. In neglected cases the danger of perforating a colonic ulcer must be considered. Digital removal of stool from the rectum is often the safest and most effective method of relieving fecal impactions.

Long-term medical management may be successful in keeping the child in good health and maintaining an adequate rate of colonic evacuation. An attempt is made to keep the stools soft by offering a low-residue diet or by the continuous administration of mineral oil. Mild laxatives may be given periodically. Many children will require regular cleansing of the colon with enemas or colonic irrigations administered through a large tube passed well up into the descending colon. Drugs that alter the activity of the sympathetic and the parasympathetic nervous systems are sometimes useful in effecting more or less regular bowel evacuations. These include Prostigmin, Urecholine, atropine, Syntropan, Mecholyl Chloride and others. Dosage must be initiated cautiously, for all of these drugs have toxic effects that must be recognized promptly. Children who can be managed successfully by medical treatment require careful attention to general hygiene and diet.

A number of surgical approaches may be considered when medical management is deemed unsatisfactory. The practice of sectioning the sympathetic nerve connections to the colon has not given very satisfactory results, since constipation usually is ameliorated but not cured. In cases where an area of constriction can be demonstrated by barium enema, sometimes a complete cure may be effected by removal of the constricted area and anastomosis of the bowel. The procedure offers the best chance of a completely satisfactory cure. Usually it is not undertaken in children under the age of two. When medical management is failing, and the preferred surgical approach cannot be done, colostomy or even complete resection of the colon may be performed. The postoperative care will depend upon the variety of procedure that is done.

Procedure for Cleansing Enema for an Infant. The equipment consists of an irrigating can and pole, rubber tubing, glass connector, stopcock, catheter (No. 10 to 12 French), lubricant, treatment rubber and towel, rubber-covered pillow, bedpan and cover, kidney basin, enema solution (105° F.) and oiled cotton for cleansing after the enema has been expelled. For a soapsuds enema, 2 drams of soap jelly to 1 pint of water is used; for a saline enema, 1 dram of salt to a pint. When giving a cleansing enema to an infant, not more than 300 ml. of solution should be used unless specific instructions have been given. After protecting the bed with the treatment rubber and towel and removing the diaper, the pillow is placed under the infant's back. Since retention of fluid is impossible for the infant, the bedpan padded with a diaper is placed under the buttocks. After the catheter is lubricated and the air is expelled, it is inserted from 2 to 4 inches into the rectum. Hanging the can not higher than 18 inches above the infant's hips allows the fluid to run in slowly. When the tube has been removed, the abdomen may be massaged gently until the solution has been expelled, if there are no contraindications. After expulsion, the buttocks should be cleansed and the diaper reapplied. In charting the procedure, the results should be noted.

Procedure for an Oil-Retention Enema. The equipment consists of a funnel, rubber tubing, glass connector, catheter (No. 10 to 12 French), lubri-

cant, bedpan and vegetable oil, from 60 to 150 ml., at 100° F. In some instances it may be necessary to inject the oil slowly into the rectum with a syringe. Pressure over the anus or adhesive strapping will prevent the oil from being expelled. After the oil has been retained for 30 minutes, a cleansing enema should be given.

INTESTINAL HERNIA

A hernia of the intestine is the protrusion of a part of the bowel through an abnormal opening in the containing walls of the abdomen. Hernia may be either congenital or acquired. The majority of acquired hernias in childhood arise from congenital abnormalities. The management of a hernia in a young child is the same, whether congenital or acquired, and no further distinction between these two types need be made. The most frequent locations for hernia are at the umbilicus and through the inguinal canals. Hernias through the diaphragm are uncommon, and those at other sites are rare.

Inguinal Hernia

In the male the testis descends from the abdominal cavity into the scrotum, carrying with it the parietal peritoneum, thus forming a tube from the abdomen to the scrotum. Normally, this tube closes completely. When it has failed to close partially or completely, descent of the intestine into it is possible, thus producing hernia. In girls, the round ligament extends from · the uterus through the inguinal canal to its attachment in the abdominal wall. In fetal life, the ligaments are surrounded by a peritoneal process which later obliterates. Weakness of the tissues about the round ligament, together with increased abdominal pressure, sometimes permits inguinal hernias in girls. However, about 90 per cent of the inguinal hernias of children occur in the male. An inguinal hernia in an infant causes no symptoms unless it becomes strangu-

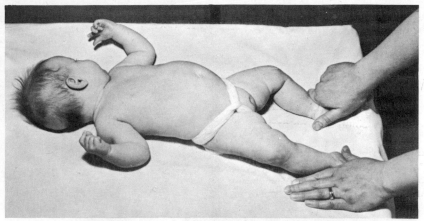

FIG. 61. A yarn truss applied for inguinal hernia.

lated, and this event is uncommon. Strangulation results when a portion of bowel becomes so tightly caught in the hernial sac that its blood supply is cut off. Severe symptoms of pain, intestinal obstruction and inability to reduce the mass occur. If unrelieved, gangrene of the bowel will result. Immediate operation is demanded.

Usually, an inguinal hernia is reduced easily. When the inguinal rings are small, reduction cannot be accomplished by pressure alone upon the herniated bowel, because the hernia then mushrooms against the external inguinal ring. In addition to moderate pressure, it is necessary to make lateral pressure on the bowel with the fingers at the base of the mass in order to elongate the bowel at this point. Sometimes reduction is made easier by having the child lie with the buttocks elevated.

If the hernia can be kept constantly reduced by means of a truss, the defect in the abdominal wall will close in many instances. Use of a truss for a year or more may be necessary. If the truss fails to hold the hernia or to permit ultimate cure, surgical repair is indicated. Even the youngest of infants stands a hernia operation well if he is in good condition.

Nursing Care. A type of truss commonly used for infants is made from a skein of yarn. Such a truss is illustrated in Figure 61. One fourth or less of a skein is rewound into a smaller skein. The size should be such that when the two sides are brought together into a single unit, it will be long enough to pass entirely around the infant's waist with an additional loop passing from the waistline in front down under the crotch and up to the waistline in back. To apply it, first the yarn is passed around the waist snugly. Then one end is passed through the loop of the other end to make a slip knot, which is adjusted to lie directly over the site of the hernia and press against it. Then the free end is carried down through the crotch and attached to the segment that passes across the back.

The advantage of the yarn truss is that in addition to being effective, it is soft, washable and easily adjusted to any size of infant. Satisfactory pneumatic trusses may be purchased. The truss treatment of hernia in an infant should begin as soon as the hernia is discovered and continue until no evidence of the hernia can be found.

When a hernia is corrected surgically the postoperative care is directed at keeping the wound clean until healing has taken place. Diapers are left open

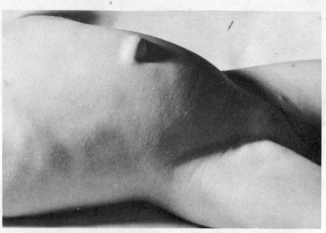

FIG. 62. An example of a small umbilical hernia.

to prevent wound contamination. Infants may be picked up for feedings and to relieve distress. Older children may be permitted activity as soon as they feel able to play. Unless bowel resection is required, feedings can be resumed a few hours after operation.

Umbilical Hernia

Umbilical hernia consists of a protrusion of a portion of the intestine or omentum through the umbilical ring, producing a bulge under the skin at the navel (Fig. 62). The size of the tumor varies but seldom exceeds that of a golf ball. Umbilical hernias are usually not apparent at birth but appear within the early months of life and enlarge during the acts of crying or straining. They are reduced easily, and strangulation is practically unknown. All but the largest hernias will heal spontaneously at least by the time the child begins to develop strong abdominal muscles—between 3 and 4 years of age. The traditional treatment of strapping or binding the abdomen of such an infant is generally unnecessary, although it improves the cosmetic appearance. Hernias that are large and fail to close spontaneously may be repaired surgically in later childhood.

OBSTRUCTION OF THE BILE DUCTS

Obstruction of the bile ducts of the newborn may be caused by congenital stenosis or atresia, or absence of any part of the duct system; it may be caused also by a plug in the larger ducts of thick viscous biliary secretion somewhat similar to the material that obstructs the pancreatic duct in cystic fibrosis of the pancreas.

When the bile ducts are obstructed, bile does not enter the intestinal tract; it accumulates in the liver. Bile pigments enter the blood and are carried to all parts of the body with resulting jaundice, which increases in intensity. Usually, obvious jaundice from obstruction does not appear until the age of 2 weeks, often after icterus neonatorum has disappeared.

Continued unrelieved obstructive jaundice ultimately leads to death. A baby so affected may live for as long as several years. During the early weeks or months, nutrition and general health seem to be little affected, but soon evidences of illness appear. Because of absence of bile from the intestinal tract, absorption of fat and the fat-soluble vitamins is poor. Deficiencies of vitamins A, D and K result unless special precautions are taken. Absorption of calcium is impaired. Eventually, cirrhotic changes occur in the liver, and liver function becomes impaired.

When a baby with obstructive jaundice comes under care, a dietary regimen adapted to his condition and physiologic capacity is established. The diet is low in fat and generous in protein; the remaining energy needed is supplied by carbohydrate. The fat-soluble vitamins are supplied in water-miscible form.

Obstruction of the bile ducts from congenital malformation cannot always be distinguished from jaundice caused by plugging with thick mucus or from infectious hepatitis acquired *in utero* from the mother. The distinction is an important one to make because an infant with mechanically defective bile ducts will eventually die unless surgical correction can be carried out. However, exploration under general anesthesia is to be avoided in any form of liver disease whenever possible. Hence, surgical exploration might retard a spontaneous recovery from either of the other two entities. Clinically, there is sometimes intermittent pigmentation of the stools when either of the latter conditions is present. Various tests of liver function may also be employed to assist in differentiation. Recently the technic of punch biopsy of the liver under local anesthesia has been developed to a point where it offers a fairly reliable guide to the diagnosis of infectious hepatitis. Occasionally, mucus plugs can be dislodged by the use of cholagogues such as 25 per cent magnesium sulfate instilled into the duodenum or Decholin given intravenously. When the suspicion of bile duct atresia is strongly substantiated, operation should be undertaken. Many wait until 3 to 4 months of age in order to give ample time for spontaneous remission of symptoms. Surgical reconstructive procedures are possible in less than one fifth of the infants with atresia.

Usually at least some preoperative preparation is necessary. If vitamin K has become deficient, the prothrombin level of the blood may be low, and hemorrhage may result, either spontaneously or from surgical manipulation. The prothrombin level is brought within the normal range by giving vitamin K parenterally. Often a short period of good nutritional care, including hydration, is given before operation.

Nursing Care

Postoperatively, shock-preventive measures should be instituted. Rate and quality of respiration should be noted. Pulse rates in infants fluctuate so rapidly that they are not accurate guides to the infant's condition. Before and after operation these infants tend to be lethargic and slow in physical movements; therefore, they need help in adjustment of their position. They should be moved carefully to prevent wound injury. Frequent inspection of the abdominal wound should be made, for these babies have impaired healing power, and evisceration and bleeding may occur. An abdominal binder fastened tightly for support is desirable. Distention due to accumulation of peritoneal fluid or paralytic ileus is a possible complication, and observation to detect its onset is an important nursing responsibility. Gastric suction often is begun immediately after operation and is continued until peristalsis is heard. Elbow restraints to prevent the infant from removing the tube should be applied at the time the tube is inserted. Irrigations of the tube with small amounts of warm saline keep it patent.

Until adequate feeding can be resumed, fluids are administered parenterally. When feedings are begun, they should be given slowly from a medicine dropper. These infants may be picked up for feeding and bubbling, but it must be done with care.

If an anastomosis has been performed successfully, change in the color of the stools will be noted postoperatively, and their description should be charted accurately.

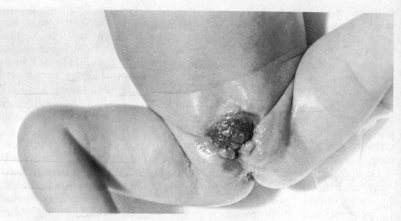

FIG. 63. Exstrophy of the bladder.

GENITO-URINARY TRACT

THE KIDNEYS

Anomalous formation of the upper urinary tract is quite common and is found in approximately 10 per cent of all autopsies performed on children. Many of the malformations are of no consequence to the child, but when they result in stasis of urine flow, they are prone to become chronically infected or to produce pain from obstruction. Such conditions as hydronephrosis, double kidney or ureter, dilated ureters and hypoplastic kidneys are identified only during the course of urologic examination in the search for a focus of urinary tract infection. This subject and its management are considered in a later chapter.

On occasion renal anomalies are discovered during the newborn period. *Renal agenesis* which implies total failure of the kidney to develop is unimportant when it is unilateral, but fatal to the infant within a few hours after birth if the condition is bilateral. Infants with this disorder have a characteristic facial appearance with low-set ears and widely spaced Mongolian eyes. Treatment is impossible even when the condition is recognized at once. Severe

degrees of polycystic kidney may produce early renal failure and abdominal enlargement. The condition is due to a failure of the kidney tubules to make normal connection with the developing glomeruli. The number and the size of the fluid-filled cysts which result determines the effect upon kidney function. Although serious malformation of this type leads to early death, milder degrees may pass unrecognized until adult life. No treatment is effective.

THE BLADDER

Exstrophy of the Bladder

This condition is caused by failure of union between the two sides of the lower abdomen, a failure which produces a fissure in the mid-line from the umbilicus to the genitalia. The defect includes the abdominal wall, the anterior wall of the bladder, the symphysis pubis and the urethra (Fig. 63). The posterior and the lateral surfaces of the bladder are exposed, and the ureteral outlets are visible. The condition is more common in boys than in girls. In boys, usually a groove is present in the anterior surface of the penis; in girls the clitoris is divided, and the labia may be separated. Other congenital malformations may be associated.

Treatment consists of operative removal of the bladder, the ureters first having been transplanted to the colon. A suitable age for the operation is 3 to 4 years after the child has acquired bowel control and can learn to hold urine within his rectum.

Bladder Neck Obstruction

Congenital valvelike folds in the posterior urethra or bladder neck may seriously hamper passage of urine through the male urethra and lead to enlargement of the bladder, hydronephrosis and progressive loss of renal function. The difficulty is often present even before birth, but it takes an alert observer to recognize that a small male infant is not voiding a sufficiently forceful stream. Prompt urologic examination and relief of the destructive back pressure upon the kidneys may save the child from a lifetime of crippling disease.

THE MALE GENITALIA

Preputial Adhesions

Adhesions of the prepuce to the glans are very common and should be broken up at an early age. After this procedure, a small amount of antiseptic ointment should be applied, particularly if bleeding has occurred, and the prepuce should be retracted daily for cleansing and to prevent reformation of the adhesions.

Phimosis

Phimosis signifies a narrowed outlet through the foreskin of the penis. It is to be distinguished from the term "redundant" prepuce, which is applied to an unusually long foreskin irrespective of narrowing and also from the term "adherent" prepuce, in which condition adhesions exist between the foreskin and the glans. Phimosis rarely is sufficiently severe to obstruct the outflow of urine and is not a cause of symptoms, either local or general. Phimosis is undesirable chiefly because it does not permit suitable cleanliness. In some instances the content of the preputial sac is invaded by bacteria to the extent of causing a local infection (balanitis). Phimosis may be corrected either by circumcision or by stretching. Preputial adhesions usually are present. When stretching is the procedure employed, the subsequent management is similar to that for preputial adhesions. Care must be taken not to permit paraphimosis, which is a condition in which the tight ring of foreskin formerly in front of the glans is left posterior to the glans, resulting in severe edema of the distal parts and requiring prompt attention and possibly surgical relief.

Circumcision consists of surgical removal of that part of the foreskin which covers the glans. The preferable time for circumcision is on the sixth or the seventh day after birth. At a later age the procedure may require the use of a local or a general anesthetic.

After the procedure is completed, the cut edges are covered with gauze impregnated with petrolatum. The postoperative treatment consists in keeping the wound clean.

The necessity for circumcision is seldom one of medical urgency. Since it may create considerable emotional disturbance in the young child, the operation should be undertaken in early infancy if the parents wish it done. When the child is left uncircumcised and the parents change their minds at a later date, it is preferable to wait until the boy himself can have some part in the decision and has an understanding of its implications.

Hypospadias

Hypospadias is a malformation in which the urethra opens on the under surface of the penis proximal to the usual site. Minor degrees of hypospadias are very common and require no treat-

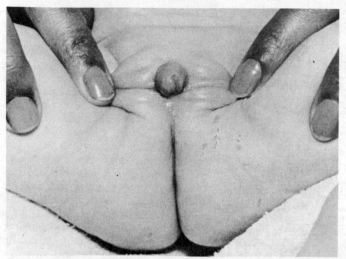

Fig. 64. The "adrenogenital syndrome," showing the enlarged clitoris and absence of the vagina.

ment. When the urethral opening is back on the shaft of the penis or at its base, surgical correction will ultimately be required. It is deferred until after infancy and sometimes until puberty when advantage may be taken of the full growth of the structures.

Epispadias

A much less common anomaly is epispadias in which the urethra is open on the dorsal surface of the penis. It likewise is corrected surgically when the defect is pronounced.

Undescended Testis (Cryptorchidism)

The testes which originate within the abdominal cavity have usually descended into the scrotum by the time the infant is born. Absence of one or both is not necessarily a cause for immediate concern since late descent often takes place during infancy or early childhood. The management of undescended testis is presented in more detail in Chapter 21.

THE FEMALE GENITALIA

Malformations of the female genitalia are so infrequent that no extensive discussion is warranted. With anal atresia in the female there may be an abnormal entrance of the rectum into the vagina so that meconium escapes through it. An imperforate hymen may lead to accumulation of secretions with the formation of a mass which is visible bulging out between the labia. Simple incision permits discharge of the retained contents.

Pseudohermaphroditism

When structural abnormalities of the genitalia of the newborn are discovered, prompt study is indicated. Many varieties of genital configuration intermediate between the male and the female may occur. One of the most common aberrations is due to the masculinizing effect of cortical adrenal hormones upon the developing female genitalia, resulting in enlargement of the clitoris and sometimes in sequestration of the vaginal opening (Fig. 64). The overproduction of androgenic hormone by a hypertrophied adrenal may be accompanied by insufficient output of other adrenal hormones so that the infant may simultaneously suffer from addisonian adrenal insufficiency. This type of adrenal dysfunction can be identified by determining the rate of excretion of 17-ketosteroids in the infant's urine and by measuring the blood levels of sodium, potassium and chloride. Treatment with cortisone can be expected to correct the excessive excretion of androgens and prevent the abnormal masculinization which otherwise would occur early in childhood. If electrolyte disturbance is also present, desoxycorticosterone and salt are usually indicated.

Not all abnormalities of the genitalia are associated with the "adrenogenital syndrome" described above. It is equally important, however, to attempt to arrive rapidly at a decision concerning the infant's proper sex through hormonal and anatomic studies, for it is psychologically very disturbing to both the child and the parents when uncertainty exists or when attempts are made to shift the child's way of life from one sex to the other after the period of infancy.

RESPIRATORY TRACT

CONGENITAL LARYNGEAL STRIDOR

Congenital laryngeal stridor is a noise produced on inspiration because of obstruction to air flow. It is due to any one of several laryngeal conditions, all of which are the result of immaturity of the larynx or persistence of fetal characteristics. The larynx may be soft and collapsible, large tissue folds may be present between the larynx and the epiglottis, the epiglottis may be soft and flaccid. In any of these conditions the parts are brought together on inspiration to cause obstruction and noise; they are pushed apart on expiration, and no symptoms are present. During inspiration also the soft parts of the chest are pulled in.

The noisy breathing appears in the first few days after birth and persists from 1 to 2 years, by which time the larynx has grown and matured sufficiently to permit normal breathing. The stridor is worse during periods of crying and excitement. At such times cyanosis is likely to appear. During quiescent periods no cyanosis is present, and the baby appears to be in no distress. Rarely, if at all, is congenital stridor dangerous to life, though there are occasions when the appearance and the behavior of the baby are alarming to the parents. By means of laryngoscopy the diagnosis can be confirmed, and a more serious abnormality excluded. No treatment is indicated.

CHOANAL ATRESIA

Choanal atresia is a congenital obstruction of the posterior nostril where it enters the nasopharynx. It may be complete or partial or occur on one or both sides of the nose. The symptoms are restricted to difficulty in breathing through the nose and consequently in feeding. In complete bilateral obstruction, early surgical relief is almost imperative because of the great difficulty in feeding an infant which cannot breathe through its nose. The condition is identified by passing a soft rubber catheter into the nostril and encountering obstruction which makes it impossible to guide the tip into the nasopharynx.

CARDIOVASCULAR SYSTEM

Congenital malformations of the heart are treated in Chapter 18.

CENTRAL NERVOUS SYSTEM

SPINA BIFIDA

Spina bifida is a malformation of the spine in which the posterior portion of the bony canal containing the spinal cord is completely or partially lacking because of failure of the vertebral laminae to develop or to fuse. Some degree of this defect is relatively common, especially in the lumbar region. When it exists without associated changes in the cord or the meninges, it is known as spina bifida occulta and, being symptomless, it is not discovered unless sought.

A more serious condition is a protrusion of the cord and its membranes (myelomeningocele) or the cord membranes alone (meningocele) through the defect to form an external cystic tumor, which is present at birth. The tumor is rounded, fluctuating, more or less compressible, and contains cerebrospinal fluid. It is commonly about the size of half of a small orange and most frequently is located in the lumbar or the sacral region. The wall of a meningocele is made up of spinal membranes and skin. In a myelomeningocele (Fig. 65), a portion of the cord is spread out and embedded in the cyst wall. Commonly, the condition is associated with increased pressure of the cerebrospinal fluid, so that the tumor tends to increase in size, the wall becoming thinner. With continued enlargement the tumor may rupture spontaneously, or more commonly it is the seat of ulcerations, often perforating, consequent on the poor blood supply. Rupture or ulcerative perforation usually leads to meningitis. Spina bifida with meningocele causes no symptoms. If the cord is included in the cyst wall, urinary and fecal incontinence and paralysis of the legs are likely to result.

Treatment

The treatment of simple meningocele is surgical removal of the sac with plastic reinforcement of the tissues over the fissure. Operation usually is not advisable for myelomeningocele when paralyses are present, except for the purpose of avoiding infections or at times for cosmetic effect.

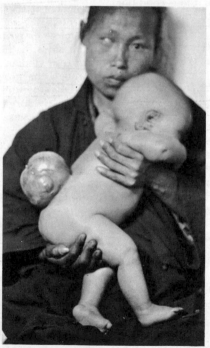

FIG. 65. Myelomeningocele.

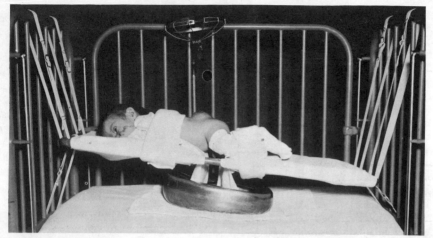

FIG. 66. A baby with spina bifida, illustrating also a method of care on a frame.

Prognosis

The only instances of favorable result from operation are those of simple meningocele in which hydrocephalus is not present or does not develop after operation. Hydrocephalus is a common accompaniment of spina bifida with tumor, in some instances developing spontaneously and in others as soon as the sac is removed. Hydrocephalus occurs or increases with such frequency after operation that the operative results are most discouraging. However, hydrocephalus associated with spina bifida is more amenable to treatment than that from other causes.

Nursing Care

When the covering over the tumor is very thin, the surface must be kept clean and protected from pressure. In the period preceding operation, nursing measures to prevent or to clear infection must be carried out. Placement on an infant Bradford frame facilitates care, exposes the tumor and prevents pressure on it (Fig. 66). To keep the infant in position over the frame opening, ankle and chest restraint is necessary. Diapers folded as cravats can be placed around the chest and also around one ankle, under the frame and over the other ankle. To prevent deformity, a small pillow made of abdominal pads should be placed under the lower portion of the legs to keep the toes and the feet from pressing into the hard surface of the frame.

When the spinal cord is included in the tumor wall, urine and feces are excreted constantly. Therefore, care to prevent excoriations around the perineum becomes necessary. Folded diapers under the abdomen and under the legs, over the edge and into a receptacle beneath the frame opening protect the frame covers and permit easy change to keep the infant dry. Cleansing the perineum and the groins with oil each time the diapers are changed will keep the skin in good condition.

When an infant is kept in this position for long periods of time, attention to the skin of the face and the knees becomes imperative if excoriation is to be prevented. If paralysis of the lower extremities is present, abrasion of the knees does not occur frequently, but if the infant's motor development is normal, frequent knee movement may cause skin irritation. Stockings prevent skin irritation in many instances. Good

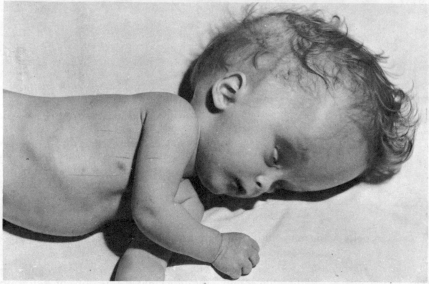

FIG. 67. An infant with hydrocephalus.

care of the knees and the skin of the face with applications of zinc-oxide ointment to the tip of the nose, the chin and the cheeks will prevent abrasions.

Various methods to prevent or to clear infection of the tumor mass may be used. Cleanliness with exposure to light may be all that is necessary. Alcohol, antibiotic or petrolatum gauze dressings may be desired. If used, they should be changed frequently enough to keep them sterile and the area free of exudate.

During the preoperative period the infant should be held for feedings. It gives him needed position change and affection and facilitates feeding and bubbling. The infant should be handled gently, for the tumor area is sensitive. The tumor should be covered with a sterile towel, and the infant held in such a way that pressure on the area can be eliminated. Observation as to his weight and his behavior before and after feedings will serve as a guide to his need for food. Optimum nutritional state is necessary before surgical intervention, and more frequent feedings

may be necessary to satisfy his needs.

The sac may be excised, or the meninges may be folded in to preserve the absorbing surface of the sac before the skin is closed over them. In either type of operation the principles of postoperative care remain the same. In the period immediately after operation, symptoms of shock should be watched for, and appropriate treatment given if they occur. The dressing must be kept clean and free from feces, and the prone position must be maintained by the same method as is used in the preoperative period. No covering directly over the infant should be used, as it will become soiled.

If the infant's temperature is subnormal, a light should be placed over the infant, and the bed should be covered with blankets, encasing the child in a heated unit. When the infant's temperature is subnormal and unstable, care in an incubator may be indicated. A Bradford frame may be simulated by pinning firm material across the frame of the bassinet inside the incubator. Temperature of the incubator should be regulated according to the individual needs of the infant.

Nursing measures used preoperatively should be continued, with the exception of the position used to feed the infant. Until sutures are removed, the baby should be fed on his frame, which is now hung so that his head is from 3 to 5 inches lower than his body. The chest restraint can be loosened, and the infant may be turned slightly to make feeding less difficult for him. The same method should be used to bathe the undersurface of his body.

During the postoperative period, observation as to whether or not the head circumference is increasing guides the physician and the nurse in the type of advice that the parents will need upon the baby's discharge from the hospital. Many times, operation is performed in the neonatal period. Therefore, the mother will require help in understanding the total needs of her child. The infant has been born with an anomaly: the development of wholesome attitudes toward it can be influenced by the nurse.

HYDROCEPHALUS

Hydrocephalus (Fig. 67) is a condition in which the amount of cerebrospinal fluid is increased greatly above normal, resulting in increased size of the head and characteristic pressure changes in the brain.

In the older child whose skull sutures have united, lesions which would cause hydrocephalus if they occurred in infancy result fatally before gross changes in the brain occur. Increased intracranial pressure in the older child is not referred to commonly as hydrocephalus.

Etiology

Cerebrospinal fluid is secreted by a network of veins (choroid plexus) situated in each of the lateral ventricles. From the ventricles it passes downward and posteriorly by way of the foramina of Monro, the aqueduct of Sylvius, the fourth ventricle and the foramina of Luschka and Magendie. At the base of the brain the fluid passes into the subarachnoid space which completely surrounds the brain and the spinal cord. From this space it is reabsorbed into the large venous sinuses on top of the brain. Normally, a balance exists between secretion and absorption.

Noncommunicating Hydrocephalus. If all or any large part of the subarachnoid absorbing space is shut off by any cause so that fluid from the ventricles does not circulate, the rate of absorption cannot keep pace with the rate of secretion, and noncommunicating hydrocephalus results. The obstruction may be in the path between the ventricles and the base of the brain from occlusion of the aqueduct of Sylvius.

Communicating Hydrocephalus. In some instances, obstruction is caused by adhesions between the meninges about the base of the brain. The adhesions may be from some unknown prenatal cause; they may be secondary to intracranial hemorrhage from birth injury or they may occur as a result of recognized meningitis after birth. The adhesions may obstruct the foramina at the base of the brain completely, so that no absorption can take place, or they may surround the foramina without obstructing them so that fluid can enter the spinal subarachnoid space freely, but not the cerebral space. The latter event gives rise to what is termed communicating hydrocephalus. By this is meant that communication exists between the ventricles and the spinal space and that fluid can be obtained freely by spinal puncture. Even though hydrocephalus may be communicating, it is still obstructive.

In cases of spina bifida, the medulla and part of the cerebellum may be pulled into the foramen magnum because of attachment of the cord at the site of the spine defect. The tissues are pulled into the foramen by growth in the length of the bony spine and are changed characteristically in shape and position (Arnold-Chiari deformity). It is the obstruction of flow over the cortex that causes the hydrocephalus so common in those with spina bifida.

Symptoms

The progressive accumulation of unabsorbed fluid distends the ventricles and causes the head to enlarge and the brain cortex to become thin. With continued enlargement of the head the skull sutures separate. The infant becomes increasingly helpless, first because of inability to support the large head, later because of damage to the brain and because of malnutrition which always accompanies severe degrees of hydrocephalus. During the late stages, pressure sores are frequent unless most carefully avoided by changes of position and protecting pads. Death finally occurs from either progressive malnutrition or intercurrent infection.

Diagnosis

The head may be larger than normal at birth, but more often no change is noticed until several weeks after birth. The finding that the head is larger than normal is strongly suggestive of hydrocephalus. Question as to diagnosis arises only in the early stages when the head size is not greatly in excess of normal. The diagnosis can be made certain by encephalogram (skull roentgenogram taken after the spinal fluid in the ventricles has been replaced with air), which shows the dilated ventricles. Increase in head size of an inch or more a month is also good evidence of hydrocephalus.

Occasionally, hydrocephalus is caused by meningovascular syphilis. This variety is not obstructive in a mechanical sense and never becomes extreme. Because of its failure to progress beyond a moderate degree and because of the characteristic cerebrospinal fluid changes, syphilitic hydrocephalus seldom would be confused with the usual obstructive types.

Treatment

In a few instances, hydrocephalus undergoes spontaneous arrest, a balance between secretion and absorption having been reached by some means. When the hydrocephalus is of moderate degree, it is well to defer radical surgical treatment until the rate of head growth can be determined. Operation may be unnecessary.

Since the cause of hydrocephalus is entirely mechanical, not much is to be expected of any kind of treatment except mechanical. Surgical treatment offers the only hope of cure and occasionally is effective. However, the operative mortality is high, and unfortunately the results are frequently disappointing or only temporarily successful. Procedures which are used include: (1) removal or destruction of the choroid plexus to decrease the production of spinal fluid, (2) shunting operations which attempt to lead off the accumulated fluid through artificial openings in the ventricular system or through catheters to absorbing areas such as the tissues of the neck, the mastoid antrum, the peritoneal cavity or the ureter and (3) removal of a portion of the occipital bone and the vertebral lamina in the presence of the Arnold-Chiari deformity to provide decompression and improve the circulation of spinal fluid.

Nursing Care

Preoperatively, the chief nursing problems are concerned with the maintenance of nutrition and the prevention of pressure sores on the head. Babies with hydrocephalus often have increasing nutritional failure as the hydrocephalus progresses. Important are feeding schedules which avoid vomiting and at the same time permit an adequate intake of food.

As the head increases in size the

baby becomes more helpless. He cannot hold up his head to assume a sitting position and ultimately cannot move the head much while lying in bed. The head must be moved for him, and this must be done often enough to prevent pressure sores. Special care of the scalp and the use of a lamb's-wool pillow are measures suggested. Unless the head is enormous and heavy, holding the infant for feedings will relieve pressure for short periods.

After operation, the temperature and the pulse and the respiration rate should be observed every 15 minutes until the child is fully conscious. In children over 2 years of age blood pressure readings should also be taken. Subsequently, until the vital signs become stabilized, they should be taken hourly for a 2-day period. During the first day the child's temperature may be subnormal or markedly elevated. Nursing measures must be adapted to the child's vital signs. When the rise in temperature is marked, alcohol sponges (35% alcohol), minimal clothing and bedcovering, aspirin by rectum, a water mattress, or the use of a fan directed away from the child's body may help to control it. Fluids are given continuously by the intravenous route until fluid, electrolyte and nutritional needs can be satisfied orally. A suction set should be in readiness, for mucous secretions may cause respiratory difficulties. Convulsions after operation may occur and should be watched for.

When operative procedures have been used to remove or destroy the choroid plexus to decrease the production of spinal fluid, the infant should be placed on the unoperated side to prevent pressure from within being exerted on the bone flap. Because positions are limited, every precaution should be taken to prevent pressure sores from developing. The ear may become the site of a pressure ulcer, and before the head bandage is applied cotton should be placed behind and over the ear.

When intravenous fluid therapy is discontinued the infant may be held for feeding, but the position on the unoperated side should be continued until healing of the wound site is complete. Spinal punctures to remove cerebrospinal fluid to lessen symptoms of intracranial pressure may be necessary at periods after operation. The nurse's functions in this procedure are described in Chapter 22.

Nursing care after operations to shunt spinal fluid from the lateral ventricle of the brain or from the lumbar subarachnoid spaces into the urinary system after the removal of a kidney includes additional details which are of utmost importance for recovery. In these operations a long rubber catheter is inserted into the lateral ventricle or lumbar subarachnoid space, fastened to the dura and led down through subcutaneous tissues of the back where it is joined to a polyethylene tube which is passed through the paraspinal muscles into the ureter of the removed kidney. The position of the child postoperatively is based upon the amount of fluid that is draining through the catheter which is used to shunt the fluid from the ventricular system to the ureter. Observation of the anterior fontanel and the amount of fluid excreted from the urinary tract will give the nurse the information she needs to determine the position in which she should place the child. Children who have ventriculo-ureteral shunts usually have a depressed fontanel after the operation. When the anterior fontanel is depressed, the child should be kept flat in bed or with his head lowered slightly. Children who have a lumbar subarachnoid-ureteral shunt often have slower drainage of cerebrospinal fluid into the urinary tract. Their anterior fontanel shows no signs of depression during the first postoperative day. When the anterior fontanel appears to be normal, the child is kept flat or with his head elevated to a moderate degree.

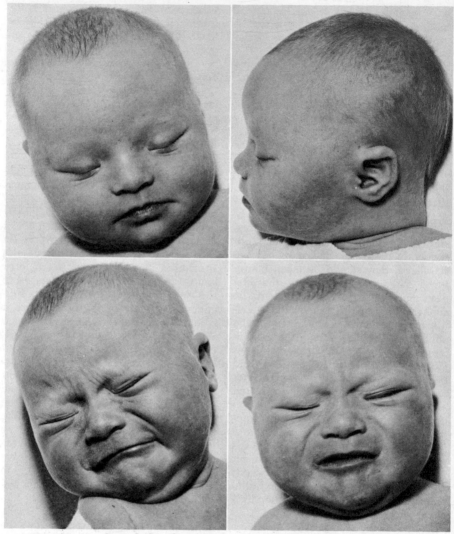

Fig. 68. Newborn baby showing the facial characteristics of mongolism. (Potter, E.: Pathology of the Fetus and the Newborn, Chicago, Year Book Pub. Co.)

Whether the child's head is kept elevated or lowered, he should be turned at 2-hour intervals to prevent pressure areas and hypostatic pneumonia from developing.

Because salt and fluid are being lost by drainage of the cerebrospinal fluid into the bladder, intravenous fluid ad-ministration and total intake and output measurement must be done with the greatest of accuracy. When losses of fluid and electrolytes are not replaced by a corresponding intake, the volume of plasma may drop abruptly, causing peripheral vascular collapse and death. In most instances 24-hour

FIG. 69. A 2-year-old infant showing the facial characteristics of mongolism which are now defined more clearly than in the newborn.

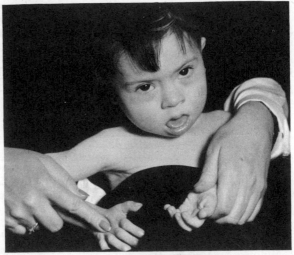

collection of urine is essential. Details concerning this procedure will be found in Chapter 20. Fluids are given orally as soon as the child shows evidence of a capacity to tolerate them. At first small amounts of 5 per cent dextrose and saline solution are given. Gradually, milk formula is introduced, followed by solid foods in accordance with the child's age and tolerance for it. After the fourth postoperative day, the child may be held for feeding. Because the infant loses sodium in the spinal fluid drainage, 2 Gm. of ordinary table salt are added to the daily amount of formula and continued indefinitely.

Watching for untoward symptoms and prompt reporting of them to the doctor are additional details of care. Vomiting, signs of infection, abdominal distention, symptoms of dehydration and salt loss and bulging of the anterior fontanel are danger signals. Fullness or bulging of the fontanel betokens inadequate drainage of cerebrospinal fluid; vomiting may evidence increased intracranial pressure or intolerance for the amount of food and fluid prescribed; apathy and loss of tissue turgor spells impending peripheral collapse which may quickly lead to shock if the body stores are not replaced immediately.

Antibiotics are usually prescribed for prophylactic purposes during the first few postoperative days.

Teaching the mother the care of her child after operation must be done prior to discharge. She will need thorough understanding of the operation and the changes that the operation produced so that she will see the importance of adding the prescribed quantity of salt to the child's total formula and of preventing illness and watching for earliest prodromal signs of impending ill health. Illnesses which prevent the child from taking fluids and foods or which cause vomiting or diarrhea are a great threat to the infant who has had a ventricular or spinal subarachnoid shunt. In addition to teaching the mother methods of preventing illness, she must be cautioned to notify her pediatrician immediately, for the infant will require intravenous therapy to prevent excess salt and fluid loss. This teaching must be done carefully to ensure caution but without instilling abnormal fears which prevent the mother from following her intuitive feelings of motherliness. These babies can be handled as other babies are cared for. The only significant differences are those cited above.

MONGOLISM

One group of mentally defective children usually can be recognized at birth by virtue of the associated physical defects which they present. The facial characteristics simulate those of persons of Oriental races, hence the name (Figs. 68 and 69). The face is round, with close-set eyes which slant upward at their lateral extremities. Epicanthus is usually present. The head is small in circumference and grows at an abnormally slow rate. It is flattened in the anteroposterior diameter. Posteriorly, the infant has a flat occiput with broad and pudgy neck. Anteriorly, the nose is flat, and the cavities of the nasopharynx and the mouth are shallow in the anteroposterior diameter. The tongue is often large and protruded constantly. There may be marbling of the irides of the eyes. The muscles are lax, and the joints are loose, so that hyperextension is possible with the assumption of bizarre postures without apparent discomfort to the child. The hands are usually broad, with short and incurved fifth fingers and abnormalities of the creases of the palm. The great toe of the foot often is separated from the other toes by a wider space than normal through which runs a deep skin crease. Other abnormalities may include congenital malformations of the heart and umbilical hernia.

Mongolism (also called Mongolian idiocy or Mongolian imbecility) occurs with greatest frequency in the children of women who are approaching the end of their child-bearing period. The Mongolian child is very often the product of the last pregnancy possible for the individual woman. In a minority of the cases, the Mongolian child occurs first in the sequence of pregnancies of a young woman. Under these circumstances the subsequent children are almost always normal. Rarely, Mongolian children may appear in the middle of a succession of pregnancies or twice in the same family. The cause is unknown, but it is presumed to be due to a wide-

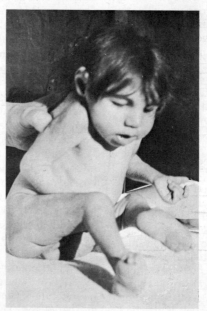

FIG. 70. Microcephalic idiocy.

spread defect in the early development of the embryo.

Mongolian children develop slowly, generally have placid dispositions and can be expected to perform menial tasks only. They seldom reach a developmental level greater than 7 years. They are unusually prone to infections that carry an increased risk for them. In spite of modern antibiotic therapy their prognosis for life is less than that of the normal child.

MICROCEPHALY

An uncommon variety of mental deficiency which can be recognized at birth is microcephaly (Fig. 70). The newborn microcephalic infant has a skull that is obviously smaller in volume than it should be and measures less in circumference than does the chest. The skull usually is flattened in the frontal region and sometimes comes to a point on top. The primary defect is in the brain itself, which has failed to develop properly. The skull size is merely a reflection of the abnormal size of the brain beneath. Such infants are retarded severely and seldom learn to talk. Sometimes their motor development is within reasonably normal limits.

AMYOTONIA CONGENITA

Two forms of this disorder are recognized; both may be observed in the same family. The outstanding feature is generalized weakness of muscles without loss of intelligence. In the congenital form (Oppenheim), weakness is present from birth and prevents the child from learning to hold up his head, to sit or to make any forceful voluntary movements. Because of his difficulty in coughing and clearing his respiratory passages he eventually succumbs to aspiration pneumonia, usually within the first 2 years of life. Nursing care can prolong life by attention to his accumulating pharyngeal secretions, but any illness is likely to be fatal. In the acquired (Werdnig-Hoffman) type of the disorder, early development for most of the first year may be normal but followed by progressing weakness which terminates fatally for the same reasons. Whether or not there is a real distinction between these two disorders is debated.

ORGANS OF SPECIAL SENSE

THE EYES

Retrolental Fibroplasia

This disorder of prematures is the most common cause of blindness among infants. It is actually a postnatal toxic disorder rather than an anomaly and is discussed in Chapter 10.

Cataract

Cataract is a condition in which part or all of the lens of the eye is opaque. The affected part of the lens appears white. Any cataract that is present at birth or appears early in life is included in the congenital group. In some instances, cataract is familial; in others, it is nutritional in origin; in still others it is traumatic, perhaps from birth injury in some cases. The occurrence of rubella in the mother during the first trimester of pregnancy is known to cause congenital cataract in a high proportion of babies. Partial cataract may be anterior, central or posterior in the lens. The only symptoms of cataract are those pertaining to interference with vision. The only treatment is surgical. Needling of the lens causes it to be absorbed, leaving the path of vision clear but also leaving the eye without power of accommodation.

Cataracts affecting the entire lens require operation. Whether or not operation is indicated in partial cataract depends on the amount of useful vision present. Most partial cataracts do not progress, but a careful watch must be kept to detect those that do increase, in order that appropriate surgical treatment may be given when indicated.

Nursing Care. There are differences of opinion as to the amount of restraint that is necessary for the child postoperatively. Some surgeons feel that attempts at restriction result in more tension and attempted movement than does complete freedom. They suture adequately and eliminate the need for body restraint, recommending only the use of elbow restraints to prevent the child from removing the dressings. Other surgeons feel that immobilization is essential. They recommend the use of jacket and elbow restraints to prevent the infant from disturbing his dressings and to keep him from sitting up or turning onto his abdomen. Often sandbags are used on each side of his head to immobilize it completely.

The infant must be fed on his bed until orders that permit him to be moved into a sitting position are given. Fluids should be given in small amounts until tolerance for larger quantities is noted. Every measure should be taken to prevent vomiting, which may result in aspiration and increased intra-ocular pressure.

Care should be taken to prevent startling the infant when he is approached. Talking pleasantly to him before the cribside is lowered lessens the danger of frightening him with an abrupt approach to his bedside.

The infant who requires immobilization will miss the comfort he formerly felt when he was held for feedings, for play, and for parental enjoyment. Substitute satisfactions must be provided during the period when immobilization is necessary. Stroking the infant's head, talking to him in gentle, soothing tones and carrying out all measures that ensure physical comfort will lessen his need for sedatives, which are required when he is restless, tearful and irritable.

Squint (Strabismus)

Squint is a condition in which the eyes cannot be used at the same time for looking at an object; such a person is said to be cross-eyed. Normally, the lines of vision (visual axes) of the eyes are parallel when the object is at a distance of 20 feet or more. When looking at a nearer object, the visual axes converge to meet the object. In squint, the visual axis of only one eye goes to the object. The other eye is the squinting eye.

Many varieties of squint exist. Squint from prenatal causes may become apparent at any time from birth to the sixth year. Development of squint after this time usually is caused by disease. Sometimes the muscles that move the eye outward or those that move the eye inward are overactive or underactive, and the resulting condition may be referred to as paralytic squint. When squint is caused by underaction of the muscles of one eye, the affected eye does not have as full ocular movements as the fellow eye. In nonparalytic squint the squinting eye moves with the eye used for vision, but always with a visual axis not corresponding to that of the seeing eye, a condition known as concomitant squint. Concomitant squint may be either monocular or alternating. In monocular squint, one eye is used constantly for vision and the other eye is turned either inward (convergent squint) or outward (divergent squint). In alternating squint, either eye is used for vision, and the other eye becomes the squinting eye.

Concomitant squint usually is due to errors of refraction. When the eyes change fixation from a distant to a near object, the pupils contract, the lenses change power for an exact focus, and the eyes converge. The error of refraction may be such that the focus (accommodation) is not accurate at the same time that both eyes are able to fix accurately on the object. The child must choose between accurate fixation with poor vision and accurate accommodation with double vision. The choice resulting in squint may be made at any time in early infancy.

When both eyes cannot be brought to bear on an object, double vision (diplopia) results, and the images in the eyes differ. The person with squint quickly learns to disregard the image in the squinting eye. As a result, vision in the squinting eye may be reduced markedly. Usually the false image of the squinting eye is suppressed by the time the child comes under care.

Because of danger to vision, as well as for cosmetic effect, treatment for squint should be undertaken as soon as the condition is observed. Usually, the earlier the treatment is undertaken, the better the results, and, conversely, the later the treatments, the slower the progress and the less satisfactory the final status. The objectives of treatment are to improve the vision of the poorly functioning eye, to produce or restore single vision when both eyes are focusing together and to correct the deformity.

In early infancy the better eye should be occluded by a patch or a cover until the baby is old enough to wear glasses, which may be at the age of from 12 to 14 months. With use of the poorer eye the vision should improve, and often it can be brought to normal. Correction of the refractive error helps to restore single vision and is fully effective in many instances. For some children, correction of the deformity by operation may be necessary, but operation is not indicated until maximum improvement by glasses and training has been attained, usually not before 3 or 4 years of age. Correction of the deformity early, particularly before the child goes to school, is important for psychological reasons. Otherwise, the child is taunted, becomes embarrassed and is likely to develop personality changes with an inferiority or a defense complex. After operation, if this has been necessary, further treatment must be given in the use of the eyes together.

Spurious Squint. During the early months of life, infants are not expected to maintain parallel vision at all times. Brief periods of convergent or divergent squint usually have little significance. Frequently, too, parents and relatives may be misled by an optical illusion which causes them to believe that the young infant with a broad nose and epicanthal fold is suffering from convergent squint, when actually he is using parallel vision. The explanation lies in the fact that during lateral gaze, the eye that is turning toward the nose appears to go too far inward because the epicanthal fold obscures more of the white sclera than the observer thinks that it should. The superficial conclusion of squint is drawn easily. A simple test will permit a distinction between real and spurious squint. If a bright point of light is directed into the infant's eyes, the reflections from the two corneas should be seen in the same relative position with respect to the center of the pupil in each eye. If the eyes are not parallel there will be an obvious difference between them.

Nursing Care. When operation is necessary to correct strabismus it is advisable to hospitalize the child a few days before it is performed. The child needs to become adjusted to the hospital and to the nurses who will attend him postoperatively. Some surgeons have ceased to use eye dressings postoperatively to prevent psychic trauma. They feel that it must be terrifying to receive a general anesthetic and awaken blinded by eye dressings. Other surgeons feel that eye dressings are essential postoperatively. In these instances the child needs to become accustomed to the feeling of elbow restraints and to dressings that completely occlude his vision *before* he is anesthetized. His nurse also must anticipate the fears that he may experience after operation (of awakening in the dark and of permanent loss of vision, for instance) and give him preparation to meet them.

When nausea has ceased, a regular diet can ·be introduced. Children with eye dressings enjoy having their food described as they are being fed. They also enjoy the feeling of independence that comes when their restraints are removed and they are permitted to feed themselves the finger foods provided on their trays.

In most instances longer visiting periods are necessary for the child who has had an operation on his eyes. This is especially true when eye dressings have been applied. Temporary loss of vision produces panic in many children. The child's mother can allay his fears more effectively than the nurse because the latter has had too short a time to establish a relationship that gives the security and the satisfactions that he needs.

During the period when dressings cover both eyes, the child can be entertained by music and stories. Radios, which are a great source of pleasure and entertainment, should be provided when eye dressings make play activities impossible.

Fortunately, the period of blindness is short, but unless nurses safeguard the child from frightening experiences during the period of hospitalization by permitting his mother to be with him, a feeling of insecurity may develop. Insecurity may last beyond the time when successful correction of the deformity has been achieved.

When exercises are recommended postoperatively, the nurse should assist the mother in understanding their importance. If the child is attending school at the time of operation, it is advisable to notify the school nurse so that she may follow the child's care and ensure continuation of the orthoptic training.

The Ears

Minor variations in the formation of the external ear are very common among newborn infants. These usually consist of supernumerary projections of skin with or without cartilage beneath, projections which are easily removed surgically when they are large enough to be unsightly. Less common is an anomaly in which the external auditory meatus fails to canalize and the underlying bony portion of the ear is imperfectly developed. When this anomaly is unilateral it presents mainly a cosmetic problem, since hearing will be adequate from the other, normal ear. However, if the defect is bilateral, the infant will have defective hearing, and measures must be instituted to perform a plastic repair and establish a connection with the bony internal ear if function is present.

SKELETAL SYSTEM

Both localized and generalized abnormalities of the skeletal system are seen in the newborn. The variations are too numerous to describe in a short text. Their management falls within the province of the orthopedic surgeon.

THE CHRONICALLY HANDICAPPED CHILD

When an uncorrectible defect is discovered in a newborn infant the physician in charge has the unpleasant responsibility of relating the news to the parents. In the authors' opinion it is important that this be done promptly, completely and in a forthright manner whenever circumstances will permit. Too often the natural tendency to delay notification or to conceal the extent of the defect in a well-meant effort to "let the parents down easily," has unfortunate long-range consequences. It creates an aura of mystery about the defect and either confirms the parents' guilty suspicions that they are somehow responsible for the outcome or points an unjustifiably accusing finger at the obstetrician who delivered the infant. Since the unhappy outcome is no one's fault, it should be treated in a matter-of-fact straightforward manner. The parents may well react to their disappointment with an emotional outburst or temporary depression, but they usually regain their composure rapidly and are then ready to make realistic plans for the child's care. The support and the professional advice that they require is better accepted from a person who has been completely honest with them from the start than from one who has practiced deception, however well-meant. When the responsible physician does not consider this approach to be a wise one the nurse must, of course, regulate her conduct with the parents in accord with his wishes.

The nurse has opportunities to help shape the attitudes of parents toward their defective children. Since the parents provide the environment in which the child will develop, their feelings about him are usually crucial to his adjustment. Guilt feelings must be dispelled not only for the parents' comfort but also to prevent them from rearing the child in a too compassionate or too permissive way which fails to develop his character assets and leaves him poorly prepared to compete in the outer world. Excessive parental guilt may also have a devastating effect upon other normal children if the mother does penance by devoting herself exclusively to the abnormal offspring.

The attitude which parents adopt toward the handicapped child will also influence his acceptance by friends, relatives and other members of the community. Frank acceptance of the defect as a misfortune which requires him to modify his way of life but does not necessarily bar him from all constructive and satisfying pursuits is a healthy entrée into the life of the community and the school. Details concerning the nurse's functions in relation to the handicapped child and his parents are discussed in Chapter 8.

Mary was born with an abnormal, fingerless hand which her parents were able to accept in a healthy fashion. No attempt was made to conceal the deformity. Relatives, friends and neighbors soon satisfied their curiosity about the *hand* and accepted the *child* as the attractive person she was. When Mary entered nursery school she held out her hand for all to see, explaining that this was the way she was born. After due inspection the children's curiosity was appeased, and she promptly became a "normal" member of the group.

Chronic handicaps frequently require special facilities for prolonged medical care and training. Most states recognize the excessive financial drain which this imposes upon the average family and provide free clinics and hospital care through a division of services to crippled or handicapped children. Other community organizations provide similar or supplementary services. States also provide institutions for the permanent placement of those children whose handicaps are too severe to permit their continued care at home. The nurse should familiarize herself with the resources of her local community and learn the methods by which referral to them can be made.

SITUATIONS FOR FURTHER STUDY

1. A 3-week-old infant with a cleft palate has been discharged from the hospital after repair of a cleft lip. If you were to supervise this infant's care at

home, how would you proceed in helping the mother?

2. Investigate community facilities available for speech training of children with cleft palates. Visit a speech clinic to observe methods of speech training and to learn ways in which a nurse can help parents to continue speech training in the home.

3. In a young infant what symptoms would suggest a strangulated hernia?

4. What symptoms would lead you to believe that a baby had hydrocephalus?

5. In bathing a newborn baby, what observations would lead you to believe that the baby had an atresia of the esophagus?

6. At what age should a mother seek medical attention for her infant with strabismus?

7. What care is necessary after operation to correct strabismus?

8. How would you help a 3-year-old child to accept eyedrops without untoward emotional response?

9. If a 3-year-old child who had repair of strabismus had his restraints but not his dressing removed, what diversion could you suggest that required no sight?

10. How do you imagine a 3-year-old child feels when he awakens from an anesthetic in a strange place, with strange people, with painful eyes and blinded from the application of dressings over both eyes?

BIBLIOGRAPHY

Battersby, J. S., and Greve, M. L.: Modern treatment of atresia of the esophagus, Am. J. Nursing 50:158, 1950.

Blake, Florence G.: Role of the nurse in the care of newborn infants who deviate from normality in The Child, His Parents and the Nurse, p. 87, Philadelphia, Lippincott, 1954.

Campbell, Meredith: Clinical Pediatric Urology, Philadelphia, Saunders, 1951.

Ford, F. R.: Disease of the Nervous System in Infancy, Childhood and Adolescence, ed. 3, Springfield, Ill., Thomas, 1952.

Gilson, Martha, and Matson, Dónald D.: Care of a child after an arachnoid ureteral shunt, Am. J. Nursing 56: 1429, 1956.

Gross, R. E.: The Surgery of Infancy and Childhood, Philadelphia, Saunders, 1953.

Ingraham, F. D.: Spina Bifida and Cranium Bifidum, Cambridge, Mass., Harvard, 1943.

Lancaster, W. B.: Crossed eyes in children, Am. J. Nursing 50:535, 1950.

Lemmer, K. E., and Watson, S. R.: Inguinal hernia, Am. J. Nursing 53: 471, 1953.

Lis, E. F., Pruzansky, S., Koepp-Baker, H., and Kobes, H. R.: Cleft lip and cleft palate, Ped. Clinics of North America 3:995, 1956.

Potter, E. L.: Pathology of the Fetus and the Newborn, Chicago, Year Book Pub., 1952.

Ryan, Elizabeth K.: Nursing care of the patient with spina bifida, Am. J. Nursing 51:28, 1951.

Weiss, M. O.: Psychologic aspects of nursing care for eye patients, Am. J. Nursing 50:218, 1950.

West, Jessie Stevenson: Congenital Malformations and Birth Injuries, Ass. for the Aid of Crippled Children, New York, 1954.

Wishik, Samuel M.: How To Help Your Handicapped Child (pamphlet), Public Affairs Pamphlets, New York, 1955.

Wright, Lucille, and Prince, C. L.: Hypospadias: nursing care in surgical repair, Am. J. Nursing 46:686, 1946.

The Child With a Cleft Palate (pamphlet), Washington, U.S. Govt. Printing Office, 1953.

Nursing Care of the Sick Child

CHAPTER SEVENTEEN

Diseases of the Respiratory System

ACUTE UPPER RESPIRATORY INFECTIONS

Infections of the upper respiratory passageways are by far the most common diseases among children. Clinical classification is hampered by the lack of precise knowledge about etiology and by the confusing overlap of the symptoms produced by different infections and by their complications. A number of terms such as coryza, acute rhinitis, nasopharyngitis, "virus infection" and undifferentiated respiratory disease, have been applied to illnesses of this sort. The respiratory infections with clear-cut clinical pictures and accepted etiology (influenza, measles and streptococcal pharyngitis, etc.) are considered in later chapters.

It is desirable for the nurse to have some idea of current theories concerning the manner in which these infections arise and spread, and of the factors that determine the amount of damage they do. Newer methods for studying these infections make it probable that these ideas will be modified in the near future through the accumulation of more precise knowledge about etiology and epidemiology.

EPIDEMIOLOGY

The agents that produce upper respiratory infections are passed around from one individual to another mainly through the air. From the nose and the

372

throat of an infected person they are discharged into the surrounding atmosphere where they remain suspended for a time on minute drops of water vapor or particles of dust. During the act of breathing the nose and the throat of the child is continually sampling this atmosphere several times a minute. When it is contaminated by infectious agents they lodge on the mucous membranes of the nose or the throat during inspiration and, if they find a favorable climate there, proceed to multiply rapidly and produce disease in the new host. The newly infected child then serves as a fresh point of dissemination to the air about him.

Since the infectious agents die off more rapidly in outdoor air when exposed to unfavorable temperatures and to the action of ultraviolet light from the sun, the chain of transmission becomes more difficult during the summer months when children spend much of their time out-of-doors and when windows are open and houses are well ventilated. At the fall opening of school, children are congregated into enclosed rooms containing warm air and are brought into close range of each other. Introduction of an infectious agent into one member of such a group is readily followed by its dissemination to others. Consequently, it is the usual experience to find that after a period of grace, respiratory infections begin to make the school rounds during the late fall and continue to do so until spring. Exclusion of infected children from the school group has only a partial effect in breaking up the chain of spread, for each victim serves as an unwitting dispenser of germs for a day or two before obvious symptoms of his disease are present. Isolation is thus imposed a bit too late to provide complete protection for the group.

Age is an important factor in epidemiology. From long experience it seems clear that the older the child the better he is able to resist infection. He appears to develop immunity from repeated experience with the infecting agents. This accounts for the high incidence of disease among children who are having their early school experience in kindergarten or nursery school and for the much lower incidence among the teenagers. In a general way it seems as though most children must spend one or two bad winters before they begin to combat infections successfully. Individual exceptions are noteworthy, for each class has a few children who never seem to be affected by the illnesses of the group, and a few others who acquire immunity at such a slow rate that they continue to have trouble at short intervals for several years.

ETIOLOGY

Certain bacteria can be cultivated regularly from the noses and the throats of healthy children. Staphylococci, micrococcus catarrhalis, probably alpha-hemolytic streptococci and some varieties of pneumococcus fall within this group. This "normal flora" of the respiratory passages presumably is held in check by the natural body defenses. Other bacteria, notably the beta-hemolytic streptococcus, certain varieties of pneumococcus and the influenza bacillus are associated more regularly with respiratory disease and are considered to be at least potential pathogens. Perhaps at times upper respiratory infections are initiated entirely through a loss of resistance to those bacteria comprising the normal flora. But a more generally accepted mechanism is that a virus agent invades first, establishes an infection which lasts only 2 or 3 days, but in so doing breaks down the local resistance to bacteria so that they are able to infect tissues which normally resist their activity. The later symptoms of upper respiratory infections and of many of the complications are blamed upon such a secondary bacterial invasion of the tissues.

A number of virus agents have been

isolated which are capable of producing the symptoms of early respiratory disease in monkeys and in human volunteers. New technics of cultivating viruses have yielded a group of agents known as adenoviruses which are now under intensive study to discover what role they play in the initiation of the respiratory infections of children.

The popular lay idea that wet feet, fatigue and exposure to cold can initiate respiratory infections probably has some basis. Reflex changes in the nasal mucous membrane are known to occur when the body is suddenly chilled. It is likely that temporary loss of local tissue resistance follows and permits the invasion of bacteria or viruses which are already present in the passageways.

SYMPTOMS

The symptoms of acute upper respiratory infection are too well known to require elaborate description. The common cold begins with sneezing, clear nasal discharge and general malaise, but little or no fever. Conjunctivitis may be present, due to the invasion of the mucosa of the eye. Headache usually is due to the distention of the paranasal sinuses with fluid. Cough may be due to the irritation of the larynx by posterior nasal discharges or to primary infection of the laryngeal tissues. Upper respiratory infections may also begin with fever, headache, cough or sore throat. The clinical picture of the disease is not necessarily reproduced exactly in the succeeding victims to whom it is passed.

After the early catarrhal stage of the infection, bacterial invasion is apparent in the purulent character of the discharge from nose and sinuses and in the complication of otitis media which may follow retrograde extension from the pharynx up the eustachian tube.

PROGNOSIS AND PREVENTION

The strictly viral phase of upper respiratory infections is a brief affliction with uniformly good prognosis. However, the bacterial complications may protract the symptoms and lead to annoying complications such as sinusitis, bronchitis and otitis media. In small infants or children with debilitating disease or those with poor general resistance, bacterial invasion initiated by an apparently mild upper respiratory infection may progress to serious or even fatal disease such as pneumonia, bacteremia or meningitis. In this latter group it is essential to protect them by isolation from known infections and in certain instances by prophylactic administration of antibiotics when exposure cannot be foreseen. Prevention of respiratory infections in the school population is a difficult problem only partially solved by exclusion of infected children. In general it is probably best to permit the child to attend school as regularly as possible in order to acquire immunity through exposure, since no effective vaccination is yet available. Delicate children or those whose upper respiratory infections precipitate bronchitis or asthma may require protection with small doses of antibiotics taken regularly during the winter months. The problem of tonsillectomy and adenoidectomy is discussed in a later section.

TREATMENT AND NURSING CARE

In the treatment and the nursing of uncomplicated coryza in infancy, the most important measure is to keep the nose clean in order that the infant may breathe and suckle. Babies cannot suckle satisfactorily unless they breathe through the nose. Nasal breathing is more comfortable for the older child also, but it is not so important for him as for the infant. Freeing of the nose for breathing can be accomplished in the early stage by dropping into the nose a very small amount of a solution of ephedrine (½ to 1%) or Neo-Synephrine Hydrochloride (¼%), which decreases the swelling of the mucous membrane and permits drainage. Drops of the solution should be put into the infant's nostrils from 5 to 10 minutes before his food is given to him.

When dropping solutions into the nose for the purpose of treatment, the head should be held backward until it is below the level of the shoulders. After 3 or 4 days, when the discharge has become purulent, suction may be used for the removal of the secretions.

Solutions containing oil should not be used in the nose, since they are known to pass unchecked through the larynx and into the trachea. Their accumulation in the lung may be responsible for lipid pneumonia.

When the nasal secretion is profuse and irritating, the nostrils and the upper lip should be protected with cold cream or petrolatum. If symptoms are acute, and if the infant is irritable and uninterested in his food, no attempt should be made to encourage him to take the usual amount of food. When fever accompanies the cold, infants often reduce their own diet, a procedure that tends to prevent gastro-intestinal disturbances. Water should be encouraged between feedings. The infant's position should be changed frequently. Increasing the humidity of the room helps to keep secretions fluid and relieves cough.

There is no essential difference in the treatment and the nursing care of the older child. Nose drops will be accepted more readily if the need for proper position is explained to him and if he is given opportunity to press the dropper bulb that releases the solution into the nostrils. Rest in bed is necessary as long as fever persists and should be continued for 48 hours longer. When the child's temperature becomes normal, he will feel much improved. Unless interesting play materials are provided for him, bed rest will be difficult to maintain in the home. In the home, cribsides are not high enough to prevent the child from leaving his bed to go where playthings are accessible. In order to prevent the spread of infection into the eustachian tube, children should be taught a safe method of clearing their nasal passages. They never should be directed to "blow hard." Instead, they should be taught to keep their mouths open while they ease the secretion from both nostrils at the same time.

Sedative or antipyretic drugs are often used to decrease discomfort in both infancy and childhood. In infancy they also decrease restlessness. The drugs used include aspirin, codeine and the barbiturates. Although sulfonamides and antibiotics are widely used in the treatment of colds, they probably should be reserved for use in complications or to terminate a protracted infection. In premature or debilitated infants the immediate administration of antibiotics is rational.

CHRONIC RHINITIS

CAUSATIVE FACTORS

Chronic rhinitis may be due to any one of a number of causes. In infancy, it may be a manifestation of inherited syphilis. At any age, but especially in infancy, it may be the result of nasal diphtheria. A foreign body in the nose gives rise to a chronic purulent discharge from the same side as that in which the foreign body is located. Allergy to pollens is a cause of chronic discharge in hay fever. Allergy to other materials, such as feathers and animal hair, often causes chronic rhinitis that is not seasonal. All the causes enumerated are relatively uncommon as compared with chronic pyogenic infection unassociated with any of the conditions mentioned. Chronic rhinitis of this character usually is caused and maintained by an abnormality in and about the nose. Such causative factors may be enlarged adenoids, hypertrophy of the turbinate bones, marked deviations of

the septum and disease of the paranasal sinuses.

TREATMENT

When examining a child with chronic
rhinitis, the causative factors enumerated should be considered as possible
agents, and those not responsible excluded by appropriate tests and special
examinations. The treatment depend
altogether on the nature of the cause
When the rhinitis is due primarily t
pyogenic organisms, any associated ab
normal conditions should be correcte
in so far as this is possible. Diseased tor
sils and adenoids should be removed
and sinusitis, if present, should receiv
appropriate treatment.

PARANASAL SINUSITIS

The paranasal sinuses are cavities,
normally filled with air, which are outlying portions of and communicate with
the nasal chambers. Clinically, they are
of little importance until they become
diseased. The sinuses are only partially
developed at birth and do not attain
their maximum size until maturity. The
maxillary and the ethmoidal sinuses are
sufficiently developed at birth to be of
clinical importance. The sphenoidal
sinuses have relatively little development before 5 years. The frontal sinuses
develop later than the others and are
not of clinical importance until the latter part of childhood.

ETIOLOGY

The paranasal sinuses are invaded by
every generalized intranasal infection,
such as the common cold. If the mucosa of the upper respiratory tract is
normal, and if no anatomic anomalies
are present, any such infection usually
will subside completely. However, if
for any reason drainage from the sinuses is impeded, or if the mucosa loses
its ability to combat the invasion, the
inflammatory process in the sinuses may
persist and become firmly established.
Adenoids or deviated nasal septum may
produce obstruction and thus serve as
a causative agent in continued sinus
inflammation. Sinus disease disappears
spontaneously in a considerable proportion of cases when such obstructions
have been removed. Repeated or persistent infections may lead to alteration
in the mucosa: it loses its ciliated structure, and polypoid degeneration occur
These changes favor persistence of th
infectious process. Swimming and div
ing is often reputed to be a frequen
cause of sinus infection.

SYMPTOMS

Sinus disease may present itself in
variety of forms. It may be acute o
chronic, and it may involve any or a
of the sinuses. Most instances are char
acterized by the presence of exudate
which may be serous, mucoid or puru
lent. In some cases the changes ar
chiefly hypertrophic. The symptoms o
sinus disease vary with the acutenes
of the infection, its extent and distribu
tion, and the adequacy of the drain
age of the exudate. If the drainage
blocked, the retention will lead to loca
pain and to absorption of toxic proc
ucts with resultant generalized effect
Chronic sinusitis may be associated wit
low-grade intermittent fever. The ac
companying symptoms seem to be ir
relevant, but they suggest continue
absorption of toxic products. Anorexia
lassitude and weakness, with vagu
muscle stiffness and pain, are presen
especially in the early morning. Pallo
may be marked, out of proportion t
the decrease of hemoglobin, and th
ears often appear waxy and translucen
During certain stages of the attack
mental acuity may seem to be impaired
Many types of disease, both local an
remote, have been attributed to sinu
infection. In conditions such as chroni
bronchitis and bronchiectasis the cause

relationship is definite; in others, it is largely circumstantial.

DIAGNOSIS

Although the existence of sinusitis may be suspected from the history, the diagnosis is made on the basis of objective findings. In the presence of chronic sinusitis, the lymphoid tissue of the oropharynx is usually hyperplastic and somewhat reddened. The tonsils, if present, usually show some evidence of inflammation. The soft palate may appear reddened and slightly granular. Pus may or may not be seen in the posterior pharynx. Often the discharge is swallowed by the child without his being conscious of its presence. Regional lymph glands usually are enlarged and may be tender.

Examination of the nose by both the anterior and the posterior nasoscope may reveal the presence and the location of nasal discharge. During acute sinusitis, no discharge may be visible because of acute retention. When chronic maxillary sinusitis is suspected, aspiration of the sinus is considered useful as a diagnostic procedure. Roentgenograms of the sinuses are usually reliable, and when operative procedures are contemplated they provide information about the size, the location and the degree of development of the sinuses. Transillumination as a diagnostic aid in children has not proved to be wholly reliable and satisfactory.

TREATMENT

In the treatment of sinusitis in children, conservative measures should be employed. One of the primary requirements of treatment is drainage of the sinuses. Often this may be accomplished by intranasal medication. Ephedrine or Neo-Synephrine solutions applied frequently during the day by dropping, spraying or nasal packing cause a decrease in swelling of the mucous membrane of the nasal cavities, thus freeing the natural opening of the sinuses.

In the presence of sinusitis the tonsils and the adenoids, especially the latter, are likely to be hypertrophied and chronically infected. Their presence often serves to continue and aggravate the sinus infections. Removal of the tonsils and the adenoids is followed in a considerable proportion of instances in childhood by gradual disappearance of sinusitis.

When the maxillary sinuses are inflamed and contain pus that does not drain adequately with the conservative treatment mentioned, they may be washed out at intervals, or the opening from the nose into the sinuses may be enlarged. In the great majority of cases in childhood, more radical procedures than these are neither necessary nor indicated.

EPISTAXIS (NASAL HEMORRHAGE)

Epistaxis may occur as a symptom of heart disease, typhoid fever, whooping cough and diseases of the blood, such as purpura and leukemia. It may be due also to inflammation within the nose. Frequently recurring nasal hemorrhage in the absence of systemic disease is usually due to an ulceration of the anterior part of the septum. Very commonly, hemorrhage results from injury: an external blow, as from a ball, or internal trauma—picking the nose or inserting an object into it.

In the common variety of nasal hemorrhage, the bleeding is from the anterior and inferior portion of the nasal septum. Such a hemorrhage is controlled easily. If the child remains quiet, the hemorrhage may stop spontaneously in a few minutes. Pressure on the bleeding point by pinching the nose is accomplished easily and usually is effective. In case the hemorrhage persists, it always can be stopped by packing into the anterior part of the nose a small piece of cotton or strip of cloth, either plain or moistened with thromboplastin or a vasoconstrictor such as epinephrine or ephedrine. In case of the more severe and less common type of hemorrhage from some other part of the nose, posterior packing may be necessary.

TONSILS AND ADENOIDS

The term *tonsils,* when used without qualification, usually refers to the faucial tonsils which are located anteriorly in the oropharynx, one on each side. The term *adenoids* refers to a mass of lymphoid tissue of the same general structure as the faucial tonsils located in the nasopharynx posteriorly. Adenoids are known also as the pharyngeal tonsil. The lingual tonsil is located at the base of the tongue. The tubal tonsils are situated near the eustachian tube, one on each side of the pharynx. All these lymphoid tissues as a group are referred to as Waldeyer's ring.

Acute inflammation of any of these lymphoid tissues may be catarrhal, follicular or membranous, depending on the severity and the type of infection. The lingual, the pharyngeal or the faucial tonsils may be involved separately, or all may be affected at the same time. Similarly, any of these tissues may be the site of chronic infection or may be abnormally hypertrophied.

Relatively normal faucial tonsils vary considerably in size, the pillars are not adherent, the crypt mouths are open and show no inflammatory products on pressure, and the color of the tonsil is the same as that of the mouth.

Chronic disease or abnormality of the faucial tonsils may manifest itself in several ways. The tonsils may be large and ragged from hypertrophy. They may be small and fibrous, and, in addition, they may be buried between adherent pillars. The crypts on pressure may exude pus or cheesy material. The surface of the tonsil may be redder than normal and have the appearance of being subacutely inflamed. Enlargement of the cervical lymph glands is corroborative evidence of chronic tonsillar inflammation.

Chronic infection of the lymphoid tissues of the pharynx may be a factor in the occurrence of rheumatic fever, pyelitis, arthritis, otitis media, partial deafness, cervical adenitis, recurrent colds and infections of the nasopharynx, unexplained fever, periodic gastro-intestinal and metabolic upsets, and other conditions.

TONSILLECTOMY

Chronic disease in the tonsil, repeatedly recurring acute disease and hypertrophy to the extent of interference with breathing are indications for tonsil removal.

Antibiotic treatment of chronic and acute respiratory disease has been responsible for a considerable decrease in the number of tonsillectomies performed.

While there is no question about the benefits of tonsillectomy for properly selected children, it does not necessarily follow that all children are better off without their tonsils and adenoids. So long as these structures remain healthy they provide a first line of defense against respiratory infection. They also probably limit the spread of such diseases so long as they function normally. The decision to remove tonsils and adenoids must also take into consideration the risks of anesthesia, silent bleeding in the small infant, and the psychic trauma to a young child who is unable to comprehend what is being done to him. During the period of the year when poliomyelitis is prevalent, tonsillectomy should be avoided, because there is good reason to believe that a child with a recent tonsillectomy wound runs a greater risk of the bulbar type of poliomyelitis if exposed to the virus.

When tonsillectomy and adenoidectomy are indicated, the nurse in the doctor's office or in the clinic should assist the mother in learning how to prepare her child for his hospital experience. Frequently, erroneous information is given children prior to hospitalization. One constantly sees the result of it in the admitting room and in the hospital wards. It increases the adjustment problems for the child; it complicates his postoperative nursing care; and it indicates to him a lack of parental honesty. The period of hospitalization before surgery frequently is too brief for the nurse to establish the type of relationship that gives the child a sense of security and confidence in her. Preparation that relieves fear and anxiety should be given by someone in whom the child has faith, security and confidence; therefore, it is the parent who should prepare the child for his new experience. However, the nurse should function by helping the parents to gain insight into the necessity for preparation and by imparting the knowledge that serves as a basis for truthful child-teaching. In instances where the mother has not prepared the child, the nurse will need to do it for her. This is essential because the child should know what he will experience before and after operation.

POSTOPERATIVE NURSING CARE

When the child returns from the operating room, he should be placed in a prone position with a pillow under his chest and abdomen to facilitate drain-age and to prevent aspiration of blood or secretions. When the child becomes fully conscious, he can be turned on his back and supported in a sitting position. Fluids should be given cautiously until vomiting ceases; then they can be increased as rapidly as they are tolerated. Cold and sweetened synthetic fruit juices and milk drinks usually are tolerated a few hours postoperatively. The child's pulse rate and behavior should be observed at frequent intervals to detect early signs of bleeding. Restlessness, frequent swallowing, clearing the throat and vomiting often accompany bleeding. Apparatus for suction and materials necessary for checking hemorrhage should be in readiness for use. In some instances, throat icebags relieve the pain; in others, they tend to annoy and to increase restlessness. Aspirin may be indicated for relief of discomfort.

Before the child leaves the hospital the mother should be instructed to provide soft, warm, nonirritating foods for her child until the soreness of the throat has subsided. Also, she should understand the necessity for keeping him in bed for a few days and for providing daily rest periods for a short time subsequently. Earache, not accompanied by fever, sometimes occurs after tonsillectomy, and the mother should be forewarned of this to prevent anxiety should it occur. Also, she should be told of the importance of any mild or sudden bleeding during the convalescent period.

ACUTE TONSILLITIS AND PHARYNGITIS

Acute faucial tonsillitis is caused most commonly by streptococci but may be caused by any of several pyogenic bacteria. It is less common in the infant than in the older child.

SYMPTOMS

Tonsillitis or pharyngitis commonly has an acute onset with fever, head-ache and malaise. The onset may be accompanied in the older child by a chill and in the younger on rare occasions by a convulsion. Pain on swallowing usually is present. Gastro-intestinal symptoms, chiefly vomiting and diarrhea, are frequent and are more pronounced in the younger child. The lymph glands receiving the drainage from the inflamed area, the submaxillary and the cervical glands, are frequently enlarged and tender. Though tonsillitis usually causes marked constitutional symptoms, some children may have an acute infection with only few and mild subjective symptoms. Sometimes acute and sharply localized abdominal pain accompanies tonsillitis, presumably caused by inflammation of the mesenteric lymph glands. The symptoms may be of such a nature as to lead to the suspicion, or even the diagnosis, of an acute abdominal condition, such as appendicitis.

COMPLICATIONS

The most common complications of acute tonsillitis or pharyngitis are otitis media and cervical adenitis. Under modern treatment, adenitis seldom progresses to the point of suppuration. If the initial infection is caused by a hemolytic streptococcus there may be recurrent fever and mild adenitis over a period of weeks or months, due either to incomplete treatment or to the relatively feeble resistance of a young child. Peritonsillar abscess is seen occasionally in an older child following tonsillitis. The relation between acute tonsillitis and a number of systemic diseases is considered under the discussion of the etiology of rheumatic fever, nephritis, arthritis, purpura and scarlet fever.

TREATMENT

Chemotherapy is usually effective. The choice of drug should be determined from a knowledge of the causative agent, but often this is not done because of the lack of adequate facilities. Most infections will respond promptly to penicillin; a little more slowly to the sulfonamides. Oxytetracycline (Terramycin) and chlortetracycline (Aureomycin) are required sometimes when the infecting agent does not respond. Aspirin is useful to relieve fever, headache and general malaise. Gargles, compresses, sprays and local applications to the pharynx have very limited usefulness for children. The diet should be light and nonirritating, and the fluid intake should be kept high.

RETROPHARYNGEAL ABSCESS

A retropharyngeal abscess arises from suppuration in the lymph glands back of the posterior pharyngeal wall. Infection in these glands is preceded by infection elsewhere in the upper respiratory tract. Often the primary infection is a common cold. Retropharyngeal glands are present at birth and tend to atrophy and disappear after a few years. For this reason, retropharyngeal abscess occurs most frequently under 3 years of age.

SYMPTOMS

As the abscess develops, the child becomes restless and is found to have fever, which, though variable, is often high. Prostration frequently is out of proportion to the obvious physical findings. Swallowing is painful, and attempts to swallow may give rise to choking. Sometimes the taking of food is impossible. The head may be held retracted toward the affected side, the abscess usually having a unilateral origin. A swelling may be visible externally on the affected side. When the swelling in the pharynx increases sufficiently, obstruction to breathing occurs, and stridor and dyspnea result. Respiratory obstruction may be great enough to threaten life unless promptly relieved.

DIAGNOSIS

Examination of the throat is difficult because of the small size of the child, difficulty in opening the mouth, and the resence of frothy mucus in the harynx. Usually the diagnosis must be erified by palpation. By palpation the resence of swelling is determined. It nay have a boggy feeling, and sometimes fluctuation will be observed. The se of a laryngoscope usually is of coniderable assistance in the diagnosis beause of the better opportunity for dequate inspection.

The condition must be distinguished rom peritonsillar abscess and from bscess resulting from tuberculosis of he cervical vertebrae. Peritonsillar bscess (quinsy) is an abscess about he tonsil resulting from tonsillar inammation and is located farther forward than a retropharyngeal abscess. It s rare in childhood. A tuberculous bscess is a cold abscess, i.e., not assoiated with acute inflammation. There nay be little or no fever and no prostraion except that which might be assoiated with respiratory obstruction. A oentgenogram will show erosion of he underlying vertebrae.

TREATMENT

The treatment of retropharyngeal bscess is incision and drainage, always without an anesthetic. If respiratory obstruction is present, an anesthetic prevents the use of accessory muscles of respiration. As a consequence, respiration may cease from obstruction as soon as the anesthetic is given and before the abscess can be drained. An anesthetic will abolish the cough reflex, and, as a result, pus may be aspirated. The incision should be small, and, if necessary, the opening should be enlarged by inserting closed scissors or forceps and then spreading and withdrawing them. Incision through a laryngoscope has several advantages. A better view of the incision site is obtained. The head is held downward while the abscess is lanced, and suction for removal of pus can be applied immediately through the laryngoscope. After operation the wound should be spread each day until drainage ceases. After drainage the healing may be prompt. In other instances, inflammation with its accompanying fever and prostration may not subside completely for several weeks.

NURSING CARE

Immediately after incision specific nursing care consists of maintaining the child in a position suitable for mouth drainage. He may be placed in a prone position with the foot of his bed elevated, or a pillow may be placed under his chest and abdomen to facilitate drainage. A "mummy" restraint is required when the incision is made and when the abscess is spread daily. After operation, the taking of fluids should be encouraged as rapidly as ability to swallow develops. Observation to detect signs of hemorrhage should be made as long as the infection continues.

OTITIS MEDIA

ACUTE OTITIS MEDIA

Etiology

The middle ear is a small air-containing cavity interposed between the drum, which separates it from the external ear, and the inner ear which is set into the temporal bone and contains the organs of hearing and equilibrium. The ear drum is a sensitive curtain hung between the air of the external and the middle ear. It transmits the minute changes of pressure created by the sound waves through a chain of small bones (the ossicles) to the oval window of the inner ear. The middle ear communicates through a long narrow channel (eustachian tube) with the pharynx. During health the eustachian tube is closed most of the time by its external muscular coating but opens briefly during the acts of swallowing, yawning and crying to permit rapid equalization of air pressure between the middle ear and the pharynx. (Except during violent nose-blowing, the pressure in the pharynx is automatically the same as that of the air on the external surface of the ear drum.) The symptoms of mild pain in the air and blurred hearing which are experienced during air travel are due to imperfect equalization of air pressures on the two sides of the drum. The middle ear also communicates with the mastoid antrum and its ramified system of air cells within the temporal bone.

Infection of the middle ear almost invariably arises from the pharynx by way of the eustachian tube. Consequently, the bacteria usually involved are the same ones responsible for pharyngitis and tonsillitis—hemolytic streptococci, pneumococci and influenza bacilli. A wide variety of other organisms may be implicated under the special circumstances of specific diseases, such as diphtheria and tuberculosis, or during debilitating illness or prolonged treatment with antibiotics which sometimes changes the flora of the respiratory tract.

The mechanical changes that occur during otitis media usually begin with obstruction of the mouth of the eustachian tube due to swelling of the mucous membrane. Complete or partial obstruction prevents air exchange between the pharynx and the middle ear, and the air within the middle ear is slowly absorbed. The ear drum bulges inward due to the unopposed external air pressure, and tension of the drum results in pain and blurring of hearing. If the obstruction persists, the air in the middle ear is replaced by fluid which may produce outward bulging of the drum. If the fluid is not infected, the process is called catarrhal otitis media. When infection has spread up the tube to the middle ear the accumulation of fluid is more rapid, and the drum bulges outward tensely, becomes exquisitely painful and not infrequently ruptures, permitting the accumulation of pus in the middle ear to

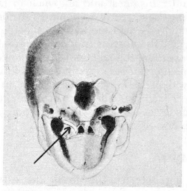

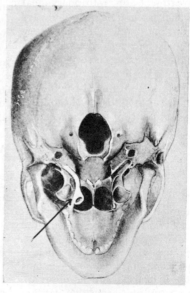

Fig. 71. Schematic representation of the eustachian tube in the infant and the adult, showing relative position and direction.

discharge into the external canal.

Infants are more prone to middle ear infection than are older children or adults. The eustachian tube is shorter, wider and straighter in the infant (Fig. 71) so that infected material is carried more readily from the pharynx to the middle ear. Infected adenoid masses in the vicinity of the mouth of the eustachian tube are often responsible for recurring blockage of the tube or otitis media.

Symptoms

The child who is old enough to communicate complains of pain in the ear and blurred hearing. The severity of the pain depends upon the rapidity with which fluid accumulates in the middle ear. Fever, headache and vomiting are also present in variable degree. Smaller children and infants cannot localize their symptoms. The source of their fever, irritability, discomfort and vomiting may be disclosed only through a comprehensive physical examination. In small infants there may be convulsions, diarrhea, refusal of food and rolling of the head from side to side.

Complications

With almost any acute inflammation of the middle ear there is some extension of the infection into the mastoid antrum and air cells. When treatment is delayed or ineffectual, mastoiditis may occur. From the mastoid area there may be spread of the infection to the venous sinuses within the skull (sinus thrombosis and septicemia) or to the meninges (meningitis) or to the brain (brain abscess). These complications are now rare since the antibiotics have made treatment simple and usually successful.

Prevention

The prevention of otitis depends upon the rapid and accurate treatment of pharyngitis and tonsillitis in most instances. Some children who are unusually prone to otitis media benefit from the removal of hypertrophied or infected adenoid tissue.

Treatment and Nursing Care

Antibiotics are indicated to combat the infection. At the beginning of treatment the appropriate drug may not be known, because the bacteria responsible for the infection have not yet been determined. Penicillin is effective in most instances and usually is given initially. One of the tetracycline antibiotics or sulfonamides may be used when the response to penicillin is inadequate or when bacteriologic study indicates that they will be more effective.

Often symptomatic relief of pain may be obtained by giving nose drops to shrink the nasal mucous membranes and promote drainage from the blocked eustachian tube. Neo-Synephrine (0.26%) or ephedrine (2%) may be used every 2 or 3 hours until relief is obtained. Sometimes drops containing phenol and glycerine are instilled into the external ear. Their effect is variable, and they have the disadvantage of preventing accurate observation of changes in the ear drum. Occasionally, when the drum is extremely tense, incision (myringotomy) may be indicated to relieve pain and promote drainage. Aspirin and sedatives with the barbiturate drugs will give temporary relief of pain until the other measures have had time to take effect.

When there is drainage from the middle ear, the ear canal must be kept clean. The nurse's hands should be washed thoroughly before cleansing the canal to prevent mixed infection of the middle ear. Sterilized cotton should be made into pledgets and used to cleanse the canal of all drainage. Hydrogen peroxide is useful in preventing the exudate from caking. In cleansing the ear canal of the young child, the ear lobe should be pulled down and back to straighten the canal; in the older child, the ear lobe should be pulled up and back. Ear wicks should be small and inserted lightly; packing them in tightly prevents free drainage and may cause extension of the infection into the mastoid process. When drainage is profuse, zinc oxide ointment or petrolatum should be applied to the external auricle to prevent excoriation of the skin.

Chronic Otitis Media

In some instances, the ear discharge persists and becomes chronic. If the condition is untreated, the discharge may continue for years. The usual result of chronic discharge is impairment of hearing, even to almost complete loss in some instances. A less common result is, soon or late, an inflammatory invasion of the surrounding temporal bone, with perhaps serious results such as meningitis or brain abscess. Sometimes chronic ear discharge will cease when adenoids have been removed and the nose and the throat are brought to a relatively normal state. In other instances, it is necessary to give postauricular drainage to such inflammation as exists in the mastoid process. Tuberculosis of the middle ear is also a cause of persistent discharge.

MASTOIDITIS

Mastoiditis is a term used, somewhat colloquially, to designate inflammation of and in the mastoid process of the skull. It occurs almost exclusively as a complication of otitis media. It is probable that some inflammation and pus are present in the mastoid antrum in every case of otitis media, since the middle ear and the antrum are connected directly. However, unless more than this minimum inflammation is present in the antrum, mastoiditis cannot be diagnosed, and such inflammation as is present is of no great clinical significance. In the majority of instances, it clears up with adequate drainage from the middle ear. When the pus has no outlet for drainage, the symptoms become more severe, and the consequences more serious.

Modern treatment with antibiotics has greatly reduced the incidence of mastoiditis in children. Occasionally, it appears when treatment of otitis media has been too long delayed or when the presence of unusually thick pus hampers drainage from the mastoid cells back into the middle ear.

Symptoms

Mastoiditis occurs at all ages, even in earliest infancy. In most instances, fever is present, and often it is high. Sometimes the temperature is constantly at a high level, while at others it fluctuates widely at short intervals. Tenderness over the mastoid process is frequent, especially in older children. Often when tenderness cannot be elicited on pressure, it becomes manifest when the area is tapped with a finger or a percussion hammer. In some instances, the inflammation extends exteriorly through the bone. External extension produces a swelling back of the ear which lifts the external ear away from the skull and pushes it forward. The swelling may be caused by edema alone, or pus may break through the periosteum to form a superficial abscess.

Treatment

When chemotherapy has failed to improve the patient's condition, it may be necessary to establish drainage from the infected cells by mastoidectomy. This operation consists of removing the bone overlying the mastoid cells or antrum to permit direct drainage to the exterior.

DEAFNESS

Bilateral complete deafness is a very serious handicap to a child. It may be due to congenital abnormalities of the external or the internal ear, of the auditory nerve, or of the auditory centers within the brain. It sometimes results from the effects of disease such as congenital syphilis, erythroblastosis fetalis, meningococcus meningitis, mumps, encephalitis or extensive infection of the middle ear. Complete deafness in early infancy may go unrecognized until the child's failure to develop speech and to relate himself normally to his parents or other children stimulates an investigation of the acuity of his hearing. Loss of hearing should be suspected in infancy if the child fails to blink at loud noises. A similarly objective test must be used in the preschool child in order to distinguish between an inability to hear and an unwillingness to pay attention. Children who grow up without the ability to hear require special training or hearing aids in order to develop speech and to learn lipreading. Without such help the child becomes socially isolated and is unable to pursue a normal school career.

Complete deafness that is unilateral may be caused by the same disorders enumerated above. It is a relatively minor handicap if hearing is normal in the other ear.

Bilateral partial deafness may be responsible for poor school performance or for various types of behavior disorders. It is most commonly the result of chronic or recurring infections of the middle ear or blockage of the eustachian tube. It may be the forerunner of more serious hearing loss in later life. The detection of impaired hearing is an important responsibility of school health personnel and always should be a part of health examinations. Thorough treatment of acute otitis media can be expected to prevent hearing loss in most instances. When the defect is due to eustachian tube blockage without infection, the services of a skilled otologist are required to determine what measures are needed to maintain the patency of the tube.

OTITIS EXTERNA

Pain in the ear is sometimes due to the extension of inflammation of the wall of the external auditory canal backward to the region of the drum. The disorder is comparable with furunculosis or cellulitis of the canal and is caused by the bacteria which inhabit the cutaneous lining of the canal. Treatment is by local application of heat and antibiotic solutions and ointments.

CROUP

Croup is a general term for inflammations of the larynx that cause hoarseness, barking cough or obstruction to breathing, or combinations of these. The term *membranous croup* has been used as a synonym of laryngeal diphtheria. In many young children, catarrhal inflammation of the larynx causes spasmodic contraction of the larynx, which results in respiratory difficulty. This latter condition at present is commonly referred to as croup and is the condition discussed here. It is known by a variety of names: for example, catarrhal croup, spasmodic croup and spasmodic laryngitis.

Symptoms

Croup is a mild, acute infection, of low communicability, occurring chiefly in children under 5 years of age. It is associated with little, and often no, fever. There is a laryngeal cough, hard and barking, usually spoken of as "croupy." Attacks of spasm of the larynx occur chiefly and often only at night. They may last from ½ hour to between 2 and 3 hours. They may recur once or twice the same night. The attacks recur on the second night, and often on the third, after which time spontaneous recovery from the affection occurs. Except for hoarseness and occasional croupy cough, the child seems to be completely well between the attacks of spasm.

During a spasmodic attack, there is very difficult inspiration and an inspiratory stridor. Expiration is little disturbed, and there is no expiratory stridor. The child sits up in bed, brings the accessory muscles of respiration into use, and on inspiration there is retraction of the soft tissues above the clavicle and between the ribs and retraction of the ribs at the attachment of the diaphragm. In a severe attack, the whole picture is very alarming because of the appearance of impending asphyxia. However, croup rarely is fatal.

DIAGNOSIS

The diagnosis of croup usually is not difficult. Diphtheria may be excluded by examining the larynx and finding an absence of membrane. The obstruction due to diphtheria is both inspiratory and expiratory; it gradually increases in severity and does not occur in spasmodic attacks, although occasionally in diphtheria, spasm is superimposed on the typical clinical picture. Streptococcic laryngitis may cause swelling and membrane formation which give symptoms similar to those described for diphtheria. In laryngospasm of tetany, other signs of tetany usually are pres-

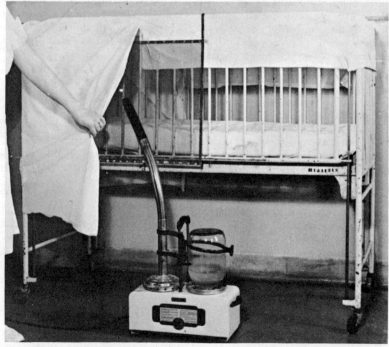

FIG. 72. A croup tent and a croup "kettle." A wire screen protects the child from being burned.

ent, and the chemical changes in the blood are diagnostic.

TREATMENT AND NURSING CARE

Treatment and nursing care of croup are directed chiefly toward relief of laryngeal spasm. Breathing warm moist air often gives complete relief. Various volatile drugs, such as benzoin, may be employed along with "steam," but the essential part, and usually the only necessary part, of the inhalation is the water vapor. Various methods may be used to supply moist air. The most commonplace is a "croup tent" kept filled with moist air by a "croup kettle." Croup tents may be made by draping a sheet and a bath blanket over the crib. The spout of the croup kettle should point upward and away from the child to prevent the condensing steam from dropping and scalding him. Unless the child can have a nurse with him constantly, a jacket restraint must be used to prevent the child from moving toward the apparatus and being burned. An alternative is to provide a wire screen to be attached to the bed between the child and the steam outlet (Fig. 72). When constant nursing is available, it should be provided, because restraining a child with respiratory infection keeps him in one position and increases the incidence of complications. In addition, constant attendance is necessary to alleviate anxiety. Respiratory distress is frightening. The young infant cannot tolerate this distress without the support of a comforting mother or nurse.

Provision for a constant supply of fresh air to the tent should be made. A good plan is to have the bottom of the tent at the same level as the highest portion of the child's face when lying down. Then the tent should be kept filled with visible water vapor down to this level. There is then space for ventilation beneath the tent.

In the home, croup tents may be made by draping a sheet and a blanket over the crib or the baby carriage or over an umbrella in bed. The steam may be led into the tent from a croup kettle heated by an alcohol lamp or a gas or electric plate. A lead-in pipe may be improvised from rolled paper or cardboard. Sometimes in institutions rooms are equipped specially with steam outlets, and steam is delivered in such quantity that a tent is unnecessary.

Devices which mechanically vaporize water are used in many hospitals to humidify a tent or a room. They are equally as effective as steam and provide more comfortable working conditions for the personnel.

Several antispasmodic drugs are useful in preventing or relieving the muscle spasm of the larynx. If ipecac is used, the preparation known as syrup of ipecac is the one commonly employed. For a child of several years or older in the midst of an attack, the syrup may be given in teaspoonful doses every 15 minutes until emesis occurs, or until 3 doses have been given. Administration in subemetic doses may be useful in preventing an attack. Antipyrine also is useful, especially in preventing attacks. A proper dose for the age, given at night on retiring, and perhaps repeated during the night, may serve to prevent an attack entirely. A wet compress on the neck is often useful for control of both laryngeal spasm and the inflammation.

The larynx of the infant and the young child is relatively smaller than that of the older child. It is more flexible and susceptible to spasm, and when infection of the larynx is present, respiratory difficulty may become marked and prostrating. In caring for the child with croup, the nurse should be constantly alert for signs of respiratory embarrassment. If cyanosis develops and the child becomes increasingly prostrated from labored breathing, tracheotomy may be indicated. For such children specific nursing care is required.

FOREIGN BODIES IN THE RESPIRATORY TRACT

Foreign bodies of small size and wide variety may be aspirated into the lower respiratory tract, especially by children. These may remain in the pharynx or pass into the bronchi. Seldom do they lodge in the trachea. In the larynx they are the cause of immediate and acute distress with violent coughing and with stridor due to obstruction or to spasm of the larynx. If the foreign body remains fixed in one place in the larynx, coughing subsides, but usually an inflammation occurs, the edema of which obstructs respiration, and operative relief becomes imperative.

When a foreign body passes into a bronchus, the effects vary with the size and the nature of the foreign material. If the bronchus is completely occluded, the air in the lung beyond the obstruction is absorbed, and the lung collapses. If a large or primary bronchus is affected, the resultant pulmonary collapse may give rise to alarming symptoms, including cyanosis and dyspnea. A foreign body of any variety in a bronchus causes inflammation; but certain kinds, especially nuts, more easily induce inflammatory changes which are of a serious type. In a child who survives the immediate effects of a foreign body, the late result is likely to be a lung abscess or chronic pneumonia and bronchiectasis, unless the foreign body is removed early. The primary indication in treatment is removal of the offending material by laryngoscope or bronchoscope, as the need may be.

Nursing Care

After the foreign body has been removed by laryngoscope or bronchoscope, the child should be placed in a ventilated "croup tent" or other source of moist air. The child should be observed closely for signs of respiratory difficulty. Trauma during laryngoscopic or bronchoscopic examination may produce edema of the larynx with accompanying respiratory embarrassment. Increased, labored respirations, crowing hoarseness, retraction of the soft part of the chest on inspiration, cyanosis and restlessness are danger signals that should be reported immediately. If respiratory embarrassment occurs, tracheotomy may be necessary.

Care of the Child with a Tracheotomy

After tracheotomy, the child should be placed in a warm bed in a room at 80° F. to prevent chilling. Respiratory difficulty exhausts a child, and often after tracheotomy he is prostrated. Elbow restraints should be applied immediately to prevent the child from removing the tracheotomy tube.

Normally, air is filtered, warmed and moistened in the upper respiratory tract before it is breathed into the lungs. After tracheotomy, nursing measures must provide warm, moist and filtered air for the child to breathe. A croup tent or humidifier is usually employed. Two thicknesses of gauze saturated with normal saline solution placed over the opening of the tracheotomy tube, filter and moisten the inspired air. The gauze should be changed as it becomes dry and soiled with drainage.

A tray with the following sterile equipment should be at the child's bedside: duplicate tracheotomy tubes, with tapes attached, obturator, scissors, 2 curved clamps, pipe cleaners, medicine dropper, gauze dressings, tongue depressors, applicators and a catheter (No. 8 or 10 F.) which has additional holes near the tip to facilitate aspiration. Other necessary equipment includes 2 covered jars of sterile normal saline solution, a jar of hydrogen peroxide, a jar of sterile petrolatum and suction apparatus.

Constant nursing care is required for the infant or child after tracheotomy has been done. He cannot cry or call, and respiratory embarrassment results when aspiration does not keep the cheotomy tube free from mucus and ainage. The child must become accstomed to breathing through the oe. In the adjustment period, the rse should be in constant attendance soothe the infant and allay the anxy of the older child. During the first hours after tracheotomy, the tube ust be cleaned frequently by aspiran. The frequency is dependent on : amount of drainage and the needs the individual child. Before aspiran, a few drops of normal saline solun should be put into the tracheotomy oe with a medicine dropper. The ops of normal saline moisten dried acus, stimulate coughing, loosen the acus and make it easier to aspirate. piration tends to produce excitement, er and coughing. Until the child rns that the procedure brings him ief, reassurance is necessary. After : lock of the tube has been turned ward toward the face, the inner anula should be removed and placed the jar of hydrogen peroxide. To oirate, the catheter should be comessed and inserted through the outer anula opening until it reaches approxiately the end of the tube. Then comession on the tube should be released aspirate the secretions. The catheter ould be removed, flushed with normal ine solution and reinserted until all ainage has been removed. After oirating, the inner cannula should be ansed with pipe cleaners and hydron peroxide and, before it is reinserted o the outer cannula, it should be exined carefully to ensure complete anliness. If aspiration and cleansing the inner cannula does not relieve the ild's respiratory difficulty, the phyian should be notified at once. The dressing around the tracheotomy

tube should be changed frequently. Applicators dipped in hydrogen peroxide should be used to cleanse the area around the incision, and a tongue depressor should be used to coat the area with sterile petrolatum. A gauze square cut to the center should be placed around the tube and under the tapes that hold the tube in position. Any bleeding from or signs of infection in the wound should be reported. Before the dressing is changed and before aspirating the tube, the nurse's hands should be washed thoroughly. If the tube should be coughed or pulled out, the nurse should establish an airway at once by spreading the incision with a curved clamp.

Fluids and food may be given the child as he tolerates them. In the early period after tracheotomy, the child may be fearful of swallowing lest he have pain. However, as he finds that it causes him no discomfort, he will begin to take fluids and food more eagerly. Any coughing associated with swallowing should be reported.

When drainage and respiratory difficulty have ceased, a cork plug is inserted in the inner cannula to obstruct the tube partially. Gradually, the opening is obstructed completely, and breathing takes place entirely around the tube, the trachea being much larger than the tube. If no respiratory embarrassment occurs during the ensuing 24 hours, the tracheotomy tube is removed, and the wound is closed and covered with a sterile dressing. The tray containing the duplicate tracheotomy tube and obturator should be kept at the bedside until respiratory difficulty has subsided completely. Continued observation is imperative always during this period.

ACUTE LARYNGOTRACHEOBRONCHITIS

ETIOLOGY

The causative organism is variable d sometimes not determined. Hemoic streptococci, influenza bacilli and eumococci at times appear to be re-

sponsible, but frequently no bacteria other than those normally expected in the pharynx can be isolated. Infection with a virus has been suspected and recently proved. The disease appears to depend more upon the low resistance of the individual child than upon the specific infecting agent. It is much more common in infancy and early childhood than at later ages.

SYMPTOMS

The symptoms depend in part on the severity of the infection, but in larger measure on the character of the exudate. The temperature tends to be high. The inflamed tissues are edematous, but the edema does not cause special difficulty except as it may affect the vocal cords and the region immediately below them and produce obstruction to respiration. In all instances the inflammatory exudate is a major cause of symptoms. It is so thick and viscous that it cannot be coughed up. The normal reflex for cough is incited by movement of foreign material in the respiratory tract. If the material is exudate that is too thick to move, no cough occurs. Thus the cough reflex may be abolished. Respiratory obstruction may occur from accumulation of the exudate. A large bronchus may become plugged with exudate, and so atelectasis of the part of the lung supplied by the bronchus results. Air passing partial obstruction causes stridor. Dyspnea and cyanosis also result from respiratory obstruction. The mortality is high. Death may be due to respiratory obstruction, to secondary pneumonia, to general sepsis or to exhaustion.

TREATMENT

Immediate treatment includes full dosage with one of the broad-spectrum antibiotics such as oxytetracycline (Terramycin), tetracycline (Achromycin) or chloramphenicol and placement of the child in an atmosphere saturated with water vapor. How much additional treatment is given will depend upon individual circumstances and often requires astute clinical judgment. The administration of oxygen may give immediate relief of cyanosis and dyspnea but unless the oxygen is well humidified, ultimately it may aggravate the disease by drying out the thick secretions and making it more difficult for the child to cough them up from the respiratory tract. When obstruction at the larynx is severe, tracheotomy must be done. Sometimes the decision to do a tracheotomy is delayed too long; at other times the tracheotomy increases the inspissation of mucus in the bronchial tree and leads to generalized obstruction of bronchioles. Sedatives must be used with caution, and atropine derivatives are contraindicated. When the child is struggling to maintain his respirations, food and oral fluids should be avoided and hydration preserved through subcutaneous infusions.

NURSING CARE

Careful observation is essential in all cases of acute laryngotracheobronchitis. A close watch must be kept for evidence of increasing respiratory obstruction or fatigue. Advancing cyanosis, restlessness, tachycardia, or pyrexia are danger signals which should be called to the attention of the physician. If a tracheotomy has been done, the care of the patient is similar to that described in the preceding section. Even when the tube is in place, continued watchfulness must be maintained to detect evidence of obstruction at the end of the tube or deeper in the branches of the bronchial tree. General reassurance and adept attention to the patient's needs without disturbing him unnecessarily are important factors in maintaining comfort and preserving his strength.

BRONCHITIS

ACUTE BRONCHITIS
Etiology and Symptoms
Acute bronchitis is one of the common illnesses of infancy and childhood. It is somewhat more frequent before 2 or 3 years of age than after. It may be

primary or secondary. When primary, it has much the same causes as the common cold; when secondary, it is a complication of other diseases.

The mild and common variety of acute bronchitis usually has a gradual onset. For the first 2 or 3 days the temperature may be from 100° to 102° F., after which time it becomes approximately normal. Prostration is not great and is of short duration. The appetite is decreased, and lassitude and headache are present. During the first few days the cough is dry and nonproductive. The usual resonance to percussion over the chest remains unchanged. Auscultation reveals rales which are variously described as dry, sonorous and whistling. Moisture gradually appears in the bronchi, and after a few days the rales become bubbling. The cough becomes looser and productive. Cough is often started by change in position. It is increased in the morning on awakening and on first lying down at night. The cough is variable in severity in different cases. In some instances, repeated paroxysms of cough disturb sleep through the night. In the average child bronchitis may be expected to last from 7 to 10 days.

In the more severe type of bronchitis the smaller bronchi are affected. This type is more common in infants than in older children. The rales are smaller, and fever and prostration are greater than in cases of bronchitis of the larger tubes. Pneumonia is much more likely to result. The cough is tight, and dyspnea and cyanosis may be present. In infants, diarrhea and vomiting are common.

In many instances, bronchitis in infancy and early childhood is associated with asthmatic symptoms. In these cases, wheezing respiration is prominent, and difficulty in getting sufficient air into and out of the lungs may be experienced. The asthma disappears along with the symptoms of bronchitis.

Treatment and Nursing Care

Children with bronchitis should be kept in bed while fever is present. In mild bronchitis this period will be only a few days. They should be kept in the house in inclement weather for a week. The clothing need be no different from that worn by the children when they are in health, either day or night. It is desirable to have sufficient clothing to maintain a more or less normal skin temperature.

In the acute stage of bronchitis, inhalations of "steam" with or without the addition of benzoin or creosote are useful. These may be given for periods of from 15 to 30 minutes every 3 to 6 hours, or as ordered. The air of the room should be kept fresh but warm and preferably moist. A good room temperature is from 68° to 70° F.

Drugs other than those used for chemotherapy accomplish little except symptomatically. If cough is distressing, a sedative is indicated. Expectorant mixtures are commonly employed, but their usefulness is doubtful. Chemotherapy is indicated when bronchitis is severe, but usually not when the illness is mild, especially in the older child.

OBSTRUCTIVE BRONCHITIS OF INFANCY (CAPILLARY BRONCHITIS, BRONCHIOLITIS)

Etiology and Symptoms

Sometimes infants are afflicted with a type of diffuse bronchitis which blocks the egress of air from the air sacs and results in overdistention of the lungs, dyspnea, cyanosis and exhaustion. The disorder has no specific bacterial etiology. It may result from any process that produces widespread inflammation of the bronchial mucous membrane in a small infant. The swollen mucosa and the sticky exudate within the lumen of the tiny bronchioles may permit air to enter the alveoli during inspiration, but the orifice closes and traps air within the lung tissue during expiration. Each breath thus adds more to the volume of air within the lung without permitting an equivalent amount to escape. As the lungs become progressively distended many of the alveoli lose their normal function of aerating the blood, since they are unable to exchange the air from which oxygen has already been absorbed. Small areas of pneumonia may also be present within the lungs.

The infant with obstructive bronchitis displays an overdistended chest which collapses poorly on expiration and retracts during inspiration. The respiratory effort is labored, rapid and shallow. As the process advances, varying degrees of cyanosis appear. The infant is restless, has a hacking cough and eats and sleeps poorly. Fever may be absent, intermediate or high. In fatal cases the child dies from exhaustion and inability to oxygenate his blood. Usually the severe stage of the disease is limited to a period of two or three days.

Treatment and Nursing Care

Antibiotic therapy is usually given at once, although its effectiveness is variable. In some instances the response is prompt; in others the drug selected has no effect. Measures similar to those used in laryngotracheobronchitis should be employed to keep the bronchial secretions fluid and as mobile as possible. The air should be completely saturated with moisture, and oxygen must be used cautiously because of its drying effect. Infants often get some relief from being placed on their abdomens, since this fosters better drainage of secretions from the trachea and permits the weight of the back to assist in compressing the distended lungs during expiration. The fluid intake should be maintained by subcutaneous infusion if necessary. Feedings may be omitted temporarily if the infant finds the process of eating too tiring. ACTH, cortisone or meticortin will often give dramatic relief during this alarming disease.

CHRONIC BRONCHITIS

Bronchitis that lingers or recurs over a period of several weeks usually is associated with persisting infection of the paranasal sinuses or adenoids. The symptoms are cough which is worse at night and on arising, and a sensation of tickling in the throat or the trachea. Fever is usually lacking. Treatment must be directed at the focus of infection in the upper respiratory tract. Chronic bronchitis also accompanies other conditions such as cystic fibrosis of the pancreas, asthma and bronchiectasis. The possibility of tuberculosis or heart disease must be entertained when other explanations are lacking.

BRONCHIECTASIS

Bronchiectasis is an extreme form of chronic bronchitis in which branches of the bronchial tree are enlarged or sacculated as a result of the distorting effects of infection which has penetrated beyond the mucous membrane.

Etiology

Certain of the contagious diseases—whooping cough, measles and influenza—are sometimes complicated by a type of pneumonia that damages the structure of the bronchial wall and fosters prolonged infection. Long-standing sinusitis or foreign bodies that have lodged in the bronchi may also be responsible for perpetuating the infection that results in bronchiectasis. No specific bacteria are responsible.

Symptoms

The chief symptom of bronchiectasis is chronic cough that produces purulent sputum. Fever is not usually present except during bouts of superimposed pneumonia or acute sinusitis. If the disease is extensive the breath may be malodorous, the child's nutrition poor, and there may be enlargement of the ends of the fingers and the toes (clubbing). Usually there is some degree of nasal obstruction due to the chronic sinus infection which is a common companion of bronchiectasis.

Diagnosis

The disease should be suspected when there is a history of chronic cough and sputum production over a period of months or years. Ordinary chest roentgenograms do not provide conclusive evidence of the deformity of the bronchial tree. Films taken after the instillation of an opaque oil such as Lipiodol are required to outline accurately the location and the extent of the disease (Fig. 73).

Prognosis and Treatment

With the possible exception of mild bronchiectasis in which the dilatation is slight, the disease tends to progress very slowly because the abnormal structures never can quite clear themselves of the infected secretions. Medical treatment attempts to clear up sinus infection when present and to provide regular systematic drainage of secretions from the bronchial tree by postural drainage. In the latter procedure the child is placed head down over the side of the bed and kept in this position for increasing periods of time several times a day to let the infected portions of lung completely discharge their contents by gravity. Antibiotic therapy and periodic aspiration through a bronchoscope may supplement this procedure. Sometimes antibiotics are given in the form of an aerosol which the child inhales for a quarter or a half hour 2 or 3 times a day. When it is apparent that medical measures are not stemming the progress of the disease, surgical removal of the diseased lobe or lobes of lung must be considered. If the disease involves only the lower portion of one lung, successful operation usually results in a permanent cure.

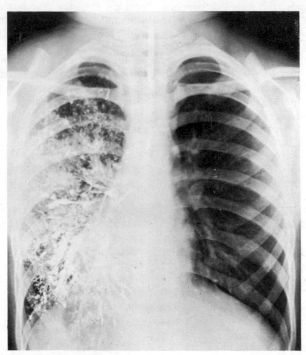

FIG. 73. Bronchiectasis of the lower lobe of the left lung shown by "mapping" the left lung.

PNEUMONIA (PNEUMONITIS)

Pneumonia or pneumonitis is an inflammation of the lung. It may be caused by any pyogenic bacterium or, in some instances, by a virus. It may occur as a primary disease or it may be a secondary or complicating infection in association with some other illness. As a primary infection with pneumococci, the inflammation may be massive in one lobe of a lung and involve all the alveoli of the lobe. In such case the disease is designated as lobar pneumonia. Pneumonia may be disseminated in various parts of the lungs, not be confined to a lobe or not involve a whole lobe completely, and in such case the disease is designated as lobular pneumonia or bronchopneumonia. Regardless of the cause or the type of pneumonia, the function of the lungs is affected in a characteristic manner.

In pneumonia, the affected portions of the lungs are not aerated because the air spaces (alveoli) are filled with exudate. This factor, together with the shallow breathing of this disease, causes poor oxygenation of the blood. Blood that passes through the affected portion remains unaerated and venous in character and later mingles with the blood from the aerated portions of the lungs. Blood passing through the aerated portions cannot be oxygenated sufficiently, even with oxygen therapy, to compensate for the lack of oxygenation in the affected portion. Thus the oxygen saturation of arterial blood is always reduced in pneumonia. The average reduction in lobar pneumonia is approximately 15 per cent. It is greater in bronchopneumonia. Symptoms of anoxia (oxygen want due to defective oxygenation) appear when the blood has reached about 85 per cent oxygen saturation. The mortality rate increases as the saturation decreases. The rate is high with saturation less than 80 per cent.

The shallow breathing of pneumonia is caused in part by the inflammation of the lung, a reflex mechanism. Often, in addition, the breathing is shallow because of pain on breathing, as when pleurisy is present. This effect on the breathing is increased by the effect of anoxia on the respiratory center; the greater the anoxia the more shallow the breathing.

Anoxia produces cyanosis, dyspnea and cerebral symptoms, including delirium and inability to sleep. These symptoms increase as anoxia increases. Anoxia is also a cause of failure of circulation.

Pneumonia occurring as a complication of some other illness is called secondary pneumonia and is of the lobular pneumonic or bronchopneumonic type, regardless of the age of the child. It may be caused by almost any pyogenic bacterium. Primary pneumonia (caused by pneumococci) is of the lobar type in the older child and the adult, but in the infant it is of the lobular type. Lobular pneumonia or bronchopneumonia of the primary type behaves differently from that of the secondary type. However, primary pneumonia of infants resembles secondary pneumonia in many of its symptoms and signs, and by many authors these two conditions are classified in the one group of lobular pneumonia or bronchopneumonia. One reason for considering these two conditions together is that clinically in the early stages of the disease it is not always possible to distinguish one from the other. Some authors choose to classify pneumonia according to the infecting organism. Each classification has its advantages. It is chosen here to discuss pneumonia from the standpoint of its clinical appearance.

PRIMARY BACTERIAL PNEUMONIA

As a primary disease pneumonia is likely to appear suddenly, without warning, or with only mild preceding symptoms, such as those accompanying a common cold. It classifies easily as a communicable disease, although predisposing factors are important. Anything that lowers resistance, such as a chill, predisposes to pneumonia when pneumococci are present. In most instances, primary pneumonia is not caused by organisms commonly found in the mouth. A few types of pneumococci are found only with pneumonia.

Primary pneumonia of infants is a disseminated inflammation in the lungs in contrast with lobar pneumonia, the primary pneumonia of the older child, which is localized and sharply limited in extent. The same conditions of infection produce these two quite different types of lesion. Presumably, the difference is due to immunologic and structural changes with age. The infantile type is found chiefly in the first 2 years after birth, and after this time with decreasing frequency. Lobar pneumonia is seldom observed in the first year, but it occurs with increasing frequency with advancing age and becomes the predominant type after 3 or 4 years of age.

Primary Pneumonia in Infants

Symptoms. The onset of primary pneumonia in infancy is likely to be sudden, with fever and prostration. Vomiting is frequent, and convulsions may occur at the onset. The temperature is high and usually irregular, with fluctuations of from 3° to 4° F. The respirations are rapid, from 60 to 70 or more to the minute, and associated with effort and with retraction of the soft parts of the chest on inspiration. The alae of the nose move laterally with each inspiration. The pulse rate increases to 160 or more and is likely to be irregular. Cough is frequent, persistent and annoying. Moderate diarrhea usually is present. Leukocytosis is high (20,000 to 50,000). Blood culture grows the pneumococcus occasionally and with greater frequency than in lobar pneumonia. In the milder illnesses and without chemotherapy, improvement occurs in approximately a week. In the more severe illnesses, improvement, if it occurs, may not be observed for as much as 2 weeks or even longer.

Certain exceptions to the clinical course as described are to be encountered. On rare occasions a hyperacute form occurs, with stormy onset, high temperature and extreme prostration. Death may occur in from 12 to 48 hours after the onset and before any physical signs have developed in the chest. In some instances of primary pneumonia in infancy severe enough to cause death, the temperature may remain low. This type of illness occurs especially in young, delicate and malnourished infants. Also in delicate infants, pneumonia, although it may have the usual course at first, may spread from one area to another, thus prolonging the illness, increasing prostration, causing emaciation and usually terminating in death. This course is not so likely with the use of modern chemotherapy.

Diagnosis. The correct diagnosis is often suspected by an experienced person merely from observation of the infant's respiratory behavior. Physical examination of the chest discloses areas of moist rales in the involved portions of lung. When the patches of consolidation are large enough there may be typical changes in the quality of the breath sounds heard through a stethoscope. Roentgen examination is frequently conclusive, but if the consolidated areas are small, interpretation of the shadows which they cast is sometimes difficult. The etiologic diagnosis is important as a guide to proper antibiotic therapy. Cultures of the nose, the throat, or sputum when it is available, always should be made. Blood cultures may yield the invading organism in some instances. Once isolated, the organism should be tested for sensitivity to the various antibiotics in order to speed selection of the most effective drug.

Complications and Prognosis. Otitis media and fibrinous pleurisy are common complications of pneumonia; usually they are not serious and they respond to the treatment being given for the pneumonia itself. Rarely, an infant develops meningitis, peritonitis or empyema. These serious complications increase the mortality of the disease and require special measures of treatment as described under the sections that deal with them.

Primary pneumonia of infancy is a serious disease if it remains untreated or is treated inadequately. Before modern antibiotic treatment was available the mortality rates ranged as high as 30 to 50 per cent. The outlook is very much better today, but pneumonia in the small infant is not a disease to be regarded lightly.

Treatment and Nursing Care. Most of the cases of primary pneumonia in infancy are caused by pneumococci or hemolytic streptococci. These organisms respond promptly to penicillin, which should be given intramuscularly in full dosage. Other types of antibiotic may be necessary when the pneumonia is shown to be due to organisms other than the above or when a resistant strain is encountered. Ordinarily, if treatment is effective the infant's temperature will approach normal levels within 24 hours. A delay in response beyond 48 hours should raise the suspicion that the wrong antibiotic has been selected. Immediate testing of the sensitivity of organisms isolated from infants with pneumonia will greatly assist in directing the choice of drug.

Oxygen is administered when there is cyanosis or other evidence of anoxia. Methods of administration and nursing care are described in the next chapter.

In a large measure the nursing care of the infant with pneumonia is symptomatic and geared to his individual requirements. He requires rest and relief of his physical and psychological discomforts. Nursing procedures should be organized in such a way as to disturb the infant as little as possible. Frequently, feedings are omitted until the expected improvement from antibiotic therapy has taken place. Usually fluids are administered by mouth when possible; by subcutaneous infusion when necessary. The infant's position may influence his comfort to some extent. He may be more comfortable in a semierect posture or when lying with the affected lung down.

Abdominal distention from paralytic ileus is a common and distressing aspect of pneumonia in infants. It is both painful and embarrassing to the respiratory effort and should be relieved by enemas or by the external application of turpentine stupes. Turpentine and sweet oil are used in a proportion of 3 cc. of turpentine to 30 cc. of sweet oil. The two ingredients should be mixed thoroughly, and the mixture should be applied to the skin of the abdomen with cotton balls before and during the procedure. The warmth of the wet flannel stupes should be tested on the back of the hand before they are applied to the abdomen. Oiled silk and dry flannel should be applied over the wet stupes. The wet flannel should be changed every 3 minutes for a period of from 15 to 20 minutes. During the procedure a rectal tube should be kept in place to facilitate the passage of flatus. Children burn easily, and the condition of the skin should be observed very carefully each time the procedure is repeated. Oiling the skin after the stupe has been completed tends to keep the skin in good condition.

Temperatures up to 104° F. usually require no special measures for their control. Excessive fever is best controlled by hydrotherapy or by placing the child on a cool water mattress. Hydrotherapy is useful also for restlessness, nervousness and insomnia. Since pneumonia is a communicable disease, isolation precautions must be taken.

Lobar Pneumonia

Symptoms and Diagnosis. Lobar pneumonia is abrupt in its onset, any preceding indisposition being not more than a few hours in duration. Vomiting is frequent among the symptoms of onset, and, especially in young children, diarrhea is common. The temperature elevation is rapid, sometimes rapid enough to cause a chill or a convulsion, although chills are much more frequent in adults than in children. The temperature rises to 104° or more and remains elevated continuously with relatively little remission throughout the course of the marked symptoms. Along with the temperature rise, the pulse and the respiration rates increase, the respiration out of proportion to the other two. The nasal alae move laterally with each inspiration. Very quickly after the onset the child appears to be acutely ill, becomes apathetic and weak and loses his appetite. Restlessness and marked thirst are common. Cough appears a day or two after onset and persists, although seldom is it annoying.

When chemotherapy is not used, the disease runs a rather typical course. Although the child may be somewhat more comfortable after 4 or 5 days, little change in the symptoms is to be observed until the crisis, which may be expected about the 6th or the 7th day. Sometimes the temperature drops temporarily and briefly the day preceding the crisis. This drop has been termed the pseudocrisis. The crisis represents termination of the acute symptoms. The temperature drops rapidly to normal, as do also the pulse and the respiration rates. The child becomes comfortable, loses his apathy, regains his appetite and recovers rapidly and completely.

The physical signs of lobar pneumonia consist chiefly of those produced by a massive area of consolidation in a lung. With typical involvement of an entire lobe, dullness on percussion and tubular breathing on auscultation over the affected lobe are easy to determine. Rales are seldom prominent. After the crisis, however, when the exudate is liquefying, rales are characteristically present. Early in the illness the consolidation may involve only part of a lobe, perhaps only the periphery. In such case, when no continuity of consolidated lung between the stethoscope and a large bronchus exists, tubular breathing is not heard. Without a roentgenogram the diagnosis of pneumonia or at least its localization may be difficult.

The diagnosis of lobar pneumonia is accomplished in the same way as that described for primary pneumonia of infants. Typical findings of lobar pneumonia almost always mean that the infecting agent is a pneumococcus. Sometimes roentgen examination will disclose a shadow which cannot be detected by physical examination; conversely, the physical findings may precede the appearance of consolidation which is visible in the roentgenogram.

Prognosis. Uncomplicated lobar pneumonia in the child of 3 years or over carries a very good prognosis. Even before antibiotics were available the mortality was as low as 3 to 5 per cent. Today the response to therapy is almost invariably prompt, and few children succumb unless the disease is complicated by myocarditis, empyema or meningitis.

Treatment and Nursing Care. This differs in no essential point from that given for primary pneumonia of infants.

SECONDARY BACTERIAL PNEUMONIA (BRONCHOPNEUMONIA, LOBULAR PNEUMONIA)

Secondary pneumonia is lobular, or bronchopneumonia and is similar in many respects to primary pneumonia of infants. It may occur at any age as a complication of any acute illness. It is a more frequent complication in infancy than in late childhood. It is especially frequent as a complication of measles, pertussis, diphtheria, influenza and bronchitis.

Etiology

Any one or several of a variety of organisms may be found associated with the disease as the cause. In a large measure, secondary pneumonia is caused by the ordinary bacteria of the pharynx and the upper respiratory tract which gain entrance to the lungs by aspiration or during inspiration. Hemolytic streptococcic pneumonia, such as occurs in measles, must be considered as communicable.

Symptoms

The onset of secondary pneumonia is usually gradual, with subsequent increase in the severity of the illness. The amount of fever varies with the severity of the illness and the general condition of the child. In general, it tends to be high and irregular or intermittent in type. Prostration is present. The symptoms and signs are the same as those described for primary pneumonia of infants. Clinically, secondary pneumonia differs from primary pneumonia chiefly in its persistence. In the absence of modern chemotherapy, the course of secondary pneumonia tends to be protracted and, as a rule, lasts for a period of from 3 to 6 weeks. Sometimes during this period new areas of inflammation develop while older ones may be subsiding. The symptoms end by lysis in nearly all instances of spontaneous recovery. Recovery is slow, and relapses are relatively frequent. Pleurisy is seldom a striking feature in secondary pneumonia, except when streptococci are the cause. Occasionally, streptococcic empyema occurs.

Prognosis

Secondary pneumonia is a much more serious disease than primary pneumonia. Several factors contribute to its relatively bad prognosis. Many of the victims are already weak and poorly nourished from the effects of a protracted illness or from convalescence following a surgical procedure. Their resistance is consequently poor. If the original illness is characterized by vomiting or immobility, some of the pulmonary changes may actually be due to lipid pneumonia from aspiration of milk or to atelectasis from failure to clear the secretions from the bronchi. The type of secondary pneumonia which follows acute contagious diseases, such as pertussis, measles and influenza, may respond adequately to antibiotic therapy but may invade the structure of the lung to set the stage for bronchiectasis as described in a preceding section. The bacterial etiology of secondary pneumonia is often mixed or composed of organisms which are less easily influenced by the available antibiotics.

Treatment and Nursing Care

The same measures are required as in the case of primary pneumonia. Some prevention of secondary pneumonia is possible if its occurrence is anticipated. Chronically ill or immobile patients should be isolated from contact with respiratory infections among the patients around them. They should have their positions changed frequently to avoid imperfect ventilation of portions of the lung. Sometimes prophylactic administration of antibiotics is warranted when the risk of secondary pneumonia is great.

SPECIAL TYPES OF PNEUMONIA

Staphylococcus Pneumonia

Pneumonia that is due to infection with the staphylococcus is mainly a disease of small infants. Occasionally, it is seen as a complication of staphylococcus bacteremia in the older child or the adult. The disease is characterized by a tendency to form multiple abscesses throughout the lungs. Even in small infants the contents of these abscesses may be apparent in purulent sputum or vomitus. Abscesses that form on the surface of the lung often create an empyema or pneumothorax by discharging their contents into the pleural cavity and at the same time establishing a communication between the pleural cavity and the bronchial tree. The diagnosis is made by culture of sputum and by the discovery of characteristic abscess shadows in the roentgenogram of the chest. Treatment is complicated by the fact that increasing numbers of staphylococci are becoming resistant to the older antibiotic drugs such as penicillin. The newer antibiotics, such as erythromycin or chloromycetin, are more regularly effective than penicillin, but the sensitivity of each individual strain of staphylococcus must be tested in order to guide treatment. When empyema is present, the mechanical principles described in the next section should be used. Untreated, staphylococcus pneumonia is almost universally fatal. Even with early and adequate treatment by antibiotic drugs the mortality is likely to approach 25 per cent. Small infants may die before the nature of the disease is recognized.

Primary Atypical Pneumonia

This is a type of pneumonia, presumably caused by a virus, which produces symptoms of cough, fever and general malaise. Its course is likely to be protracted to 2 or 3 weeks in length, but the child is seldom alarmingly ill, and the prognosis is universally good. Diagnosis is made by exclusion of bacterial pneumonia and by the discovery of various types of pulmonary consolidation in the roentgenogram of the chest, often in the absence of physical signs in the chest. The treatment is entirely symptomatic. Chlortetracycline (Aureomycin) has been considered as effective in shortening the course of the illness, but its worth is debated. There are no complications of this type of pneumonia.

Kerosene Pneumonia

Small children in the toddling age occasionally swallow kerosene which is carelessly left around the home. Frequently, an extensive pneumonia ensues due to the irritant effect of kerosene which has been aspirated or is being excreted from the body by way of the lungs. Immediately after ingestion of kerosene the child may feel well except for nausea. Respiratory symptoms and fever appear during the first 48 hours and pursue a variable course, depending upon the amount of kerosene taken. In mild cases there may be little or no pulmonary irritation and no fever. When large amounts are taken and retained, hyperpyrexia, dyspnea and convulsions may ensue. The roentgenogram of the chest usually demonstrates large areas of pulmonary consolidation extending out from the central portion of the lung fields. In the absence of hyperpyrexia and convulsions, the child usually recovers completely after a few days of dyspnea and cough. Diagnosis can be made from the characteristic odor of kerosene. Early treatment probably demands gastric lavage to recover as much of the kerosene as possible from the stomach. Treatment of the pneumonia, once it is present, is mainly symptomatic and directed at control of hyperpyrexia.

Lipid Pneumonia

Lipid pneumonia is pneumonitis produced by oils or fatty material aspirated into the lung. It occurs chiefly in small, weak infants, seldom in older children, unless the cough reflex is diminished. The aspirated fat may be nose drops, cod-liver oil, mineral oil or fat from the milk formula that has been vomited. Fats of animal origin have more severe effects than those of vegetable origin. A very few fats have no ill effect; for example, the poppyseed oil used in the preparation of iodized oil for diagnostic purposes.

Lipid pneumonia tends to occur in the posterior dependent portions of the lung, more often on the right side. The onset is insidious, often without symptoms. In such instances it is diagnosed by x-ray examination. Small infants develop dry, nonproductive cough and rapid respirations. They usually show impairment of growth. Older children also have chronic cough and, in addition, are subject to repeated attacks of bronchitis. Occasionally, bronchiectasis results. Evidences of inflammation, such as fever and leukocytosis, vary according to the amount of associated infection. Often no infection is present.

Diagnosis is made chiefly by exclusion. Always more of a lesion is present than is indicated by physical examina-

tion. The distribution of the lesion x-ray examination and its chronicity a helpful in diagnosis.

No special treatment exists. T milder forms may persist for as long a year before recovery occurs. Seve forms produced by some of the anim fats may become complicated by a scess or bronchiectasis and persist for much longer time.

Prevention is highly important. O nose drops should not be used in i fancy. The giving of oils to young weak infants must be done with cautio care being taken to see that they a swallowed.

PLEURISY

Pleurisy is an inflammation of the linings of the pleural cavity, i.e., the inside of the chest wall and the outer surface of the lung. It usually produces pain in the chest on respiration. Sometimes the pain is referred to the shoulder or to the abdomen. If the accumulation of inflammatory exudate is large, there may be embarrassment of the respirations and cyanosis.

The accumulation of exudates within the pleural space is seen in a wide variety of conditions. The term pleural effusion is used when the exudate is bacteriologically sterile. Effusion may be seen during nephrosis and with heart failure. It is rarely found in other conditions such as nephritis and over the lesions of pulmonary metastatic tumors. A variety of pleural effusion which is not really sterile is seen with early tuberculosis. During the course of pneumonia, fibrin is often deposited upon the surface of the lungs and produces pleural pain with pneumonia caused by staphylococci or hemolytic streptococci, or when adequate treatment of pneumococcus pneumonia is delayed, significant collections of infected purulent exudate may accumulate in the pleural space, forming an empyema that requires special attention.

EMPYEMA

Genesis

The onset of empyema after pneu monia usually is not very obviou Pneumonia may end by crisis, and the the temperature gradually rises agai or the temperature may not fall at th time recovery from pneumonia is to b expected. At first the pus in the pleur sac is thin. It increases in amount an allows the lung on the affected side t collapse increasingly. Finally, it cause the heart to be displaced toward th opposite side of the chest. As the flui increases in quantity, increasing cardia and respiratory difficulty occurs. Th child lies on the affected side. With drawal of the pus by aspiration is de sirable to relieve these symptoms. I the course of several days, in the cas of pneumococcic infection, the pus be comes thick, often so thick that it is no easily withdrawn through a needle.

Diagnosis

Increased dullness on percussion anc altered breath sounds on auscultatior are present in empyema. These shoulc lead one to suspect that empyema i present. Roentgenograms are very help ful and often make the diagnosis almos ertain. The diagnosis is made definitely y removal of pus through an aspirating needle.

Course and Prognosis

Pus present in the pleural cavity in arge quantity is not likely to be absorbed, although in some instances it may be. Rarely, it may drain spontaneously by making a way for itself through the soft tissues at some point between the ribs or through the lung tissue into bronchus. Thus, in some cases empyema may terminate by spontaneous recovery. On the other hand, death may occur from wasting which accompanies chronic infection, from the spread of infection to the pericardium, or from compression of lung space to the point of insufficiency. Continuance of underlying pneumonia also may be a cause f death. The mortality rate from empyema is much higher in infancy than in later childhood. Also, it is higher in those cases in which radical surgical treatment is undertaken early than when more conservative early treatment is used. This is especially true in infancy and in those cases of pneumococcic empyema in which the pus has not yet become thick.

Treatment and Nursing Care

The chemotherapy that has been used through the course of preceding pneumonia should be continued. Otherwise, the early treatment, especially in infancy, should consist of nothing more radical than withdrawal of pus by aspiration. In many instances such treatment will be followed by absorption of the remaining pus and complete recovery. Recovery may be hastened by injecting from 50,000 to 100,000 units of penicillin in saline into the pleural cavity once or twice daily after aspiration. When empyema persists despite these measures, surgical drainage is indicated. Surgical drainage through the chest wall is greatly preferable to spontaneous drainage through a bronchus,

since the latter may lead to chronic pneumonia and bronchiectasis.

Sometimes pus is not generally distributed throughout the pleural cavity but is encapsulated between the parietal and the visceral layers of pleura. In such case also the treatment is the same as that already discussed. If the empyema is wholly interlobar, conservative treatment without operation is usually indicated.

Thoracentesis may be done for diagnosis, for relief of dyspnea caused by pressure of fluid, for the obtaining of exudate for culture or for the instilling of penicillin into the pleural cavity. Sterile equipment required for thoracentesis consists of: 50-cc. syringe, 2-cc. syringe, hypodermic needles, 3-way stopcock with short piece of rubber tubing attached, aspirating needles, procaine 1 per cent, curved clamp, lumbar puncture drape sheet, cotton balls, small gauze squares, graduated receptacle, gloves and medication as ordered by the physician. Unsterile equipment consists of a skin preparation tray, culture media, test tubes and adhesive plaster. Epinephrine should be ready for use in case of need.

One of several positions may be required for successful thoracentesis. The child may be placed in a sitting position with his arms and trunk brought forward, or he may be placed on his unaffected side in a semirecumbent position. Whatever the position, care must be taken to ensure maximum comfort for the child. An overbed table and pillow to lean on may lessen exertion and provide a degree of comfort when a sitting position is desired for an older child. One nurse will be required to hold the child in the desired position, to prepare him for the procedure, to give him emotional support and to observe his response to treatment. A second nurse will be needed to assist with the skin preparation and to collect specimens of aspirated fluid. During the procedure the nurse should watch for changes in the child's respiration and pulse rates, for changes in his color and for any increase in coughing.

After the treatment the child should be kept warm and observed for changes in his general condition. Charting should include a description and the amount of the aspirated fluid, amount and kind of medication instilled, any symptoms of shock or syncope and the child's physical and psychological response to the treatment.

SITUATIONS FOR FURTHER STUDY

1. What help do parents need to prevent common colds in their children during the period of infancy and childhood?

2. What feelings do you think a hospitalized infant experiences when he is hospitalized for laryngotracheobronchitis? How can a nurse eliminate feelings of anxiety? Why is constant attendance of a mother or a nurse essential in his care?

3. In what diseases might a tracheotomy be necessary? How would the nursing care of those patients differ from the care necessary for a child who had had a tracheotomy after a foreign body had been removed from the respiratory tract?

4. A 3-year-old child with papilloma of the larynx required a tracheotomy. After the child had been hospitalized for a period of 6 weeks, the physician recommended that he be discharged from the hospital with the tracheotomy tube in place. What help would the child's mother require to take care of him at home? How could you relieve his mother's fears and build up her confidence in her capacity to take care of her child at home?

BIBLIOGRAPHY

Bellam, G.: Tonsillectomy without fear, Am. J. Nursing 51:244, 1950.

Conley, J. J.:Tracheotomy, Am. J. Nursing 52:1078, 1952.

Cutler, H.: Otitis media, Am. J. Nursing 53:573, 1953.

Gibson, F.: Laryngotracheobronchitis, Am. J. Nursing 52:174, 1952.

Hall, J. T., and Sadler, J. B.: Nursing care in tonsillectomy, Am. J. Nursing 47:537, 1947.

Lewis, D. K.: Deafness, Am. J. Nursing 52:575, 1952.

Neffson, A.: Acute Laryngotracheobronchitis, New York, Grune, 1949.

Seitock, B. B.: The deaf child, Am. J. Nursing 56:594, 1956.

CHAPTER EIGHTEEN

Diseases of the Circulatory System

ANATOMY AND PHYSIOLOGY

The circulatory system consists of the heart and the blood vessels. The latter include the arteries, which carry the blood away from the heart, the capillaries, which are very small and numerous and connect the terminal branches of the arteries with the veins, and the veins, which carry blood back to the heart. The capillaries are the points of exchange between the blood stream and the tissues. All other divisions of the circulatory system serve only to maintain circulation of the blood through the capillaries.

The circulating blood has two great circuits: one of these is the pulmonary; the other, the systemic circulation. The heart is divided into two parts, known as the right and the left hearts. Each acts independently of the other, although they act synchronously. The right heart receives blood which is returning from the body tissues and pumps it into the capillaries of the lungs for aeration. The blood returns from the lungs to the left heart, which then propels it to the various parts of the body (Fig. 74).

In the normal child, blood which is returning from the body by way of the great veins (venae cavae) and fills the right side of the heart and the branches of the pulmonary artery, is venous or unoxygenated blood (dotted line in the diagrams). Its relatively low oxygen content gives it a dark purple color. Once the blood has passed through the lung capillaries and becomes fully oxygenated, it is a bright red in color. Oxygenated blood (solid lines in the diagrams) normally is found in the pulmonary veins, the left side of the heart and all the branches of the aorta and the arterial system.

The heart, the arteries and the veins are made up of involuntary muscle surrounded by a supportive layer of fibrous tissue and lined by a thin membrane composed of endothelium. In the heart, these divisions are spoken of as myocardium, pericardium and endocardium, respectively. The integrity of each is essential for the normal functioning of the heart.

The capillaries consist of the endo-

403

thelial layer alone. Their walls are very thin and are permeable to water, electrolytes and other small molecules of the blood but not to the plasma proteins and cellular elements.

HEART CHAMBERS

Each side of the heart is divided into 2 chambers, the auricle and the ventricle. The former receives blood from the veins and serves as a reservoir for the supply of the ventricle. The latter serves to propel the blood through the arteries, the capillaries and the veins. The endocardium is so arranged that it forms 2 valves in each side of the heart. One of these is between the auricle and the ventricle; the other, between the ventricle and its artery. These valves serve to prevent backward flow of blood.

ACTION OF THE HEART

The action of the heart is proportioned to the amount of work that it must do. When a person is at rest, the heart contracts with a rate and a degree of force exactly sufficient to supply the tissues adequately with fresh blood. If the requirements of the tissues are increased by activity, the heart can increase its output by increasing either the rate or the strength of contraction. Usually it does both. The rate is the first to change; then the cardiac muscle re-

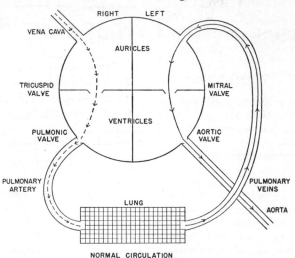

Fig. 74. Diagram of the normal circulation of blood. Unoxygenated, or venous, blood is indicated by the dotted line from its entrance into the heart through the vena cava, thence into the right auricle, through the tricuspid valve into the right ventricle, out the pulmonic valve into the pulmonary artery and thence into the lungs, where it becomes oxygenated. The solid line indicates the course of the oxygenated blood through the pulmonary veins, the left auricle, the mitral valve, the left ventricle, the aortic valve and the aorta. The last distributes oxygenated blood to all the body tissues, where it loses oxygen in the capillary circulation, is collected by the veins and returned to the heart by way of the vena cava for recirculation. (Adapted from Cassels, D. E., and Morse, M.: Blood volume in congenital heart disease, J. Pediat. 31:485)

sponds with greater strength of contraction. Repeated demand for increased blood flow leads to strengthening of the cardiac musculature, so that it needs less increase in rate when called on for extra work. In athletes, the heart may become slightly larger than in an untrained person. This type of enlargement is known as cardiac hypertrophy and is a form of compensation or adjustment to environmental requirements. The rate of the heart beat is governed largely by the autonomic nervous system, while the force is more inherently a myocardial function. Less work is required to propel blood through the pulmonary circulation than through the systemic. As a result, the left heart is much more muscular than the right.

Diseases of the heart may be considered in relation to the effect on the heart and to the way in which they modify the heart's function. Acute cardiac diseases may be classified as myocarditis, endocarditis or pericarditis, depending on the type of tissue chiefly affected. Often, all are involved simultaneously. Seldom does endocarditis or pericarditis occur without co-existing myocarditis.

DIAGNOSTIC PROCEDURES

Several special methods of examination are now in use which yield information about the anatomic and the physiologic state of the heart—information which in cases of congenital malformations is often essential to an exact diagnosis and to the decision to attempt surgical amelioration. These procedures are highly technical ones; only the general type of information sought can be discussed here.

Fluoroscopy

By watching the action of the heart under a fluoroscopic x-ray screen, its size, position and contours can be determined. In addition, the degree to which various portions of the outline of the heart pulsate and the amount of disten-

tion of the auricles and of the pulmonary vessels can be observed. Knowing the normal appearance of the heart, often abnormal increases in size or activity of the various chambers of the heart can be detected. Conversely, too, the lack of normal pulsation or distention also can be detected. Sometimes barium is given by mouth while the child is observed under the fluoroscope. By this method the normal indentation of the esophagus by the aorta and abnormal indentations by constricting vessels, by a right aortic arch or by a distended left auricle or ventricle can be seen. Similar information is obtainable from ordinary roentgen films of the chest, but the motion of the various portions of the heart and the great vessels cannot be observed.

Angiocardiography

In this technic the actual course of the blood through the heart and the great vessels is visualized by injecting radiopaque material into the veins and following its course through the heart by roentgenograms taken at brief intervals and in specially determined projections. Abnormal communications between various portions of the circulation may be detected in this fashion. Since the child must be held still and in proper position, usually it is necessary to use a general anesthetic.

Aortography

In this technic the radiopaque material is injected in a retrograde fashion through a needle inserted into the left brachial artery. The objectives are to outline the region of the branching of the left subclavian artery from the aorta and to determine the presence of a coarctation of the aorta, an open ductus arteriosus or both.

Cardiac Catheterization

With the child anesthetized, the right brachial vein is dissected out, and a small radiopaque catheter is inserted into it and pushed up into the right auricle. By manipulation under the fluoroscope, the tip of the catheter can be directed into the right auricle, the right ventricle and the pulmonary artery. Readings of the pressure in each of these locations are made, and blood samples are obtained for chemical examination to determine the degree of oxygenation of the blood. When congenital abnormalities are present, such as an opening in the septum between the two auricles, sometimes it is possible to demonstrate these communications by probing with the tip of the catheter.

Electrocardiography

The electrocardiogram measures differences in the electric potentials of various leads taken from the heart. It often gives information about the relative activity of the 2 ventricles and about the state of health of the cardiac muscle. These inferences are drawn from an analysis of the tracings obtained. The terms "left axis deviation" or "left ventricular preponderance" indicate a relatively more vigorous activity of the left ventricle compared with the right.

MALFORMATIONS OF THE HEART
(CONGENITAL HEART DISEASE)

In early embryonic life the heart consists of a straight tube which receives blood at one end and pumps it out at the other. Through a remarkable and complicated series of changes, the tube folds upon itself, forms internal septa and valves, modifies its connections with the large blood vessels which enter and leave it and transforms into the complex organ which we recognize as the fully developed heart. Nearly all the stages in this transition are completed within the first 2 to 3 months of embryonic growth. Any interference with their normal sequence of full completion results in a malformed heart.

Undoubtedly, there are many conditions of the mother which may interfere with cardiac development. Thus far, only one—rubella (German measles) during the first trimester of pregnancy—has been definitely incriminated as a cause of abnormal development.

A great variety of malformations of the heart are known. Many of these have little clinical significance, since they either do not interfere with the child's welfare or are so serious that the newborn infant is able to survive only a short time. A few types are important because they permit survival yet interfere with the child's general welfare. During recent years the technical pro-

cedures described above have been developed. They permit accurate diagnosis of many types of congenital heart disease and surgical amelioration of some. Dramatic technics are being developed which permit operations even within the opened heart. By lowering body temperature (hypothermia) the patient's metabolic rate is reduced so that anoxia is less dangerous to vital tissues. Various devices are used as temporary pumps while the heart is excluded from the circulation and opened up. Understandably, such procedures require a great deal of complicated apparatus and the close collaboration of a large team of specialists.

The classification of cardiac abnormalities is based upon their capacity to produce cyanosis. Cyanosis results from the contamination of arterial blood circulating in the systemic arteries by venous blood which enters through an abnormal channel.

ACYANOTIC CONGENITAL HEART DISEASE

A few types of malformation of the cardiovascular system are incapable of producing cyanosis because there is no abnormal communication between the pulmonary and the systemic circulations. If symptoms are present they are due to abnormalities in the course or the caliber of the vessels leaving the heart.

Coarctation of the Aorta

Coarctation is a narrowing of the aorta in a short segment just distal to the point of emergence of the left subclavian artery. The severity of symptoms depends upon the degree of constriction. When the narrowing is slight, the disorder may go unrecognized until late in childhood or adult life, when hypertension is found in the arms and low blood pressure in the legs. Sometimes the child will fail to grow at the proper rate or will be unable to play normally, due to weakness in the legs. Severe degrees of constriction place a burden upon the heart, which is trying to pump blood through the narrow channel. Cardiac failure and death may result during early infancy.

The diagnosis is suspected from the observation of discrepant blood pressures—high in the arms and low in the legs. It can be confirmed by visualization of the aorta by roentgenogram after injection of radiopaque material (aortogram).

Treatment requires the surgical excision of the constricted segment and anastomosis of the free ends thus produced. Whenever possible, it should be performed in early childhood, since the adult cardiovascular system does not tolerate the necessary manipulations so readily.

Other Types of Acyanotic Malformation

Reduction in the caliber of the aorta may take place closer to the heart than in the usual site of coarctation.

Hypoplasia of the Aorta. This malformation is a general narrowing of the aortic arch.

Subaortic Stenosis. This is a more localized narrowing directly below the emergence of the aorta from the heart. Neither of these conditions is amenable to surgical correction.

Aortic Valvular Stenosis and Pulmonic Stenosis. When there is isolated narrowing of the aortic or the pulmonary valves alone, recently developed instruments and technics are available for enlarging the passageway through these valves. These conditions are known as congenital aortic valvular stenosis and pulmonic stenosis.

Double Aortic Arch. A double aortic arch may occur, with the two branches encircling the esophagus, the trachea or both in such a way that swallowing or respiration is compromised. The diagnosis can be made by careful roentgen examination with opaque dye in the esophagus and the trachea. Surgical relief of symptoms may be obtained by dividing one of the encircling branches of the aorta.

POTENTIALLY CYANOTIC CONGENITAL HEART DISEASE

In the potentially cyanotic group of malformations an abnormal communication exists between the pulmonary and the systemic circulations, but the pressure relations are such that the blood flows through this shunt from the arterial side to the venous side so that no cyanosis results. Under unusual stress, such as superimposed disease or myocardial failure, it is impossible for the flow in the shunt to reverse its direction and produce cyanosis by admixing venous blood with arterial. When reversal of flow occurs, it is usually a terminal phenomenon; consequently, this group of disorders also is called the late cyanotic type of congenital heart disease.

Patent Ductus Arteriosus

The ductus arteriosus is a fetal connection between the pulmonary artery and the aorta. Ordinarily, this channel spontaneously constricts, closes its lumen and atrophies shortly after birth. In some infants this change fails to take place, and the fetal communication between the pulmonary and the systemic circulations persists. Symptoms result when the opening is large, because there is leakage of blood from the aorta back into the pulmonary circulation (Fig. 75). No cyanosis results, but the volume of blood which the heart must pump in order to meet the requirements of the peripheral tissues is increased. A small channel has no effect upon growth or physical activity, for the heart can hypertrophy enough to meet the slightly increased burden. When the volume of blood flowing through the ductus is large, both physical activity and growth may be hampered.

Diagnosis. The diagnosis is suspected from the presence of a typical machinerylike murmur over the pulmonary artery. It is confirmed by the presence of a low diastolic blood pressure and by various roentgen maneuvers which dem-

onstrate enlargement of the pulmonary artery and increased blood flow to the lungs or by actual visualization of the ductus itself after injection of opaque dye (angiocardiography).

Surgical Treatment. The surgical treatment consists of ligation and division of the abnormal channel. Usually it is performed after the age of 2 or 3 years. Even if symptoms are lacking, the ductus usually is closed, because its continued patency carries a risk of subacute bacterial endocarditis. In skilled hands the operative mortality is very low, and relief of symptoms can be confidently expected.

Nursing Care. Usually the child with a patent ductus arteriosus comes into the hospital several days prior to opera-

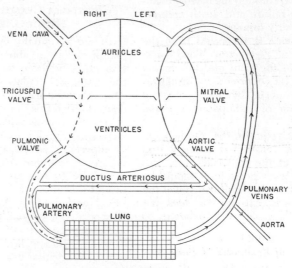

PATENT DUCTUS ARTERIOSUS

Fig. 75. Diagram of the circulation in patent ductus arteriosus. This is similar to that in Figure 74 except that oxygenated blood in the aorta can leak back through the open ductus into the pulmonary artery, thus adding to the volume of blood circulating through the lungs. Cyanosis does not develop, because the pressure relations are such that the blood in the ductus flows from the oxygenated side to the unoxygenated side, except under unusual circumstances. (Adapted from Cassels, D. E., and Morse, M.: Blood volume in congenital heart disease, J. Pediat. 31:485)

tion for diagnostic tests and preparation. The nurse to whom he is assigned needs to establish a friendly, trusting relationship with the child to help him adapt to hospitalization and to prepare him for all the new experiences that he will have both before and after operation. Usually the child is placed in oxygen for the first 24 hours after operation. He and his parents need to see the tent and the chest Wangensteen suction apparatus which will be used postoperatively and to know why they are necessary to keep him comfortable. During the preoperative period the child is guarded carefully against infections, is served a nutritious diet and is encouraged to take an adequate amount of fluids.

A sedative is given, and a blood pressure reading is taken before the child goes to the operating room. After the permanent ligature or division is made, blood pressure reading discloses a rise in diastolic pressure. Blood pressure remains high for 4 to 5 days postoperatively and then stabilizes at a new level.

While the child is in the operating room, the necessary equipment for postoperative care is assembled—oxygen tent, chest Wangensteen suction and a suction machine to aspirate mucus from the respiratory passages. In the first 48 hours postoperatively, the nurse must be alert for evidence of bleeding and respiratory distress. She also must keep careful watch of the suction apparatus to see that no kinking of or pressure on the tube occurs. If there is kinking or pressure on the tubing, clot formation may occur and prevent drainage. The effectiveness of the drainage apparatus also must be noted. If there is regular fluctuation of the fluid level which corresponds to the respiratory rate, it is indicative of a patent drainage system. The amount of water in the chest Wangensteen apparatus also should be noted. If the water runs to a low level, the doctor should be notified.

When chest suction is not used, vigilance to detect signs of respiratory distress is imperative. Dyspnea arises from a collection of fluid in the pleural cavity. Often, dyspnea is relieved by raising the head of the bed and by turning the child onto the affected side. If dyspnea is not relieved by a change in position, and the pulse and the respiration rates remain high, the nurse should notify the doctor and prepare immediately for thoracentesis.

The child should be turned every 2 hours and kept comfortable with sedatives, fluids and food as tolerated, and supportive measures should be taken to relieve his anxiety pertaining to all that he sees going on around him. Hospital personnel will view him frequently to check the oxygen tent, the suction apparatus, the dressing and the intravenous therapy apparatus, if it is utilized. Unless the personnel's interest is interpreted to the child, he will grow anxious, wondering about the meaning of all their activities.

On the second day, when the child is given a trial period out of oxygen he will require careful observation. His pulse and respiration should be noted. Observation to detect dilatation of the alae nasi and flushing of the face should be made. Usually the child is put back into the tent for another 24 hours, after which time it is discontinued.

On the third day postoperatively the child is usually ready for quiet activity. In another few days he may be up in a wheel chair. Activity should be increased gradually and planned in accordance with the child's capacities. Usually, by the end of 10 days he can resume normal activities.

Ventricular Septal Defect

An opening in the septum between the right and the left ventricles of the heart is perhaps the most common type of congenital heart disease. Fortunately, the defect is frequently small, and no obvious interference with cardiac function results. The flow of blood from the left to the right ventricle does not produce cyanosis, but a loud harsh murmur is usually present. Accurate interpretation of this murmur is desirable to prevent unnecessary concern or unwarranted restriction of the child's activity. For most children with this defect, no treatment is required. In rare instances the placement or the size of the defect may lead to cardiac enlargement and restriction of function. At the present time surgical repair of an interventricular defect is hazardous, since it requires operation upon the open heart.

Auricular Septal Defect

Openings in the septum between the right and the left auricle may occur. Oxygenated blood flows from the left to the right auricle through the defect and then is recirculated through the lungs (Fig. 76). A disproportion between the amount of blood circulating in the pulmonary and the systemic circulations ensues, producing enlargement of the right heart and distention of the pulmonary vessels. It has been postulated that the relatively meager flow to the rest of the body may lead to the slender delicate habitus which sometimes is observed. Susceptibility to pneumonia and rheumatic fever is increased. The diagnosis may be suspected from the presence of a loud murmur in the area of the pulmonary artery, with enlargement of the heart and roentgen evidence of congestion of the pulmonary circulation. It may be confirmed by insertion of a catheter into the right auricle

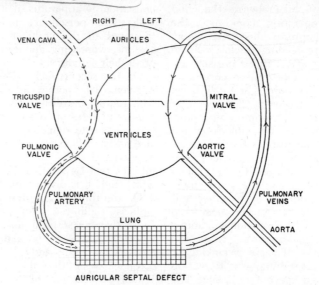

AURICULAR SEPTAL DEFECT

FIG. 76. Diagram of the circulation in auricular septal defect. This is similar to that of Figure 74, except that oxygenated blood returning to the left auricle can flow through the defect in the auricular septum into the right auricle, thus decreasing the volume of blood sent to the left ventricle and increasing the volume in the right side of the heart. No cyanosis develops unless the distention of the right side of the heart becomes excessive and reversal of the flow through the auricular defect takes place. (Adapted from Cassels, D. E., and Morse, M.: Blood volume in congenital heart disease, J. Pediat. 31:485)

and through the defect into the left auricle (cardiac catheterization). Technics for the surgical closure of the defect are difficult and carry a high mortality at the present time.

CYANOTIC CONGENITAL HEART DISEASE

In cyanotic congenital heart disease there is a communication between the pulmonary and the systemic circulations in which the blood is flowing continually from the venous to the arterial side. The blood delivered to the periphery of the body by the aorta never is fully saturated with oxygen, and the tissues take on a bluish hue instead of the normal pink. Cyanosis may be apparent at birth and persist or it may be inapparent at birth but develop during the first year of life. In either event it tends to become more marked during the early years of life. In part this is due to an increase in the number of red cells per unit volume of blood (polycythemia), which represents an attempt of the body to improve the oxygen-carrying power of the blood. When polycythemia is marked, the peripheral capillaries of the skin and the mucous membranes become distended with purple blood, the fingers and the toes may take on a clubbed shape (Plate 2), body growth is delicate

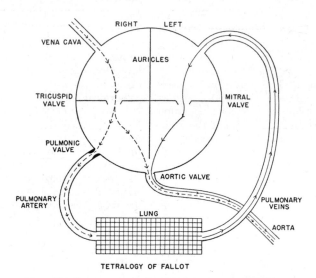

RIGHT   LEFT

VENA CAVA

AURICLES

TRICUSPID VALVE

MITRAL VALVE

PULMONIC VALVE

AORTIC VALVE

PULMONARY ARTERY

PULMONARY VEINS

LUNG

AORTA

TETRALOGY OF FALLOT

FIG. 77. Diagram of the circulation in tetralogy of Fallot. Venous blood entering the right ventricle is diverted from the pulmonary artery because of the narrowed orifice at the pulmonic valve. Some of it escapes through the defect in the interventricular septum into the left ventricle and almost immediately into the abnormally placed aorta. Partly because of anatomic relations and partly because of hypertrophy of the right ventricle, the venous blood is able to flow into the aorta. A decrease in the volume of blood sent to the lungs and a continual contamination of the stream of oxygenated blood from the left ventricle result. Cyanosis is present, and an increased volume of blood is present in the greater circulation. (Adapted from Cassels, D. E., and Morse, M.: Blood volume in congenital heart disease, J. Pediat. 31:485)

and retarded, the capacity for exercise is reduced, and the child runs the hazard of complications due to spontaneous clotting of the thickened blood within his vessels. All of these symptoms are subject to considerable variation in degree in the individual child.

Tetralogy of Fallot

The most common variety of cyanotic heart disease which permits survival consists of a combination of abnormalities. Blood leaving the right ventricle toward the lungs encounters an abnormally narrow opening into the pulmonary artery (Fig. 77). In the same vicinity there is an opening in the interventricular septum which provides a ready diversion of blood into the left side of the heart and particularly into the aorta. Cyanosis arises because of the contamination of the aortic contents by venous blood. The direction of flow through the shunt is determined in part by the position of the aortic opening and in part by the fact that the right ventricle has hypertrophied because of its excessive task and thus is able to overbalance the pressure of the left ventricle. Poor oxygenation of the tissues is furthered also by the fact that the rate of blood flow through the lungs is decreased. Diagnosis is made from fluoroscopic examination of the heart, which demonstrates enlargement of the chambers of the right side, decrease in size of the pulmonary artery and decrease in blood flow through the lungs.

Usually the physical activity of the child with tetralogy of Fallot is impaired. He walks or plays for a few minutes, grows tired and gets into a squatting position which relieves his dyspnea for some unknown reason. In spite of the fact that these children have a chronic circulatory disturbance to the brain with some degree of relative anoxia, many of them are of average or above-average intelligence. Fainting spells and occasionally convulsions may occur when the degree of anoxia is increased temporarily.

The child with tetralogy of Fallot is usually irritable, overdependent and prone to emotional instability. It is understandable why he reacts in this way. From birth his parents have been concerned about his defect, his physical health and his prognosis for survival. The child with tetralogy of Fallot grows blue when he cries. Therefore, his parents prolong gratification when normally he should be learning to tolerate frustration. He refuses to do things for himself, partly because he fatigues easily and partly because his mother feels that she must protect him from all experiences which are difficult or frustrating. The child with a congenital heart defect starts life under adverse circumstances, both physically and psychologically. Empathy with the child is an essential quality in his nursing care.

Surgical Treatment. The original "blue-baby operation" of Blalock and Taussig was designed to ameliorate this abnormality. In this operation a branch of the aorta is anastomosed to the pulmonary artery. In older children the subclavian artery is used. In children under 2 years of age the subclavian artery is too small to be used, and the innominate artery is selected to achieve the shunt. The Blalock and Taussig operation does not correct the original defects but adds a compensating one by connecting a systemic artery to the pulmonary artery. This increases the blood flow to the lungs, reduces cyanosis and improves the tolerance for exercise.

The Potts operation also achieves the above result. The Potts operation makes a direct connection between the aorta and the pulmonary artery. The aorta has higher pressure and forces blood into the pulmonary artery, from whence it will flow through the lungs for oxygenation.

Nursing Care. During the preoperative period the child should have a nurse who can accept him with his individual personality patterns and needs. He will need a great deal of help in becoming familiar with the hospital, his nurse, the doctors and the routines. He will be subjected to diagnostic procedures—oxygen saturation and exercise tolerance tests, roentgen pictures and barium swallow and fluoroscopic examination. He will adapt himself more readily if time is spent letting him stir up the barium and chocolate syrup and permitting him to discover that the drink is similar to cocoa. Permitting him to examine the fluoroscopic machine while the lights are on will do much to eliminate the frightening aspects of an examination in the dark.

The child with this type of defect is undernourished, underdeveloped and susceptible to respiratory infections—especially to pneumonia. For this reason he needs protection from patients and personnel with respiratory infections. He also needs an adequate diet and fluid intake. These children usually have capricious appetites. Serving small quantities in an attractive fashion in an atmosphere of friendliness brings infinitely better results than urging.

The child's parents also will need help in the preoperative period. The doctor explains the operation, the complications that may occur and the prognosis. However, there will be many questions directed toward the nurse and many signs which indicate the parents' need for preparation, support and hope. Sometimes their overprotectiveness may be difficult to bear. However, if the nurse can visualize imaginatively what they have experienced in the months or the years before, she will understand why overprotectiveness and anxiety have become a habitual response to the problems that they have had to bear.

The parents not only will need answers to their questions but also they should be prepared for what they will see when their child returns from the operating room. They should know the length of time that the operation will take. Waiting for one's child to return from the operating room is tedious and anxiety-provoking—and especially so when the parents know that the prognosis is unpredictable. Informing them of the child's condition at intervals relieves anxiety, supports them at a critical time and gives them hope.

When the child returns from the operating room, he must be placed in an oxygen tent. When intratracheal anesthesia is used, the child must be watched for signs of tracheal irritation. It is manifested by cyanosis, increased pulse rate, labored breathing or restlessness. When signs of tracheal irritation develop, steam inhalations must be provided to bring relief from dyspnea. If edema of the larynx develops, a tracheotomy may become necessary. Vital signs are taken every hour. If the Blalock-Taussig operation has been performed, blood-pressure readings must be taken from the arm opposite to the operated side. The child must be turned at frequent intervals. Sedatives are given freely to keep the child at rest. Penicillin is administered to prevent infections. Observation to detect postoperative hemiplegia is necessary. It is not a common complication but it can occur from spontaneous clotting of blood during dehydration after operation. Coramine, adrenalin and a thoracentesis tray should be in the room for emergency use. An accumulation of bloody fluid in the chest may cause listlessness, diminished breath sounds and increased pulse rate. If a thoracentesis is done, the amount of fluid withdrawn and the child's response to the treatment should be noted on the chart. The child's color should be noted, and changes recorded. Fluids may be given as tolerated, followed by a soft to general diet. Mouth and skin care gives comfort. Encouraging the child to cough up mucus prevents atelectasis and should be suggested at intervals.

When the operation is successful, the child recuperates rapidly. Usually oxygen is needed for 4 or 5 days. Then the child is ready for graduated amounts of activity. Marked changes in behavior will become evident. The operation increases his vigor, and often he begins to assert himself, to become aggressive and to demand to do things for himself. These changes are striking and often frightening to the parents who repeatedly have responded with fear when the child became active.

The nurse will need to help the parents to accept their child's increased need for independence and self-assertion. With reassurance and insight they will learn to observe his increased capacities and see that soon he will be ready for many new kinds of socializing experiences. The parents will need help to change their feelings about their child before they can institute new methods of guidance. This takes time, along with advice and direction that are given understandingly. Gradually, they will see and feel that their child has become more nearly normal. The nurse can increase their powers of observation by pointing out his enjoyment of self-directed activity and his freedom from signs of untoward reactions during periods of activity.

Other Varieties of Cyanotic Heart Disease

Eisenmenger Complex. This is similar to the tetralogy of Fallot except for the absence of narrowing of the pulmo-

nary artery. Operative procedures will not improve this type of defect at the present time.

Pulmonary Stenosis With Auricular Septal Defect. This can be improved markedly by new measures which are designed to enlarge the pulmonic opening. In general, shunting operations are not effective for this abnormality. Most of the other cyanotic types of congenital heart disease do not permit survival for more than a brief period of time.

Nursing Care

The type of nursing care required will vary considerably, depending upon the degree of functional incapacity. Infants or children with severely handicapping malformations require the type of care described later in this chapter for children with heart failure or with chronic valvular heart disease. Those in whom the malformation is mild should be encouraged to utilize their exercise capacity to the limit of tolerance. For many this will mean a normal life; for some it may require diversion of interests from competitive sports to more sedentary pursuits. Often the problem for the child lies mainly in convincing the parents to let him participate in activities commensurate with his functional capacity instead of overprotecting him and regarding him as a cardiac invalid.

FUNCTIONAL HEART CONDITIONS

FUNCTIONAL MURMUR

Murmurs heard over the heart in the absence of organic disease of the heart are known as functional or accidental murmurs. In some instances, functional murmurs are dependent on anemia. These murmurs disappear when the hemoglobin has been brought to a normal value. Accidental murmurs not related to anemia are very common in childhood. Their cause is not well understood, and they have no significance or

importance. Accidental murmurs are of only moderate intensity, are heard usually in systole and when the child is lying down. The intensity of the murmur varies with the heart rate, the murmur disappearing with a rapid rate. A child may have an accidental murmur over a period of years without related symptoms.

The only importance of the functional murmur is in relation to the diagnosis and the decision that it is functional rather than organic.

SINUS ARRHYTHMIA

Under normal conditions the heart rate is determined by the sino-auricular node. In embryologic life this is known as the sinus. Sinus arrhythmia is a change in heart rate produced by reflexes acting on the sino-auricular node. The usual reflex cause of this change in rhythm is respiration. In the presence of sinus arrhythmia, the heart rate increases with inspiration and decreases with expiration. This type of cardiac irregularity is very common in childhood, so common that it is considered as a normal condition. It disappears in the presence of tachycardia from any cause.

TACHYCARDIA

Tachycardia, or rapid heart rate, may be an accompaniment of heart disease or it may occur from various causes when the heart is entirely normal. Increased heart rate occurs with fear, excitement, exercise and fever. When tachycardia is functional and fever is not present, the heart and the pulse rates become normal during sleep. They do not become normal during sleep in hyperthyroidism, rheumatic carditis or in the condition known as paroxysmal tachycardia. When a child first comes under medical or nursing care for any reason, he may have tachycardia from fear and excitement incident to the occasion. In order to obtain a satisfactory and significant pulse rate, the child must be calmed, or one must wait until he is asleep.

If the heart rate is increased from any cause above 150 to the minute for a protracted period, the myocardium becomes weakened, and severe damage may result. Paroxysmal tachycardia is a condition which is relatively rare in childhood; the heart rate is increased often to 200 or more to the minute for no known reason. An attack may last a few minutes or for several days. The drugs Quinidine and Mecholyl are used to prevent the attacks or to stop them when they occur.

ACUTE RHEUMATIC CARDITIS

The term "rheumatic carditis" is used in preference to "rheumatic endocarditis," which was employed formerly, for the reason that the changes in the heart never are limited to the endocardium in the acute stages of the disease. The myocardium always is affected, and often the pericardium also. Rheumatic carditis is an inflammation of the heart which occurs as a part of rheumatic fever, not as a complication.

ETIOLOGY

The mechanism that causes rheumatic carditis also causes rheumatic fever and is discussed under the latter disease.

Fully nine tenths of all the heart disease that occurs in the first 4 decades of life is rheumatic, and in nearly three fourths of these cases the cardiac disease has its onset before 15. It is rare in the first years of life, common after 5 and has its greatest incidence of onset between 7 and 10. Its distribution between the sexes is approximately equal. The frequency of its occurrence varies with the geographic location. In surveys of hospital admissions, the proportion has varied from 0.1 to 5.5 per cent. Among college students, a mean average of 1.2 per cent has been found. The seriousness, as well as the frequency, of the disease is indicated by mortality statistics, which are more accurately known than is the morbidity. The mortality formerly varied from 5 to more than 9 for each 100,000 population, according to the area of the country. In the last year for which reports are available (1954), the mortality rate in the United States as a whole dropped to 1.9 per 100,000 for children in the age range of 1 to 14. During the last decade deaths from rheumatic fever and heart disease have fallen from third to fifth place as a cause of death among children.

PATHOLOGY

In the beginning of rheumatic carditis and during its exacerbations, rheumatic nodules (see Rheumatic Fever) form in the various heart structures. Subsequently, some localized endothelial proliferation takes place, and frequently small excrescences, consisting largely of fibrin (vegetations), occur on the heart valves and the chordae tendineae. The left auriculoventricular (mitral) valve is the one most often affected; the aortic valve is the next. The vegetations interfere with good closure and function of the valves, thus throwing an added load on the heart muscle in order to maintain circulation. The function of the myocardium is disturbed directly by the inflammatory changes within its structure. Thus, frequently the work demanded of the heart muscle exceeds its capacity, with the result that the heart may increase in size by dilatation. The circulatory inadequacy which results is reflected in the symptoms exhibited by the child.

SYMPTOMS

The symptoms of rheumatic carditis are proportionate quantitatively and qualitatively to the severity of the carditis. In cases of mild disease, the symptoms are in part those of a prolonged low-grade infection. The usual picture is one of irregular low-grade fever, pallor, moderate anemia and poor nutrition, with a history of preceding poor appetite, loss of weight and easy fatigue. All these symptoms are vague as far as indicating carditis is concerned. If other rheumatic manifestations are present, the significance of the symptoms may become apparent, but mild carditis easily may escape recognition when a careful physical examination is lacking. On closer observation one may find slight dyspnea on exertion and pulse and

respiration rates out of proportion to the temperature. A soft systolic murmur usually is to be heard over the apex of the heart, the point where murmurs produced by lesions of the mitral valve are heard best. Often epistaxis occurs in the early stage of the disease.

When the carditis is more severe, the child is definitely ill. He prefers or finds it necessary, to remain in bed. Usually the face is flushed, with perhaps some cyanosis. The temperature may be high in the very acute disease or range up to 101° or 102° F. with disease of moderate severity. The temperature is always irregular. The white-blood-cell count is increased definitely and sometimes greatly. Cardiac damage is severe, and pain over the precordium is frequent. Abdominal pain also is often present. Because of the myocardial weakness and the concomitant valvular lesions, the heart dilates, and evidences of inadequate circulation appear. Failure of the heart in this manner is known as decompensation. Decompensation causes very rapid pulse and respiration rates, dyspnea, pallor and cyanosis. It also permits a back pressure of the blood in the venous system, which causes enlargement of the liver and, in more severe decompensation, edema and ascites.

When the cardiac valves are involved, the sounds produced by the heart are modified, causing murmurs. From the timing and the location of the murmur one may determine the valve affected; from the character of the murmur the condition of the valve may be estimated. The stronger the action of the heart and the greater the scarring of the valve, the louder and rougher the murmur will be. The amount of myocardial inflammation is indicated by the weakening, the spacing and the rapidity of the heart sounds, as well as by the amount of dilatation. Enlargement of the heart may be caused by stretching of weakened heart muscle, or it may be the result of hypertrophy consequent to cardiac damage by preceding attacks of carditis. An associated pericarditis may cause accumulation of fluid around the heart, simulating cardiac enlargement.

PROGNOSIS

The normal healing powers of the body tend to check the cardiac inflammation, particularly if outlying infections subside and cardiac work is kept at a minimum. Thus, children may become cured after a period of several months. Recovery from the first attack is usual. However, carditis, like other rheumatic manifestations, has a strong tendency to recur. The child may die as a result of failing circulation in the midst of one of these attacks, or, if he recovers from the illness, the summation of damage to the valves with associated scarring may lead to permanent valve deformity and dysfunction with its consequent invalidism because of inability to withstand the effects of even moderate exercise. On the other hand, from apparently severe valvular lesions in the absence of further recurrences he may recover ultimately to the extent that no dysfunction exists and even the murmurs largely disappear.

TREATMENT

The treatment of active rheumatic carditis attempts to spare the heart as much work as possible until the acute inflammatory reaction in its muscle has subsided completely. The measures which reduce cardiac work include (1) continuous and absolute bed rest, (2) the relief of pain, fever and anxiety insofar as possible and (3) appropriate treatment of cardiac failure when it is present. The success of these aspects of treatment depends in large measure upon the nurse and the other persons who care for the child. Details of nursing care are considered in a separate section at the end of this chapter. The treatment of cardiac failure also is considered in a separate section.

Measures that suppress the rheumatic inflammatory process are an important adjunct to the treatment outlined above. Salicylates or cortisone or ACTH, when used in proper dosage, will terminate fever and pain and reduce cardiac activity in most instances. What effect these measures have in limiting the ultimate degree of cardiac damage is still a matter of dispute. Their withdrawal before the end of the usual period during which spontaneous subsidence of rheumatic activity might be expected results in an immediate return of symptoms. Whether suppression of rheumatic activity does or does not limit the ultimate damage to cardiac valves and muscle, it is an important temporary expedient which lessens cardiac work by the reduction of fever and the relief of pain, anxiety and discomfort.

Both the salicylates and the hormones have undesirable side effects which must be recognized and eliminated before the disturbances which they create add to the burden of cardiac work. High dosage of salicylates may result in gastro-intestinal upsets, ringing in the ears, headaches or disturbances of mental state. Stimulation of respiration can cause alkalosis through hyperventilation. Acidosis also may occur when there is excessive accumulation of salicylates in the blood. The manner in which children respond to salicylate dosage is a highly individual matter. Some can tolerate large doses without disturbance; others are easily upset by relatively small quantities.

Administration of cortisone and ACTH also is restricted by toxic manifestations. The bodily appearance may change through the rounding of facial contours (moon face), localized fat deposits, the appearance of acne or excessive hair and by weight increase with linear marks appearing in the stretched skin (striae). More serious to the child with rheumatic carditis are hypertension and the tendency to accumulate salt and water within the tissues. The latter may be counteracted by restricting the dietary intake of salt and by the periodic administration of mercurial diuretics. When mental or emotional disturbances occur during hormone therapy, they must be regarded as a serious complication which probably demands withdrawal of the drug.

During the acute stage of rheumatic carditis the maintenance of nutrition presents a serious problem. The sick child eats poorly, yet needs essential nutrients to combat his disease. Hormone therapy usually is attended by an increase in appetite which is superior to that observed when salicylates are used. Blood or plasma transfusions in small amounts are sometimes very helpful in improving nutrition.

As the acute stage subsides and the heart becomes compensated, less rigorous restriction of activity is required, but confinement to bed is continued for as long as any evidence of activity of the disease persists or for as long as compensation is incomplete. The criteria for determining persistence of activity of the disease are stated under rheumatic fever. After the child has been permitted out of bed for brief periods and has been given bathroom privileges, the pulse rate is a fairly good criterion as to the degree of compensation of the heart. Other tests of cardiac function may be applied, such as noting how quickly the pulse rate returns to its former level after a brief period of exercise. Restriction of bodily activity for many months has been a common custom. Such radical restriction is unnecessary, provided that all evidence of infection, including laboratory evidence, has disappeared and provided that the state of nutrition is excellent because of previous close attention to it. In most instances, unlimited activity may be allowed 6 weeks after the child has been permitted to be out of bed. When heart damage persists, the activity of the child always should be restricted within the limits of easy tolerance, as discussed subsequently.

The general measures which are discussed in Chapter 26 for the prevention of recurrences of rheumatic episodes are most important for children who have suffered from carditis.

CHRONIC VALVULAR DISEASE

Damage to the heart valves, usually produced by rheumatic carditis, leads to changes which alter the normal functioning of the valves. When the child has recovered from the active or the acute inflammation of carditis, the residual heart damage with scarring of the valves is termed chronic valvular disease. It results in changes in the remainder of the circulatory system to compensate for the valvular changes.

Two types of valvular damage may be produced. One of these consists of a puckering or a partial destruction or a binding down of the valve leaves, which results in an inability of the valve to close tightly and so allows a leakage of the blood in the circulation in the direction opposite to that in which it normally goes. This type of defect occurs most frequently at the mitral valve. At this site the condition is known as mitral insufficiency, and the backward flow of blood is spoken of as mitral regurgitation.

The other type of valve damage consists of a narrowing of the valve orifice by scar contraction or fusion of valve leaflets so that the leaflets cannot open completely. Such a lesion constitutes a stenosis and prevents easy passage of blood through the heart.

As a result of these changes, the heart must do more work. This goal is accomplished usually by increase of musculature or hypertrophy. If hypertrophy is insufficient, the heart rate also is increased.

SYMPTOMS

When compensation is adequate, chronic valvular disease produces no symptoms. Examination will reveal cardiac murmurs and an enlarged heart. Symptoms arise when for any reason compensation is inadequate. Decompensation is discussed subsequently. In the absence of cardiac insufficiency or decompensation, children with chronic valvular disease need only to avoid exertion beyond their cardiac capacity and to guard against further cardiac damage.

MANAGEMENT

It is necessary for some children with heart disease to lead a guarded and restricted life. However, it is always desirable that they lead a life as nearly normal as possible. Such children should be examined at suitable intervals to determine whether the regimen followed is adequate or unnecessarily restrictive. They should have such supervision as would detect at their onset any deleterious conditions. Not only the habits of life but the mental attitude toward life needs careful consideration and adjustment. The chief function of childhood is preparation for adult life, and an important part of the preparation is formal education. A lack of understanding between medical supervisor and educator may result in unnecessary neglect of the child's education.

Too often the instruction to the parent or the child is of a negative type with admonition as to what not to do, for example, "Do not run up the stairs and do not play hard." Instruction of this type may well produce psychological harm. What is needed is advice as to constructive use of time. The child should be told what to do rather than what not to do. Let him have his unrestricted periods. For such restriction as is necessary, definite rest periods should be prescribed.

MYOCARDITIS

Under the term "myocarditis" are included acute and chronic inflammations and degenerations of the heart muscle. In childhood, myocarditis is encountered most frequently as a manifestation of rheumatic fever. It occurs also with diphtheria that is severe or has been treated late and with other severe acute infections.

PECULIARITIES OF HEART MUSCLE

Disorders of the myocardium are understood more easily if the peculiarities of heart muscle are kept in mind. This tissue has the ability to contract; it holds itself in constant readiness to contract—a condition termed "tonicity." It has the ability to stimulate itself to contract and thus is automatic. Its contractions follow each other in orderly sequence or rhythm. Stimulation produced or applied at any point is conducted to all parts of the myocardium and causes a contraction of the whole heart. If the heart contracts at all, it contracts completely.

SYMPTOMS

Myocarditis may cause disturbances of any or all of the stated properties of the heart. One common manifestation is weakened contractility, necessitating a more rapid heart rate. The pulse becomes noticeably weaker. On auscultation the first heart sound is faint, the two heart sounds become of almost equal intensity at the apex, and the spacing between the first and the second sounds becomes approximately equal. What is termed a gallop rhythm frequently develops. A splitting of the heart sounds results in a rhythm that sounds like a galloping horse.

The ability of the heart muscle to transmit a wave of contraction to all its parts may become impaired. Such disturbances of conduction may result in irregular pulse, and sometimes the heart chambers cease to contract synchronously. One type of conduction difficulty is known as auricular fibrillation or flutter and is characterized by very rapid and ineffective contractions of the auricles with occasional irregular ventricular contraction. In some instances, a blocking of conduction from one part of the heart to another occurs. This also leads to lack of synchronism and may result in complete independence of contraction in the auricle and the ventricle. The latter is much slower than the normal rate, often from 30 to 40 to the minute. The ventricular rate may be determined by counting the pulse or the auricular rate, from pulse tracings made from the external jugular vein and from the electrocardiogram.

TREATMENT

The treatment in cases of myocarditis is similar to that in rheumatic carditis. In addition, there is an attempt to remove or relieve the causative factor. If cardiac failure should occur, the treatment is as described subsequently under cardiac decompensation. Some varieties of myocarditis, such as that secondary to diphtheria, have a high mortality rate associated with them. With other varieties (e.g., rheumatic) the chances for recovery often are excellent.

PERICARDITIS

The pericardium is a thin layer of serous tissue which forms a double-walled sac, the inner layer covering the heart and the outer layer lining the space in which the heart lies. The free surfaces are moist and smooth.

Pericarditis or inflammation of this membrane may be of various types and may come from several causes. It is not common in infancy or early childhood. When it does occur at such an early age, it most frequently results from the extension of a pneumonic or a pleural infection. This produces commonly a suppurative type of pericarditis which causes a high mortality rate, particularly in infancy. Occasionally, pericarditis caused by tuberculosis is encountered. Though pericarditis occurs from these and other causes, by far the most frequent factor in the production of this disorder in childhood is rheumatic fever, especially after 4 or 5 years of age.

RHEUMATIC PERICARDITIS

This type is characterized early by an exudate of fibrin and cells on both free surfaces of the pericardium. With movement of the heart the two roughened surfaces rub together, producing what is heard on auscultation as a scratching sound. Subsequently, the exudate consists also of fluid, which is clear or only slightly cloudy. The quantity of fluid usually is small, though at times it may be large, producing pericarditis with effusion.

Symptoms

Rheumatic pericarditis always is accompanied by myocarditis with its associated symptoms. Local pain and tenderness usually are present. As the inflammation subsides, a strong tendency exists to form adhesions between the two pericardial layers. The adhesions may be only slight or they may be sufficiently extensive to obliterate the entire pericardial sac. The adhesions do not seem to interfere seriously with cardiac function, especially if the inflammation and the adhesive process have not extended to structures beyond the parietal pericardium. Adhesions which fix firmly to the parietal pericardium are more frequently dependent on other than rheumatic disease. Such massive adhesions interfere greatly with the heart action. Because of the increased work, the heart is compelled to hypertrophy. If hypertrophy is insufficient, decompensation results.

Treatment

The treatment of rheumatic pericarditis is that of rheumatic carditis. Rarely is drainage of pericardial fluid necessary. Suppurative pericarditis may require surgical drainage, but usually, no matter what is done, the outlook is poor.

CARDIAC DECOMPENSATION

A damaged heart or one subjected to excessive strain is said to be compensated when it has hypertrophied and adjusted its performance sufficiently to overcome its handicap completely. If it fails to maintain an adequate circulation, it is decompensated.

ETIOLOGY

The work of maintaining a high blood pressure may exceed the heart's capacity, although this is an infrequent cause of decompensation in children except during nephritis. The most frequent cause is active rheumatic carditis with its attendant myocarditis and myocardial weakening. Chronic valvular disease may be sufficiently severe to be in itself a cause of decompensation, although, more often than not, decompensation occurs in this condition only with a recurrence of the infection.

SYMPTOMS

When the circulation is inadequate, blood accumulates in the venous system. In the lungs, the congestion of the vessels causes symptoms resembling bronchitis. Small amounts of blood may appear in the sputum. Congestion of the systemic venous system causes digestive disturbances, enlargement of the liver and accumulation of fluid in the tissue spaces (edema) and in the serous cavities (ascites). Nausea and vomiting may be the first outstanding symptoms of decompensation. The congestion of the liver may lead to dysfunction sufficient to cause jaundice. Only rarely does the ascites become great enough to embarrass respiration or heart action.

An adequate gas exchange between the blood and the tissues is impossible in the presence of circulatory failure. Cyanosis and dyspnea result. Cyanosis is noted best in the lips and the fingertips; dyspnea may be so severe as to require the child to maintain a sitting posture.

TREATMENT

The treatment of decompensation consists of reducing to a minimum the amount of work required of the heart, administering cardiac stimulants to help the heart meet the circulatory needs and, finally, when compensation has been attained, providing favorable conditions for the heart to recover as much reserve as possible. The child should be in bed, absolutely at rest and lying flat unless dyspnea prevents it. Not only rest but also an abundance of sleep is necessary. Sedative drugs usually are strongly indicated, and no hesitancy need be shown in the use of morphine. In fact, morphine is a very important drug in this condition. The early administration of oxygen is very valuable. In cases of most severe decompensation, removal of blood from the circulation may be desirable unless anemia is present. However, removal of blood is seldom necessary when the other measures mentioned are carried out appropriately.

Digitalis

This drug is the cardiac stimulant used. Digitalis serves to slow the heart rate by prolonging diastole, thus allowing more cardiac rest and at the same time permitting better ventricular filling. Digitalis increases cardiac tone. It increases the extent of ventricular contraction and relieves or prevents dilatation beyond the physiologic limit, making possible maximum cardiac output. Digitalis should be given in large doses for the first day or two. After that its administration should be continued in smaller amounts. A period of a day or two is required for the drug to become fully effective. The administration of the large dosage for the initial period is designated as digitalization. Precise dosage varies with the preparation of digitalis and the speed with which an effect is desired. The initial saturating dose must be computed carefully to avoid toxic symptoms when the delayed effects appear. The benefits of digitalis may be erased by such symptoms.

Great care must be exercised in the digitalization of children who have had previous treatment, in order to avoid overdigitalization. Moderate excess of digitalis causes premature heartbeats and vomiting. Other irregularities of conduction of the impulse in the heart may be observed. In more severe digitalis intoxication, heart block is likely to occur. In the event of overdosage, administration of the drug should be discontinued temporarily, then resumed at a lower dosage than previously. The administration should be discontinued when compensation is well established. A few children may require the continued administration of digitalis over a long period in order to maintain compensation.

The heart does not respond sufficiently to the preceding measures in all instances. In the presence of edema and ascites, certain other measures may be indicated. One of these is the administration of a diuretic in an attempt to cause elimination of some of the excess fluid. Theophylline is valuable for this purpose. Mercurial diuretics are in common use. A diet containing little salt and considerable carbohydrate, limited in fluid, with most of the fluid in the form of milk, has been found to be useful for many of these children.

After all signs of decompensation have disappeared, the child should refrain from activity until some cardiac reserve has been attained. Then activity should be permitted gradually. If the pulse rate becomes much accelerated or remains increased after exercise, the exercise has been too severe or too prolonged. It may be that the child never will have the normal degree of cardiac reserve and that his activities always must be somewhat restricted. Any noteworthy recurrence of decompensation is an indication for renewed convalescent care for weeks or months and calls for prolonged restriction of activity. It is to be remembered that in rheumatic heart disease, decompensation is brought about most frequently by active rheumatic infection. Recurrences of decompensation usually depend on recurrences or exacerbations of the infection. A primary duty to the children is to find and treat all infectious foci and to make every attempt to help them learn to manage their lives in such a manner that respiratory infections are avoided.

NURSING CARE OF THE CHILD WITH HEART DISEASE

Since reduction of the load carried by the heart is of primary importance for the child with active heart disease, all nursing care is directed toward that goal. The child in severe decompensation presents a typical picture: his pulse is rapid; respirations are fast, shallow and labored; his color ranges from pallor to severe cyanosis; he usually has a hacking cough and a chest which pulsates with a visibly enlarged heart; he is alert, restless and apprehensive.

NURSING CARE DURING THE ACUTE PHASE

Rest is the first requisite in acute cardiac decompensation. The child should have rest in bed, should be moved as little as possible and should do nothing for himself which causes fatigue. The nurse's movements should be sure, smooth and unhurried. The child should be told when the nurse is going to insert the thermometer, lift him in bed, roll him to his side or perform any other act, as quick, unexpected movements startle him and increase his apprehension. Elevation of the head rest often relieves dyspnea. Support of the arms at the sides by pillows takes the weight of the arms from the shoulders. This also helps to overcome the tendency to fold the arms over the abdomen, which causes undesirable pressure and hampers chest expansion. Poor muscle tone and fatigue predispose the child to postural defects, and measures to support the body help to prevent poor posture.

Every possible measure should be taken to alleviate anxiety and to inspire confidence, as emotional calm is as essential as physical comfort and restriction of exercise. All nursing care should be planned carefully to provide for maximum amounts of rest. By thoughtful organization of essential nursing care the hypnotic effect of sedative drugs administered may be prolonged greatly. This includes careful recording of the temperature and the pulse and respiration rates. The pulse rate indicates the progress of the child and, to obtain an accurate measure, it should be observed for a full minute before the thermometer is inserted. When sleeping pulses are requested, the nurse must be sure that the child is not wakened.

A high temperature, increased perspiration and edema make care of the skin a prime requisite. The back and the buttocks need particular care and should be washed and rubbed with alcohol 3 times daily. Rubber rings or cotton "doughnuts" are useful in preventing pressure areas which develop easily, especially in edematous children. Change in position is essential for good skin care and it also helps in aeration of the lungs. When joints are painful and swollen, a cradle to raise the bedclothing from them will give added comfort.

Good mouth care needs to be given, especially if the child is receiving limited fluids or is dyspneic and is breathing through his mouth. Lemon juice and glycerine, half and half, is a good lubri-cant for dry tongue, gums and lips after they have been cleaned.

Recording the intake and the output of these children also requires the careful attention of the nurse. When intake is limited, a schedule should be made which will give the child a proportion of the total amount ordered at short intervals during the day and during the night when he wakes up feeling thirsty.

The nurse is responsible also for the nutrition of the child, often a serious problem, for these children have poor appetites and often their capacity is limited because of heart enlargement and decompensation. In the acute stage, a liquid diet of high caloric value usually is given. Later, as the child's physical condition and appetite improve, a high-protein, high-vitamin diet is introduced gradually.

These children are especially susceptible to infections, and association with other sick children should be avoided. Visitors and personnel with sore throats never should be permitted near the child with heart disease. Usually the child will be receiving prophylactic antibiotics, but this does not obviate the necessity for shielding him by isolation.

Administration of oxygen is usually the next remedial measure after rest is instituted. This is performed most satisfactorily by an oxygen tent; as it is less confining, the child can see the personnel, and a good concentration of oxygen is assured. A temperature of between 65° and 70° F. should be maintained in the tent, and the child should be protected with appropriate body covering. Explaining the purpose of the tent to the child before he is put into it will allay fears so frequently associated with confinement in a small, enclosed space.

Paracentesis of the pericardial sac gives immediate relief to the heart if a great amount of fluid has collected because of pericarditis. Paracentesis of the abdominal cavity likewise may be in-

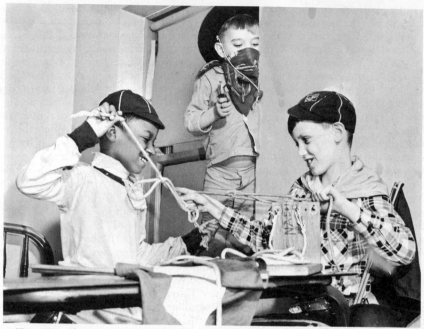

Fig. 78. The play of boys with cardiac disease is similar to the play of normal children. (La Rabida Jackson Park Sanitarium for Children with Cardiac Disease, Chicago, and The Chicago Daily Sun Times)

dicated for relief of respiratory difficulty caused by ascites.

The drugs prescribed are chiefly digitalis and salicylates. Digitalis slows and strengthens the heart and so improves circulation. Before each dose of this drug is given, the pulse rate should be observed. If it has gone down markedly or has changed in quality, the doctor's approval should be secured before the next dose of the drug is given. Anorexia, nausea and vomiting are the chief toxic symptoms.

The toxic manifestations of overdosage with salicylates, cortisone and ACTH have been described under acute rheumatic carditis. The nurse should be thoroughly familiar with these untoward reactions, which may demand a change in therapeutic plans.

CONVALESCENT CARE

The child convalescing from heart disease offers a real challenge to the nurse. She must provide experiences which foster the child's personality growth but at the same time help him accept the limits imposed by cardiac involvement. Carrying out the order for bed rest in a way which protects the child's mental health is a skill of great import. The child who has spent long periods in bed feels no need for rest and therefore has little or no interest in it. In fact, he usually has a desire and a need to give up his dependency, to become active and to express the resentment he acquired during the period when he was forced to turn over the physical care of his own body to other persons.

Children respond to illness, treatment and hospitalization with varying degrees of anger. They feel a driving need to strike out at those who frustrated them. The offenders are often represented by the physician, the nurse, the roommates

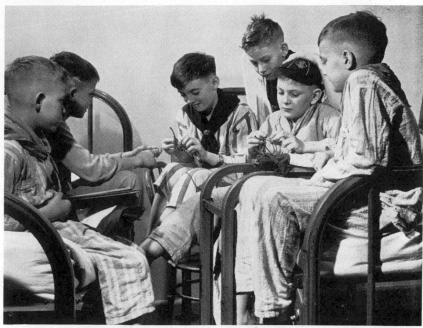

Fig. 79. Scout activities are a part of the activity program at the La Rabida Jackson Park Sanitarium. (La Rabida Sanitarium, Chicago, and The Chicago Daily Sun Times)

and the parents. These feelings are frightening. Some children express their feelings of resentment overtly with or without accompanying feelings of guilt. The temper outbursts, the torrents of growling and explosive language, the pillow fights and throwing of water which occur in wards of children with long-term illnesses are safety valves. It is the child's way of ridding himself of intolerable tension which has been building up within him. Other children are so afraid of their feelings that they hold them in. The accompanying feelings or inner unrest become manifested by an inability to keep quiet or by withdrawing into themselves.

In wards of convalescent children the nurse will see children with varying needs. She will see children who are restlessly moving about during all of their waking hours and are completely unable to control their activity. Scold-

ing, criticism and nagging increases their resentment, anxiety and tension because it adds to the reservoir of disruptive emotions they are already feeling. The nurse will also see children who are nearly mute. They sit placidly as if they were afraid to move. They rarely talk; they respond to questions with nothing further than "Yes" or "No" and manifest their anxiety with damaging apathy. These children are inhibiting their feelings and are in a dangerous emotional state. In giving up their fear they often give up everything else as well, including hope which is absolutely essential for successful rehabilitation. The apathetic child is easier for some nurses to accept than the child with an explosive, volatile, tempestuous temperament but he is infinitely less healthy. Openly expressed anger and anxiety is much easier to handle. The child who expresses his feelings overtly gets reassurance from having someone listen to his tirade and accept his need to explode occasionally. The withdrawn child needs hope and trust. It can come only from relationship experiences which prove that his life is less threatened and his feelings are less dangerous than he suspects.

The understanding doctor and nurse recognize the genesis of resentment and anger and care for their patients with a minimum of enforced bed rest. They observe the child carefully. They notice what is physiologically and psychologically best for him and modify the prescribed activity accordingly. The understanding doctor and nurse use the word "don't" as little as possible because they know its use calls attention to the child's handicapped body, increases his anxiety, arouses antagonism and influences the development of personality problems as devastating as his disease.

Teaching the child about his disease and guiding him into quiet activities which are of absorbing interest *to him* helps him to accept the limitations which recuperation requires. Little by little through the use of artful, positive direction and teaching which increases his understanding of his disease and his need for rest, the nurse gradually can build up in the child a sense of responsibility for his own actions. The acutely ill child may be told stories, shown pictures, read to—anything that requires no effort on his part. As he recuperates he may hold the book, turn the pages, cut pictures from magazines and direct the placement of them in a scrapbook. Later he can color, fingerpaint, mold clay, work simple puzzles, use paper dolls, dress dolls and do schoolwork.

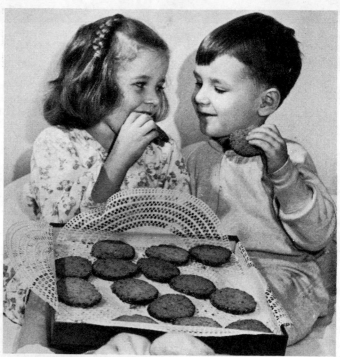

Fig. 80. Two children with cardiac disease enjoying party food and the company of each other. (La Rabida Jackson Park Sanitarium, Chicago, and The Chicago Daily Sun Times)

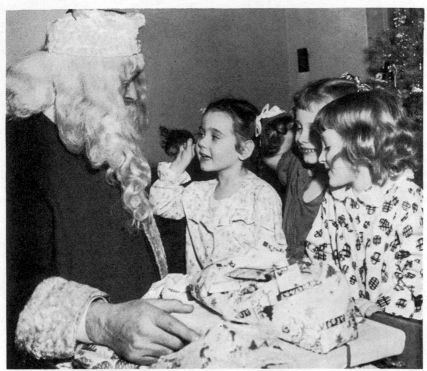

FIG. 81. Christmas festivities are important for children in hospitals. (La Rabida Jackson Park Sanitarium, Chicago, and The Chicago Daily Sun Times)

Play periods should be of short duration. His play should eliminate emotional strain and be interspersed with periods of music, stories and movies which have been planned to provide relaxation and rest.

A graduated program of activity with gradual increase in exercise should coincide with the rate of his physical progress. A period of a few weeks to many months is required, depending on the course of the disease and the return of cardiac efficiency.

Time out of bed should be increased gradually. When the child first is permitted to be up, a chair without wheels should be provided to prevent overactivity. A child who has been bedridden for a long period cannot be expected to maintain quiet when he is tempted with a chair that can transport

him to places he has long wanted to explore. At first, he should be placed in a chair near a window with play materials that interest him and ensure quiet activity. Then, when the nurse can be in constant attendance, excursions in a wheel chair will revive his spirits and give him something more constructive to think about. Later, when his condition has improved, he can be placed in a wheel chair and given limited freedom to move about.

The pulse rate should be observed before he is lifted into the chair and again when his position has been made comfortable. If his pulse does not return to normal within 5 minutes, he should be put back into bed. If his temperature rises in the evening, if his sleep seems to be disturbed, or his behavior indicates undue fatigue, it probably means that a longer rest period is required.

A study of the child's physical and psychological needs, his home and family circumstances should be made to determine the appropriate location for convalescent care. This is one of the many services that a social service department can give to a hospital to increase its usefulness to its child patients. When the child's own home can provide individualized care, convalescent care there is to be preferred. A child thrives best in his own family when the home provides the security necessary for personal and social adjust-

ment in addition to satisfying his physical needs for food, clothing and shelter.

During the convalescent period, whether the child is being cared for in the convalescent hospital, in his own home or in a foster one, consideration must be given to the promotion of his normal development. His environment must provide emotional security, opportunities for play, work and group life as well as continued supervision of his physical health. The continuation of his schoolwork will prevent a feeling of inadequacy when he returns to school and has to compete with his former

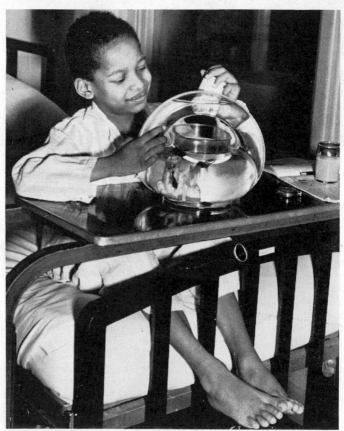

FIG. 82. Confinement to bed is more tolerable when interesting projects are available. (La Rabida Jackson Park Sanitarium, Chicago, and The Chicago Daily Sun Times)

classmates. In some cities, the board of education provides visiting teachers for children unable to attend school. There exist for severely handicapped children schools which meet their needs of transportation, special classes and a program planned in accordance with their individual capacities.

When school opportunities are not available or the home is found to be lacking in the essentials necessary to satisfy a child's needs, care in a convalescent hospital or a foster home may be considered advisable. The convalescent hospital provides association with other handicapped children. In many instances such an environment helps the child to adjust himself more easily to limited activity and to face his problems in a more wholesome way. Schoolwork and group activities appropriate to his capacity and interests can be supplied more easily (Figs. 78 to 82). The group provides friendship and a sense of belonging and stimulates his interest in school and play activities. It also helps the child master his fear lest he be different from other children. Because one of the commonest fears of the school age child and the adolescent is that he is different from every other child, he must have constant reassurance from his parents and nurses. This is best provided through provision of opportunities to mix with age-mates. With them he can get first-hand experiences which help him to learn that his difference from normal children is only temporary but that he has many things in common with his age-mates. This is the reason why the sick child needs contact with age-mates as soon as it is possible.

In a convalescent home or a hospital, a child's physical condition can be supervised more adequately. When the earliest signs of respiratory infection are detected, bed rest can be resumed, and thereby recurrences can be minimized.

Care in a foster home is sometimes necessary for either of two reasons: because convalescent-hospital care is unavailable or because study of a child indicates his need for the type of nurturing that is supplied by a smaller and more intimate family group. The latter is especially true of the child whose previous home background has not been sufficiently stable to give him the affection and the security that he needed for normal personality development. When plans for foster-home care are being made, participation of the child should be encouraged so that he can master the experience. Placing an unprepared child in a strange family setting tends to increase insecurity and in some instances might signify to him rejection by those whom he needs the most. Visits by foster parents prior to discharge from the hospital give the group opportunity to become acquainted and build up the child's sense of security which facilitates adjustment into a new family situation. Continued supervision of the foster home is required to observe the child's response and adjustment to it. The child's family should be encouraged to maintain relations with him. As soon as adjustments which suit the child's needs can be made in his own home, he should be returned to that environment.

Re-establishing independence after a long period of helplessness requires thoughtful guidance. He should have supervision, but those who are entrusted with this responsibility must give it without crippling him psychologically. There are children who find it difficult to give up the privileged position they enjoyed during the acute phase of illness. When this characteristic is observed in a child, it indicates his need for motivation toward participation in normal activities. He needs to discover the rewards of getting well. He also should be given freedom to enjoy activities with other children. Sometimes nurses and parents unknowingly keep children dependent upon them. They do things for children that they are able to do for themselves.

They reward dependence and provide too little freedom for them to develop relationships with their age-mates.

Those who care for children who are convalescing from heart disease need an understanding of their developmental needs, an appreciation of their capacities and limitations and the ability to help them accept their handicaps in a realistic way. Personnel who supervise the health of these children must be convinced of their capacity to live normal, useful lives. They must keep these children in contact with their parents and provide an environment which fosters emotional, social, mental and spiritual growth. Without a wholesome environment which recognizes children's need for continuity in their relationship with parent figures, psychological crippling will impose a second handicap which may be infinitely more self-limiting than the physical disease.

Preparation for Home-going and Follow-up Care

Discharge from the hospital or the convalescent home is frequently associated with feelings of concern and anxiety. Discharge terminates an experience which has been different from those the child has known before. It has been an experience which necessitated dependence and produced some regressive tendencies. Going home confronts the child with a need to change his pattern of living. Feelings which were repressed during hospitalization often come to the surface when he is reinstated in his own home. Readjustment to home is often difficult even though he has resented the hospital experience. Often children are depressed, withdrawn and weepy when they first go home. This is a state of affairs which can cause both children and parents great concern unless they are prepared for it. These children often show ambivalent feelings upon return home; they are happy to be at home yet they miss the hospital to which they had to become adjusted.

Often they feel apprehensive about starting something new.

Parental and teacher insight is necessary to help the child become readjusted to life at home and at school. It is important that teachers and parents neither push the child before he has readiness to adjust nor retard his forward progress because he has had cardiac disease.

Teamwork between the personnel in the hospital, the family physician or the physician in the division of services for crippled children, the school nurse, the teacher and not by any means of least importance—the child and his parents—is essential in the follow-up care of the child who has cardiac disease. The school nurse and the teacher must have information which will assist them in understanding the child's individual requirements and in carrying out the health plan in the school situation. The advantages and the disadvantages of a special class or special school for the child who has had cardiac disease are often discussed. The child who has had heart disease is different, but this difference is usually temporary. When the difference becomes lessened or absent, most authorities believe his development is furthered if he learns to adjust himself to life with children who never have had cardiac disease. Many teachers will need help in handling their fear of children who have been hospitalized with heart disease. This is accomplished best if the school nurse encourages the teacher's expression of feeling toward her responsibility in teaching a child who has been hospitalized. Unless her concerns are expressed and she is helped to handle her feelings about the child, interpretation of the doctor's recommendations will have little impact upon the ways she responds to the child.

Continued health supervision is imperative to prevent recurrences. Parents, and children who have been hospitalized, need to understand the necessity for frequent clinic visits, for adequate dental care, for prophylactic medication and for a regimen of living which provides adequate rest, diet, school activities and play and protects against infection. Both the child and his parents need to know the earliest symptoms of a respiratory infection and to accept his need for extra rest and medication during periods of illness.

SITUATIONS FOR FURTHER STUDY

1. What are the symptoms of tetralogy of Fallot?

2. How do you imagine a 5-year-old child feels when he learns that he is going to have his heart repaired? What do you think he needs to know before going to the operating room?

3. Prepare a child with patent ductus arteriosus for operation. Write a report of your approach, your verbal preparation, the child's response to you and all you were saying and your reactions to this experience. Include your observations of the child's response to going to the operating room, to having the anesthetic and to the experiences of the immediate postoperative period.

4. Write a description of a child who has tetralogy of Fallot. Describe his physical appearance, his behavior, his response to nurses, doctors and the tests that he has had in the hospital. Include your observations of his behavior after operation. In what ways is his behavior different from that which you observed in the preoperative period? Describe his parents' response to his change in behavior? How did you help them to see that operation had changed his physical condition and made it possible for him to lead a more nearly normal life?

5. What symptoms in a school-age child would lead you to suspect that the child was in the beginning stages of rheumatic fever?

6. What are the social and the emotional needs of the school-age child who is convalescing from heart disease?

7. What anxieties might a school-age child with rheumatic carditis feel? How might the nurse function in alleviating his anxiety?

8. What might be possible reasons why a school-age boy with rheumatic fever would show resistance to the order for absolute bed rest? What would you do if you noticed this kind of resistance in one of your patients?

BIBLIOGRAPHY

Bauer, Irving L.: Attitudes of children with rheumatic fever, J. Pediat. **40**: 796, 1952.

Blake, Florence: Development and care during the school-age period *in* The Child, His Parents and the Nurse, p. 301, Philadelphia, Lippincott, 1954.

Brazelton, T. B., and Holder, R.: Emotional aspects of rheumatic fever in children, J. Pediat. **43**:339, 1953.

Clark, Hazel V.: Music, mobiles and cardiac catheterization, Am. J. Nursing **57**:1026, 1957.

Dodds, Maryella: Have fun . . . get well! (pamphlet), New York, Am. Heart A., 1953.

Flemming, Mildred: Rheumatic fever and cortisone therapy, Am. J. Nursing **56**:728, 1956.

Gross, R. E.: Surgery of Infancy and Childhood, chaps. 60-64, Philadelphia, Saunders, 1953.

Hansen, A. E.: Rheumatic fever, Am. J. Nursing **53**:168, 1953.

Jetter, L. E.: Some emotional aspects of prolonged illness in children, Pub. Health Nursing **40**:257, 1948.

Josselyn, Irene M., Simon, Albert, and Eells, Eleanor: Anxiety in children convalescing from rheumatic fever, Am. J. Orthopsychiat. **25**:120, 1955.

Nadas, A. S.: Pediatric Cardiology, Philadelphia, Saunders, 1957.

Nurse, Amy G.: But why can't I get up? Am. J. Nursing **53**:172, 1953.

Overholser, M. T.: The congenital cardiac program, Am. J. Nursing 53: 1478, 1953.

Pierson, D. E.: Nursing care of a child with tetralogy of Fallot, Am. J. Nursing 47:301, 1947.

Potts, W. J.: Tetralogy of Fallot, Am. J. Nursing 47:298, 1947.

Sadler, Sabra: Rheumatic Fever Nursing Care in Pictures, Philadelphia, Lippincott, 1949.

Sadler, Sabra, and Seibel, Elizabeth: The child with acute rheumatic fever and his nursing care, Am. J. Nursing 46:170, 1946.

Smith, E. M.: A nursing staff prepares for cardiac surgery, Am. J. Nursing 49:589, 1949.

Wallace, Mildred: Care of the child with tetralogy of Fallot, Am. J. Nursing 52:195, 1952.

Yasumura, Michi, and Baldwin, J. S.: Occupational therapy for the rheumatic and cardiac children, Am. J. Occup. Therapy 1:62, 1953.

Convalescent Care for Children (pamphlet), Chicago, Nat. Soc. Crippled Child., 1946.

The Child With Rheumatic Fever (pamphlet), Washington, D.C., Dept. Health, Education and Welfare, 1955.

CHAPTER NINETEEN

Diseases of the Blood

PHYSIOLOGIC CONSIDERATIONS

Blood consists of a fluid portion known as plasma and of formed components or cells. The plasma comprises slightly more than 50 per cent of the volume of the blood. Among the many functions of the plasma are the carrying of food materials to all parts of the body and the carrying away of waste products for excretion.

The plasma contains the elements necessary for blood clotting. A blood clot is formed by conversion of fibrinogen of the plasma to fibrin, which forms the coagulum. Fibrin is formed under the stimulus of thrombin. Thrombin is formed from the prothrombin of the blood through the action of thromboplastin derived from damaged blood platelets and from injured tissues. The calcium of the blood also is necessary for clot formation. That part of the plasma which remains after the fibrin is separated is serum.

The formed components of the blood consist of red cells (erythrocytes), white cells (leukocytes) and platelets (thrombocytes). (Plate 3.)

In fetal life and earliest infancy the red cells are formed in the liver, the spleen, the bone marrow and other lymphatic structures; after birth they are formed in the bone marrow. The mature red cell has no nucleus, but a nucleus is present in an early stage of its formation. In fetal life, nucleated red cells are common in the blood, and some may be found in the early days after birth, particularly in prematurely born babies.

After the earliest period of life, the finding of nucleated red cells means an abnormally rapid formation of red cells to supply a demand, as in the case of some of the anemias of infancy. A lesser degree of immaturity of red cells is shown by persistence in the cell of material known as reticulum, which is identified easily in a specially stained preparation of blood. Normally, red cells are being destroyed constantly and

433

being replaced by new ones. As evidence of normal speed of generation and replacement, approximately 1 per cent of the red cells of the blood are reticulated (reticulocytes). An increase above this proportion indicates rapid cell generation. Conversely, a paucity of reticulocytes connotes abnormally slow formation of red blood cells. Thus in the anemias, a knowledge of the proportion of reticulocytes is important for diagnosis and prognosis.

The chief function of the red cells is to carry hemoglobin, and the chief purpose of hemoglobin is to take oxygen to the tissues and remove carbon dioxide for excretion by way of the lungs. Hemoglobin is formed by the reticulo-endothelial cells of the bone marrow. In the normal disappearance of red cells from the blood, the cells are removed by the reticuloendothelial tissues, especially those of the spleen. The hemoglobin of the cells is broken down. The iron of the hemoglobin is split off and is largely reused. The pigment is changed to bile pigment and is excreted.

The white cells of the blood consist of granular leukocytes or granulocytes, lymphocytes and monocytes (large mononuclear leukocytes). The mature lymphocytes and monocytes have no important subdivisions. Granular or polymorphonuclear leukocytes are of 3 varieties: neutrophils, eosinophils and basophils. The granular leukocytes are formed in the bone marrow, the lymphocytes develop in the spleen, the lymph nodes and other lymphatic tissue, and the large mononuclear leukocytes have their origin in the reticuloendothelial lining of the blood sinuses of the spleen, the bone marrow, the liver and the lymph nodes (Plate 3).

In the course of development of granulocytes, the type of cell immediately preceding the mature cells is known as a myelocyte. Myelocytes differ from mature cells in their appearance and staining characteristics when a stained preparation is examined microscopi-

cally. The presence of myelocytes in the blood indicates an unusually rapid formation of granulocytes. The abundance of myelocytes characterizes the disease myelocytic leukemia.

The mature lymphocyte is small in comparison with the larger and more deeply staining immature form. The immature forms are found abundantly in lymphatic leukemia.

Plasma cells are infrequent but important units of the lymph nodes and bone marrow which are also found in the circulating blood at times. Their special significance is due to the belief that they form the gamma globulin of the plasma. This is the blood fraction which contains the antibodies.

The white blood cells seem to have no physiologic function in health other than to serve as a part of the defense mechanism of the body against infections. They are actively motile and penetrate tissues, especially at the site of infection. An increase in the number of neutrophils in the blood is often evidence that an infection is present and is stimulating the increase. After these leukocytes have migrated to the site of infection, they ingest and destroy many, though not all, varieties of bacteria. The so-called pyogenic infections stimulate an increase in the polymorphonuclear leukocytes. Other types of infection cause an increase in the lymphocytes of the blood. The eosinophils are increased especially in parasitic infestations.

The blood platelets or thrombocytes are formed in the bone marrow. The chief function of the platelets concerns blood coagulation. Platelets adhere to injured surfaces. In a wound, they quickly become damaged. Damaging of platelets releases thromboplastin, which initiates clot formation. When platelets are decreased greatly in the blood, spontaneous bleeding or purpura results. While platelets are important in the prevention of spontaneous bleeding, they are of less importance than the

PLATE 2

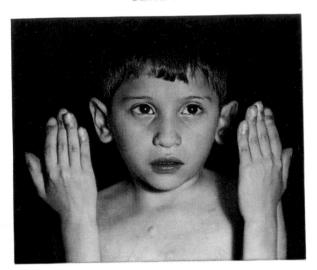

Cyanosis and clubbed fingers in a boy with
tetralogy of Fallot.

PLATE 3

ORIGIN AND DEVELOPMENT OF BLOOD CELLS

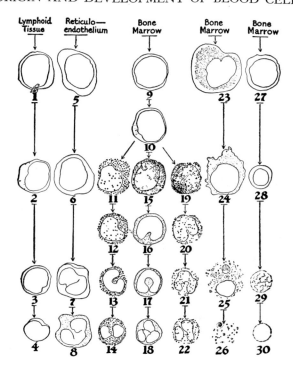

1. Lymphoblast
2. Large lymphocyte
3. Intermediate lymphocyte
4. Small lymphocyte
5. Monoblast
6. Large monocyte with azure granules
7. Monocyte with a few granules
8. Mature monocyte with azure granules
9. Myeloblast
10. Premyelocyte
11. Eosinophilic myelocyte
12. Juvenile eosinophil
13. Band eosinophil
14. Segmented eosinophil
15. Neutrophilic myelocyte

16. Juvenile neutrophil
17. Band neutrophil
18. Segmented neutrophil
19. Basophilic myelocyte
20. Juvenile basophil
21. Band basophil
22. Segmented basophil
23. Megakaryocyte (bone marrow)
24. Later megakaryocyte (bone marrow)
25. Megakaryocyte (peripheral blood)
26. Thrombocytes (platelets)
27. Megaloblast
28. Normoblast
29. Reticulocyte
30. Normocyte (erythrocyte)

PLATE 3

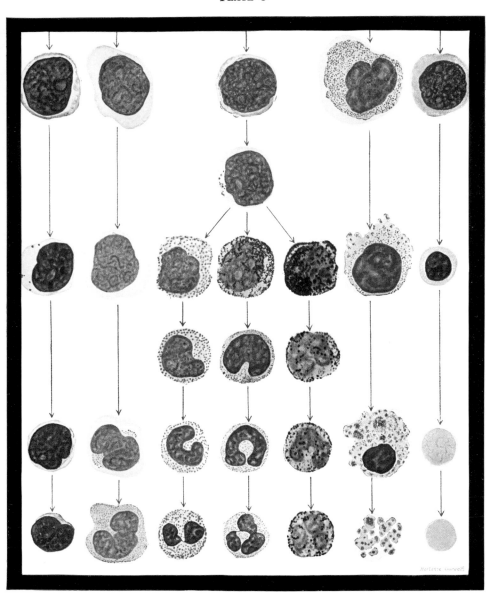

Blood cells.
(Kracke, Roy: Diseases of the Blood and
Atlas of Hematology, Philadelphia, Lippincott)

TABLE 8. NORMAL BLOOD VALUES AT DIFFERENT AGES

	BIRTH	12 WKS.	6 MOS.	2 YRS.	12 YRS.
Red cells (millions/cu. mm.)	4.5-5.5	3.5-4.5	4.0-4.5	4.3-4.7	4.5-5.0
Hemoglobin (grams/100 cc.)	15.5-18.5	10-12	11-13	12-13.5	13.5-15
White cells (average/cu. mm.)	20,000	12,000	12,000	10,000	8,000
Platelets (average/cu. mm.)	350,000	300,000	300,000	300,000	300,000

injured tissues in stopping hemorrhage from a wound. Injured tissues are a more important source of thromboplastin in these circumstances. Another important function of platelets is associated with their tendency to agglutinate. Thrombi in blood vessels sometimes consist mainly of agglutinated platelets. Agglutination of platelets in the terminal vessels of a wound assists in stopping bleeding.

The number of red cells at birth varies from 4.5 to 5.5 million for each cubic millimeter of blood. The number decreases rapidly in the first 7 to 10 days, the resultant accelerated hemoglobin breakdown often causing the so-called physiologic jaundice. Subsequently, the decrease is slower. The lowest number (3.5 to 4.5 million) is reached at from 6 to 12 weeks. Then the number gradually increases and at 6 months averages between 4 and 5 million. Subsequently, the number increases to a mean value of approximately 5 million, where it remains permanently.

The amount of hemoglobin at birth varies, with an average value of 17 Gm. for each 100 cc. of blood. The amount decreases for a period of from 10 to 12 weeks to 10 to 12 Gm., with subsequent increase of the lower values to approximately 12 Gm., where it tends to remain during infancy. The value rises through childhood. The rise is more rapid early in childhood and less rapid later. Adult values are reached at about 16 years of age. These values are from 14 to 16 Gm. for boys and as much as 2 Gm. less for girls. Average values vary geographically, the variation being dependent chiefly on the iron content of the soil and its vegetation.

The total number of white cells (exclusive of platelets) may be 20,000 or more for each cubic millimeter of blood on the day of birth. The number decreases rapidly to a total of from 10,000 to 15,000 by 2 weeks. Thereafter the decrease is slow. The number is between 9,000 and 14,000 at 1 year, between 8,000 and 13,000 at 2 years, and between 7,000 and 12,000 thereafter in childhood. The large mononuclear cells, the eosinophils and the basophils maintain a small but fairly constant proportion of the total white cells throughout infancy and childhood, ranging from 1 to 4 or 5 per cent. The chief variations with age are in the relative proportions of lymphocytes and polymorphonuclear leukocytes and in the numbers of immature white cells. The proportion of immature cells may be as high as 20 per cent in the early days of life, but very few, if any, are to be found after 6 months of age. The polymorphonuclear leukocytes predominate at birth but decrease to equal the lymphocytes between 1 and 2 weeks of age. Thereafter the lymphocytes predominate until late in the second year, when the two are again equal. Subsequently, the polymorphonuclear leukocytes permanently outnumber the lymphocytes during health.

The number of platelets varies, but

the variations with age are not remarkable. The number tends to be slightly higher in the first year than later. A normal value after the first year is between 200,000 and 350,000 for each cubic millimeter.

ANEMIA

GENERAL DISCUSSION

Anemia literally means without blood. Sometimes the term is used in this sense in relation to organs of the body, such as anemia of the brain, a condition in which the supply of blood to the brain is greatly reduced. More commonly the word "anemia" is used to designate a condition in which the concentration of red blood cells or of hemoglobin or of both in the circulating blood is reduced below normal. Usually, in childhood anemia the level of hemoglobin is the more important figure to consider.

Classification

Normally, red cells and hemoglobin are formed at the same rate at which they are destroyed. Anemia occurs whenever formation is decreased or destruction is increased. In the growing child the rate of formation also must keep pace with the demands of a body which is increasing in size. Except for the circumstance in which blood is lost from the body by hemorrhage, these two mechanisms are the sole fundamental causes of anemia. However, in many conditions there is a combination of the two mechanisms (or even of three mechanisms if we include blood loss) taking place, and a strict classification of anemias on this basis is not made easily. In the outline that follows, the principal mechanisms of anemia are outlined with examples of specific disorders in which these mechanisms operate as the main cause of the resulting anemia.

Principal Mechanisms Producing Anemia in Childhood

Blood loss (hemorrhage)
  Acute (trauma, operation, purpura, hemophilia)
  Chronic (ulcerative colitis)
Inadequate rate of blood formation (hypoplasia)
  Poor hemoglobin synthesis (prematurity, iron deficiency)
  Delayed red cell maturation (megaloblastic anemia, scurvy)
  Combination of above factors
  Infection (chronic respiratory, nephritis, rheumatic fever)
  Drugs (tridione, folic acid antagonists, nitrogen mustard)
  Poisons (lead, benzol)
  Bone marrow invasion (leukemia, tumors)
  Other (idiopathic anemia, hypersplenism, radiation injury)
Increased blood destruction (hemolysis)
  Antibody reactions (erythroblastosis, transfusion reaction)
  Hereditary trait (congenital hemolytic jaundice, sickle-cell anemia, Mediterranean anemia)
  Drugs (sulfanilamide, acetanilid)
  Poisons (naphthalene, fava bean)
  Infections (malaria, septicemia)
  Other (acquired hemolytic anemia, Lederer's anemia)

Symptoms

The symptoms of anemia are similar regardless of the cause. Lassitude, listlessness and fatigability are the early manifestations. As the severity increases, pallor, weakness, tachycardia and palpitation may occur. It is surprising how well a child with chronic anemia can get along. Compensations for the low level of hemoglobin often permit fairly normal activity when the concentration is reduced to a third of the normal value. However, persistence of such levels results in mental sluggishness, irritability and cardiac enlargement. Fatal anemia is a consequence of the inability of the heart to perform its normal work.

General Treatment and Nursing Care

The management of anemia will depend upon the severity and upon the presumptive cause in the individual case. Transfusion is the obvious and most widely applicable method of correction. It is imperative and often lifesaving when acute blood loss or severe chronic anemia has progressed to the point of interfering with cardiac function. It also may be useful in supplying missing blood elements other than red blood cells and hemoglobin (coagulation factors in hemophilia and platelets in purpura, for instance). Even in anemia of lesser severity it often provides the child with a sense of well-being and permits better appetite and a more active existence. In some forms of anemia it is the only possible method of ameliorating the failure of an inactive bone marrow. The nursing management of transfusion has been considered in Chapter 9.

Anemia which is due to insufficient intake of iron or to loss of the body stores of iron through hemorrhage requires an increase in the iron intake. This supplies the missing elements necessary to build new hemoglobin and also stimulates the activity of the bone marrow. Iron may be given by mouth in a number of ways. Ferrous sulfate, ferric ammonium citrate and ferrous glycinate are some of the compounds in common use. In infants particularly, it is desirable to start with a small dose and work up to the desired level gradually because it sometimes irritates the gastro-intestinal tract, and vomiting and diarrhea may result. When adequate dosage is achieved the stools usually assume a dark-green or black pigmentation. In occasional circumstances iron is given intravenously. Sometimes copper and cobalt salts are added to the iron medication in the hope of augmenting its erythropoietic powers.

Vitamin B complex factors such as folic acid, vitamin B_{12} and liver or liver extracts are essential adjuvants in treating some of the anemias associated with a megaloblastic bone marrow. In scurvy the correction of the deficiency by treatment with vitamin C rapidly helps the associated anemia.

Splenectomy is usually curative in congenital hemolytic jaundice and sometimes is used to advantage in Mediterranean anemia and other forms associated with tremendous enlargement of the spleen.

In nursing the older child with anemia, supportive measures are essential. Good general hygiene to build up resistance to intercurrent infections is important. Anorexia is a common symptom, and encouragement is often necessary to help the child to eat foods that are high in vitamins, calories and iron. Observation to note symptoms of fatigue should be made during the meal periods. Often these children are too weak to feed themselves and yet they resent being completely dependent during this routine. Allowing the child to begin feeding himself, giving him help when fatigue is apparent and then, after a rest, giving him an opportunity to finish independently often will influence his acceptance of larger quantities of food and satisfy his desire for independence.

In play, overfatigue must be guarded against. Some children stop playing when they are tired, but more of them become absorbed in play and do not react to fatigue until they become overstimulated. Redirection of play into less strenuous activities, such as doing puzzles or molding clay, should take place before injurious overstimulation develops.

When periodic transfusions require hospitalization, the nurse and the parents should help the child to meet the problem of frequent separations which involve procedures difficult for a young child to face. As a child grows old enough to understand, his interest and co-operation can be won by showing him a blood smear under a microscope and demonstrating to him the way in which a transfusion set gives him blood to increase his ability to do the things that other children are capable of doing. It is not uncommon to see a child with anemia accept his transfusion happily because he has learned from experience that co-operation reduces pain, brings recognition for his achievement and provides an increased amount of energy which is necessary to satisfy his need for activity. Emotional trauma produced by necessary blood counts can be lessened if the technician will give the child opportunity to investigate the apparatus, to cleanse the area and to assist in manipulating the equipment.

If an individual child's personality characteristics and interests have become known during hospitalization, helping him to adjust on subsequent admissions is facilitated greatly. When a child is greeted by a head nurse and a doctor who know and understand him, it gives him a sense of security and lessens the discomfort he feels when he returns to the hospital. A favorite toy may be in readiness, and in some instances it may be feasible to allow the child to select his own bed location. Encouraging the child to make his own preparations for the hospital trip may bring satisfactions that compensate in part for the uncomfortable aspects of the experience.

Anemia Due to Blood Loss

When there is sudden loss of blood from the body as from a severe epistaxis, a freely bleeding wound or a gastro-intestinal hemorrhage, the disturbance in body physiology is not related to the loss of blood cells alone, but in addition there is a loss of the plasma portion of the blood with reduction in the circulating blood volume. Thus, in addition to the effects of anemia, the child also may be suffering from shock. Treatment consists of transfusion and, of course,

appropriate measures to terminate the hemorrhage.

The common causes of excessive blood loss vary with the age of the child. In the newborn the common causes are an improperly tied umbilical cord, birth injury from a difficult delivery and free bleeding from the gastro-intestinal tract. In the infant, bleeding from the bowel is most common. In the older child it is more commonly the result of a traumatic accident or a defect in the clotting mechanism of the blood, such as hemophilia or purpura.

When blood loss occurs at a slower rate, as from chronic ulcerative colitis or bleeding from an intestinal polyp, the reduction in blood volume does not take place, and the symptoms are due chiefly to the resulting anemia. Treatment is directed at the underlying cause and may include transfusion as a temporarily supportive measure.

Nutritional Anemias

Hypochromic or Iron-Deficiency Anemia

The most common form of anemia in infants is that which develops from a failure of the child to take in enough iron in his diet to supply building material for the new hemoglobin which he needs for his expanding size. The anemia is characterized by a relatively normal production of red blood cells. The cells are smaller than normal in size and very deficient in hemoglobin content, so that each may contain less than half the normal quantity. This type of anemia is called hypochromic or microcytic. It occurs between the ages of 9 months and 2½ years. Almost invariably the infant is one who has developed an inordinate fondness for milk, consuming 1 or 2 quarts per day and refusing most other foods. In spite of rather severe degrees of anemia, there is little interference with activity. The child is usually pale, irritable and obstinate about his refusal of solid foods. Treatment consists of the addition of one of the iron preparations to his daily milk ration. This usually produces a rapid improvement in anemia and at the same time increases the appetite for foods other than milk so that gradually the child can be encouraged to accept a diet which is better balanced nutritionally. Restoration of normal blood values can be expected in 4 to 8 weeks' time. If the anemia is so severe that the circulation is embarrassed or if the child is otherwise ill, it may be necessary to effect a more rapid correction by transfusion.

Megaloblastic Anemia

During fetal life the bone marrow contains very large cells (megaloblasts) which are the precursors of the fetal red blood cells. Normally, these large cells disappear from the bone marrow during the last weeks of intra-uterine life and are replaced by a smaller type of cell (erythroblast) which is the precursor of the adult type of red blood cell. Under certain clinical conditions megaloblasts may persist in the bone marrow after birth or may return to it. Their presence in the bone marrow can be detected only by marrow aspiration, but it may be suspected when the circulating blood contains red cells which are larger than normal (macrocytes) or when anemia is accompanied by a sharp decrease in the number of red blood cells in the circulating blood in addition to the reduction of hemoglobin. In hypochromic anemia, as described above, each red blood cell carries an abnormally small quantity of hemoglobin, but the number of cells is close to normal. In megaloblastic anemia the number of cells is decreased, but each cell may carry a normal quantity of hemoglobin (normochromic) or even an increased quantity (hyperchromic), due to its large size. A variety of clinical circumstances may precede the development of megaloblastic anemia. These have in common a disturbing effect upon the normal metabolism of folic acid, folinic acid

(citrovorum factor), vitamin B_{12} or vitamin C. These disturbances in turn interfere with the synthesis of nucleoproteins which are necessary for the maturation of the red blood cells. The clinical conditions which may result in megaloblastic anemia are not very common. Among them are scurvy, dietary deficiency of folic acid, pernicious anemia, celiac disease and certain varieties of liver disease. Treatment depends upon the exact nature of the metabolic disturbance, but in most instances correction can be achieved by giving liver extract, vitamin B_{12}, folic acid or vitamin C.

ANEMIA OF INFECTION

With repeated acute infections or with chronic infection of long standing, some degree of anemia usually is found. Increased red cell destruction is sometimes a factor, but the more severe effect of infections is on the blood-forming tissues. The formation of hemoglobin is retarded in most instances, with a secondary effect of decreased formation of red cells. In other instances, in addition the blood generative cells are affected adversely, a condition known as hypoplasia when the decreased formation is partial and as aplasia when it is complete. Hypoplasia may outlast the infection. In many instances, the hypoplasia does not affect the generation of white cells; rather, a leukocytosis occurs. A few infections cause deficient generation of both white cells and platelets. If aplasia of granular leukocytes (agranulocytosis) occurs, the condition becomes serious, and death is likely to result. In the case of most of the infections, the anemia is neither severe nor serious.

HYPOPLASTIC TYPES OF ANEMIA

Under this heading are included those forms of anemia in which the *main* abnormality is the inability of the bone marrow to manufacture new red blood cells and hemoglobin at a rate which will support a normal concentration of these substances in the circulating blood.

Anemia of Prematurity

At the time of his birth the premature infant usually has average normal values of hemoglobin and red cells. Likewise, he has a store of iron from his mother which is appropriate for his small size. However, since he grows at a very rapid rate during the first few months of life and since his diet contains very little iron, his bone marrow is frequently unable to keep pace with the demands for new blood cells, particularly with the demand for more hemoglobin. In consequence, an exaggerated decline of the red blood cell count and of the hemoglobin level of the blood takes place. This is similar to the fall in values suffered by the full-term infant but is more exaggerated in degree. The smaller the premature at the time of his birth, the more severe his anemia is likely to become during these first few months.

Usually, iron is given to prematures routinely in an attempt to prevent or to lessen the degree of fall in hemoglobin. Success in this type of therapy is not always achieved, for it now seems to be true that the premature is not able to absorb and utilize iron very well for the first 6 to 8 weeks of his life. Usually the hemoglobin can be permitted to fall as low as from 6 to 8 Gm. per cent. A more marked degree of anemia may demand transfusion. Iron preparations for intramuscular use are now available which can be administered early during prematurity.

Drugs and Poisons

A number of substances which are used in treatment of childhood diseases or are ingested accidentally by children may interfere with the formation of red cells and hemoglobin by the bone marrow. Tridione, chloromycetin, arsphenamines, the folic acid antagonists used in the treatment of leukemia and nitrogen mustards are examples of ther-apeutic agents which must be monitored by periodic blood examinations. To this list the effects of radiation from roentgen therapy or from the use of radioactive compounds in the treatment of neoplastic diseases must be added. Lead and benzene derivatives are the most common types of poison that may depress bone-marrow activity.

Bone-Marrow Invasion

In leukemia and in some of the tumors of childhood which have widespread metastases (neuroblastoma of the adrenal, for instance) there may be so much replacement of normal marrow tissue that an insufficient quantity remains available to form new blood cells. This type of anemia also is called myelophthisic anemia.

Miscellaneous Causes

Congenital and idiopathic types of hypoplastic and aplastic anemia are known to occur. In the congenital variety the failure to form sufficient red cells is present at birth. In the idiopathic variety the deficiency appears later in life for unknown reasons. Hypoplastic anemia implies that the rate of formation of red cells is slowed; aplastic anemia implies that the formation of red cells has stopped altogether. Usually there is an associated defect in the formation of the other elements of the blood, such as the platelets and the white blood cells. Stimulation of the sluggish bone marrow is sometimes possible through the administration of ACTH or cortisone. Where this fails, repeated transfusions must be given in the hope that a spontaneous remission will occur.

Certain disorders associated with splenic enlargement may be accompanied by anemia. Both the excessive destruction of red cells by the spleen and a depressant effect upon the bone marrow by unknown substances produced in the spleen have been blamed. In some instances removal of the spleen causes improvement in the anemia. In other instances the splenic anemia is part of a more widespread disorder which cannot be treated in this fashion.

HEMOLYTIC TYPES OF ANEMIA

In the hemolytic varieties of anemia the predominating mechanism is too rapid destruction of the red blood cells. The speed at which excessive destruction takes place determines the nature of the symptoms. Very rapid destruction takes place in the types of hemolytic anemia which are mediated by antibody reactions. These include erythroblastosis fetalis and transfusion reactions. Under these circumstances a large quantity of pigment resulting from the breakdown of hemoglobin from destroyed red cells is presented suddenly to the liver for excretion. Since the liver is unable to clear the blood of this pigment, jaundice develops. The process is acute, often serious and usually limited to a brief time. In congenital hemolytic jaundice a slower degree of hemolysis takes place continuously, with superimposed "crises" during which the rate of hemolysis is accelerated temporarily. A similar but less marked phenomenon may occur with sickle-cell anemia, but in Mediterranean anemia the hemolysis tends to be slow and steady. Jaundice in these latter disorders is ordinarily difficult to detect except during a crisis. However, increased levels of bilirubin are present in the circulating blood. In all varieties of hemolytic anemia the bone marrow responds to the demands for a more rapid production of red cells. It hypertrophies and occupies a larger than normal share of the inner structure of the bones. Microscopic examination of a sample of bone marrow obtained by aspiration reveals evidence of great acceleration of red blood-cell formation. Reticulocytes and in some cases nucleated red blood cells appear in the circulating blood in increased numbers.

Transfusion Reaction

When mismatched blood is transfused there is rapid agglutination of red blood cells, due to admixture with agglutinins of the same type as the agglutinogens of the transfused cells. Once agglutinated, the red cell masses are destroyed rapidly, and their hemoglobin is released. Jaundice results. No aggravation of the pre-existing anemia takes place, since only the transfused cells are being destroyed.

Erythroblastosis Fetalis

This disorder, also known as acute hemolytic anemia of the newborn, is discussed in Chapter 10.

Congenital Hemolytic Jaundice

This disease occurs only in the white race. The outstanding clinical features are mild jaundice and enlarged spleen. Anemia may be only moderate. In the typical case, the red cells show increased fragility when suspended in salt solution of decreasing concentration in a series of test tubes. Hemolysis normally begins when the concentration has been decreased to 0.42 per cent and is complete with a decrease to 0.32 per cent. In congenital hemolytic jaundice, hemolysis may begin before the salt concentration has been reduced to 0.50 per cent and is complete at concentrations higher than that required for normal blood. The increased fragility in the test tube does not explain the increased fragility in the body, because similar osmotic conditions do not exist. In some instances in which the disease cannot be otherwise distinguished from congenital hemolytic jaundice, the fragility in the test tube is unaltered from the normal. Other evidence that the red cells of this disease are abnormal is shown when a preparation of fresh blood is examined under a microscope. Many of the red cells are more or less spherical in shape (spherocytes) instead of being the usual biconcave disks.

The disease makes its appearance at any time after birth and persists indefinitely. Often the health apparently is unaffected. In other instances, severe anemia may develop. An acute hemolytic crisis may occur abruptly with fever and chill and it may last for several days or weeks. Recovery is usual.

The treatment consists of splenectomy. Removal of the spleen always causes improvement and often apparent cure. Increased phagocytic activity for red cells has been demonstrated in the spleen. Immediately after splenectomy, a major increase in red cells and hemoglobin equivalent to an autotransfusion occurs. However, the red blood cells retain their abnormal shape and increased fragility to laboratory tests.

The classic variety of congenital hemolytic jaundice depends upon a hereditarily transmitted abnormality of the red blood cells. Transmission is through the passage of a dominant gene. Other members of the child's family, including at least one parent, will show the same abnormality in fragility. The extent to which the abnormality bothers an individual is variable, since some have no symptoms while others may have recurring severe hemolytic crises. In the classic form of the disease, splenectomy is curative. When hereditary transmission is not apparent or other features are missing, the disorder may not be affected by splenectomy.

Sickle-Cell Anemia

This disorder occurs almost exclusively in the Negro race. The red blood cells tend to assume a crescentic or sickle shape, due to the presence of an abnormal hemoglobin which is designated as hemoglobin S. The tendency of the cells to sickle can be demonstrated by the following test: A drop of blood on a slide is mixed with a drop of normal saline, covered with a thin cover-slip which is rimmed with petrolatum and allowed to stand 24 hours at room temperature. The number of cells which sickle depends upon the proportion of hemoglobin S as compared with normal hemoglobin in each cell. When the dominant sickling trait is inherited from one parent alone (heterozygous state) it does not cause an anemia. But when it is inherited from both parents (homozygous state), an anemia develops as a result of the rapid breakdown of red cells carrying a large proportion of hemoglobin S, and the child shows all of the signs of a chronic hemolytic anemia, i.e., enlargement of the spleen, jaundice and fragility of the bones which develops as a result of the widening of the marrow spaces. The active disease may start during the first year but seldom before 3 to 4 months of age. Its onset may be gradual or by the sudden appearance of a crisis with fever. Treatment is symptomatic and directed at reversing the agglutination of sickled cells within the small blood vessels. This latter is accomplished to a degree by the administration of oxygen and by expanding the blood volume through hydration with fluids low in electrolyte content. ACTH may be used to decrease pain. Transfusions are avoided whenever possible, for they add to the iron content of the body and in time may lead to abnormal deposition of iron in the tissues of the body (hemosiderosis).

Mediterranean Anemia (Cooley's Anemia, Erythroblastic Anemia, Thalassemia)

This hemolytic anemia is both hereditary and racial. It occurs in families whose national extraction can be traced to the races inhabiting the Mediterranean Sea, predominantly Greek, Italian and Sicilian. It is congenital and often familial. Although congenital, the signs of the disease are rarely present in the newborn period but develop within the first few months of life. The anemia progresses slowly and is severe; it is characterized by marked distortion of the shape and the size of the red blood cells and the presence of large numbers of nucleated red cells (erythroblasts and normoblasts) in the peripheral blood. Hemoglobin formation is faulty, and the bone marrow continues to make fetal type hemoglobin as a compensation. Like sickle-cell disorder the condition may occur as a mild, heterozygous trait (thalassemia minor) or as the homozygous, full-blown disease (thalassemia major).

The characteristic feature of the disease is the extreme activity of the blood-forming organs, which produce large numbers of immature and defective red cells which are destroyed rapidly. The distinctive clinical signs—enlargement of the spleen and the liver and thinning of the long bones of the skull and the face —result from the combination of excessive blood formation and destruction. The physical appearance of severely affected children is similar; physical growth is stunted, the pallor is muddy, the faces are broad with high malar prominences and shallow orbits, the abdomen is enlarged, the posture is poor, and the musculature is flabby. Roentgenograms of the bones reveal progressive evidence of dilatation of the medullary cavity and atrophy of cortical and cancellous bones. The anemia eventually becomes severe and causes death. No satisfactory treatment is known. Transfusions are necessary to support life but cannot correct the anemia adequately or indefinitely.

Other Types of Hemolytic Anemia

Drugs, poisons and infections may produce an accelerated rate of red blood-cell destruction which eventually leads to anemia. Sulfanilamide, acetanilid, naphthalene and fava beans are examples of substances whose ingestion may lead to hemolytic anemia. During the course of malaria the parasites disrupt the red blood cells and produce hemolysis which eventually leads to anemia. In various types of septicemia, notably that caused by the hemolytic streptococcus, acute hemolysis may occur. Lederer's anemia is a severe acute form of hemolytic anemia seen among children. Its mechanism is not entirely understood, but it frequently appears to be the result of an acute infection. Ordinarily, it does not recur.

LEUKEMIA

Leukemia in childhood is an acute, rapidly progressive and fatal disease in which the essential pathologic lesion is an overproduction of any one of several types of white blood cells. The most common types seen in children are (1) acute undifferentiated or stem-cell, (2) acute myeloblastic and (3) less commonly, the acute monoblastic type. The subacute and the chronic forms of lymphatic and myelogenous leukemia are extremely rare in children.

PATHOGENESIS

In all of the 3 types of acute leukemia, immature white blood cells or blast forms are produced in large numbers in the blood-forming tissues throughout the body, while the production of normal cells is reduced progressively. The immaturity of the leukemic blasts may limit their identification by any of the specialized hematologic technics, and it is often impossible to distinguish among the different types of cells involved in the acute forms of the disease. However, certain characteristics are common to all of the blast cells typical of leukemia: (1) they multiply rapidly, (2) they fail to develop into the mature cells of the strain which they represent and (3) therefore they are unable to function as mature white blood cells. The factors which stimulate production of these cells and limit their maturity are unknown, but at the present time it is felt that leukemia has many of the features of a neoplasm. The immaturity of the blasts and the infiltration of these cells into tissues outside of the centers of blood formation support this concept of the disease.

Although it is true that an overproduction of a single cell type always occurs in leukemia, the number of leukemic cells which circulate in the blood is not always high. When the white blood count is high, the blasts are present in high percentage, and the blood picture is said to be "leukemic." When the count is low, with a low percentage of blasts, it is spoken of as "aleukemic." In the latter case it may be necessary to confirm the diagnosis by a study of a sample of the bone marrow, which is obtained by aspiration of fluid marrow.

Anemia develops rapidly in the early course of leukemia in children. It is a hypoplastic type of anemia in which the hemoglobin and the red cell count are reduced proportionately, and a low reticulocyte count reflects the failure of red-cell formation.

Platelet production is impaired, and the level of platelets in the blood is reduced severely. The hemorrhagic manifestation of the disease is due largely to the lack of platelets and the consequent oozing of blood from the smaller blood vessels.

The lymph nodes throughout the body enlarge, and the liver and the spleen may grow to great size unless the development of the leukemic tissue can be controlled. The bony skeleton may be involved as a result of widening of the medullary spaces and infiltration of the periosteum with leukemic cells.

The peak of the age incidence of leukemia occurs in children between 3 and 8 years. This curve is similar to that of the acute communicable diseases. However, to date, no relationship has been demonstrated between leukemia and infections. The disease may occur at any age; several cases are recorded of congenital leukemia recognizable at birth. It occurs throughout childhood, adolescence and young adult life. The acute leukemias are rare in people over 30.

SYMPTOMS

In general, the symptoms of the acute leukemias are the same regardless of the cell type involved. The onset may be gradual or rapid. Common first

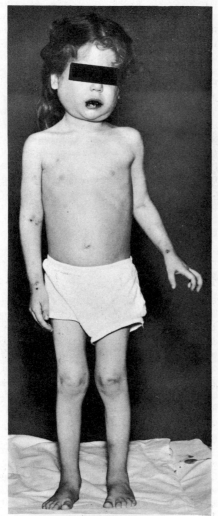

FIG. 83. A child with leukemia, showing parotid and cervical gland swelling, mouth and skin lesions.

symptoms which date the onset of the disease are low-grade fever, pallor, tendency to bruise, enlargement of the lymph nodes, pain in the legs or the joints and lassitude. When pain in the bones occurs early, the condition may be confused with rheumatic fever. The early symptoms must be differentiated from many of the acute infectious diseases which involve the peripheral

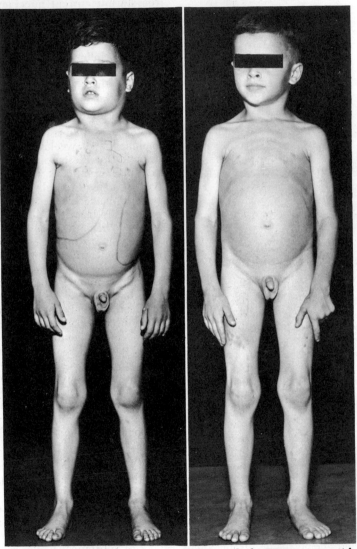

Fig. 84. (*Left*) A child with leukemia before treatment with ACTH. Note enlargement of cervical and inguinal lymph nodes and the penciled outline of liver and spleen. (*Right*) Same child after treatment with ACTH, showing decrease in size of lymph nodes of neck and groin.

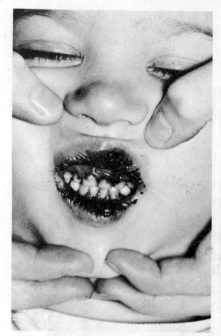

Fig. 85. The mouth lesions of leukemia.

lymph nodes and the spleen. As the disease progresses, fever of a relapsing type, hemorrhagic manifestations, increasing pallor and enlargement of the liver and the spleen develop. The symptoms vary greatly in individual cases, as might be expected in a disease which affects not only the blood-forming organs primarily, but all of the tissues of the body, either by infiltration or indirectly by the changes in the blood which is brought to them. In the natural course of the disease, the complications which develop from a lack of normal white blood cells are usually fatal; ulcerations of the mouth and the pharynx form as a result of bacterial invasion of the buccal mucous membrane, and hemorrhages from these sites are common. The low level of blood platelets causes purpuric and petechial hemorrhages in the skin and elsewhere throughout the body (Fig. 83). Intracranial and visceral hemor-

rhages are not uncommon. Anemia is progressive, and although it can be supported with transfusions temporarily, the child becomes weaker, and death results either from the disease itself or from an intercurrent infection. Prior to 1948, when certain drugs became available for treatment, the course of the disease averaged 3 months. Death sometimes followed within 3 weeks and rarely was postponed until 6 months following the onset of symptoms.

DIAGNOSIS

Leukemia often is suspected from the combination of weakness, pallor, hemorrhagic manifestations and enlargement of lymph nodes, the spleen or the liver. If immature cells are present in the peripheral blood, the diagnosis is made easily from the differential blood smear. When there is doubt, microscopic examination of bone marrow is usually conclusive. In some instances the suspicion of leukemia may arise through histologic study of a lymphnode biopsy.

Sometimes leukemia is confused with other disorders which produce an increase in the number of circulating white blood cells or an alteration of their appearance. Pertussis, severe infections, infectious mononucleosis and occasionally the iron-deficiency anemia of infancy may cause temporary confusion until study of the bone marrow eliminates the possibility of leukemia.

TREATMENT AND NURSING CARE

Although leukemia is an invariably fatal disease, recent medical advances have improved the methods of palliation and offer hope that eventually a cure may be discovered. Two general types of substances which can produce a remission are now available—the adrenal cortical hormones and the folic acid antagonists. The duration of life after the discovery of leukemia has been extended for many children to periods up to and even beyond 2 years. ACTH, cortisone and hydrocortisone all have been found capable of initiating a complete or partial remission of the symptoms, together with a change in the appearance of both the peripheral blood and the bone marrow (Fig. 84). The duration of improvement is variable, from a few weeks to several months. In some cases a second or third effect can be obtained by retreatment. The usual manifestations of hormone therapy can be expected as side effects when heavy dosage or prolonged administration is used. In addition, these children must be protected from intercurrent infection by continuous administration of antibiotic drugs because of their lowered resistance.

Similar effects may be obtained by the administration of the folic acid antagonist drugs—Aminopterin and A-methopterin. These drugs presumably interfere with the metabolism of folic acid, which is necessary to the synthesis of the nucleoproteins required by the rapidly multiplying white cells. Remissions obtained by these substances are often longer than those initiated by the steroid hormones, but the drugs themselves are quite toxic and may produce severe depression of the bone marrow and gastro-intestinal irritation and bleeding. With this form of treatment the child also requires protection against casual infection.

Recently another drug, 6-mercaptopurine, has proved to be effective in producing remissions of the disease. It acts differently from the folic acid antagonists but also interferes with the metabolism of the nucleoproteins of leukemic cells by inhibiting their use of the purine, hypoxanthine.

Antibiotics have played a large role in prolonging the course of leukemia by controlling the tendency to intercurrent infections. However, there is no indication that the use of any one antibiotic has been effective against the disease itself.

Transfusions are required to correct severe degrees of anemia when the leukemic process is not in remission or to stem the bleeding which may result from toxic effects of the folic acid antagonists.

Bone-marrow aspiration is a necessary part of the diagnosis and the control of the treatment of leukemia. To obtain bone marrow for study, a special Turkel bone-marrow needle is inserted through a nick in the skin into the sternum or the iliac crest. Procaine is used to anesthetize the area, and pressure is necessary to get the needle into the bone from whence the marrow is aspirated. The procaine anesthetizes the area, but the child feels the drug on his skin, the first injection, the pressure of the needle as it penetrates his tissues and the immobilization which is necessary to carry out the procedure effectively. Therefore, the child needs to have these details anticipated for him. He also should know that the doctor is going to get a tiny bit of tissue and blood from his chest or hip bone to help him find ways to make him more comfortable. He will feel supported if he knows that his nurse will be there to assist him in finding ways to help the doctor. The equipment listed is necessary for a bone-marrow aspiration: Turkel bone marrow needle, 2-cc. syringe, No. 25 gauge needle and procaine 1 to 2 per cent for local anesthesia, 20-cc. syringe and No. 22 gauge needle to obtain heparin from the vial to prevent clotting, 50-cc. syringe, No. 11 scalpel blade and handle, sponges, iodine and alcohol, eyedropper, 3 towels, gloves, gauze dressing and adhesive tape.

The symptomatic nursing care of the child with leukemia is not unlike that which is necessary for one with anemia. Frequently, the child with leukemia comes into the hospital not once but many times. He comes in for diagnostic procedures and treatments which are painful. For this reason it is especially important that he have help in making a constructive adjustment to the hospital experience. Many of these children need their mothers with them to alleviate anxiety and to make the experience more tolerable. With the nurse's assistance, the mother can help the child adapt himself to routines and to become acquainted with other children and the personnel. With the use of the newer drugs, many children experience long periods of remission. When they are hospitalized during these periods, they need to participate in an activity program which keeps them happy and growing emotionally.

In the terminal stage of leukemia, more intensive nursing care is necessary to give the child the maximum amount of physical and emotional comfort. Often the child with leukemia is miserably uncomfortable. He is irritable and demanding; it is understandable why he is perpetually dissatisfied with all that is done for him. His gums may be sore and bleeding (Fig. 85), his arms and legs may be painful to touch, he may be dyspneic, and the mucous membrane of his rectum often is inflamed, painful and, in some instances, necrotic. He may be nauseated, yet thirsty; he is lonely, yet fatigues easily and becomes irritated by those who attend him. He is apprehensive and fearful and is apt to be irritable when any change in routine is anticipated for him. He acts as if he senses the advent of danger. Part of that feeling comes from his parents' response to his rapid failure and part from sensitivity to bodily changes that he cannot help feeling.

Both the child and his parents need gentleness, sympathy and understanding. Although the parents have known perhaps for months that their child could not live, hope usually remains until the last. When death is imminent, it often seems unbearable to them. An ability to feel with the parents and to accept the way in which they express their grief is a quality which is needed

in the nurse who must minister to a dying child and his family. This quality takes time to acquire. It necessitates facing one's own feelings toward death as an inevitable part of life. This must be done before the nurse becomes able to handle her own tensions in a way which permits her to be helpful to dying patients and their parents. It must also be done before the nurse becomes ready to be of help to children in the ward who have been made apprehensive by the tension of the staff and by an awareness that something unusual is happening to a child whom they have known. For help in working through the nurse's feelings toward this important aspect of her work, the reader is referred to the references at the end of this chapter by Norris, Richmond, Wolff and Blake.

During the terminal stage of the child's illness, the nurse gives him a degree of comfort when she carries out procedures to keep his mouth and nose clean, his lips and tongue moistened, when she administers sedatives regularly, bathes his feverish skin, changes his position when she sees that he is becoming fatigued and stays with him to minimize the anxiety which he is experiencing. When the child's parents cannot be with him, the nurse must remain to support him when pain is acute and to give him the security of knowing that someone is with him.

Although the child may lapse into unconsciousness, a nurse's presence is a great comfort to the parents. They need to see that everything possible is being done for their child. They also should have the sympathetic understanding of the staff.

Leaving them alone with their grief indicates disinterest; it also may be interpreted as rejection—especially is this true if the parents manifest their grief overtly. The nurse who possesses the capacity for empathy can support the parents and make the experience more tolerable for them.

MALIGNANT LYMPHOMA
(HODGKIN'S DISEASE, LYMPHOSARCOMA, RETICULUM-CELL SARCOMA)

The several types of malignant lymphoma are closely related neoplastic disorders affecting the lymph glands and the related lymphatic tissue. Differentiation among the 3 types is made by the histologic appearance of the tissue in the enlarged lymph nodes which are characteristic of the disease. All of the types are progressive but at a variable rate. In Hodgkin's disease the progression may be very slow; in reticulum-cell sarcoma, very rapid.

The cause is unknown. In some respects, the lesion appears to be neoplastic in much the same manner as does lymphoid leukemia, except that a different type of cell is involved in the hyperplasia. The disease runs a much slower course than leukemia of childhood, from 2 to 4 or more years, but the outcome usually is the same.

In the beginning, only a few glands are affected. Often these are in the neck, where the increase in size becomes obvious. Later, other groups of glands are involved. The spleen usually is enlarged. Lymphoid tissue of the bone marrow increases and gradually replaces blood-forming tissue.

SYMPTOMS

At first symptoms are meager or absent. As the various groups of glands enlarge, pressure symptoms are likely to appear. Glands in the mediastinum may press on the trachea and the bronchi, causing respiratory embarrassment. Other groups may press on blood vessels, causing edema or ascites. Many types of pressure symptoms are possible.

After the disease has progressed sufficiently, constitutional symptoms appear. Fever of remittent and intermittent type is present. Anemia of hypoplastic type gradually increases. Weight loss occurs. Death occurs eventually from general weakness if it does not occur sooner because of disturbance of some vital function from gland pressure.

DIAGNOSIS

Diagnosis is made with certainty only by histologic examination of a lymph gland and the finding of cells characteristic of the disease.

TREATMENT

In a few fortunate instances the process may be discovered early when it is limited to a few lymph nodes which can be completely removed surgically. More often by the time the diagnosis is made, widespread changes are apparent. Roentgen therapy is effective in reducing the size of the nodes, but there is a limit to the amount which can be given safely to any one area or to the body as a whole. Usually, such treatment is given to nodes which are causing pressure symptoms by impinging on adjacent vital structures. The nitrogen mustard compounds are also effective in reducing the size of lymph nodes by destroying the more rapidly growing cells. The frequency and the dosage of administration must be regulated carefully, since these compounds also have a depressing effect upon the bone marrow in general.

INFECTIOUS MONONUCLEOSIS
(GLANDULAR FEVER)

This mildly contagious disease presumably is caused by a specific virus, although the agent has not been identified. It is characterized by fever, sore throat and swelling of the lymph nodes in the cervical region. The peripheral blood contains large, atypical white blood cells of the lymphocytic series. For these reasons, the disorder sometimes is confused with leukemia. However, its course is benign and self-limited. No treatment is effective. Diagnosis depends upon the recognition of the abnormal cells in the blood and the appearance of heterophile antibodies during the second week of the disease.

INFECTIOUS LYMPHOCYTOSIS

Infectious lymphocytosis is also a contagious disease, the cause of which is unknown. Symptoms are mild or even absent. Its importance lies in the fact that a very great increase in the number of normal lymphocytes in the blood occurs. Often it is discovered during the course of routine blood examination and may cause unnecessary concern. No treatment is required.

PURPURA

Purpura is a condition in which spontaneous hemorrhages occur. They are mostly in the skin but sometimes in the mucous membranes, on serous surfaces and in internal organs. The hemorrhages may be minute (petechiae) or up to several centimeters in diameter.

Etiology

The hemorrhages of purpura occur from blood capillaries. Capillaries are extremely fragile structures, more so than thin tissue paper. The capillaries, especially those of the skin, are subject to injury with almost every motion of the body. When the capillary wall is broken, bleeding into the surrounding tissue would occur were it not for normal and prompt blood clotting. One of the key parts of the clotting mechanism is the blood platelet. Platelets adhere to injured tissue, disintegrate and release thromboplastin, which starts the clotting process and stops the bleeding. Also, platelets tend to agglutinate in the injured capillaries and thus aid the control of bleeding. So it is that purpura may occur in association with any condition which decreases the number of platelets in the blood (thrombocytopenic purpura or thrombopenic purpura). In some instances, the cause of platelet decrease is apparent (symptomatic thrombopenic purpura); in others, the cause remains unknown (idiopathic throm-

bopenic purpura). Any condition which causes hypoplasia of bone marrow causes platelet decrease. These conditions include certain infections, certain chemical intoxications and leukemia.

In some instances, purpura occurs despite a normal number of platelets. In all such instances damage has been done to the capillary walls in excess of the capacity of the platelets to take care of the situation. In some instances, the platelets seem to be abnormal in structure, in that they appear unusually stable. Even when platelets are normal in structure, their number is very small, and the normal number is only one twentieth that of red cells. The thromboplastin available is inadequate when capillary walls are made defective by disease or when extraordinary stress is placed on them. Defective capillary walls are present in scurvy, in cachectic or wasting states caused by disease and in some toxic states caused by infection. Petechiae occur in some infections in which the organisms are present in the blood and lodge in the capillaries. Petechiae from this cause are common in bacterial endocarditis and epidemic meningitis.

Petechiae occur in association with certain allergic reactions. In these instances, it seems likely that the purpura is the result of a localized specific tissue reaction which causes capillary stress, a reaction comparable in some respects with hives.

CLINICAL SIGNIFICANCE OF PURPURA

Most of the purpuras dependent on defective capillary walls (purpura simplex) are of no great importance clinically. The purpura of cachectic states is mild and is limited to the skin. The condition causing the wasting requires attention, but usually not the purpura. The same can be said for the purpuras of bacterial endocarditis, meningitis and other septicemic states. The management of the symptomatic thrombocytopenic purpuras is largely that of the underlying disease. It is desirable to discuss idiopathic thrombocytopenic purpura and allergic purpura separately.

IDIOPATHIC THROMBOCYTOPENIC PURPURA

This disease has wide variation in severity of symptoms. In the mildest form, the constitutional disturbance is only moderate, and the purpuric lesions are limited largely to the skin. When more severe, the purpura involves both the skin and the mucous membranes. The skin lesions are larger and more extensive than in the milder form. Fever and moderate or great prostration are present. The mucous membrane lesions frequently are the site of hemorrhage (purpura haemorrhagica). Bleeding may occur from the nose, the gums or the mouth. Blood may be vomited or passed in the feces and rarely it may be present in the urine. Rarely, hyperacute purpura occurs (purpura fulminans) with sudden onset, high fever and great prostration, with delirium, stupor, coma and death. Usually, cerebral hemorrhage is present.

Except for the few instances in which death occurs, a single attack of purpura runs a course of from 1 to 5 weeks and gradually subsides. Recurrence of the attacks is common. In the course of an attack, the lesions appear in crops, a phenomenon easily observed in the skin. The color at first is bright red and it does not disappear with pressure, which distinguishes the lesions from erythematous eruptions. The color of the lesions becomes darker and gradually fades. The color changes are familiar to all those who have had a bruise.

Because of the decreased platelets, the bleeding time from a skin puncture is prolonged. When blood is drawn into a test tube, the clotting time is normal, but the clot fails to retract in the normal manner. A tourniquet applied to the upper arm causes petechiae to appear in the skin below the constriction.

Treatment

Treatment is not required for the mildest variety of purpura. When the disease is more severe, transfusions are indicated. The adrenocortical hormones may be effective in restoring the platelet level to normal. If the disease is recurrent or chronic and does not respond to hormone therapy, a splenectomy should be done. The favorable effect of splenectomy on the disease is not understood completely, but removal of the spleen is followed in most cases by an improvement in the bleeding tendency and a rise in the level of platelets in the blood. Even if the platelet level of the blood does not rise, the rate of their destruction appears to be retarded, and the disease is made milder.

ALLERGIC PURPURA
(SCHÖNLEIN-HENOCH PURPURA)

This is a condition in which purpura is only one of several symptoms, often a minor one. In some instances, a prominent feature is pain in several of the large joints (purpura rheumatica, Schönlein's purpura); in others, acute abdominal symptoms predominate (Henoch's purpura). It is possible for both the abdominal and the joint symptoms to be present in the same child.

The purpura of this condition may be associated with other skin manifestations of allergy, such as urticaria and erythematous allergic lesions. Sometimes the urine contains albumin and at times blood. Bleeding may occur in the intestinal tract. The blood contains a normal number of platelets, and the tourniquet test is negative.

The abdominal symptoms are likely to be severe, and the diagnosis may be difficult. Intense colicky pain is present. The abdominal wall is held rigid. Nausea is common. Fever may be present. The arthritis may be confused with rheumatic fever. Even though the pain is often intense, other local signs tend to be meager. The attacks last several days. Recurrences are common, and at times the interval between attacks is very short.

The responsible allergen is not easy to determine. Skin tests are not often helpful. In some instances, the disease may depend on bacterial allergy and a focus of infection. Perhaps more often food allergy is responsible. In the search for the cause, it is useful to keep a food diary, noting what foods were ingested preceding an attack.

HEMOPHILIA

Hemophilia is an inherited disease in which a congenital defect in blood coagulation leads to a severe bleeding tendency. It is a disease of males only. The genes of the disease are carried by the females and transferred to their male offspring, yet the female herself has no symptoms of disease. A male hemophiliac will transmit the latent form of the disease to his female children but will not transmit the disease to his sons if he marries a woman who is not a carrier of the trait.

The defect in blood coagulation is demonstrated by the increased clotting time of the blood. Normal blood will clot within 20 minutes after removal from the body. Hemophiliac blood requires a longer time—often from 60 to 90 minutes—for the clot to form. The specific nature of the defect in hemophiliac blood is not known, but it is known that normal plasma free of platelets will correct the deficiency. Bleeding from a cut or an abrasion tends to continue indefinitely. Despite this characteristic of the disease, the bleeding time is normal when tested by the standard technic, the reason presumably being that the test cut is small and smooth-edged, the cut surfaces lie in close approximation and adequate thromboplastin becomes available from damaged tissue cells.

Bleeding from even a small accidental cut eventually may become serious because of the total loss of blood with continued bleeding. At times, hemorrhage may be spontaneous or result from a slight bruise. Common sites for spontaneous hemorrhage are the nose and the knees. Repeated hemorrhage into the knee joints may lead to ankylosis and permanent crippling.

TREATMENT AND NURSING CARE

Treatment consists of use of those measures which stop bleeding. In some instances, compression may be appropriate; in others, the local application of thromboplastic substances. In any case, the bleeding usually will be stopped by transfusion of blood. The effect of transfusion is transitory, though it serves to stop the current attack. It affects coagulation time by supplying those elements which are necessary for the normal coagulation mechanism and are missing from hemophilic blood. In addition, whole blood transfusion helps to correct the anemia which has been suffered from blood loss. When bleeding has been slight, coagulation time may be controlled by administration of frozen or lyophilized plasma or antihemophilic globulin prepared from normal blood. Sometimes orthopedic measures are required for joints that have been crippled badly by repeated hemorrhage.

A diagnosis of hemophilia is frightening and evokes resentment in the parents and is potentially crippling for the child. To be faced with the responsibility of raising a child with hemophilia cannot help but evoke some feelings of resentment. An abundance of protection is essential to safeguard the child's health and life. If the diagnosis is made early in life, the infant must be protected with padded crib-sides and toys that are noninjurious. When he begins to crawl and walk, his mother must be vigilant constantly to prevent falls and to restrict potentially dangerous investigative pursuits. The care of a young child with hemophilia is a burdensome task which must be faced. If it is not faced, guilt and overprotection will result. When the child begins to seek playmates, the mother's fear of injury becomes manifested in warnings against fighting, running, falling and climbing. Every newly acquired capacity poses a potential crisis situation. Eternally the parents interrogate themselves in a manner similar to the following: "Dare I permit my child to go out to play with the neighbor's children? Will they be too rough or lure him into activities which might be dangerous? Dare I let him go to kindergarten? Should we take a chance and permit him to join the Scouts or let him take a week-end trip which is supervised by the scoutmaster?" If the child is hurt, many mothers blame themselves and feel as if they had been incompetent.

Living in a guarded environment suggested by the above comments poses problems for the child afflicted with hemophilia. Experiences which are necessary for psychological growth often are denied him. He feels his parents' anxiety and overprotectiveness, experiences frustrations unknown to normal children, experiences conflict and anxiety and searches for ways to relieve his discomfort. He may withdraw to lessen his anxiety and meet his parents'

need to overprotect or he may use his condition to control his parents. To master his fear of being an invalid or helpless he may defy his parents and do things that are potentially dangerous for him.

The child with hemophilia needs protective nursing care which meets his individual psychological requirements. Often he is faced with many hospital experiences. He comes into the hospital for blood examinations, transfusions or because he has been injured or has developed a crippled joint from repeated hemorrhage. The nurse needs to understand his background experiences within his family. She also needs to be able to understand his parents and recognize from whence their attitudes have come. When the child has been admitted because he has suffered an injury, his mother may be defensive because she expects to be labeled a negligent mother. The nurse who cares for a child with hemophilia will feel the impact of her responsibility in caring for the child 8 hours a day. She will recognize her need to scrutinize his environment and to institute protective measures to safeguard further injury without making him feel "crippled," inadequate or fearful. Her responsibility is minimal in comparison with that which a mother must face. A mother has the responsibility 24 hours a day, 365 days a year. When a nurse realizes the magnitude of the mother's responsibilities she will be able to feel with her and help her to handle her problems more effectively. It is not easy to protect in a way that eliminates feelings of inadequacy and fear. Nor is it easy to provide experiences that are both growth-producing and safe. Many mothers need help in this area of guidance. The nurse who can help a child to face his limitations and find safe constructive activities that produce feelings of inner strength will be able to give mothers the tangible help that many of them require.

SITUATIONS FOR FURTHER STUDY

1. Review fetal hemopoiesis. How does hemopoiesis of a normal infant differ from that of a baby with erythroblastosis?

2. What personal problems did you encounter in caring for a child during the terminal stages of leukemia?

3. How do you imagine a mother might feel when she discovers that her child is a hemophiliac. How might she manifest these feelings?

4. How might hemophilia affect a child's personality development?

5. What guidance does a child with hemophilia require? What would be your objectives in helping him understand himself?

BIBLIOGRAPHY

Blackfan, K. D., and Diamond, L. K.: Atlas of the Blood in Children, New York, Commonwealth Fund, 1951.

Blake, F. G.: The expansion of curiosity in The Child, His Parents and the Nurse, p. 212, Philadelphia, Lippincott, 1954.

Conley, C. L.: The anemias, Am. J. Nursing 52:957, 1952.

Cooke, J. V.: Leukemia in children, Am. J. Nursing 50:353, 1950.

Cooley, T. B.: The anemias of infancy and childhood in Brenneman's System of Pediatrics, vol. 3, Hagerstown, Md., Prior, 1948.

Hartman, John R., and Bolduc, Rose A.: Hemophilia, Am. J. Nursing 56:169, 1956.

Norris, Catherine M.: The nurse and the dying patient, Am. J. Nursing 55: 1214, 1955.

Richmond, Julius B.: Psychological management of children with malignant diseases, A.M.A., Am. J. Dis. Child. 89:42, 1955.

Smith, C. H.: Anemias of infancy and childhood, Am. J. Nursing 48:617, 1948.

Wilson, Henry E., and Price, Geraldine: Leukemia, Am. J. Nursing 56:601, 1956.

Wintrobe, N. M.: Clinical Hematology, Philadelphia, Lea & Febiger, 1951.

Wolff, Ilse S.: Should the patient know the truth, Am. J. Nursing 55:546, 1955.

CHAPTER TWENTY

Diseases of the Digestive System

STOMATITIS

Inflammation of the mucous membranes of the mouth may result from a variety of causes. It may be a part of a general disease, such as measles or chickenpox; it may be due to trauma from the teeth or too vigorous attempts to cleanse the mouth; it may result from injury by heat or chemicals or the allergic response to drugs such as sulfadiazine or penicillin or the anti-folic acid drugs used in leukemia; or it may be due to infection with bacteria (streptococci), with viruses (herpes), with spirochetes (Vincent's infection) or with a fungus (thrush). Deficiency of vitamins of the B complex such as niacin and riboflavin may also be responsible. A few of the characteristic forms of stomatitis will be described.

GEOGRAPHIC TONGUE

This condition is produced by a wandering eruption on the tongue which in appearance gives some suggestion of a map. The condition is symptomless and of no importance other than that its recognition permits reassurance of worried parents. The condition is common, and the cause is unknown. The lesion consists of a broad irregular line which travels slowly across the tongue. As the line progresses, desquamation occurs in the older parts of the lesion, leaving a bright red tongue surface. New areas of epithelial thickening appear in the older parts of the desquamated surface, and these in turn progress across the tongue in the same manner. The configuration of gray and red epithelium changes constantly. No treatment is required.

CATARRHAL STOMATITIS

This disease is characterized by a general reddening of the mucous membranes with a tendency to easy bleeding. There is pain and an increased flow of saliva. The discomfort may produce restlessness and usually interferes with the taking of food. Slight fever may be observed. Uncomplicated catarrhal stomatitis is of short duration and requires no treatment. Mechanical cleansing of the mouth should be avoided.

APHTHOUS STOMATITIS
(CANKER SORES)

In this painful but afebrile disorder of the mouth one or more ulcers appear suddenly. They presumably originate as small blisters of the membranes which break rapidly. Their cause is uncertain. Discomfort usually lasts about a week, after which the lesions heal without a scar. Gentian violet or tincture of benzoin may be applied locally.

HERPETIC STOMATITIS

This is a common disorder of children of preschool age. It is a specific infection with the virus of herpes simplex, which in the older child or adult produces a few fever blisters on the lips or may be responsible for some canker sores.

The disease is more important in infants and young children who are having their first encounter with the virus. A diffuse reddening and swelling of the gums and the mucous membranes usually is followed by superficial ulcerations. Fever and local soreness may be marked, and the lymph nodes of the jaw may enlarge. The child usually salivates more than he does when well. The discomfort from eating ordinarily limits food intake to milk or a few other bland substances. Temporary underfeeding may result. Fortunately, the disease is self-limited so that healing can be predicted in approximately 10 to 14 days. Local treatment is ineffectual. Tetracycline antibiotics sometimes appear to shorten the period of symptoms.

THRUSH (MONILIASIS)

Thrush of the mouth is found almost exclusively in small infants but may also appear during prolonged antibiotic treatment of the older child. It is due to the implantation and the growth of a yeast fungus called *Monilia albicans* or *Candida albicans*. The lesions begin as small slightly raised areas which become larger and confluent. The mycelia of the fungus grow down between the epithelial cells, making the plaque difficult to remove. Symptoms are absent except in very extensive infections. Usually the disease is acquired at birth from the mother's vaginal secretions which sometimes are infected with the fungus responsible for thrush. Later contact with the mother or spread from another infected infant through contaminated objects in the nursery or even by the medium of fungus spores floating in the air are additional means by which infection may be acquired.

Treatment is usually effective within a few days. The most common method is application of a 1 per cent aqueous solution of gentian violet to the lesions. Merthiolate in a 1:1,000 dilution or ferric chloride in a 2 per cent solution are also effective.

VINCENT'S INFECTION

When infection with the organisms described by Vincent is present mainly in the mouth, the disease is also called trench mouth or ulcerative stomatitis;

when it involves the tonsils or the pharynx extensively it may be called ulceromembranous tonsillitis or Vincent's angina. Two causative agents are found—one a large fusiform bacillus, the other a spirochete. The same organisms may be found in mouths that have no apparent infection, and now it is believed that niacin deficiency or the presence of a debilitating illness is necessary before the organisms can produce their destructive effects upon the membranes.

The early symptoms are offensive breath, increased salivation and local tenderness of the inflamed areas, whether it be gums or pharynx. Later there may be swelling and pain in the lymph nodes of the neck or the jaw. Lesions usually begin about the dental margins or opposite the teeth on the buccal mucous membrane. An ulceration appears which becomes covered with a dirty grayish or yellow membrane which bleeds when it is removed. In severe or neglected cases the teeth may loosen and fall out, or extensive areas of necrosis (noma) may result.

Treatment consists of the administration of niacin in therapeutic doses and the local application of oxidizing agents such as hydrogen peroxide, sodium perborate or potassium chlorate. Penicillin given intramuscularly is regularly effective in producing rapid healing of the lesions.

DENTAL CARIES

Tooth decay has become such a widespread affliction of man that its appearance in a child is too often regarded casually. It is a condition which is often overlooked as a contributing factor in feeding difficulties or in suboptimal health of the older child or adolescent. A great deal can be done through preventive measures and early treatment to preserve dental health and improve the child's general well-being.

ETIOLOGY

Dental caries begins with an assault upon the enamel, the hard, protective armor of the tooth which guards the softer, vital pulp beneath. While the exact role of each is still a matter of discussion, it is generally agreed that heredity, bacteria and diet play significant parts in the development of caries. Heredity may determine the chemical composition of the tooth and of the saliva which bathes it, thus increasing or decreasing its resistance to the action of the bacteria of the mouth which produce acids capable of eroding the enamel. Diet plays a role because the growth of these latter bacteria is favored by refined carbohydrates. Hence, the continuous consumption of sugar-containing foods (pop, candy, gum, cookies) between meals is regarded as an important inducement to the growth of destructive organisms. After the enamel has been etched away by the acid-producing bacteria, a channel is created through the armor which permits other bacteria to enter the pulp cavity of the tooth where they destroy its structure and set up infection. The tooth then crumbles, producing a cavity, and if infection is trapped deep in its recesses, a gum boil (apical abscess), diffuse cellulitis or even osteomyelitis of the jaw may result. Caries of the deciduous teeth is also a factor in destroying the normal alignment of permanent teeth and in preventing proper enamel formation before they erupt. Proper enamel formation in both sets requires an adequate intake of calcium and vitamin D.

SYMPTOMS

The slow progress of dental caries produces few symptoms until the major damage to the tooth has been achieved. Pain, inability to masticate food, and the occurrence of local infections of the tooth socket or the jaw are the usual means by which advanced destruction is announced.

PREVENTION

General preventive measures consist of adequate dietary intake of milk and vitamin D from early infancy, of discouraging the development of a "sweet tooth" in the growing child or at least substituting fruit and vegetable tidbits for the more popular between-meal snacks, and of hygienic cleansing of the mouth to remove the accumulated food debris and bacteria. Most important of the preventive measures is regular dental examination for the discovery and the repair of cavities while they are small. Addition of fluoride to the community water supply or direct application to the teeth is now regarded as an important means of decreasing caries. The fluorine enters into the chemical composition of the tooth and renders it more resistive to the action of bacterial acids.

CLEFT PALATE

As indicated in Chapter 16, operation for the closure of defects of the posterior palate usually is deferred until the child is at least 2 years old. When the child enters the hospital for this corrective surgery, nursing care will be of the utmost importance in his rehabilitation. Ideally, the child should enter the hospital several days prior to surgical treatment. During the preoperative period he should be helped to become adjusted to the treatment which he will require after repair has been performed. He should have an opportunity to become related to the nurse who will have to anticipate his needs when he is unable to verbalize his wants. In this period the nurse can help his mother prepare him psychologically for the operation and postoperative care if she has not already done so. Arm restraints should be applied at intervals so that he may become accustomed to the feeling of them and get to know the reasons for their use. Mouth irrigations, an important detail of postoperative care, should be introduced and the child's co-operation obtained by making them interesting and fun for him. The first time the equipment is presented, time must be allowed for the child to familiarize himself with it. He will enjoy filling and emptying the syringe. Little by little he can be taught its use. Thus fear and resistance during the post-operative period may be avoided, and effectiveness of the irrigation will be ensured.

The child must be in good physical condition at the time the operation is performed. During the preoperative period, careful observation to detect signs of infection should be made. Isolation technic, using a mask, is generally recommended to protect the child from respiratory infection. On the day before operation, frequent feedings of sweetened fluids should be encouraged as a shock-protective measure.

In the immediate postoperative period observation is necessary to prevent aspiration of mucus and blood, to detect signs of shock or hemorrhage and to prevent injury to the child's mouth.

Placing the child on his abdomen after operation prevents the danger of aspiration. Vital signs should be taken every ½ hour until the child is fully conscious and the results are within normal limits. Arm restraints should be ready for immediate application. Tongue-depressor arm restraints will not immobilize the elbows of the older child. Tying his wrists to the sides of the bed limits position change, antagonizes him and deprives him of all opportunities for independent play. Basswood splints which have been padded with sheet wadding can be used to immobilize his elbows. They must be long enough to extend from the axilla to the wrist and should be kept in place with an Ace bandage. These splints can be removed easily at bath time and for periods of play when the nurse is with him to help him to remember to keep his fingers away from his mouth.

A tray containing a bowl of sterile saline solution, a sterile rubber ear bulb and an emesis basin should be at the bedside for postoperative mouth irrigations. The mouth irrigation can be done most effectively with the child in a sitting position with his head tilted downward. Slight pressure on the bulb will produce a gentle stream of solution, which should be directed over the suture line. Teaching the child to allow the solution to run out of his mouth into the emesis basin should be done in the preoperative period when he is having his first experiences with the irrigation equipment. Every hour for the first 6 hours the suture line should be moistened with saline to give the child comfort and to promote healing.

When nausea and vomiting have ceased, the child's need for fluid and nourishment must be considered. Fluids are given by cup or from the side of a spoon; they are never given from a straw, a nipple or a syringe. For the first 3 days, clear fluids with additional carbohydrates are given at 2-hour intervals. After this period milk, eggnogs and creamed soups can supplement the diet. Sips of water should be given after the feedings to cleanse the mouth. Most children will accept their food and irrigations more readily if their arms are unrestrained and if they are allowed to hold the glass for drinking and the basin for the irrigation. A fluid diet is continued until all sutures are removed. The child should be weighed periodically to make sure that his nutrition is being maintained.

Children begin early to be aware of their handicaps and realize that they have difficulty in making themselves understood. When the speech defect is pronounced, other children laugh at them. Some teachers have difficulty in understanding them and fail to give them opportunity to express themselves because they often appear to be mentally retarded. As a result of these attitudes toward them, these children often withdraw, become shy and retiring as they see that the effort to become understood is futile. They develop a sense of inferiority and often grow overly dependent upon their mothers.

When the above children are admitted to the hospital for operation they will need additional help to feel comfortable in the ward. Opportunities for social relationships should be provided as soon as the child's physical condition permits. These children need opportunities for creative expression from which they can gain recognition and satisfaction. If a social worker is available on the hospital staff, the parents might welcome an opportunity to discuss their problems in rearing a handicapped child with her.

After the initial postoperative period, adjustment to a liquid diet is a difficult task for the child. His appetite increases, and he often begs for the food that he sees being served to other children. Substitute satisfactions are essential to prevent feelings of deprivation. If his mother cannot be with him, play and a satisfying relationship with his nurse is necessary to minimize the discomfort that he feels from the operative manipulation on his mouth, from restraint and from the limited diet that he is served.

Many times the child who has had his cleft palate repaired is discharged from the hospital before all the sutures are removed. In these instances the mother will require help in learning about his dietary requirements. In the home greater difficulty will be encountered in restricting the child to the prescribed fluid diet, since food will be more accessible and the temptation greater.

When speech-clinic facilities are available, arrangements for the child's referral should be made. If the cleft palate is repaired before speech patterns are set, much can be accomplished with skillful guidance and training. Parents may need help in understanding the value of speech therapy; otherwise, they may neglect training which is of vital importance for the child's future adjustment.

INGESTION OF FOREIGN SUBSTANCES

SOLID OBJECTS

It is common for young children to place foreign bodies in the mouth. Small foreign bodies may be swallowed and cause no difficulty. Foreign bodies that reach the stomach usually are passed through the remainder of the tract without symptoms. If they are opaque, their progression should be observed with roentgenograms. Long bodies may be expected to cause some trouble in the sharp curves of the duodenum, and therefore should be removed through the esophagus with the help of an esophagoscope, or surgically through the abdominal wall. Large foreign bodies may become lodged in the pharynx or the esophagus.

A foreign body in the pharynx may cause gagging, choking and perhaps obstruction to respiration to an alarming degree. Except in definite emergency, attempts at removal with the fingers should not be made.

A foreign body in the esophagus may cause only moderate discomfort and difficulty in swallowing. Liquid foods may pass easily. Prompt removal is important, particularly in the case of sharp-edged objects, because of the probability of perforation and ulceration and extension of the inflammation to the mediastinum or the respiratory tract.

Bezoar

Most foreign bodies that reach the stomach pass on without trouble. Certain types of indigestible material, when swallowed in large amounts, tend to accumulate in masses so large that passage beyond the stomach becomes impossible. Any such mass is known as a bezoar. The most commonly encountered bezoar is composed of hair, which usually has been pulled from the head and swallowed over a long period. The hair becomes matted in a large ball or mass. The symptoms are vague, and health and nutrition suffer little. A tumor is felt, and a filling defect is shown by x-ray studies with barium. The only treatment is surgical removal, a relatively simple procedure.

DRUGS AND POISONS

The accidental ingestion of drugs and poisons by preschool children contributes a significant fraction to the annual toll of accidental death. (In 1954 there were 2.6 deaths per 100,000 children between the ages of 1 and 4 years.) More than 400 individual substances are known to be toxic, many of them in common use around the home and on farms. The list is growing daily by the addition of new synthetic chemicals to be used as insecticides, cleaning and polishing agents, and drugs, and chemicals for the extermination of rodents and weeds. The Food and Drug Administration requires such substances to be labeled as poisons, but it cannot control their careless use or storage. The symptoms and specific antidotes of individual poisons require access to a handbook or a compendium, but certain general measures are advisable whenever a child is suspected of ingesting a poisonous substance.

Time is most important, since the drug or poison may be recovered from the stomach before a significant degree of absorption has taken place. Immediate measures to make the child vomit consist of gagging him with a finger or the handle of a spoon. If this proves to be ineffectual, he should be induced to drink as much milk or salty water as he will; then the attempts at inducing emesis may succeed. Then the container from which the poison was taken, some of the material obtained from his stomach, and the child himself should be taken at once to a clinic or a physician's office for further management. Usually, additional gastric lavage will be performed to recover as much of the material as possible. Symptomatic treatment of shock or metabolic disturbances will depend upon the type of poison absorbed. Occasionally, exchange transfusion is used to decrease the blood level of absorbed poisons.

Corrosive Esophagitis

Sometimes corrosive chemicals, particularly lye, are swallowed by young children. Such chemicals destroy tissues with which they come in contact. Usually the alimentary tissues from the lips all the way to the stomach are affected, even though only one swallow is taken. The primary symptoms of such a burn include pain, prostration and inability to swallow. The inflammation may cause sufficient edema to obstruct respiration, a condition requiring tracheotomy. If the child survives, the acute symptoms subside, and progress seems to be satisfactory until evidences of

esophageal obstruction appear within a month or two. The obstruction is due to contracture of scar tissue and may become so severe that no food or liquid can pass into the stomach.

Emergency treatment in the beginning includes neutralization of the swallowed chemical and relief of pain with sedatives. The antidote should be given much diluted, for neutralization generates considerable heat; thus an antidote given in a concentrated state may do as much harm as the original corrosive. The extra fluid used in dilution absorbs the heat of neutralization so that the tissue will not be damaged further. Gastric lavage is contraindicated. Olive or other food oil may be useful in helping to alleviate pain. Until ability to swallow returns, food and fluid must be given parenterally.

Stricture may be prevented by passage of appropriate-sized catheters at intervals, beginning within 48 hours of the accident. After stricture has occurred, usually it is possible to dilate it, but the process is slow. If the opening is insufficient to permit the passage of food, the child must be fed through a gastrostomy until dilatation is accomplished. Often retrograde dilatation is advantageous. It may be done through the gastrostomy opening.

EPIDEMIC VOMITING

Epidemic vomiting is a benign disorder which begins suddenly with vomiting which is otherwise asymptomatic. There is usually no fever or abdominal pain. The vomiting ceases within 12 hours ordinarily and may be followed by mild diarrhea and loss of appetite. Recovery is usually complete within 2 or 3 days. Because of its tendency to affect several members of a family in sequence, the disorder is believed to

be infectious in origin. A virus has been isolated from the stools of the victims in some epidemics. Treatment consists in withholding fluids and food until vomiting has stopped and then offering nonfatty liquids in small volume at frequent intervals. Solids are introduced gradually as tolerance for them is acquired. Phosphorylated carbohydrates such as Emetrol are often effective in decreasing the tendency to vomit.

RECURRENT (CYCLIC) VOMITING

Recurrent vomiting may be considered as a metabolic disturbance characterized by recurrent attacks of vomiting and associated with ketosis, each attack having a duration of from 3 to 5 days and terminating in spontaneous recovery.

ETIOLOGY

Recurrent vomiting occurs more frequently in the upper than in the lower economic levels. The causative mechanism is not well understood. The hypoglycemia which accompanies the condition may well be the cause of the symptoms. It is not clear in most instances why the hypoglycemia should occur. In some cases, the illness is preceded by an infection, often mild; in others, by emotional disturbance. In some children who are unusually labile in regard to the sugar content of the blood, attacks are precipitated apparently by even short periods of fasting. Liver damage, probably functional in most instances, has been assumed to be the cause of the hypoglycemia. In those rare instances in which the illness is severe enough to cause death, the liver is greatly enlarged and shows marked fatty infiltration. Furthermore, in acute infections liver function is impaired for sugar utilization.

SYMPTOMS

In its most common form, the individual attack manifests itself by a period of vague abdominal discomfort, which is followed quickly by severe vomiting. All food and drink are vomited as soon as swallowed. Prostration increases rapidly. In cases of moderately severe illness, somnolence is present, and in the most severe this may increase to coma. Some children have convulsions at the beginning of the attack, although this is not frequent. Severe thirst is a constant feature. Acetone bodies are found in the urine in large amounts. The ketosis has been reported as occurring in some instances before the onset of vomiting. The formation of acetone bodies may be sufficient to produce definite and sometimes severe acidosis. Although the child is alarmingly ill, the symptoms begin to subside spontaneously within a few days, and with the retention of nourishment recovery is very rapid. The child is free from symptoms between attacks, which occur at intervals of weeks or months. Attacks usually become less frequent as adolescence approaches, ceasing entirely at that time. Some observers associate migraine in adults with this condition.

TREATMENT

Dextrose and fluids are indicated in the management of the attacks. These materials may be given by any effective route. Because of the vomiting, oral administration is inadequate. The intravenous route is the most certain and consequently the most effective. The administration of dextrose must be repeated, preferably at short intervals in submaximum amounts. Ordinary degrees of acidosis respond quickly to the treatment with fluids and dextrose, but severe acidosis may require some alkali therapy in addition.

A certain degree of success in aborting attacks has been attained by the administration of extra sugar or sugar and alkali at the earliest indication of indisposition. Any chronic focus of infection, usually the nose and the throat, should be attended to. Every effort should be made to raise nutrition to a good standard for the individual child. Preferably, the diet should be definitely antiketogenic at all times. Usually, long intervals between meals are to be avoided, and to this end it may be advisable to offer a bedtime lunch.

ACUTE DIARRHEAL DISEASE

NONSPECIFIC DIARRHEA

Most of the diarrheas of childhood are mild and of little consequence. The exceptions such as typhoid, dysentery, ulcerative colitis and celiac disease are discussed separately. The risk of severe dehydration and acidosis is very low after the child has passed the age of 2 years. Dietary indiscretion and indigestion account for most of the cases. Treatment consists in the withholding of food and support of the fluid intake, usually by the oral route. Laxatives are sometimes used but are usually unnecessary. When the diet is resumed, simple foods of low-fat content should be offered first.

FOOD POISONING

Food poisoning is uncommon among children whose food consumption is likely to be confined to the home. Poisoning may result from the ingestion of foods containing toxic substances. Mushrooms, certain fish during the spawning season, fava and castor beans and ergot-contaminated rye bread are examples. Certain bacteria, notably *Clostridium botulinum,* staphylococci and some of salmonella organisms exude a soluble toxin which may contaminate foods and produce toxic symptoms and even death when the article is consumed. Botulism is the most serious type of food poisoning and is found only in association with the consumption of improperly canned foods. The other two types of organisms are less dangerous but are encountered more frequently. They may grow in foods such as salads, cold meats, custards and whipped cream which has been prepared in advance for social gatherings and has then been left unrefrigerated. The symptoms are sudden onset of abdominal cramps and vomiting within a few hours after eating the contaminated food. In severe cases there may be prostration and collapse. Supportive treatment is usually sufficient to tide the individual over, since the symptoms abate within a few hours as the toxin is excreted.

DYSENTERY

Dysentery results from the infection of the intestinal tract by specific microscopic agents. The most common form is produced by members of the dysentery bacillus group. However, increased travel to tropical and subtropical areas has augmented the incidence of the amebic type.

Bacillary Dysentery

Etiology. Bacillary dysentery may be caused by any one of several varieties of dysentery bacilli. The Shiga type of organism produces the most severe illness but is less common in this country than the Flexner and the Sonne types. Bacillary dysentery is a communicable infection, with the alimentary tract the portal of entry. The source is fecal, and the organism is transmitted chiefly through food. Flies have been shown to be carriers. Numerous milk-borne and water-borne epidemics are on record. The disease is more common in summer and also in warm rather than in cold climates.

The inflammation resulting from this infection is most marked in the colon and may be limited to this part of the bowel. Often the lower ileum is affected also. The extent of the inflammation varies from a simple catarrhal process in mild disease to extensive ulceration causing the passage of pus and blood.

Symptoms. After an incubation period of from 2 to 3 days, the onset of the disease usually is sudden. Vomiting and diarrhea are early symptoms. The vomiting may or may not persist throughout the attack. The usual constitutional evidences of infection are present. The white blood cells are increased. Prostration and anorexia are present early. Weight loss soon becomes evident. The temperature usually is not high and may be expected to range from 99° to 102° F., except as neglected dehydration causes it to become higher. Abdominal pain and tenesmus are common. Rectal prolapse may occur. The duration of the disease is from a few days in the mildest illnesses to several weeks in the more severe, except when the course is shortened by the use of sulfonamide drugs or antibiotics.

Complications. The most common complications are otitis media, pyuria and pneumonia. When the dysentery infection is severe, profuse hemorrhage from the bowel or perforation of the bowel wall may occur. With severe or prolonged dysentery in those already in poor nutritional state, the effects of various deficiencies may become evident, such as nutritional edema, noma and various avitaminoses. Also, skin infections, especially about the head, may appear.

Prognosis. Much of the dysentery in children in this country at present is not as severe as that observed formerly or as that which occurs in some other countries. The disease is much more serious for the infant than for the child. This is especially true of infants being cared for in a hospital because of other illness. The mortality rate among infants has ranged up to or above 30 per cent in the past. The present rate is much lower when modern therapy is used.

Diagnosis in the typical disease is not difficult. It is made definitely by identifying the dysentery bacillus in cultures of pus or other material from the stools. At times dysentery has been confused with intussusception because of bloody stools. Occasionally, meningitis has been the original impression because of meningismus.

Treatment and Nursing Care. Bacillary dysentery responds promptly to sulfonamides and to several of the antibiotics (chloramphenicol, chlortetracycline, oxytetracycline). With any of these preparations improvement may be noted within a few hours, and relative freedom from symptoms within a day or two. With these newer remedies, the average duration of the disease has been reduced from 2 weeks to a few days.

Fasting is desirable until diarrhea decreases and vomiting ceases. When food is given, it should be of a type that will not aggravate diarrhea; this could be boiled skimmed milk with added sugar. Restoration of body fluid and electrolyte content may be necessary. Pain and tenesmus may be relieved by small doses of paregoric.

The nursing care of a child with bacillary dysentery is similar to the care of a child with diarrhea from other causes, except that more strict isolation is required. The causative organisms are

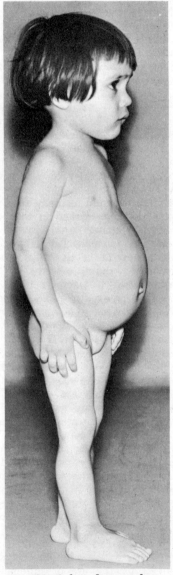

Fig. 86. Celiac disease showing protuberant abdomen.

abundant in the stools, and strict aseptic technic is necessary until stool cultures no longer show them. Effort should be made to discover the source of the infection. If the disease has been contracted because of negligence or ignorance in care, education of the family is desirable to prevent recurrence.

Amebic Dysentery

Amebiasis is a term applied to human infestation with *Endameba histolytica* whether or not diarrhea is present. This term applies to the symptomless carrier and to the carrier with mild occasional symptoms, as well as to those with acute dysentery. All these conditions are interrelated, since all these states may exist at different times in the same person. The acute disease may subside, to be followed by a carrier state and possibly by further acute attacks later.

The acute form of the disease, dysentery, is characterized by active invasion of the wall of the colon by ameba, with the formation of necrotic pockets similar to abscesses and with ultimate discharge of the necrotic material into the bowel. The acute stage is associated with nausea, vomiting, colic, abdominal pain, tenesmus, diarrhea and the passage of blood and mucus in the bile-stained fluid stool. Usually there is little or no fever. The child becomes depressed and loses strength. Spontaneous recovery may occur without special treatment.

Amebiasis is more common in adults than in children. Amebic dysentery is rare in infants in this country. Amebiasis is more common in warm than in cold climates, although probably the condition is related more to primitive sanitary conditions than to climate. The form of the parasite that causes the acute phase of the disease is not able to communicate the disease. The disease is transmitted by an encysted form of the ameba which occurs in carriers and in those with chronic forms of amebiasis. Only this encysted form can survive the passage through the stomach and the upper intestine. The disease is acquired through contaminated food and water, chiefly water which has been polluted with sewage.

The diagnosis is made by finding ameba in the stools or in scrapings obtained from an ulcer site through a proctoscope. Death from this disease is uncommon in childhood. Death may occur from dehydration, hemorrhage from an ulceration, perforation of the bowel or from an overwhelming toxemia of the fulminant infection.

Treatment usually begins with one of the tetracycline antibiotics, which effectively relieves the diarrhea and tenesmus within a few days. However, elimination of the amebae from the intestinal tract is more certain if one of the drugs containing arsenic is added to the therapy. Milibis and Thiocarbarsone are most commonly employed.

CELIAC DISEASE (CHRONIC INTESTINAL INDIGESTION)

Celiac disease is a term applied to a chronic functional disorder prevalent from the second to the fifth year, in which the chief fault lies in inability to absorb fat and digest starch. When a customary diet is ingested, bulky, frothy, foul, semiliquid stools result. The stools are composed chiefly of unabsorbed food. Continued failure to absorb sufficient food leads to failure of growth and to malnutrition, often extreme. The food deficiency is not only of calories but also of any or all nutritional essentials. Thus, deficiency diseases in addition to malnutrition may become evident.

Anatomic examination of the intestinal tract reveals nothing striking other than a greatly dilated colon, which is chiefly responsible for the characteristic protuberant abdomen (Fig. 86). When fat is fed in customary amounts, a large proportion appears in the stools, even though most or all of it has been split by digestive enzymes. These children are able to absorb and use monosaccharides, but starch is acted on by bacteria with aggravation of the indigestion. Marked and rapid fluctuations in weight due to instability of body water are commonly observed when the disease is not under dietary control.

A few children have symptoms essentially identical with those of celiac disease, in whom the fault is chiefly inability to digest starch; fats may be tolerated when starch is omitted from the diet. Such children require the same type of management as those with typical celiac disease.

TREATMENT

Although no agreement exists as to cause, celiac disease responds satisfactorily to nutritional management. Since fats and starch are not tolerated, they are omitted from the diet to as great an extent as is practical with a diet from common foods. Despite these omissions, the diet must be complete, for these children have the same nutritional requirements as healthy children. The caloric requirement is supplied by protein and simple sugars; the mineral requirement, with the exception of iron, is obtained from skimmed milk. Special attention must be given that vitamin needs are supplied. When the various requirements have been met, normal growth progress will be made.

Initial diets depend on the severity of

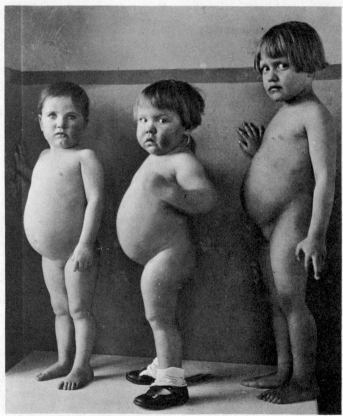

FIG. 87. Three children with celiac disease who are making good growth progress under treatment.

the symptoms and the age of the child. For an infant, an initial formula may consist of boiled skimmed milk with 10-per-cent dextrose or banana powder addition, these sugars being used because monosaccharides and invert sugars are absorbed more promptly without fermentation. Protein milk, so frequently recommended for early treatment of celiac disease, has too great a fat content to be well tolerated when the disturbance is severe. Within a day or two, finely mashed, completely ripened raw or baked banana can be added. Later, finely sieved cottage cheese and ground liver can be added in small quantities which are gradually increased.

Puréed fruits and vegetables may be added early, provided that those containing significant amounts of starch are withheld. Ground chicken and meat also may be added early. As recovery occurs, foods containing fat are added first, and those containing starch are added last. Eggs and whole milk should be included in the group of fat-containing foods. Potato and cereal foods should be the final additions in the return to a normal diet.

Since the impairment in absorption of foods extends to vitamins as well, larger than normal quantities must be fed in order to avoid deficiency. Fat-soluble vitamins A and D should be given in 3 or 4 times the usual prophylactic dose and in water-miscible form. Vitamin C is readily absorbed, and from 75 to 100 mg. per day is usually sufficient. The B-complex group is thought to be particularly important because of the similarity between celiac disease and sprue of the adult. At least 2 or 3 times the usual dose is indicated.

With this type of diet, evidence of improvement is indicated promptly by a change in the type of stools. Nervous manifestations, such as irritability and fretfulness, become less apparent, and the child begins to show a gain in weight (Fig. 87). Increase in height, which previously had been stopped or retarded greatly, begins after a period proportionate to the severity of malnutrition.

NURSING CARE

The child with celiac disease needs protection, understanding of his feelings pertaining to food deprivation and care which alleviates his symptoms of distress. He is malnourished and anemic and requires good hygiene to prevent infections. He perspires freely, tends to lie in one position and is prone to develop respiratory infections that increase his indigestion. His temperature is often subnormal, his extremities are cold, hence, he must be dressed for his protection.

When the child first comes under care, his appetite may be capricious, and he needs warm, thoughtful feeding experiences. Foods should be given to him slowly in small amounts and with no attempt to force him beyond his interest for it. As the dietary regimen is instituted, marked change in digestion and desire for food will be noted. The kinds and the amounts of food eaten and the child's behavior during feeding are observations that should be made and recorded. After the initial period when new foods are added to the diet, the stools, the degree of abdominal distention and the child's disposition should be noted to determine the tolerance to each one. Stools must be described accurately, for they are a guide in prescribing the diet. Should symptoms of indigestion be increased, the new food should be eliminated temporarily from the diet. Although appetite may be great, new foods should be introduced slowly, for unless digestion has improved, hastily introduced foods increase bulk and do little to improve the child's nutritional state.

When the child is hungry and is deprived of food, he will react to his frustration with anger or rage. Food has great meaning to a child. To be deprived of the satisfaction that comes from an adequate intake evokes feelings which may be expressed in many different ways. The child may express his feelings tempestuously or he may feel punished and withdraw. Some children completely deny their cravings, hate the impulse that strives for satisfaction and develop anorexia and vomiting. The child with celiac disease needs freedom to complain and to relieve his feelings concerning the deprivation that he feels. The infant will scream with fury when he is hungry; the older child will voice his feelings with words if he is permitted to do so. Pent-up feelings and anxiety are minimized when the child is able to express his feelings with crying or words and when he feels his nurse's understanding.

For diagnostic purposes the proportion of ingested fat excreted in the stools is determined while the child is receiving a diet with an amount of fat customary for a normal child. Such a study may be made for a period of 24 hours or longer. During the period chosen, the amounts and the kinds of foods must be recorded accurately. The beginning of the stool collection period is marked by passage in the stool of carmine given previously by mouth. The dye is tasteless and can be given in a portion of the milk; the time of ingestion of the carmine must be recorded. Beginning with the first appearance of the dye, all stools are saved until the carmine appears again after ingestion of a second capsule given exactly 24 hours, or other longer time period chosen, after ingestion of the first. The stools should be placed in a covered container in a laboratory refrigerator. The normal child excretes approximately 10 per cent of the ingested fat that is in the stool, while the child with celiac disease may excrete as much as from 50 to 70 per cent or even more.

In celiac disease, nervous instability accompanies symptoms of indigestion. The child usually is inhibited and rarely expresses his aggression overtly. His play is passive and meager. He fatigues easily and is peevish, withdrawn, depressed and precocious. Infantile habits, such as thumb-sucking and dependence on certain objects or toys, frequently are noted. The child needs study to find methods of approach that will bring him comfort. The nurse who understands his irritability, mood changes and regressive behavior and is patient gives him security and comfort. Until his physical condition improves, no attempt to divert his attention from his infantile habits should be made. When he is suffering from indigestion, he needs all the emotional satisfactions that he can get. Gradually, as he begins to gain in weight and improve generally, interest in his surroundings and a need for increased stimulation will become evident. His dependence on infantile satisfactions will decrease as he finds satisfaction in play and in his relationship with others.

The period of hospitalization and subsequent supervision is a long one, for often it is several years before a completely normal diet can be ingested safely. Before the child leaves the hospital, the mother needs to understand the child's dietary regimen, his need for general hygienic measures to prevent infection and for follow-up medical examinations. These points must be emphasized, for many of these children die because of lack of adequate supervision. On the other hand, a mental hygiene approach must be maintained. If a mother is frightened rather than helped to become more aware of her child's needs, she may protect her child so completely that changes in environment result which prevent the child from participating in normal play experiences with other children. With good supervision and care these children recover completely.

The mother of a child with celiac disease often needs help to relinquish her overprotective methods of guidance. A history of difficult feeding experiences from birth often is elicited from the mother. Frequently, the mother has responded to her crying, hungry baby with feelings of self-reproach. A crying, hungry baby disturbs the most experienced, well-adjusted mother. It is a reproach or a symbol of her failure to provide the motherliness that her infant requires. Overprotectiveness is the most natural response to such feelings. The mother of a child who has had a digestive disturbance early in life needs empathy. She needs relief from feelings of guilt and also help to find means of instituting the dietary regimen in such a way that both she and her child obtain the satisfactions that they require. A pre-school child will have feelings of resentment when he is deprived of foods that he sees his parents and siblings eating. A mother who can accept his feelings of resentment and provide delicacies which are made especially for him not only will meet her child's need but also will obtain gratification herself. Cookies can be made of dried fruit or egg whites and artificial sweetening. Ice cream and cakes can be made of gelatin. Diabetic candies are received enthusiastically, and their use minimizes the resentment against being deprived of sweets which other children receive.

CHRONIC ULCERATIVE COLITIS

Chronic ulcerative colitis is an inflammation of the colon of unknown cause. In most instances the disease is related to psychosomatic factors. It runs a chronic course but has periods of remission and acute phases of progression. The onset may be insidious, or it may be more acute, like that of dysentery. It is much more common in adults than in children, and in general is much more severe in adults.

SYMPTOMS

The child comes under care with persistent or recurrent diarrhea. The stools contain mucus, and in the acute phases there are small amounts of blood also. Fever is present in exacerbations, and often abdominal pain and tenesmus as well. Because of chronic diarrhea nutrition suffers, with loss of weight, progressive anemia, hypoproteinemia and often evidence of vitamin deficiency.

DIAGNOSIS

Diagnosis is made from the history of persistent diarrhea, failure to find causative organisms in the stools, and the finding of inflammation and ulceration on proctoscopic examination. As the condition becomes chronic, the changes in the colon are such as to cause haustra to disappear, as determined by x-ray examination with barium enema, and the colon becomes a smoothly outlined tube.

TREATMENT

No specific treatment exists. Special attention to psychogenic factors, such as emotional and environmental stresses, produces relief in many instances. Usually, psychiatric therapy is indicated. Attainment and maintenance of a good nutritive state help greatly in producing remission. The diet should be one of low-residue and high-energy value. Occasional transfusions may be indicated for anemia. Paregoric is useful during periods of more acute diarrhea. The sulfonamide drugs have a beneficial effect on the symptoms, but diarrhea usually recurs when their use is stopped. The adrenocorticotropic hormone often produces striking remission, although subsequent relapse is common. Radical surgery, which is indicated for most adults, is seldom necessary for children. Surgical treatment consists of ileostomy as the first step, with subsequent removal of the colon as the second step.

FECAL INCONTINENCE

ORGANIC CAUSES

Fecal incontinence, or lack of voluntary control of the passage of stools, is a normal feature of infancy until bowel control is achieved during the second or third year of life. General disorders which may account for the symptom during later life are mental deficiency, coma, extreme debility, or very severe diarrhea. In addition, lesions of the spinal cord such as spina bifida, myelitis and cord tumor, may interfere with nervous control of the sphincters and hamper voluntary control.

ENCOPRESIS AND PSYCHOGENIC CONSTIPATION

Encopresis is a term generally used to imply that fecal incontinence is based upon psychic rather than organic factors. It may arise from failure to establish bowel training at a reasonable age, and under such circumstances it is sometimes but not invariably associated with enuresis. It may also appear in emotionally disturbed children who had once gained bowel control.

Among small children encopresis commonly follows withholding of stool beyond the appropriate time of passage. The withholding is usually initiated by fear of pain because of a previous experience with abnormally large or hard stools. In order to prevent recurring discomfort the child suppresses the urge to defecate and retains his stool in the lower bowel where it dries out and becomes progressively more difficult to pass. Eventually, accumulated gas and liquid behind the fecal mass either force the involuntary extrusion of a painful stool or work their way around the side of the mass and escape through the anus in spite of the child's efforts to retain them. Because his lower bowel is always distended the child gradually loses the ability to appreciate the normal signals which urge him to defecate. This vicious circle may be interrupted by prolonged oral administration of mineral oil or some other substance which will keep the stools soft until the child has conquered his fear and regained the ability and the willingness to respond to the usual impulses.

At times withholding may be based upon irrational subconscious fears, fantasies or anger directed at the parents. If encopresis persists beyond 3 or 4 years of age and cannot be controlled by the measures outlined above, the services of a pediatric psychiatrist should be sought in order to explore and modify the emotional and environmental factors. Unlike enuresis, which usually

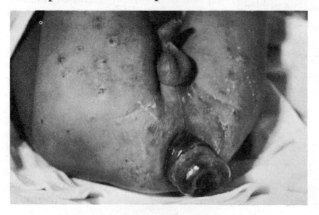

FIG. 88. Prolapse of the rectum, with beginning gangrene of the distal ½ inch of mucosa.

carries a good ultimate prognosis and is associated with relatively minor personality disorders, encopresis is most often based upon deep-seated character disturbances. Early treatment is imperative for this reason. In addition, the symptom is difficult to conceal, and the child's intrafamily difficulties soon become compounded by social inacceptability in the community. Prolonged psychogenic constipation may also lead to gradual abdominal and colonic enlargement with the symptoms and the physical findings of megacolon.

RECTAL PROLAPSE

Sometimes a distinction is made between anal and rectal prolapse. In anal prolapse, the mucous membrane immediately proximal to the anus is extruded. In rectal prolapse the large tumor is composed also of bowel wall (Fig. 88). A combination of relaxed sphincter, large hard stools and straining at stool is likely to cause moderate prolapse in children otherwise normal. Rectal prolapse is associated with weakness of the muscles of the pelvic floor. Any condition such as severe malnutrition, which brings about muscle weakness, is thus a predisposing cause. The immediate cause is straining, due either to diarrhea or constipation. It occurs only at defecation and is common in only the first 2 or 3 years.

TREATMENT

The prolapsed part of the rectum should be replaced and, as far as possible, kept replaced constantly. During defecation, the buttocks should be held firmly, either manually or with the use of adhesive strips. A tight pad or bandage may be used. Constipation or diarrhea should be managed in such a way that straining is avoided. Usually no other measures are necessary. Surgical treatment is unsatisfactory.

APPENDICITIS

Appendicitis is less frequent in children than in adults. It is uncommon under 5 years and rare under 2. In all instances the fundamental cause is the same, namely, obstruction of the lumen of the appendix. Obstruction may be due to a variety of causes.

SYMPTOMS

In the adult, the usual findings are sudden onset of nausea, vomiting, localized tenderness, leukocytosis, fever and constipation. In the older child the symptoms may be entirely similar to those of the adult; but children in general, and the younger victims in particular, often present an insidious onset with symptoms that are difficult to evaluate. The classic localization of tenderness in the right lower quadrant of the abdomen may be obscured by poor co-operation or by general hypersensitivity. Pain may be referred elsewhere or may be overshadowed by crying and restlessness. Vomiting is frequently present but is not a very helpful symptom since it is a common aspect of so many childhood ailments. Very often the diagnosis of appendicitis in a child remains in doubt until he has been observed and examined repeatedly over a period of several hours.

A number of conditions may be confused with appendicitis and lead to unnecessary abdominal exploration. The early symptoms of infectious hepatitis or gastro-enteritis often suggest appendicitis. The mesenteric lymph nodes in children sometimes enlarge and become painful during the course of acute tonsillitis. Irritation of the peritoneum may occur in rheumatic fever. Pain may be referred to the abdomen in right-sided pneumonia, in pyelitis and occasionally in meningitis. Some of the most disconcerting patients are the small number of children who suffer from recurring bouts of afebrile abdominal pain which on repeated or close examination give inconsistent or bizarre findings. Many of these children suffer from hysterical or psychosomatic disorders which are more likely to be aggravated than helped by a fruitless operation.

PROGNOSIS

The prognosis of appendicitis in children is generally good when the disease is recognized and treated. Delay in making the diagnosis or unusually rapid progression of the infection in a young child may increase the hazard to recovery, for diffuse peritonitis may occur within a short time of the initial symptoms.

TREATMENT

Once the diagnosis is made, treatment is by surgical exploration and removal of the infected appendix. Preceding the operation the child should be kept at bed rest. If postponement is necessary for some reason, an icebag will help to relieve pain and decrease peristaltic activity of the bowel. Enemas are permissible but cathartics are unwise. If operation is contemplated within a short time, usually fluids and feedings are withheld. The sulfonamides, penicillin and streptomycin are of great value in preventing or minimizing peritonitis. Postoperative care of children is usually simple, for they seldom suffer from paralytic ileus.

INTESTINAL PARASITIC WORMS

Intestinal worms have been blamed erroneously for a wide variety of symptoms such as nose-picking, restless sleep, grinding the teeth while asleep, circles under the eyes, and convulsions. Most of these symptoms are related to emotional disturbances in the child and have nothing to do with intestinal parasites. Children who do harbor worms usually have no symptoms. An accurate estimate of the frequency of worm infestations is possible only by intensive and repeated study of stools and anal swabs. Such studies usually demonstrate a remarkably high prevalence of pinworm and roundworm infestations not only in the southern climates but also in the northern cities of the United States.

PINWORM (THREADWORM, SEATWORM, ENTEROBIASIS, OXYURIASIS)

This is by far the most common variety of intestinal parasite. The worms are small white threads from ⅛ to ½ inch in length which are seen most commonly about the anus after the child has been asleep for an hour or two. Sometimes they are found on the surface of a stool. Infestation occurs when eggs are swallowed. The eggs hatch within

the intestinal tract, and the gravid female worms inhabit the cecum until ready to lay their eggs. Then they crawl out of the anus, usually after the child has gone to sleep. They either lay their eggs shortly after emerging or are broken open and scatter the eggs about the child's perineum and into his clothing. The eggs survive for several days and are the source from which the same or another individual in the environment may acquire a new infestation. The period between ingestion of the egg and appearance of the gravid female at the anus is about 6 to 8 weeks.

Symptoms

Symptoms of pinworm infestation may be entirely lacking, and the condition may be discovered only by finding the worms. When infestation is heavy there may be itching about the anus or about the vagina in the female. The scratching that results traps new eggs under the finger nails and affords an easy means of their transfer back to the mouth.

Diagnosis

Usually diagnosis is made by finding

and recognizing the worms as they emerge from the anus. The eggs may be found by swabbing the anal region with Scotch tape and examining it under a microscope. Since the females do not lay eggs within the intestinal tract, eggs are not found in the stools.

Treatment

Treatment attempts to intoxicate the worms so that they will leave the intestine before completing their maturation, and attempts to eliminate the eggs deposited in the environment before they can cause another infestation. Gentian violet in enteric-coated tablets is the standard vermifuge for pinworms. It may cause nausea and mild abdominal pain and must be used over a 10-day period to be effective. Several newer drugs have been tried with variable success. Sometimes worms are removed by repeated administration of enemas, but this is a disturbing procedure and probably no more effective than oral medication. Underclothing, night clothing and bed linen should be boiled at least twice a week in order to destroy eggs deposited therein. Careful cleansing of the perineum, the hands and the nails should be carried out several times a day. Application of a soothing ointment, such as ammoniated mercury or blue ointment, may allay the itching and reduce the viability of the eggs that have been deposited. All individuals in the family who have any suspicion of being infested must be treated simultaneously if success is to be attained.

ROUNDWORM (Ascaris lumbricoides)

The adult roundworm is a large (6 to 15 in.) white or pink parasite about the diameter of a lead pencil. It lives for periods up to 6 months in the intestinal tract, during which time the females lay enormous numbers of eggs that are discharged in the patient's stools. The eggs require from 2 to 4 weeks and a moist, shaded environment to develop into an infective stage. The

infestation is passed from one individual to another only in regions where flush toilets are absent and defecation is performed in outhouses or on the open ground.

An egg that has developed to the stage of infectivity and is ingested follows a somewhat complicated development within the child. It is transformed first into a larval stage within the intestine. The larva is able to migrate through the intestinal walls; it gains access to the portal venous system and the general circulation and then reaches the lungs, where it breaks out of the blood stream into the alveoli. From the lungs the larvae are coughed up and swallowed to complete their growth into adult worms in the intestinal tract. The full development requires from 4 to 6 weeks.

Symptoms

Roundworms produce no symptoms except when present in unusual number so as to block the intestinal tract, or through unusual migrations as into the bile duct.

Treatment

A number of highly toxic drugs are used to expel the worms from the intestine. These include hexylresorcinol, Santonin and oil of Chenopodium. The former is preferred in treatment because of its lesser degree of toxicity.

HOOKWORM (Uncinaria americana)

The hookworm is a small (¼ to ½ in.) worm that lives in the upper intestinal tract where it is attached firmly by a mouth with teethlike parts through which it derives nourishment by sucking blood from the intestinal wall. The females lay large numbers of eggs which are passed in the patient's stools. The eggs require warm sandy soil for their development into larvae within about 2 weeks. Larvae may be ingested, or more commonly they penetrate through the skin of a child who is going barefoot.

They enter the blood stream and circulate to the lungs where they enter the alveoli, are coughed up and swallowed and complete their development in the upper intestinal tract. Hookworm disease is limited to the southeastern portion of the United States and depends for its spread upon outdoor toilets and barefootedness.

Symptoms

The symptoms of hookworm disease depend upon the number of worms present in the individual. When the number is large, the loss of blood to the worms may be sufficient to cause anemia. Chronic infestations also produce anorexia, malnutrition and chronic fatigue. A sensitized child may develop itching at the site of entrance of larvae into the skin of his feet.

Diagnosis

Diagnosis is made by finding the ova in the stools.

Treatment

Treatment is effected by vermifuges such as tetrachlorethylene or hexylresorcinol. In chronic cases careful attention to the diet is required to restore nutrition.

BEEF TAPEWORM (Taenia saginata)

The beef tapeworm requires an intermediate host, the cow, for its passage from one individual to another. It is acquired by eating infested beef which has not been cooked sufficiently to kill the larvae present within the meat. A larva so ingested develops in the upper intestinal tract into an adult worm with a tenacious head which attaches itself to the intestinal wall. It grows by progressive segmentation until it reaches considerable length—10 to 12 feet or more. Segments of the worm may break off and be noticed in the stool, or the end of the worm may protrude from the anus. There are no symptoms.

Treatment

Treatment attempts to intoxicate the worm so that it will release its hold upon the intestinal wall and pass out of the tract. Oleoresin of aspidium, hexylresorcinol and atabrine are used. It is important to save all segments of the worm which are passed, for the head must be identified in order to be sure that treatment is complete. If some of the worm is broken off and the head is left behind, it will continue to grow.

DWARF TAPEWORM (Hymenolepis nana)

This is a common but unimportant tapeworm that lives only a few weeks. It requires no intermediate host and may be passed from man to man. Treatment is the same as that for the beef tapeworm. No symptoms occur.

TRICHINA (Trichinella spiralis)

This is a fairly common infestation obtained from the ingestion of uncooked pork in which the encysted larvae of the worm reside. Digestion in the stomach of the patient frees the larva from its thick capsule and permits it to develop in 3 to 5 days in the intestine into the adult form. Adults then burrow into the intestinal wall and release larvae which enter the blood stream and take up residence in the skeletal muscles. Infestation by a few trichinae may pass entirely unnoticed, but heavy infestation may produce severe or even fatal disease.

Symptoms

Symptoms of a heavy infestation may begin within a few days of the ingestion of the contaminated pork. The activity of the developing worms in the intestinal mucosa may produce diarrhea and fever. Marked constitutional symptoms of fever, pains in the muscles, swelling of the eyes and myocarditis may accompany the invasion of larvae into skeletal and heart muscle during the first 3 to 6 weeks. There is no effective treatment.

MECKEL'S DIVERTICULUM

Approximately 2 to 3 per cent of all children have a vestigial remnant of the omphalomesenteric duct remaining as a small pouch off the ileum about 18 inches from its junction with the colon. Usually this structure, called a Meckel's diverticulum, gives no symptoms. In some children there is aberrantly placed gastric mucous membrane within the pouch which secretes acid gastric juice. This juice is irritating to the wall of the ileum and may produce ulceration and bleeding. The usual symptoms are painless passage of tarry or grossly bloody stools. Diagnosis is made from suspicion when no other explanation of the bleeding can be found. It cannot be confirmed without an exploratory abdominal operation. Surgical removal of the diverticulum is simple and curative. The postoperative care is the same as that for any abdominal operation.

INTESTINAL POLYPS

Benign polypoid growths occur within the intestinal mucosa of children and lead to passage of blood in the stool. Most frequently the source is a solitary polyp in the rectum. Sometimes such a polyp on a long pedicle extrudes from the anus, but usually they must be sought by proctoscopic examination and be removed through this instrument. Less commonly polyps occur higher up in the large bowel and cause painless bleeding. They may be demonstrable by contrast barium enema, employing both air and barium to make them visible on the roentgen film. Rarely, a child has multiple polyps throughout the whole colon. This is a serious disorder which can interfere with growth and eventually may lead to malignant degeneration of the masses. When polyposis is extensive, surgical treatment becomes necessary. Total colectomy is usually required.

HEPATIC DISEASE

THE PHYSIOLOGY OF JAUNDICE

Jaundice is a symptom of various conditions. However, in all circumstances it results from one or more of 3 fundamental causes: excessive destruction of blood, impaired function of the liver and obstruction to excretion of bile. The pigment bilirubin is a product of hemoglobin breakdown. Some hemoglobin destruction occurs normally and constantly; this function is carried on by the reticuloendothelial system. The bilirubin so formed is in combination with a globulin fraction of blood protein. On passage through the liver bilirubin is freed from the protein combination and is excreted by way of the bile ducts along with bile salts and cholesterol. Bilirubin and cholesterol are waste products, whereas the bile salts, produced in the liver, aid in absorption of fat and the fat-soluble vitamins. Bilirubin is converted in the intestine to urobilinogen, some of which is excreted as such, some oxidized to urobilin, the coloring matter of the stool, and some is reabsorbed into the portal circulation, returned to the liver, converted to bilirubin and re-excreted.

When the destruction of blood within the body is excessive, combined bilirubin is formed at such a rate that the liver is unable to deal with the excess. Even though a larger quantity of bilirubin than normal is converted and excreted, the circulating level may increase and produce jaundice. The stools are not acholic, and urobilinogen is increased in the urine. Such a condition exists in icterus neonatorum, transfusion with incompatible blood and hemolytic anemias of various sorts.

When jaundice is related to impaired liver function, in the early stages of disease the liver is still able to free bilirubin from its combined form but is unable to excrete it in normal amounts. Thus retention of bilirubin occurs, producing jaundice. If liver damage progresses, the liver loses some of its ability to free bilirubin from its combined form, and both types of bilirubin accumulate in the blood. This situation occurs in hepatitis, in certain infections outside the liver and when the liver has been poisoned by phosphorus or chloroform.

When obstruction to the excretion of bile occurs, bilirubin is freed from its combined form, accumulates in the liver and overflows into the blood. The stools are acholic. Bilirubin appears in the urine, and urobilinogen disappears; if the obstruction is unrelieved, enough damage eventually occurs to impair the liver's ability to free bilirubin from the combined form, and both types of bilirubin accumulate in the plasma. Gallstones in the larger ducts, strictures of the ducts and tumors compressing the ducts are causes of obstruction which are seldom seen in childhood. Congenital atresia of the bile ducts belongs in this category.

The degree of jaundice may be stated in arbitrary units called the icterus index, which is the amount of yellow color in blood serum as determined by comparison with a dichromate standard solution. The Van den Bergh reaction offers a more precise aid to diagnosis, since it indicates both the total amount of bilirubin circulating in the plasma and the relative amounts of the free and combined forms. In the chemical determination the protein-bilirubin combination is dissolved by treatment with alcohol. Before this is done the amount of free bilirubin is first determined (direct reaction). This indicates the amount that is circulating because of obstruction. Then the serum is treated with alcohol, and the additional amount of bilirubin released from combination with protein is measured (indirect reaction). As stated above, this represents the amount produced by hemolysis under uncomplicated circumstances.

Jaundice is only a symptom. The treatment required depends upon a knowledge of the underlying causative mechanism.

INFECTIOUS HEPATITIS (CATARRHAL JAUNDICE, VIRAL HEPATITIS)

Infectious hepatitis is the most common cause of jaundice in children beyond the period of infancy. The infectious agent (a virus) is acquired by alimentary contact from an infected individual, or from direct injection into the body of human blood, plasma, or of vaccines made from plasma.

Symptoms

Symptoms may appear within 2 to 6 weeks after natural exposure but do not begin until 2 to 4 months when the infection is the result of a contaminated injection. The predominant symptom is jaundice; in mild cases it is the only symptom. More commonly there is nausea, loss of appetite, abdominal pain and vomiting at the beginning of the illness. In severe or protracted cases there may be prostration, loss of weight and permanent liver damage from cirrhosis. The urine is darkly colored from the presence of bile pigments, and the stool is light or completely white because of their absence.

Treatment

Treatment is symptomatic with a high-carbohydrate, low-fat and high-protein diet. Supplements of vitamin B complex and methionine are usually given. In children the prognosis for complete recovery without liver damage is nearly always excellent.

CIRRHOSIS

Children suffer from cirrhosis infrequently. It is the end result of scarring of the liver initiated by another disorder, often an illness which is obscure. Chronic obstruction of the bile ducts as from congenital atresia or the inspissated bile syndrome eventually leads to scarring of the liver and loss of function. Infectious hepatitis as stated above may rarely wreak such damage that permanent loss of function results. The symptoms of cirrhosis include jaundice, general lassitude, often anemia and abdominal enlargement or ascites. Treatment is palliative only and consists in providing a diet high in protein and carbohydrate and low in fat; ample intake of vitamins, particularly of the members of the B-complex; regulation of activity according to the child's tolerance; and occasionally operative procedures which have hope of relieving bile-duct obstruction or excessive pressure within the portal venous system. The disease generally advances slowly to a fatal termination, although children have a better chance to recover than do adults.

SITUATIONS FOR FURTHER STUDY

1. Visit a speech clinic to observe methods of speech training for a child who has recovered from a cleft-palate repair. What did you learn that you can use in helping parents to continue speech training in the home?

2. Study a preschool child with celiac disease. What personality characteristics did he show when he first came into the hospital? In conversation with the parents discover the symptoms that led them to seek medical assistance. Determine how these symptoms altered their guidance of the child. Compare his behavior now with the behavior observed when he first came into the ward. How has your guidance of him changed during this period? In what way have you attempted to help the mother to accept his changing needs? How did she feel about the child's illness?

3. Study a child with ulcerative colitis during the period you are giving him care in the manner suggested at the end of Chapter 8. If he is having psychiatric therapy, get recommendations concerning his emotional needs and incorporate them into your plan of care. What changes in behavior did you note as you used his therapist's suggestion in giving him care? What problems did you encounter in using the therapist's recommendations?

BIBLIOGRAPHY

Anderson, J. A.: Poisoning from drugs, metals and food in Nelson, Textbook of Pediatrics, Philadelphia, Saunders, 1954.

Babbitz, Matilda: Bobby has celiac disease, Am. J. Nursing 53:322, 1953.

Barber, W. W.: Celiac disease, Am. J. Nursing 36:660, 1936.

Dreisbach, R. H.: Handbook of Poisons, Los Altos, Calif., Lange, 1955.

Faust, E. C.: Human Helminthology, ed. 3, Philadelphia, Lea & Febiger, 1949.

Kaplan, Stanley M., and Plogsted, Helen: The nurse and psychosomatic medicine, Am. J. Nursing 57:207, 1957.

Mayo, Merle: Nursing care in bacillary dysentery, Am. J. Nursing 50:304, 1950.

Palumbo, L. T., Burnside, R., Mossholder, I., and Jensen, B.: Ulcerative colitis, Am. J. Nursing 55:311, 1955.

Parker, Mary V.: Nursing care of children following ingestion of lye, Chicago, Dept. of Photographic Reproductions, Univ. Chicago Library, 1956.

Prugh, D. G.: The influence of emotional factors in the clinical course of ulcerative colitis in children, Gastroenterology 18:339, 1951.

———: A preliminary report on the role of emotional factors in idiopathic celiac disease, Psychosom. Med. 13: 220, 1951.

Sperling, D. G., and Richmond, J. B.: Psychogenic megacolon manifested by fecal soiling, Pediatrics **10**:474, 1952.

Committee on Dental Health, Dental Caries; a survey of the literature, National Research Council Publication No. 225, Washington, D.C., 1952.

CHAPTER TWENTY-ONE

Diseases of the
Genito-urinary System

PHYSIOLOGY OF THE KIDNEY

The functioning units of the kidney are the nephrons, of which approximately 2 million exist. Each nephron is composed of a glomerulus, a convoluted tubule, a collecting tubule and a blood supply (Fig. 89). A glomerulus consists of a globular network of capillaries encased in a sac. This capillary tuft is supplied by a small artery (an afferent or entering arteriole), and blood leaves the glomerulus by another (efferent) arteriole. The capillary tuft within the glomerulus acts as a filter, fluid entering the glomerular sac from the capillaries by reason of pressure of the blood in excess of the pressure in the sac. The filtrate contains a high proportion of all the plasma contents except the protein and the cellular elements. It contains waste products as well as materials which are highly useful to the body.

The glomerular sac empties by way of a tubule which runs a very tortuous course (convoluted tubule). The first series of convolutions, lying near the glomerulus, comprises the proximal convoluted tubule. Then the tubule runs from the cortex of the kidney, where all glomeruli are located, into the medulla of the kidney and turns back (loop of Henle) to form in the cortex another series of convolutions (distal convoluted tubule). The tubule enters a collecting tubule which also collects from other nephrons. Then the collecting tubule passes through the medulla to empty into the pelvis of the kidney.

The efferent arteriole from the glomerulus supplies a capillary network which surrounds the convoluted tubule. From the convoluted tubule, materials which the body needs are resorbed into the blood of the capillary network surrounding it. Only the remaining relatively small amount of fluid containing waste products passes into the

479

collecting tubule for excretion. After performing their functions of absorption, the capillaries of the tubule become venules to carry blood away from the kidney.

In the adult, approximately 1,500 cc. of blood passes through the nephrons each minute, an amount equal to 30 per cent of the heart output and greater than that for any other organ except the lungs. Glomerular filtrate forms at the rate of approximately 125 cc. a minute, a volume one twelfth that of the blood passing through the glomeruli. By reason of loss of this filtrate, the plasma efferent from the glomeruli is concentrated approximately 25 per cent, the volume of blood cells remaining the same. As the filtrate courses through the convoluted tubules, a high proportion is resorbed, and only from 1 to 2 per cent is available finally for excretion as urine.

Resorption occurs in large part through osmosis resulting from the greater concentration of materials in the tubular than in the glomerular capillaries and because of a lower blood pressure in the tubular than in the glomerular capillaries. In smaller but important parts the filtrate is resorbed because of the presence of the

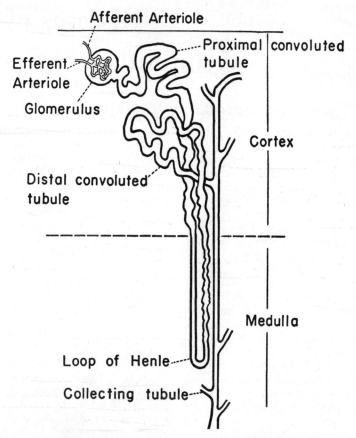

FIG. 89. Schematic representation of a nephron.

posterior pituitary antidiuretic hormone. The resorption of sodium is subject also to the influence of the adrenal cortical hormone desoxycorticosterone, this substance producing absorption. Through these various means, all the glucose, 99 per cent of the water and of the sodium and some of the urea of the filtrate are resorbed.

One of the important functions of the kidney is to excrete waste products, the chief of which are urea, carbonic and other organic acids and phosphates. An important one, present in smaller amount, is uric acid. These materials are excreted by the mechanisms which have been discussed. In addition, certain substances can be excreted into the urine selectively by the tubules.

Another important function of the kidney is to conserve basic substances for the body while excreting waste. To a considerable extent the base of bicarbonate can be resorbed, leaving the carbon dioxide in the filtrate. Most of the phosphate in the blood is dibasic (e.g., Na_2HPO_4). The dibasic phosphates can be converted by the tubules to the monobasic phosphates (e.g., NaH_2PO_4), thus conserving base by excreting an acid instead of a neutral material. Also, the tubular epithelium can form ammonia from amino acids to replace base for excretion of acids, thus further conserving base for the body.

Variations in the amount of urine produced ordinarily are the result of changes in the amount of water resorbed by the tubules. Except for disturbances in which the glomeruli are diseased, the amount of glomerular filtrate produced remains fairly constant. Rather, increases in urine volume depend upon a fall in the amount of tubular reabsorption of the filtrate. Thus, excessive water ingestion dilutes the blood and causes a decrease in production of pituitary antidiuretic hormone, and the tubules allow no water to escape; or a mercurial diuretic partially poisons the resorptive activity of the tubules, and more water escapes; or the presence of abnormal amounts of sugar, urea or other substances in the filtrate interferes with the resorption of water from the tubules.

The adequacy of renal function is measured by a variety of clinical tests. Determination of the level of urea or *nonprotein nitrogen* in the blood indicates the ability of the kidney to dispose of the waste products of protein metabolism. The *urea clearance test* is a more refined method of measuring this aspect of kidney function. The ability of the kidney to increase the *concentration of the urine* following a standard period of fluid restriction is another useful clinical test. The ability of the tubules to excrete an injected dye also may be tested by use of the *phenolsulfonphthalein excretion test*. During infancy these tests indicate that the kidney is immature and unable to perform such functions as efficiently as the kidney of the older child or the adult. After the age of 2 this functional difference is no longer apparent.

ABNORMALITIES OF RENAL FUNCTION

A number of terms are used to describe abnormalities of function of the urinary tract. Those that imply disturbance of kidney function are considered below. Others that relate to disorders of the lower urinary tract will be mentioned subsequently.

ANURIA

Anuria is the absence of urine. It usually results from failure of the kidney to excrete, but occasionally it is due to obstruction of the lower urinary tract. It occurs rather commonly in the newborn infant for periods up to 36 hours after birth and is not significant of renal disease except in the rare circumstance of congenital absence of the kidneys. In older children it usually is associated with the onset of nephritis or severe kidney infections. Occasionally, it follows mercurial poisoning, transfusion reactions, severe burns, prolonged shock or sulfonamide intoxication. In children it is generally a self-limited phenomenon which is handled best by carefully controlled administration of water and electrolytes instead of the more dramatic procedures of peritoneal lavage or the use of an artificial kidney.

OLIGURIA

Oliguria is decreased urinary flow. It is seen in dehydration and during certain stages of the several types of nephritis. The management depends upon the underlying condition.

POLYURIA

An abnormal increase in the volume of urine may result from excessive fluid intake or administration, from poorly controlled diabetes mellitus or from diabetes insipidus.

ALBUMINURIA

Albuminuria is detected by chemical examination of the urine. It results when the glomerular membrane permits passage of the smaller protein molecules from the blood stream into the glomerular filtrate and thence the urine. In a heavy or a persistent amount, albuminuria usually indicates renal disease, such as nephritis, nephrosis or pyelonephritis. It is found transiently in newborn infants and may be found in mild degree in normal children.

Postural Albuminuria

This benign condition is discovered occasionally on routine urinalysis. Albumin appears in the urine when the child is standing or exercising but not when he is recumbent. The disturbance frequently disappears after puberty and has no known relation to renal disease. It requires no treatment, but a careful exclusion of other causes of albuminuria is demanded.

CYLINDRURIA

This term indicates the presence of abnormal numbers of casts in the urine. These are microscopic plugs which form in the kidney tubules when the rate of urine flow is slow or when albuminuria is present. They often contain cellular elements which are valuable clues to the type of renal disturbance.

HEMATURIA

Hematuria signifies the presence of red blood cells in the urine. When the concentration of cells is large the urine may appear grossly bloody or may have a brown or smoky tinge. Smaller degrees of hematuria can be discovered only by microscopic examination. Hematuria usually signifies glomerular disease in the child. Bleeding into the lower urinary tract can and does occur but is relatively infrequent among children. A number of processes may alter the glomerular membrane in such a way as to permit the passage of red blood cells. Glomerular bleeding in children is most commonly due to nephritis, trauma, infection, blood dyscrasia or sulfonamide overdosage.

AZOTEMIA

This term indicates an increase of the nonprotein nitrogen constituents in the blood above the arbitrary level of 35 mg. per 100 ml. It indicates that the kidneys are unable to clear the blood of protein waste products at the usual speed. While most often found during renal disease, azotemia also may result when the blood flow to the kidneys is insufficient, as in cardiac failure or severe dehydration or to a minor extent when specimens are obtained after a heavy protein meal.

UREMIA

This term implies azotemia which is associated with severe impairment of renal function and usually is accompanied by symptoms which include nausea, headache, anorexia, diarrhea, fatigue, acidosis, anemia and bleeding tendencies. The management depends upon the nature of the underlying renal disease.

NEPHRITIS AND NEPHROSIS

In order to present the various disease conditions which should be considered under the term "nephritis," it is desirable to have a classification of the types of disease for convenience in discussion and understanding. Unfortunately, complete general agreement does not exist as to an appropriate classification. For the purpose of this presentation, a classification which at least serves as a basis for discussing the various types has been chosen.

In some respects, nephritis of children differs much from that of adults. The child's kidneys have a power of regeneration after injury far greater than do those of the adult. The commonest type of nephritis in childhood (acute glomerular) is the least common among adults and is the most benign of all the varieties. Nephritis of the older person is likely to be complicated by degenerative changes, whereas such changes are not common in childhood. Pure nephrosis that is fully reparable seems to occur only in children. Nephrosis of adults is usually a part of chronic nephritis, which ultimately leads to irreparable and fatal kidney damage. Those classifications dealing with adults largely or exclusively are likely to contain statements concerning nephritis which are wholly true for adults but do not apply to children.

ACUTE GLOMERULAR NEPHRITIS (ACUTE HEMORRHAGIC NEPHRITIS)

Acute glomerular nephritis is characterized by changes in the glomerular capillaries which permit the passage of blood cells and protein into the glomerular filtrate. The finding of blood in the urine is a constant feature of the disease. Associated changes in other parts of the body are commonly but not necessarily present. These include edema, hypertension, azotemia and the secondary phenomena which may result from them.

Etiology

The disease is dependent on a recently preceding streptococcic infection, usually in the upper respiratory tract and most frequently in the tonsils and the adjacent lymph nodes. It is one of the possible complications of scarlet fever, occurring in the second or the third week of this disease. It also may occur secondary to streptococcic infections of the skin (impetigo, infected eczema or scabies). It occurs at any age but is most frequent in midchildhood. Nephritis is a result of a toxic effect of streptococcic infection which affects all capillaries, including those of the glomeruli.

Symptoms

When the preceding streptococcic infection is recognized, a latent period of roughly 1 to 3 weeks ensues between its onset and the appearance of symptoms of nephritis. It is probable that many children have nephritis in such mild form that it goes unrecognized. Usually, the initial symptoms are puffiness of the face or grossly bloody urine or headache and vomiting. These symptoms may occur alone or in combination. Occasionally, the disease is announced by dyspnea due to impending heart failure. Oliguria is frequent but transient; anuria occurs rarely. Later in the disease, chronic fatigue, anemia and malnutrition may constitute the chief symptoms.

In the majority of affected children the symptoms rapidly reach their maximum intensity and trail off within a week or two, leaving the child symptomatically well but with evidence of the continuing disease apparent in various laboratory tests. Azotemia is seldom responsible for symptoms unless its severity is sufficient to produce uremia. The chief mechanism responsible for the symptomatology is the consequence of a general vascular disturbance which leads to edema and spasm of arterioles. Combined with hypertension, these processes lead to varying degrees of cerebral edema and myocardial insufficiency. Occasionally in children serious or even fatal complications ensue—hypertensive encephalopathy with convulsions or coma, or congestive heart failure.

Diagnosis

Usually, the history and the symptoms alone strongly suggest the diagnosis. Examination of the urine should disclose red blood cells, albumin and casts. If the casts contain red blood cells, there is no doubt about the diagnosis. Hypertension and azotemia may or may not be present.

Prognosis

Recovery from acute glomerulonephritis is to be expected in nearly all children. Even among those in whom the disease is severe enough to require hospitalization, about 85 per cent recover completely. Mild illnesses last as little as 2 to 3 weeks; in the more obstinate cases evidence of continuing renal disease may last from 12 to 18 months before recovery takes place. In exceptional instances the disease is progressive and takes on the characteristics of chronic nephritis. A small number of children succumb to the early effects of hypertensive encephalopathy or heart failure.

Treatment

Infection. Although antibiotic therapy is of no avail in the treatment of the nephritis itself, complete eradication of the beta hemolytic streptococcus infection which preceded should be assured through the use of penicillin.

Bed Rest. During the acute stage and for as long as appreciable amounts of blood appear in the urine, the child should be kept at bed rest. If the disease is prolonged and enters a subacute stage in which there are minimal findings in the urine, the child may be allowed complete activity but should be protected from further infection and from chilling, which seems to reactivate the nephritic process.

Diet. Contrary to previous belief, the diet need not be restricted in respect to protein but should contain a full complement of all nutrients as soon as the appetite returns. In the presence of edema, salt intake usually is restricted. Except during evidence of cardiac failure no fluid restrictions need be imposed.

Cardiac Failure. The management of cardiac failure is essentially the same as described in Chapter 18. Morphine, oxygen and digitalis may be required. Diuretics are contraindicated in the presence of nephritis.

Hypertension. The control of hypertension is a very important aspect of treatment. Magnesium sulfate may be given for this purpose by mouth, intramuscularly or intravenously, depending upon the severity of the cerebral symptoms. Prevention of convulsions is highly desirable, so that oral administration of a 50 per cent solution in doses of 1 or 2 ounces usually is given as soon as appreciable elevation of the blood pressure is detected. The drug has surprisingly little cathartic action during the course of nephritis. The rectal route may be substituted for the oral if vomiting is present or if the child refuses to take the medication. At higher levels of blood pressure, magnesium sulfate is given intramuscularly in a 25 per cent solution at a dosage of about 0.2 ml. per Kg.

of body weight. If symptoms are severe or other forms of administration have been ineffective, the drug may be given slowly intravenously in a 2 per cent solution at a dosage of 10 ml. per Kg. Overdosage with magnesium sulfate may produce respiratory depression, which can be counteracted by intravenous administration of a soluble calcium solution which should be readily available whenever intramuscular or intravenous treatment is being employed.

Nursing Care

The child should be dressed warmly enough to prevent chilling. While rest in bed is required, play activities should be provided to keep the child happily occupied. The blood pressure should be observed at intervals during the day and the night during the early stage of the disease. Any elevation should be reported immediately. When an elevation in blood pressure is noted, increased observation is indicated to detect signs of cerebral symptoms. When the child's blood pressure is high and he begins to show cerebral symptoms, cribsides or a crib bed should be provided for his protection. Equipment to give magnesium sulfate intravenously and intramuscularly should be in readiness in the child's room.

NEPHROSIS
(LIPID NEPHROSIS, NEPHROTIC SYNDROME)

Nephrosis is a disease which is peculiar to young children. It is characterized by generalized edema associated with a heavy loss of albumin in the urine, by a fall in the level of the blood proteins, chiefly involving the albumin fraction, and by a rise in the level of blood lipids including cholesterol. Hypertension, azotemia and hematuria are not usually present in the early stages of the disease.

Symptoms

Edema. The disease usually appears insidiously without any antecedent infection, beginning as the slow, asymptomatic accumulation of edema, which is noticed first about the eyes. As the swelling advances, it may involve the legs, the arms and the back to varying degrees (Fig. 90). Accumulation of fluid in the peritoneal cavity and the scrotum is frequent. Shifting of the edematous areas is common, depending to some extent upon the position of the child during sleep or during waking activity. With moderate stretching of the skin over the subcutaneous fluid, there is pronounced pallor which is out of proportion to the degree of anemia; with severe degrees of edema, striae may appear from overstretching—striae

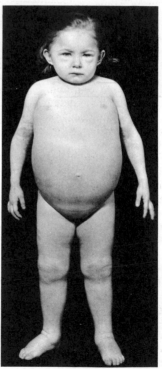

FIG. 90. Nephrosis, showing generalized edema and accumulation of fluid in the peritoneal cavity (ascites).

which simulate those seen on the abdomen of the pregnant woman.

Malnutrition. Excessive fluid accumulations impede activity and appetite and may embarrass respirations by limiting the excursion of the diaphragm. As the disease continues, inapparent malnutrition takes place, which is revealed clearly only when diuresis and loss of subcutaneous edema occur.

Anemia of moderate degree usually appears during the course of the illness.

Poor Resistance to Infection. This is characteristic. Before modern chemotherapy, death occurred in a considerable proportion of children with nephrosis because of the ravages of septicemia, peritonitis and meningitis. Formerly, streptococci and pneumococci were usually responsible for these severe infections; more recently, there has been an increasing prevalence of other organisms.

Nephrotic Crisis. A nephrotic crisis simulates peritonitis by producing abdominal pain, fever and sometimes an erysipeloid skin eruption. These events may occur without demonstrable infection. They usually subside within a few days and may be followed by a spontaneous diuresis.

When the course of nephrosis is complicated by one of the contagious diseases such as measles or chickenpox, spontaneous diuresis and loss of edema may result. Although the remission is ordinarily temporary, occasionally it is permanent.

Laboratory Findings

Urine. In the urine the constant findings are those of heavy albuminuria with casts and white blood cells. Red cells may appear transiently, in small amounts persistently, or in larger numbers when the disease is changing its characteristics toward those of chronic nephritis. The child usually retains the ability to concentrate the urine. The urea clearance test of kidney function is commonly normal, sometimes supernormal. Lipid granules are almost always present in the urine and aid in diagnosis of the disease.

Blood. The changes in the blood involve the proteins and the lipids. There is a reduction in total protein level from the usual 6 to 8 Gm. per cent to less than 4 Gm. per cent. Most of this reduction is in the albumin fraction, which may be reduced to less than 1 Gm. per cent. The levels of blood lipids, including cholesterol, are usually at least double the normal values and frequently produce a cloudy appearance of the blood plasma when it separates.

Course and Prognosis

The course of nephrosis invariably is prolonged unless death occurs from an early complication. Few children endure a course that is less than 18 months. During this period there may be fluctuations in the severity of symptoms, even to the extent of complete remission. If the child can be carried safely through the threatening infections, he has approximately an even chance between surviving with a complete cure or having his disease change its characteristics and assume the features of chronic nephritis with its invariably fatal outcome.

Etiology

Among those who deal with sick children, there is little disagreement that nephrosis constitutes an entity which is quite distinct from other varieties of renal disease. Yet there is no uniformity of opinion about its etiology and there are many points of disagreement about the mechanism of its abnormal physiology. Unlike acute glomerular nephritis, there is no relation to streptococcal infection, healing is delayed and uncertain, and renal function is usually good at the onset. Peculiarities of protein and lipid metabolism and of the distribution of electrolytes remain unexplained. The peculiar effect of acute infection in producing a remission also requires an explanation. At the present time the disease continues to be a lively topic of speculation and investigation.

Treatment

The general plan of management of the child with nephrosis varies according to the convictions of individual physicians. Some feel that it is essential to try to modify the course of the disease by active methods to induce diuresis and support blood-protein levels. Others believe that such measures have but little long-term effect upon the illness. They affirm that it is better to bank on the spontaneous healing which will occur in many children, in the meanwhile supporting the child's nutrition, combating infection and providing relief from excessive fluid accumulations by periodic abdominal paracentesis.

Diet. As in every other chronic disease, the diet should be complete. The dietary components which have received greatest attention are protein, salt and water. A generous protein allowance is desirable. To the customary need for protein must be added that which results from constant loss in the urine. Very high protein diets are not taken well and are utilized no better than those of more moderate content. A suitable allowance is from 3 to 3.5 Gm. for each Kg. Limitation of salt intake by making no salt additions to the diet is appropriate, but extreme or prolonged limitation of salt is dangerous. There is no advantage in water restriction.

Infections. Appropriate attention must be given to existing focal infections, and the child's regimen should be so regulated as to reduce his chances of acquiring respiratory disease. Prompt recognition of major infections is imperative, for antibiotic treatment must be started promptly.

Activity. Insofar as possible it is wise to permit the child freedom of activity in order to maintain his and his parents' morale during the long course of the

disease. Bed rest and confinement to a hospital should be avoided whenever possible.

Plasma Proteins. Attempts to support the level of plasma proteins by transfusion, plasma infusions or the injection of salt-free albumin have not met with impressive success. Most of the injected protein appears promptly in the urine and has no lasting effect upon the course of the illness.

Diuresis. A great variety of measures have been used to produce diuresis. Many of them are occasionally or temporarily effective. The list includes plasma and albumin injections, mercurial diuretics, calcium and potassium salts, salts which alter the acid-base balance of the blood, transmission of measles and other infectious diseases to the patient.

Currently the most widely used method of producing diuresis is by the administration of ACTH, cortisone or meticortin. A high percentage of nephrotic children will undergo diuresis following the administration of these substances for 1 to 2 weeks. Experience has not yet demonstrated whether an improvement in the over-all mortality is achieved. On one hand there is a distinct increase in the number of prolonged remissions of the disorder; but on the other hand the risk of inducing hypertension and infection is increased.

Nursing Care

This is the most important part of the management of a child with nephrosis. The illness is chronic, and effective treatment measures are few. In these circumstances, the day-to-day care becomes highly important. During the stage when edema is present, the appetite is poor. Serving small quantities of special-diet foods initially and permitting the child to help himself to additional amounts frequently stimulates his appetite. Catering to a capricious appetite is necessary to encourage the child to eat the food that is necessary for his maintenance and final recovery. The use of attractive dishes and colored straws often appeals to the child who has little or no inclination to eat.

During periods of marked edema, care of the skin is especially important. When the external male genitalia are extremely edematous, special local care becomes necessary. The genitalia should be bathed several times daily and dusted with a soothing powder. The scrotum should be supported by a cotton pad held in place by a T-binder lightly applied. Cotton to separate the skin surfaces will prevent intertrigo from developing. When the child is lying on his side, pressure on the edematous organs can be eliminated by placing a pillow between his knees. When edema of the eyelids is marked, circulation of lacrimal secretion over the eyes is impaired. Warm normal saline irrigations can be used to keep the eyes free from exudate. By maintaining head elevation during parts of the day, eyelid edema usually subsides sufficiently to give the child a greater degree of comfort.

The child with nephrosis should be weighed 2 or 3 times weekly to note changes in the degree of edema. Accurate records should be kept of intake and output. Every effort must be made to avoid respiratory infections.

When ascites is present to a marked degree, abdominal paracentesis is required to relieve the pressure symptoms. If the child is prepared in such a way that the discomfort of the procedure will be less than the discomfort from the collection of fluid in his abdominal cavity, he usually will co-operate and assist by maintaining quiet during the procedure.

Puncturing the bladder during the paracentesis can be avoided if the child is encouraged to void just prior to the treatment.

Sterile equipment required for an abdominal paracentesis consists of hypodermic syringe, hypodermic and aspiration needles, procaine (Novocain), scalpel, cannula, trocar, rubber tubing, needleholder, suture needles, sutures, forceps, gloves, towels, graduated receptacle, cotton balls, gauze squares and an abdominal dressing.

Unsterile equipment consists of a preparation tray, test tubes, a pail for the collection of fluid, a scultetus or abdominal binder and safety pins.

The child should be placed close to the edge of the examining table. Two nurses are required to assist in this procedure. One nurse prepares the area, collects samples of ascitic fluid for culture and checks the child's pulse, respirations and color during the procedure. The second nurse is responsible for maintaining the child's position. When the child's co-operation has been secured through careful preparation, no restraint is necessary. Satisfactory position usually can be maintained if the nurse stands behind the child, supports his back with her body and clasps his hands which are held at his side. By suggesting that the child close his eyes or turn his head away from the tray of equipment, fear may be lessened.

After the doctor has anesthetized the area with procaine and has made a small incision through the skin, he inserts the cannula and the trocar until fluid begins to flow from the peritoneal cavity. Then the doctor attaches the rubber tubing to the cannula, regulates the flow to prevent sudden withdrawal of fluid and directs the flow into the graduated receptacle. Sudden and rapid withdrawal of fluid reduces intra-abdominal pressure, causes the blood to distend the deep abdominal veins and reduces the normal supply of blood in the heart. If too much fluid is withdrawn, symptoms of shock develop. When sufficient fluid has been withdrawn to reduce pressure symptoms, the cannula is removed, sutures are taken, and the area is cleansed with alcohol and covered with a dressing. After a scultetus or an abdominal binder has been applied snugly, the child is returned to his bed. After the treatment, the amount of drainage from the wound and the child's condition should be observed and charted.

For most and sometimes all of the long period of illness these children have no prostration or discomfort. Play activities suitable for their age and interest must be provided. When the degree of edema lessens and the child is permitted to be out of bed, activities in a playroom will be enjoyed greatly and will contribute toward making his hospital stay constructive.

Before the child is discharged from the hospital, parental guidance will be necessary to ensure adequate continued care. The mother will require help to understand the child's diet, the measures necessary to prevent upper respiratory infections and the need for continued medical supervision.

Chronic Nephritis
(Chronic Glomerular Nephritis)

Chronic nephritis is a terminal illness which is the result of progressive destruction of nephrons, leading to severe loss of renal function. Although the clinical manifestations are fairly uniform, the avenues by which individual children enter are diverse.

Etiology

There is no uniformity of opinion about the etiology of chronic nephritis, and it is probable that the term encompasses the end result of several different disease entities. Some children are discovered to have well-advanced chronic nephritis without having suffered any recognizable renal disease previously. Others first pass through a period of nephrosis which gradually changes over to chronic nephritis. A few suffer from chronic or recurrent bacterial infection of the kidney. Rarely does the child pass directly from a classic episode of acute glomerular nephritis into the progressive form of the disease.

Symptoms

When there has been no recognized renal disease previously, the symptoms are insidious, and the onset is gradual. Fatigue, anemia, headache and mild degrees of edema of the face or the feet are the most common early symptoms. Often the disease is discovered accidentally during a routine urine examination or during a physical examination which reveals the presence of mild hypertension. In the early stages symptoms are frequently mild or intermittent, and the child is able to pursue normal activities.

The terminal symptoms are those of uremia or hypertension. Activity may be hampered by severe headache, nausea, fatigue or acidosis. In the final days of his illness the child usually passes into coma due to hypertension or uremia.

Diagnosis

The diagnosis of chronic nephritis depends upon the interpretation of laboratory tests. The earliest abnormalities are found in the urine, where albumin and casts are regularly present, together with varying degrees of hematuria. The urea-clearance, phenolsulfonphthalein and urine-concentration tests indicate marked loss of renal function. In the later stages of the disease, blood-chemical determinations show retention of nitrogen products (uremia), acidosis and the accumulation of phosphates and creatinine above their usual levels. The blood pressure, particularly the diastolic pressure, usually is elevated.

Course and Prognosis

Recovery from fully developed chronic nephritis is not to be expected. The course may last only a few weeks after discovery of the disease or may permit survival over a period of many years. In very unusual instances children have been known to reach a point of permanent stabilization of the disease.

Treatment

No treatment is known which will stem the progress of chronic nephritis toward a fatal termination. When the diagnosis has been established with certainty, the most charitable attitude is to permit the child to follow normal activities within the limits of his physical comfort. This regimen allows him the maximum enjoyment of his remaining months or years and supports his morale by tendering false assurance of favorable progress.

General hygienic measures are im-portant. The diet should be designed to maintain optimal nutrition. Salt restriction should be imposed if there is edema. Prevention and prompt treatment of all infectious illnesses should be provided. During the periods of hypertensive or uremic symptoms, hospitalization usually is required to provide comfort through such measures as sedation, transfusion, relief of heart failure and correction of acidosis.

WILMS'S TUMOR

Wilms's tumor is one of the most frequent types of neoplasm seen among children. It is an adenosarcoma arising from fetal rests in the kidney, i.e., from abnormal bits of tissue which are left behind during early embryonic life and have the capacity to begin unrestrained cancerous growth after the child is born. For this reason, Wilms's tumor is seen mainly in the first year of life and almost exclusively during the first 5 years. It appears as a mass in the kidney region which is discovered accidentally by the parent or the examining physician. Usually the mass has reached considerable size by the time it is discovered. Since the tumor has a strong predilection to extend locally through the kidney capsule or the renal vein and to disseminate to other parts of the body by the blood stream, prompt recognition is imperative. The diagnosis usually can be confirmed by intravenous pyelography, which shows displacement and distortion of the pelvis of the kidney.

Treatment consists of prompt surgical removal of the tumor, followed or preceded by x-ray treatment to the area about it. Unfortunately many Wilms's tumors already have metastasized, usually to the lungs, by the time the original tumor is discovered and treated. Irradiation of the pulmonary metastases is temporarily effective but seldom permanently curative. Even with prompt recognition and removal of the tumor, the prognosis is doubtful. Less than 25 per cent of such children survive for 3 years.

ABNORMALITIES OF BLADDER FUNCTION

DESCRIPTIVE TERMS

Several terms are employed to describe abnormalities of the manner of passing urine from the bladder.

Pollakiuria

This term refers to an increase in the frequency of urination. It may accompany polyuria when the total volume of urine is increased or may be associated with dysuria when frequent painful discharge of small amounts of urine results. In some instances there is neither increased volume nor pain, and the frequent passage of urine appears to be related to nervous tension instead.

Dysuria

This signifies painful urination. It is found most often with infections of the lower urinary tract, which are discussed in a later section. Mechanical irritants such as foreign bodies in the bladder or the vagina, burns about the external genitalia or pinworm infestations are responsible at times for painful urination.

Incontinence

Incontinence implies a lack of voluntary control over the discharge of urine from the bladder. It is a normal feature of the young infant who has not yet acquired voluntary control. It may accompany severe mental retardation; it is seen during severe prostrating illnesses and is a feature of a number of neurologic disorders which impair the operation of the lower spinal cord or the peripheral nerves that serve the bladder. The latter conditions include spina bifida, transverse myelitis, spinal cord injury and occasionally poliomyelitis.

Enuresis

Enuresis is distinguished from incontinence because it is involuntary micturition occurring in an individual, who, by reason of age, intelligence and lack of neurologic disability, might be expected to have control over his bladder function.

NEUROLOGIC BLADDER

The complexities of the nervous control over bladder function are not completely understood. Co-ordinated activity of the intrinsic musculature of the bladder is regulated in part by involuntary centers in the lower spinal cord through the autonomic nervous system and in part by higher voluntary centers in the brain. Normally, the sphincter muscle at the outlet of the bladder is kept tightly closed by involuntary signals from the spinal cord. As the bladder fills with urine, its distention beyond a certain point calls forth contraction waves in the musculature which eventually are felt by the higher centers in the brain. Through a voluntary act, the sphincter tone then is relaxed, and the bladder contracts unopposed, discharging its content of urine. Then the sphincter closes and comes back under the automatic control of the spinal cord, while the bladder refills with urine.

During sudden acute afflictions of the spinal cord such as myelitis, poliomyelitis or injury, the normal mechanism is disturbed by the loss of sensory awareness of bladder distention and by the impairment of voluntary control over the relaxation of the sphincter. The bladder distends progressively until the volume and the pressure of urine are sufficient to broach the sphincter without the mediation of voluntary relaxation. Overflow incontinence with dribbling results. The cardinal principle in the management of acute retention of this sort is prevention of infection within the stagnant pool of urine. Chemotherapy and antibiotics usually are prescribed to prevent this occurrence, and catheterization of the bladder is avoided whenever possible. When the cord injury is a temporary one, the return of normal function can be expected within a period of 1 to 4 weeks.

When the interference with nervous control is permanent, due to congenital abnormality or the persistence of an acquired disorder of the spinal cord, the clinical manifestations vary somewhat. If the spasticity of the sphincter predominates, retention persists, but usually the overflow dribbling is replaced by periodic partial emptying of the bladder, which is not under voluntary control. Under these circumstances the chronic obstruction to urine flow results in abnormally high pressures in the bladder and hence in ureters and kidney pelves which may enlarge the kidneys slowly and destroy their functioning tissue gradually.

Management of this type of chronic neurologic bladder usually requires some form of relief from chronic obstruction. This may be afforded by indwelling catheters or by artificial openings into the bladder (cystotomy). Sometimes the neurologic disturbance produces a lax sphincter which is unable to hold back urine. Under these circumstances the bladder is small and spastic and contains little or no urine.

In both varieties of chronic disorder the hazard of chronic or recurring infection of the urinary tract is so great as to be almost unavoidable. Periodic or continuous administration of antibiotics or chemotherapy may eliminate infection temporarily or reduce its severity. Although many of these patients live for years in spite of the effects of chronic infection and back pressures upon the kidneys, their prospects of reaching adult life are limited.

ENURESIS

The term enuresis is applied to instances of involuntary micturition among persons who might be expected to have urinary control because of age, training, mentality and absence of physical defects which cause incontinence. Enuresis may be nocturnal, diurnal or both.

Etiology

Involuntary micturition is normal in infancy. Many children acquire day control by the age of 2½ to 3½ and night control by 3½ to 4½. Control may be acquired earlier or later, depending upon the child's neuromuscular development and upon the guidance he is receiving. Mentally deficient children acquire control slowly or not at all. Certain organic lesions of the spinal cord, such as transverse myelitis or congenital malformations, lead to permanent incontinence. These conditions can be distinguished readily from enuresis.

In some children, enuresis may be only a continuance of the uninhibited infantile pattern of micturition. In other children, control is gained for a time and then lost. Enuresis is commonly a result of environmental factors and conflict in interpersonal relationships.

Various secondary or exciting causes have been stated. Among these may be enumerated the following: polyuria from excessive water drinking, concentrated highly acid urine, inflammation of the bladder with or without a cal-culus and numerous conditions acting reflexly, such as phimosis, preputial adhesions, narrowed meatus, pinworms, constipation and adenoids. It is doubtful if these or any other physical condition acting reflexly can cause enuresis alone. It is possible that some of them at times may be factors. It is desirable to remedy all, whether enuresis is present or not. The correction of these defects usually has no effect on established enuresis. Furthermore, the majority of children with enuresis have no such defects.

Symptoms

Enuresis does not affect the health, although at times poor health and enuresis are associated. Good habits are more difficult to acquire in the presence of poor health. Enuresis may persist up to 8 to 10 years of age. Seldom does it continue beyond puberty. With frequent voiding, a reduced bladder capacity may result and become a factor in the continuance of the habit. The longer enuresis has been established, the more difficult it is to control.

Treatment

The varieties of treatment which have been advocated are numerous. It is possible that all can be classified under the term "psychotherapy." Each clinician develops his own methods, which are adapted to his manner of practice and are successful for him. His own assurance of the effectiveness of the method employed would seem to be a large factor in its success.

A study of the child and the interpersonal relationships he has experienced within his family is necessary before any guidance of the child or his parents can begin. Obtaining a history of the training regimen that the child has experienced is important in understanding the parental attitudes to which the child has been subjected. It is the child who requires treatment. Enuresis is only a symptom of underlying conflict. In many instances, treatment in a child-guidance center is indicated and necessary.

When the services of a therapist are not available, every effort to correct the environmental factors which have produced enuresis should be made. There is no formula that will cure enuresis. The child in his family setting must be studied and treated in a way that meets his emotional requirements. The parents will need help in changing their attitudes toward the child and his symptoms. The child also needs help to change his attitudes toward his symptoms. However, this cannot be accomplished directly. It can come only through a good interpersonal relationship with his doctor—a relationship which helps him to feel that he is being guided by someone who is genuinely interested in the way he feels about himself and his intimate relationships with those within his family.

Obtaining the child's interest in acquiring increased control of his bodily functions eventually must be aroused and maintained. He needs help to feel that he can develop increased control and that the responsibility for control is his. At the same time he should be helped to feel that both the doctor and his parents are interested in and desirous of assisting him to accept the responsibility entailed in developing the controls that are appropriate for his age. Scolding and punishment accomplish nothing; they merely increase his conflicts and tension and make the symptoms more pronounced. Neither fear nor humiliation should be associated with the treatment. Humiliation tells the child he is "bad." He is not bad or inferior; he is merely the victim of interpersonal relationships that have failed to meet his emotional needs. He needs help, not condemnation.

Drugs have been used with limited success in helping the child to overcome enuresis. Occasionally, atropine and its derivatives may reduce bladder irritability and improve sphincter tone. However, reliance upon drug therapy is avoiding the main issue, which in nearly every instance is one of psychological orientation.

INFECTIONS OF THE GENITO-URINARY TRACT

Pyuria

A number of terms are employed to designate the presence of infection within the urinary apparatus. Pyelonephritis implies that the inflammation is primarily in the kidney parenchyma; pyelitis indicates the pelvis of the kidney; ureteritis, the ureter; cystitis, the bladder. The more indefinite term "pyuria" is preferable, for infection within the tract usually is not confined to a single location, nor is it possible always to localize the major site exactly.

Etiology

Pyuria is more common in infants than in older children and more common in girls than in boys. Colon bacilli are the infecting organisms in from 75 to 80 per cent of the cases; streptococci and staphylococci, in most of the remainder. The infecting bacteria may reach the urinary tract by way of the blood or from below by ascent from the exterior. Some controversy exists as to which of these routes is the more common. A widely held view is that staphylococci and streptococci reach the urinary tract by way of the blood, with the primary infection in the kidney, and that infections with the colon bacillus are chiefly of the ascending type. The wearing of diapers and the relatively short urethra of girl infants as compared with that of boys seem to be sufficient to account for the greater frequency of the disease in girl babies.

Obstruction in the urinary tract plays a highly important role in urinary infection. Once infection has occurred, obstruction aggravates the condition and is an important factor in making the infection severe and chronic. Most often, in childhood the obstruction is produced by some congenital malformation, seldom by stone. A relationship exists between urinary infection and infections of the upper respiratory tract and gastro-intestinal disturbances, particularly diarrhea.

Symptoms

The symptoms of pyuria are extremely varied. In the infant and the young child they are not localizing. In the older child they may simulate those of appendicitis, meningitis, pneumonia or other febrile illnesses. Fever is almost always present with acute attacks and frequently is marked by rapid fluctuations, with chills or convulsions during the rising portion of the fever curve. Leukocytosis is generally present.

With chronic pyuria or pyuria which persists beyond the initial attack, the systemic manifestations of fever, chills and general malaise are usually milder or completely lacking, in spite of heavy infection of the urine.

Unlike older children, the newborn infant is affected with equal frequency in the two sexes. It is assumed that such infections are the result of blood-borne bacteria. In the older infant or child, pyuria in the male is much less common than in the female, and its occurrence almost invariably means the presence of some anatomic or functional malformation of the urinary tract.

Diagnosis

The clue to diagnosis lies in the discovery of pus upon microscopic examination of the urine. Pus must be present in abnormal amount, and there must be assurance that it did not come from preputial or vaginal secretions. When there is doubt, a clean or a catheterized specimen of urine is required. The latter procedure has the advantage of permitting accurate culture of the urine in order to identify the bacterium responsible and to test its sensitivity to various chemotherapeutic and antibiotic agents.

Prognosis

The prognosis of uncomplicated pyuria is good. In many cases in which no obstruction or urinary retention exists, the pyuria and the bacilluria will cease spontaneously or with little treatment, when associated parenteral infection or gastro-intestinal disturbance has subsided. The cases of most troublesome and persistent infection are those in which obstruction exists. Obstruction alone leads ultimately to kidney failure. When infection is present in addition, kidney failure is hastened.

Treatment

Control of pyuria requires the elimination of the infecting organisms from the urinary tract. Sulfonamides are highly satisfactory in the treatment of most acute attacks; sulfadiazine and Gantrisin have the greatest popularity. Because these substances are concentrated by the kidney, an effective level in the urine can be obtained with moderate doses. In some instances the infecting organism is not readily susceptible to these substances or has acquired resistance to them. Then rational treatment must be guided by isolating the infecting bacteria and testing its sensitivity to the many antibiotic agents that are now available. In long-standing or recurrent pyuria, bacteria of the Proteus and the Pseudomonas families may be encountered. These organisms not infrequently defy the most carefully planned antibiotic attack.

With the possible exception of the initial attack of simple pyuria in girls, all cases should be studied carefully for the presence of abnormalities of the anatomy or the physiology of the urinary tract so that, whenever feasible, situations that produce stasis of urine can be corrected in the hope of forestalling future episodes of pyuria. Such studies usually begin with an x-ray visualization of the upper urinary tract by intravenous pyelography. An opaque dye such as Diodrast or Neoiopax is injected into the blood stream of the child after a period of partial dehydration and roentgenograms of the abdomen are taken at intervals thereafter. Usually the outline of the kidneys and the ureters can be discovered by this method, and some indication of the excretory power of each kidney can be obtained. The lower portion of the urinary tract may be visualized by a cystogram. This procedure involves the injection of an opaque dye into the bladder through a catheter in the urethra. Then x-ray films are taken which demonstrate the size and the shape of the bladder and sometimes reveal the ureters if their orifices are abnormally petulous. A satisfactory understanding of the abnormality sometimes requires the additional information provided by cystoscopy with retrograde pyelography. Direct visualization of the bladder and urethra is possible; urine may be collected from the two kidneys independently for study, and better x-ray visualization of the ureters and the kidney pelves can be made when cath-eters are passed up into the upper portions of the tract. Unfortunately, the procedure of cystoscopy is painful and upsetting to male children and usually cannot be done without a general anesthetic.

Nursing Care

Specimens of urine will be desired from infants and children with pyelitis. Several methods of collecting specimens are used. For the young baby the Tomac plastic urine specimen diaper* (Fig. 91) is a simple, comfortable method of obtaining a sample of urine. When the head of the bed is elevated, a specimen can be collected without restraining the infant. For girls, other devices, such as wedging a small basin between the thighs or allowing the child to be in a slightly cupped square of plastic material also may be used. A test tube or wide-mouth bottle can be attached by means of adhesive plaster to the male genitalia. A bird-seed receptacle can be used similarly for girls. Observation of the child's reactions to removal of the adhesive tape which keeps the receptacle over the genitalia shows that pain and fear are associated

* Obtainable from American Hospital Supply Corporation, Evanston, Ill.

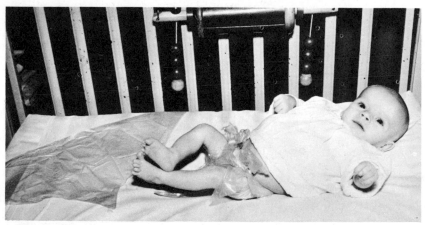

Fig. 91. Illustrating the use of a plastic specimen diaper.

with it. Therefore, it seems important to weigh these disadvantages from the child's point of view with the advantages in the use of adhesive plaster. The use of binders (Fig. 92) to keep the receptacles in place takes more time but they prevent painful removal and fear of bodily injury which are important criteria in the evaluation of their usefulness. With the use of a binder for a quiet, young infant, no restraints are necessary. For older and active infants, ankle restraints are required if the specimen is being collected during hours when he is awake. The binder with the attached test tube is pinned securely around the lower abdomen. Then the test tube is placed over the penis, and the binder tapes are brought across the perineum and pinned to the sides of the waist band (Fig. 93). The binder used for collecting specimens from babies is applied in a similar manner. The receptacle is placed above the anus and over the genitalia and held in position by pinning the center tab snugly to the back of the waist band. Elevating the head of the crib facilitates the collection of specimens. Care must be taken to prevent the contamination of the specimen with feces because it is unsuitable for examination.

Often clean specimens are desired from children with pyelitis. Before the

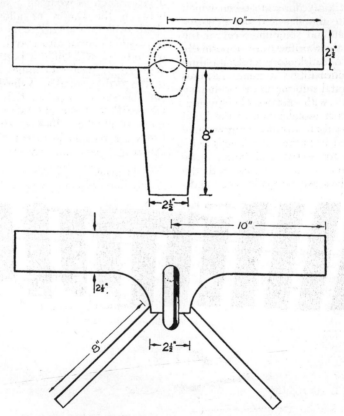

Fig. 92. (*Top*) T-binder with bird-seed cup for collection of urine from female infant. (*Bottom*) T-binder with test tube attached for collection of urine from male infant.

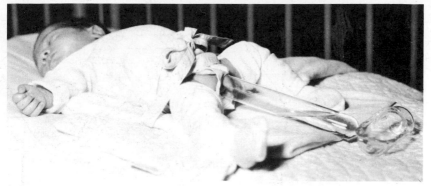

FIG. 93. Collecting single specimen of urine from male infant when binder is used. Receptacle for female also is shown.

sterilized test tube or female receptacle is applied, the genitalia should be washed with cotton and green-soap solution and rinsed with sterile normal saline solution. If the child is old enough to use a bedpan or a urinal, these receptacles should be sterilized for the collection of a clean specimen.

Twenty-four-hour urine specimens can be collected with the use of a pyrex funnel which is shaped like a lily. This can be applied to the genitalia with the use of a binder. The end of the funnel is connected by rubber tubing, the other end of which is taped just inside the bottle which is hung at the foot of the baby's crib. Gilson and Matson* devised a method of collecting a 24-hour urine specimen from the male infant which prevents the penis from being sucked down into the glass funnel each time the baby urinates. They suggest the use of a "Y" glass connection in the middle of the tubing. A piece of rubber tubing is attached to the second arm of the "Y" and secured to the top of the crib side. The second piece of tubing acts as an air vent. It breaks the suction and prevents the edema and irritation which occurs when the penis is sucked down into the glass

* Gilson, Martha, and Matson, Donald D.: Care of a child after an arachnoidureteral shunt, Am. J. Nursing 56:1424, 1956.

funnel. Jacket and ankle restraints are necessary to keep active infants in a prone position. Shock blocks, 6 inches in height, should be used to elevate the head of the bed. In this way gravity will prevent back flow and loss of the urine. During the period that 24-hour urine specimens are being collected, special back and local care should be given every 4 hours. After the infant voids, the binder and the tube can be removed long enough to bathe the external genitalia. The jacket restraint can be loosened for back care. Ankle restraints should be unpinned at intervals so that the infant may have an opportunity to exercise his lower extremities. To prevent loss of urine, the infant should be observed at frequent intervals. Movement may displace the tube and make readjustment necessary.

If a sterile specimen is required for culture, catheterization is required. The following sterile equipment is necessary for the procedure: 2 catheters (size 8 or 10 Fr.), gloves, towels, kidney basin, 1 glass with 2 drams of tr. Zephiran, basins of green soap and normal saline solution, 3 applicators, cotton balls and culture tubes standing in a round basin.

If the sterile specimen is desired from an older child who understands the pro-

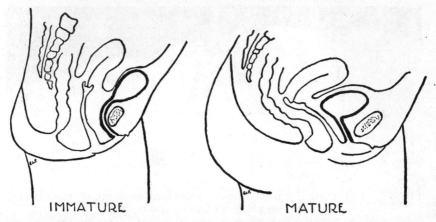

IMMATURE   MATURE

FIG. 94. Showing the relative position of the bladder and the direction of the course of the urethra (heavy lines) in the infant and the mature female.

cedure sufficiently to co-operate, the catheterization procedure is the same as for an adult. Co-operation of the child is essential, as relaxation is necessary if a catheterized specimen is to be obtained. Explaining the procedure to the child, showing her the equipment and asking her to help by breathing deeply through her mouth usually produces co-operation and the relaxation necessary to introduce the catheter into the bladder. When a specimen is required from a young child who cannot be prepared, two nurses are necessary to carry out the procedure safely. One nurse will be required to help the child lie quietly. A second nurse will carry out the procedure after she has scrubbed her hands and put on the sterile gloves. The bowl holding the standing test tubes should be placed on the sterile towel which previously had been placed in front of the perineum. One hand is used to hold the labia separated. The other hand is used to cleanse and to apply the tr. Zephiran to the meatus and the surrounding area. In cleansing the external genitalia, a cotton ball should be used only once. It should cleanse from above downward toward the anus and then be discarded. The cotton balls must be handled carefully.

The gloved hands must remain uncontaminated. After the tip of the catheter has been lubricated with saline and the wide end placed into the test tube, the catheter is passed through the meatus into the urethra until the bladder is reached and the urine begins to flow. When specimens have been collected, the catheter can be pinched off and withdrawn. If catheterization is ordered to relieve distention, the catheter is not withdrawn until urine ceases to flow. When the procedure has been completed, the test tube should be covered with sterile gauze squares, placed in a specimen bottle and sent to the laboratory.

Catheterization of the young child often produces a problem for the inexperienced nurse. In the young infant, the bladder is higher and more anterior than in the adult (Fig. 94). The bladder descends rapidly during the first 3 years, then slowly. It has the adult position at 20 years. In the female adult, the urethra is relatively short and straight; in the infant it hooks around the symphysis in a "C" shape. When the meatus is located, the catheter should be introduced and directed downward instead of in the direction necessary to reach the bladder of an adult patient.

VULVOVAGINITIS

In girls before puberty, the mucosa of the vagina and the vulva is covered with a relatively thin layer of epithelium as compared with that of the adult. The change to the adult type of epithelium occurs at puberty through increase in estrogenic hormones which stimulate growth of the epithelium, producing thickening and cornification. Also, at puberty the vaginal secretions change from neutral to acid through estrogenic activity. Both changes increase resistance to local infection. Thus it is that girls before puberty acquire vaginal and vulvar infections more easily than do those who are older.

Inflammation of the vagina or of the vagina and the vulva is relatively frequent in childhood and especially is this true among girls from the lower social or economic strata. Cases of vulvovaginitis are commonly divided into two groups: those in which the inflammation is due to the gonococcus and those in which it is not. Those of the latter group are referred to as cases of simple or nonspecific vaginitis. In both types, the child presents a more or less purulent vaginal discharge. Distinction between them is made wholly by the determination of the presence or the absence of gonococci.

Simple Vaginitis

This may be caused by any of a variety of organisms—organisms normally found in the lower intestinal tract are usually responsible. Streptococci which are simultaneously infecting the respiratory tract are occasionally isolated. Frequently, simple vaginitis is due primarily to lack of cleanliness with resultant secondary implantation of bacteria. Less often, it is due to masturbation or to insertion of objects into the vagina. Simple vaginitis is not communicable and responds readily to treatment. In some instances, a daily tub bath with local cleansing is sufficient. In other instances, a short period of treatment with simple douches produces prompt recovery. Almost any cleansing douche is satisfactory. It may be a solution of sodium chloride, boric acid or sodium bicarbonate. Sulfonamide therapy is effective and in some instances may be preferable to treatment by douches. Penicillin is effective if hemolytic streptococci are present.

Gonococcic Vaginitis

This would be rare in childhood were it not a contagious disease for girls. If the infection is newly acquired and acute, there is complaint referable to the local inflammation, especially pain on micturition because of urethritis and vulvitis. There also may be a certain amount of constitutional disturbance with fever. In some cases, proctitis also is present. After a time all symptoms disappear, and there remains only continued vaginal discharge. Periods of visible discharge may alternate with periods of latency during which no discharge is seen, although the infection is still present, as shown by culture or smear.

When untreated, gonorrhea in girls resembles the same disease in women in its chronicity and its latent periods. It is dissimilar in that secondary pelvic inflammatory disease and involvement of the glands of Skene and Bartholin and of the glandular structures of the endocervix are very rare in childhood. Although an adult may be a source of contagion to a child, the infection is not contagious in the same sense among adults.

In its chronic form, gonorrheal vaginitis in childhood seldom has any ill effect on the health nor has it usually any local symptoms other than discharge.

Intramuscular injection of penicillin in doses of 300,000 units per day or more is regularly effective in the treatment of gonorrheal vaginitis. Cure may be effected in as brief a period as 3 or 4 days. During the early stages of treatment, isolation technic must be observed to prevent the spread of infection to other female children in the environment.

INFECTIONS OF THE PENIS AND THE URETHRA IN THE MALE

Balanoposthitis

Uncircumcized males in whom cleansing of the glans and the prepuce of the penis is neglected may develop nonspecific infection of the mucous membrane of these structures. The infection yields promptly to adequate cleansing and warm applications. When edema is severe and the prepuce cannot be retracted to permit cleansing, a dorsal slit operation may be required to permit adequate drainage to be carried out.

Urethritis and Prostatitis

Occasionally, balanoposthitis may extend upward into the urethra. Gonorrheal urethritis also is known to occur in older boys and runs the same clinical course as in the adult male. Treatment is by intramuscular injection of penicillin.

A nonspecific variety of prostatitis may be seen in adolescent boys. The symptoms are those of dysuria and hematuria without fever. The disorder may be related to excessive masturbation either as a cause or as an incitant. Expectant treatment is usually sufficient, for the disease runs a brief, self-limited course of a few days.

UNDESCENDED TESTICLE (CRYPTORCHIDISM)

Early in fetal life the testicles develop within the abdomen near and below the kidneys. In most instances, they descend into the scrotum during the last 2 months. In some instances, they are still in the inguinal canal at the time of birth and occasionally within the abdomen. Those undescended at birth usually descend during the first few weeks after birth, but may descend at any time up to the period of adolescence. When nondescent is bilateral, the testes nearly always descend before puberty. When it is unilateral, approximately half descend at puberty or soon afterward. Undescended testicle is to be found in only about 0.3 per cent of men by the time full maturity is reached.

At puberty, the testes normally increase in size and develop spermatogenic and increased androgenic activity. An undescended testis develops at puberty in the same manner for a short time, but eventually the sperm-forming cells degenerate, with sterility as a result if both testes are affected. Although slight decrease in androgenic activity may occur, the body and the secondary sexual characteristics develop normally.

The temperature at which the testis is maintained seems to be the controlling factor in its spermatogenic activity, scrotal temperature being lower than that of the body.

A testicle in the inguinal canal is more subject to injury than when in the scrotum—both external injury and that from torsion and strangulation. An undescended testis produces a psychological handicap.

There is considerable divergence of opinion about the proper treatment of undescended testis. Many physicians wait until puberty before instituting treatment. Others treat at from 10 to 11 years old, a period preceding puberty development, in order to avoid the possibility of prepuberal degeneration. Normal puberty development results from a hormone produced by the anterior pituitary gland. An active principle similar in action to the pituitary hormone can be obtained from human pregnancy urine. This material, known as chorionic gonadotropic hormone, may be responsible for descent of the testis before birth. It is the hormone used in the treatment of undescended testis. The hormone is given in doses of from 200 to 500 units 2 or 3 times a week, the total not exceeding 6,000 units, and over a period not exceeding 6 weeks. Treatment in excess of these amounts is likely to produce precocious puberty. In some instances, the treatment is repeated after an interval of several months. Hormone treatment causes descent in possibly half the cases and possibly only in those instances in which the testes would have descended subsequently without treatment.

Those who fail to respond to hormone treatment require operation to bring the testis into the scrotum. Surgical treatment should be given as soon as the hormone treatment has been stopped and while the testis and its cord are still increased in size as a result of the treatment. Operation is not uniformly successful in producing a good result.

SITUATIONS FOR FURTHER STUDY

1. How does nephritis in children differ from that in adults? How can nephritis be prevented in childhood? What are the complications of nephritis?

2. Observe a child with nephrosis who has had several hospital admissions. Describe his behavior in relation to you. What is his health problem? Has he a personality problem? What is it? What do you think produced it? Describe his relationship with his mother and with other children. What is the pattern of his play? How do you think he feels about himself, about you and his mother? Has he the inner strengths you would expect in a child of his age? What inner strengths do you think he is ready to acquire? Describe the way you helped him gain increased inner strength.

3. An 8-year-old child has been brought to the children's clinic because of enuresis. Observe the doctor's interview, talk with the parents and the child and consider the following points:

How did the mother describe the child's problem? Did she talk about it in the child's presence? Has he always had enuresis? If not, when did it begin? What was the family situation when enuresis began? How did the mother attempt to help the child establish control? When did she begin to institute training? What problems developed at that time? What was the mother's reaction to the child's enuresis? How has she attempted to help the child overcome it? What was the child's reaction to his problem? Did he feel ashamed, guilty, or did he seem anxious to be helped to overcome it? What type of parent-child relationship existed? Were any physical abnormalities found on examination? How did the child respond to the examination? What guidance did the doctor suggest? Do you feel that the mother received sufficient insight to utilize the doctor's recommendations? What further help will the parents and the child require?

BIBLIOGRAPHY

Campbell, Meredith: Clinical Pediatric Urology, Philadelphia, Saunders, 1951.

Gerard, M. W.: Enuresis: a study in etiology, Am. J. Orthopsychiat. 9:48, 1939.

Heyman, Walter: Renal disorders in infants and children, Am. J. Nursing 48:436, 1948.

Kaplan, Sol A., and Collison, Cornelia: Nephrosis in children, Am. J. Nursing 56:300, 1956.

Rubin, M. I.: Disturbances of the kidney in Nelson, Textbook of Pediatrics, ed. 6, Philadelphia, Saunders, 1954.

CHAPTER TWENTY-TWO

Diseases of the Nervous System

The nervous system consists of an intricate complex of nerve centers and pathways (the brain and the spinal cord) which is confined within a protective bony shell (the skull and the vertebral column) and sends out branches (the peripheral nerves) to all parts of the body. Through the anterior motor nerves, the brain and the spinal cord control the activity of muscles and organs; through the posterior sensory nerves they receive sensations from them and also from the skin and the organs of special sense. Intellect, mind, memory, feeling and personality are all related intimately to the function of the brain.

Structural or functional disturbances of the central nervous system occur in bewildering numbers. Their complexities can be understood only with the aid of an extensive knowledge of the anatomy and the physiology of the nervous system. In a brief text of this sort it will be possible to mention only a few of the representative types. For more detailed consideration the reader is referred to the texts suggested in the bibliography.

MENTAL DEFICIENCY

ETIOLOGY

The failure of a child to develop normal intellectual capacity nearly always is due to structural defects within the brain. These defects may be the result of gross malformations of brain structure. However, more often, they depend upon the loss of brain cells through injury, anoxia or infection or upon the congenital absence of such cells. Since the cells of the brain are susceptible to a wide variety of noxious influences, mental deficiency is seen as an accompaniment of, or sequel to a similarly large number of disorders. It will be possible to cite some representative examples only.

Heredity

Heredity can be responsible for mental deficiency, for its occurrence may, in

502

some instances, be traced through other members of the family. The genetic basis is not entirely limited to the degenerative disorders described later in this chapter.

Maternal Infection

Maternal infection during pregnancy (rubella) may be responsible for maldevelopment of the brain.

Prenatal Infection

Prenatal infection with syphilis is sometimes responsible for brain damage.

Birth Trauma

Birth trauma with the associated anoxia and hemorrhage is regarded as a frequent cause and may result in additional motor disorders.

Anoxia

Anoxia after birth may occur during severe atelectasis or anemia.

Toxic Effects

The "toxic effects" of bilirubin or other substances produced during the course of erythroblastosis fetalis may damage the brain and result in the condition known as kernicterus.

Phenylketonuria (Phenylpyruvic Oligophrenia). A hereditarily transmissible defect in the metabolism of one of the amino acids—phenylalanine—leads to the excretion of an abnormal substance in the urine which can be detected by a simple chemical test. The accumulation of the products of incomplete metabolism of the acid lead to mental deficiency in most of the afflicted children. They are usually blonde and blue-eyed and a high percentage suffer from eczema. When recognized, the defect may be partially controlled by a diet low in phenylalanine. The extent to which this type of control will preserve normal mentality is now under test. Unfortunately, the diet is expensive and not very palatable. Although

relatively uncommon, this cause of mental deficiency might be discovered with increasing incidence if the urines of all newborns were regularly tested for phenylpyruvic acid.

Infection of the Central Nervous System

Beyond the newborn period infection of the central nervous system is the most common precursor of mental deficiency. Meningitis and the several varieties of encephalitis are the most frequent causes of acquired mental deficiency.

Degenerative Diseases and Thyroid Deficiency

Mental deficiency is a part of the degenerative diseases such as Schilder's or Tay-Sachs disease and accompanies some metabolic diseases such as thyroid deficiency. A spurious type of mental retardation is seen among children with severe emotional disturbances.

SYMPTOMS

The cardinal symptom of mental deficiency is failure to reach the normal developmental milestones at the appropriate age. The appearance of symptoms depends in large measure upon the severity of the defect. A few types, such as mongolism and microcephaly, are identifiable at birth, due to the presence of characteristic physical defects. However, usually the disorder is not suspected during the early months of life unless the defect is quite severe. The first inkling of abnormality comes with delay in grasping, sitting, standing and walking. Slowness to talk and difficulty in self-feeding and toilet training appear later. The infant's behavior may be very placid, so that he is regarded as a "good" baby, or he may present the opposite extreme of restlessness, hyperactivity, irritability and sleep disturbances. Drooling of saliva is common. Convulsions, feeding difficulties and spasticity of muscles are sometimes the first indications of defective development.

When the defect is of lesser severity

the child may pass through infancy and the preschool years without showing obvious symptoms. The difficulty may become apparent only when he attempts to cope with the abstract concepts of his school work.

DIAGNOSIS

As indicated above, only the more severe grades of mental deficiency can be diagnosed with confidence in infancy. Caution is necessary in the interpretation of delay in motor performance, for there is a wide variation from the average among intellectually normal children. It is important to be sure that delay in motor achievement is not due to associated physical disability, to the effects of chronic illness or to severe malnutrition. Poor hearing or vision may complicate the diagnosis by hampering the development of normal skills in an otherwise competent child.

Beyond the period of infancy, standardized mental tests permit an estimate of the severity of the intellectual defect. The intelligence quotient or "I.Q." is computed by dividing the child's mental age as measured by the test by his chronologic age and multiplying by 100. Mental deficiency is classified on the basis of such tests into the following general types:

Idiot	0 to 24 I.Q.
Imbecile	25 to 49 I.Q.
Moron	50 to 74 I.Q.
Borderline	75 to 90 I.Q.

The interpretation of intelligence tests is not a simple matter, as was stated in Chapter 4. Whenever the results are doubtful, repeated testing in 6 to 12 months is desirable as a confirmation. The test always must be regarded as a minimum measure of the child's intelligence, since any interfering factors tend to depress his achievement.

PROGNOSIS

Except in the severe degrees of mental deficiency or those associated with disturbances of motor control, the prognosis for life is about the same as that for normal children. The outlook for the child's adjustment in society will depend in large measure upon the degree of his deficiency and the degree to which his parents and others can help him to utilize the mental resources he possesses. Idiots and imbeciles require permanent care and supervision. Morons are generally able to make a living; those of borderline intelligence ordinarily get along quite well in jobs suited to their capacities.

MANAGEMENT

With a few exceptions (thyroid extract for cretinism, dietary control in phenylketonuria) there is no useful treatment which will alter the underlying defect. Some improvement can be expected from adequate control of convulsions when these are present and from the removal of unwarranted pressures applied to the child by parents or teachers who have an unrealistic concept of his ability.

Lacking any effective treatment, the objectives of management are to arrange an environment for the child in which he can utilize his limited powers to the best advantage.

During the past 3 years the Children's Bureau has made grants to State Departments of Health for pilot projects in the field of mental retardation. The states to which funds have been granted have set up special diagnostic centers in connection with a pediatric program where a diagnosis and plans for each individual child's care and education can be made. The team's plans include follow-up visits to special clinics and the use of community resources for nursery and elementary school education, for social services and public health nursing supervision. It is estimated that from 75 to 80 per cent of the children diagnosed as mentally defective have the capacity to learn self-care and partially support themselves in adulthood. The staff of the Children's Bureau is working

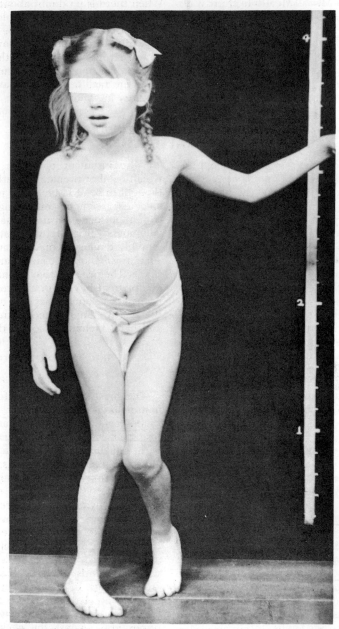

FIG. 95. Girl with spastic paralysis, showing spasticity of
the legs, with abductor spasm.

with the Division of Social Services of the Children's Bureau and with the Office of Education and the National Institute of Mental Health to study ways in which the available resources can be improved and expanded to meet the needs of the parents of young retarded children and of the children themselves.

Discussion of the problem with parents is often a difficult and delicate procedure. Whenever there is reasonable doubt about the diagnosis of mental retardation, the parents must be spared the anguish which the diagnosis creates. When there is no doubt about the diagnosis the parents must be told in order that reasonable plans can be made for the child. Such plans will have to vary somewhat, depending upon the parents' reaction to the child's handicap and upon the facilities that are available in the area in which they live.

MOTOR DISABILITIES OF CEREBRAL ORIGIN (CEREBRAL PALSIES)

"Cerebral palsy" is commonly but unwisely used as a comprehensive diagnostic term for children who have difficulty with voluntary muscle control. It erroneously implies that such children suffer from a specific disease entity which has some uniformity of etiology, symptomatology, prognosis or therapy. Such is not the case. On the one hand, the use of an all-inclusive label may unnecessarily stigmatize the child who has a mild disability and a good prognosis; on the other hand, it may encourage the parents of a hopelessly disabled child to pursue the chimera of recovery because of the knowledge that others with the same diagnosis have improved under treatment or have made a good adjustment in society.

ETIOLOGY

In a few children with motor disability the etiologic mechanism is clear and not subject to debate. In such children the symptoms begin after a specific postnatal illness. The most common cause is encephalitis, either primary or as a complication of one of the contagious diseases. Other precursors of motor disability are brain damage due to lead poisoning or to severe febrile illness, such as pneumonia, complications of meningitis, head injury, and kernicterus, the cerebral complication of erythroblastosis fetalis.

However, more numerous than these are the instances of motor defect in which natal or prenatal disturbances are thought to be at fault. There is considerable disagreement concerning the relative importance of abnormal brain development during fetal life and the potentially damaging mechanisms of birth —narcosis, anoxia, trauma and hemorrhage. The presumptive mechanism may be apparent in certain children, but it is necessary to admit that in a great many the relative importance of the prenatal and natal factors cannot be designated.

CLINICAL MANIFESTATIONS

Spasticity

The most frequent manifestation of motor disability is spasticity (Fig. 95). In this condition the voluntary muscles lose their normal fluidity and respond with difficulty to either the voluntary efforts of the child or the passive efforts of the examiner to alter their position. Abnormally strong tonus of certain muscle groups keeps the extremities and other portions of the body in characteristic attitudes which are altered jerkily by voluntary efforts. Spasticity is most often apparent in the lower extremities, where it tends to point the toes and cross the legs. In the arms it usually produces some clenching of the fist, flexion of the forearm and adduction of the upper arm against the chest wall. In severely affected children there may be an involvement of the muscles of the trunk which keep the back arched and the head extended.

All degrees of severity of the symptom are observed. Severe generalized spasticity results in a rigid, physically helpless child. Very mild degrees may not be apparent to casual observation and can be detected only by a careful neurologic examination. In some instances spasticity may be limited to one side of the body or to one extremity. The eye muscles may participate with the production of a convergent squint. In severely affected infants and children, swallowing may be difficult or impossible, due to the involvement of muscles of the face, the tongue, the jaw and the pharynx.

Weakness

Localized and diffuse weakness of muscles often is mixed in with the more obvious symptoms of spasticity. In some children the signs of brain damage are exclusively those of general or local weakness without associated spasticity.

Involuntary Movements

Several varieties of involuntary movement may be seen, usually in conjunction with other manifestations of brain damage.

Chorea consists of quick, brief movements of a localized portion of the body, most commonly an arm or the face.

Athetosis is a slow, prolonged, writhing movement of the extremities.

Choreo-athetosis. Frequently, athetosis is combined with chorea, and the resulting motions are designated as choreo-athetosis.

Tremor. A persistent vibration of an extremity is called a tremor.

Associated Disturbances

Children with motor disability frequently have the additional problems of convulsions or mental retardation or behavior disturbances. These aspects are probably a concomitant of the brain damage which has produced the motor disturbance and the parents' reactions to it. They are of varying importance to individual children and have no necessary relationship to the severity of the motor disturbance. A child with severe choreo-athetosis may have normal or even superior intelligence; one with mild spasticity may be severely retarded. Their management must be considered in relation to the child's total problem and his and his family's response to it.

Diagnosis

Motor disability of cerebral origin may be recognized shortly after birth when the symptoms are severe. The early appearance of afebrile convulsions, feeding difficulties or spasticity in the first few months of life may raise the suspicion of brain damage which is confirmed by the subsequent failure of the child to follow the normal pattern of motor development. Except for the milder and the localized varieties of motor disability, all manifestations, such as spasticity, weakness and involuntary movement, interfere with the achievement of sitting, walking, talking, feeding and other co-ordinated muscle activities. Often it is the failure in such performance that first attracts attention to the possibility of brain damage. While the presence of motor disability is an adequate explanation for developmental failure, it does not necessarily imply that the more complex functions of the brain are damaged. It is imperative to evaluate the intellectual capacity of the child separately in order to guide his management. This is often a very difficult task, because the motor disability may hamper his ability to communicate and vitiates many of the performances required by the standard intelligence tests.

Treatment and Nursing Care

No form of therapy can be expected to restore the cerebral defect. Appropriate management must be based upon a realistic appraisal of the individual child's assets and ultimate potentialities. If convulsions are present they should be controlled by the measures discussed in the next section.

In the period of infancy, the child with cerebral palsy may show difficulty in sucking, swallowing and learning to eat solid foods. A hyperactive gag reflex often initiates vomiting. The whole body tightens up, and when feedings are not given slowly enough, vomiting and aspiration may result. Gradually, he will need to be taught to eat solid foods. At first, swallowing them will produce difficulties, but patience and calmness when they are refused, spit out or vomited eventually will help him to learn to eat them.

Respiratory difficulties and body spasticity in early life are not uncommon. The changes in respiration may be due to mucus or to the cerebral lesion. Often, the infant lies with his back arched, and spasticity may make movement difficult. Frequent change of position lessens his irritability and discomfort.

In the management of the child with cerebral palsy, one of the first objectives is the prevention of contractures. If contractures develop or seem to be imminent, the baby should be provided with corrective splints. For most babies these may be worn only at night. A back support or a corset may be needed to enable the baby to sit. Leg splints usually are used in the daytime if the Achilles group of muscles go into spasm whenever the baby is placed on his feet.

During this early period in the child's life, the parents will require help to accept the child and to gain security in their ability to satisfy his needs. Details concerning supportive help are discussed on page 164 and the pages immediately following.

Many times parents hesitate to hospitalize the child for the correction or the prevention of further deformity. Economic factors may influence their feelings, and when this is the case, the help of a community agency, such as States Services to Crippled Children, should be enlisted. However, many times fears exist because of a lack of knowledge as to procedure, period of hospitalization, outcome or adjustment of the child outside the home.

The nurse who understands the problems of parents of handicapped children, can help them gradually to feel a need to secure medical care for their child. She also can allay fears that prevent them from utilizing community resources that function to provide the handicapped child with opportunities equal to those of the normal child. Often the nurse will need to initiate the co-operation of community agencies when she observes the child's need for continued medical care.

Several periods of hospitalization may be required. Often those periods are long ones, and opportunities for psychological growth, as well as good physical nursing care, must be provided. A child recuperates quickly from surgical operation. If a Sprengel operation to sever the nerves leading to the spastic extremities has been performed, the child will be in a cast that covers the lower half of his body. If he has not matured to a stage of bowel and bladder control, care on a Bradford frame will be indicated. If an operation has been performed to lengthen the Achilles tendon, casts from below the knee over the foot will be applied. If this operation has been performed, more play opportunities can be provided, for the child can be placed in a chair where he can enter into group activities. Other surgical procedures are employed to overcome the adductor spasm that produces the "scissors" gait so frequently seen in the child with the spastic type of cerebral palsy.

The child's mental capacities should be known. It is not the intelligence quotient but a knowledge of his potentialities that will assist the adult in planning an environment that will ensure optimum individual growth. A true picture of his mental ability is an intricate task, because the cerebral defect interferes with both verbal and motor expression. However, a test given by an experienced psychologist tells far more than casual observation.

Emotionally, the child with cerebral palsy seems to be unstable; there are reasons why this is so. Some of the instability may be due to inherent factors, but much of it results from the kind of guidance he has had during the formative years of his life. It is much more difficult for the child with cerebral palsy than for the normal child to get his basic human needs satisfied. He has a drive to explore, to master himself and his environment, but his physical limitations often prevent him from having the normal experiences of childhood. It takes imagination and ingenuity to help him find ways to learn. Unless his mother faces his handicaps and finds ways for him to have play experiences, intense frustration and insecurity from lack of mastery and self-fulfillment will result. Often the need for recognition is unsatisfied because of his unattractive appearance, which may be grotesque. Many parents, siblings and playmates find him difficult to accept. He becomes the object of ridicule and jests by his playmates and schoolmates and he is incapable of doing the things that other children can do. They see his body and its abnormal functioning instead of his person. As a result he is deprived of a vital ingredient for emotional growth— the responsiveness of others. Frequently, he is unable to express himself creatively, which is another basic need for personal satisfaction. Often he has speech difficulties and is limited in his ability to communicate verbally with others. He also may have eye defects which produce reading difficulties and prevent him from having vicarious experiences through the media of movies, television or books. Learning to write presents problems because of muscular in-co-ordination. Sometimes his need for

affection is completely unsatisfied because his parents and others are unable to accept him as he is. Many times he is overprotected rather than guided in a way that meets his individual changing needs.

Assisting the child to a stage of greater independence is a slow process but a very possible one in most instances. He must be helped to do things that he shows readiness to learn, yet too much must not be expected of him. The child with cerebral palsy can learn to feed himself. Feeding him is a skill; teaching him to do it himself is an art. It requires patience, faith in his ability, an understanding of his limitations and ingenuity in finding suitable equipment and methods of teaching that make the process of eating an easier and more enjoyable experience. The child also can learn to do many other things. Observation of skilled nursery school teachers as they teach children with cerebral palsy to do things for themselves, to express their inner creativeness and to learn to communicate with others will provide unlimited educational opportunities for the inexperienced nurse.

Helping the child to relax and take frequent rest periods is important because he fatigues easily. Soft music in a room with few stimuli, with a person who talks quietly in a reassuring manner and leads him to feel that she is trying to help, produces the desired effect. Excitement of all types immediately before bedtime and technics that produce resistance should be eliminated. Discipline must be redirective and given with understanding. Irritation and impatience create tension that makes self-control almost impossible. The child needs to feel that his mother, nurse or teacher is truly interested in him. Although his speech is difficult to understand, it will increase his self-esteem and sense of security if the adults in his environment learn to understand his attempts to communicate verbally with them. Responsiveness on the part of the adult lessens tension, increases relaxation, provides emotional comfort and efficient use of all his powers.

Many of the child's needs can become satisfied in play. His interests should be encouraged from the time they first are manifested. The child needs encouragement to feel that his interests are important. If the nurse uses ingenuity in finding play materials, and if the child is helped to use them constructively, he will acquire belief in his powers. With help he may excel to such a degree that his need for recognition becomes satisfied. Self-expression also can become possible.through careful selection of materials and guidance in their use.

Play experiences should assist the child to recreational productivity and provide opportunities for socialization. Play within a group is necessary. It will satisfy his need for friends and for normal social play experiences. It will help him to identify himself with a group outside his home, a need that must be fulfilled in the school-age period if wholesome emotional development is to occur.

The nurse's attitude toward the child with cerebral palsy will influence the group's acceptance of him. In the beginning, the nurse may have to direct the activity in a way that provides opportunity for him to participate in it. If she prevents him from meeting defeat, the group eventually will plan ways to utilize his abilities.

Educational opportunities should be provided in accordance with the child's abilities. The advantages of schools especially adapted to deal with his physical handicaps and to provide physiotherapy and muscle re-education are indicated. The child who is mildly incapacitated may be expected to attend a regular school but may require guidance in the selection of an occupation which is commensurate with his potentialities. Education which is commensurate with his mental ability is essential for the normally intelligent child. Through it he

can develop his interests and eventually find ways of losing himself in an all-absorbing life task. With education and wisely directed guidance he can learn to excel in some realm. Succeeding is a necessary factor in eliminating feelings of inferiority that underlie attitudes of self-pity, the most injurious of all emotional feelings.

During childhood, growth-producing experiences which provide opportunities for satisfaction in the growing-up process must be provided. It is possible for the child with cerebral palsy to have normal personality development if environmental influences are conducive to it. Whether or not maladjustment occurs depends upon the number and the severity of the problems that he must face. The child is severely limited only insofar as he has accompanying personality limitations. If opportunities for growth are denied him, he will suffer untold misery from feelings of inadequacy and incompetency, which will produce disturbances in his relationships with other people.

Guidance that helps the child face reality must begin in infancy and grow in proportion to the child's capacity to utilize it in finding constructive modes of adjustment. Denying his handicap impedes his progress toward self-understanding. When the adult recognizes the child's problem *with him,* he can approach it with the feeling that he has help and support to overcome it. He must recognize his problem and deal with it if he is to understand and learn to cope with it in a constructive manner.

The period of adolescence is a volcanic experience for a normal child, but for the child with cerebral palsy, surmounting the development tasks of the period is infinitely more difficult. Finding himself and accepting his sexual role, emancipating himself from his family and selecting and preparing for a career pose problems of great magnitude. In adolescence the social aspects of his handicap take on new proportions. If he has not been helped to accept the reality of his handicap prior to adolescence, he may show signs of acute emotional distress. He should be encouraged in social activities with both sexes to grow emotionally, to give him opportunities to emancipate himself from his parents and to prevent introversion.

The nurse's responsibility extends to those in the school and the community. She can explain the cause of the child's disability to the teacher, increase her insight into his psychological and physical needs and interpret his prognosis for future adjustment. She also can influence the attitudes of lay people toward the child with a motor handicap. The nurse who recognizes that the crippled child's basic needs are like those of the normal child will utilize her insight to help others accept him and find ways to meet his educational needs and accept his problem.

SEIZURES (CONVULSIVE DISORDERS)

The term "seizures" is used to encompass a number of varieties of episodic disturbance of brain function. Most seizures are accompanied by loss of consciousness; many of them, by abnormal muscle tone. In children the most common variety of seizure is a convulsion, but other varieties of spells, attacks, fits and abnormal states also are seen. These phenomena of diverse and uncertain etiology are grouped together because of the conviction that they all represent periods of disorganization of the normal physiologic state of the brain.

Seizures create two general types of medical problems—the management of an acute convulsion and the study and the control of recurring attacks.

SINGLE CONVULSIONS

Symptoms

Convulsions usually are sudden in onset, though in some instances their imminence may be suspected by the general behavior of the child. In a typical case, the entire body becomes stiff, and consciousness is lost. More or less skin pallor is present. The eyes tend to be fixed in some one position, perhaps rolled up or crossed. As a part of the general tonic state, the head is held backward, the back is more or less arched, the arms are flexed, and the hands are clenched. Immediately after the general stiffening of the body, twitching or clonic movements occur. These may be generalized in the beginning or may start in some part and extend to all parts of the body. The clonic movements consist chiefly of quick, jerking to-and-fro movements of the extremities and similar spasmodic movements of the muscles of the face. The spasm includes the muscles of respiration, so that breathing is irregular and ineffectual, and cyanosis results. Inability to swallow saliva may produce frothing at the mouth and rattling in the throat. The pulse becomes weak and often irregular. Convulsions may be very brief or may last a half hour or more. Usually after a few minutes the convulsive movements become weaker and finally cease. The body relaxes, and consciousness returns. If the convulsion is severe, the child may remain somewhat stuporous, and at times certain parts appear to be paralyzed temporarily.

A convulsion may not be repeated or it may recur in a few minutes or hours. In some cases, convulsions may recur frequently over a period of several days. All are not so severe as the preceding description indicates. They may be lacking in several of the described features and may be of very short duration. In some instances, convulsions may involve only part of the body; in other instances of repeated convulsions, one part may be affected during one convulsion and other parts during other convulsions.

Partial involvement of the body in this manner is not necessarily evidence of a localized intracranial lesion.

Etiology and Prognosis

A convulsion is a symptom of an underlying disorder and not itself a disease. The prognosis both for life and for the patient's mental and neurologic future depends upon the setting in which the convulsion occurs. Often the significance of an acute convulsion can be determined only in the light of future developments.

Febrile Convulsions. Some infants and young children have convulsions at the onset of infectious diseases when the temperature is beginning to rise. These are commonly but somewhat inexactly called febrile convulsions. The phenomenon is somewhat analogous to the chill that takes place in adults under similar circumstances of disease but it depends upon the susceptibility of the individual patient to convulse. The infection itself may be a trivial one; a rapidly rising or excessively high fever triggers the convulsion without necessarily implying that the disease is a serious one. Children who have such a tendency ordinarily lose it as they grow older, so that febrile convulsions generally are not observed in children beyond the age of 4 or 5. Such convulsions are alarming but rarely fatal. When they are occasional, brief and limited to the period of early childhood and feverish illnesses, they probably have no adverse effect upon the child's ultimate development.

Infection of the Central Nervous System. In the presence of fever, an acute convulsion sometimes announces the presence of infection of the central nervous system. Meningitis, encephalitis, rabies, cerebral sinus thrombosis and brain abscess are examples. The prognosis will depend upon the particular variety of infection and the adequacy of treatment that can be marshaled to combat it.

Increased Intracranial Pressure. Acute convulsions may be seen associated with an increased intracranial pressure from causes other than infection—intracranial bleeding, brain tumor, uremia, lead encephalopathy. Here the immediate prognosis for life and the later prognosis for complete recovery of function are relatively poor.

Toxic and Metabolic Disorders. Many toxic and metabolic disorders can be listed as causes of acute convulsions. Kernicterus in association with erythroblastosis of the newborn, rachitic or parathyroid tetany, insulin reactions, asphyxia and inhalation anesthesia, alkalosis, hypertension and prolonged treatment with ACTH are some of the disturbances which may have convulsions associated. Prognosis depends upon the ability to recognize the precipitating disorder and to bring it under control.

No Associated Disturbance. Many acute convulsions have no associated disturbance. Some of them represent the first in a series of recurring episodes which are considered in a following section.

Treatment

Most acute convulsions are the unexpected harbinger of an illness. The majority are brief and self-limited and subside spontaneously, no matter what is done. When they are brought to medical attention, immediate sedation usually is indicated to ensure their termination. Many drugs have been used in the past, but the safest and easiest to administer is sodium phenobarbital by subcutaneous injection. Doses from ½ to 3 grains may be used, depending upon the size of the infant or the child. If the fever is high, the use of a tepid bath or sponging to reduce the temperature gradually is rational.

If simple measures fail to terminate the convulsion within a period of ½ to 1 hour, rectal anesthesia with Avertin may be employed. Search for associated disease requiring independent treatment always is indicated, whether the convulsion ceases spontaneously or not.

Nursing Care

Protection of the child from injury is one of the first considerations during a convulsion. Regardless of age, a crib bed is essential. If the convulsions are severe the crib sides should be padded. Inspection of the child's toys to remove those that might produce injury during a seizure should be made. To prevent suffocation, soft pillows should not be allowed. A padded tongue depressor should be in readiness to place between the teeth to prevent biting of the tongue. If convulsions produce increased secretion from the pharynx, a suction set should be kept in readiness. In some instances, oxygen may be necessary for extreme respiratory difficulty produced by muscular in-co-ordination.

Placement of the child where continued observations may be made is important for the protection of the child and for recording behavior that is helpful in making a diagnosis. Prior to the convulsion there may be an aura. The older child may tell the nurse of the experience. He may complain of tingling sensations, of seeing light, of hearing sounds or of dizziness, or he merely may utter a shrill cry. The young child is not able to express his sensory experience in words but instead may show changes in his behavior. He may become more irritable and restless or more destructive or he may become apathetic and listless. Whenever changes in behavior occur, keener observation should follow.

There is nothing that a nurse can do to stop a convulsion; her duty lies in observing and recording it in all its detail and in protecting the child from injury. In describing the movements, the term "twitching" should be used when the movements are clonic or jerking and "contraction" when the child holds himself in a tonic or a contracted and stiffened state. Observations as to the following should be made: behavior state preceding onset; length of the seizure in minutes; the site where the twitching or the contraction began and the parts of the body involved; eye movements and pupillary changes; types of movement; degree of perspiration; incontinence before, during or after the seizure; pulse and respiration rates; posture of the body; color; secretions from the mouth; the first and the last areas to relax; behavior at the end of the convulsion. If the child is old enough to talk, the state of consciousness can be observed. Degree of memory for recent events, type of speech and amount of co-ordination are observations that are needed to detect the extent of cerebral dysfunction produced by the seizure. After the convulsion the child should be placed in bed if he is not already there. Usually he will sleep for long periods, the time depending on the severity of the seizure.

After one convulsion the child should be protected against recurrence by continuing administration of sedatives until the danger of recurrence seems to be past.

RECURRENT SEIZURES

Persons who have recurring seizures of one sort or another often are said to be victims of epilepsy. To the average lay person this ancient appellation connotes a disease that is hereditary, incurable, socially disgraceful and a precursor of mental deterioration. While it is true that some unfortunate sufferers are so fated, it is manifestly unjust and undesirable to stigmatize the much larger number who have infrequent seizures or are able to control their seizures completely. These individuals may have normal or even superior intelligence and may lead useful and productive lives. Epilepsy does not denote a specific disease entity. It is preferable to avoid the use of the term entirely and to speak of individual varieties of recurrent seizure patterns.

Nearly three fourths of those who eventually suffer from recurrent seizures do so in childhood; a significant number begin to have seizures before the age of 5. Untreated seizures tend to become more frequent and more severe. However, if a therapeutic regimen can be discovered which will keep the child free of attacks over a long period of time, it is often possible to withdraw the drugs gradually without return of symptoms.

Varieties of Recurrent Seizures

Recurrent seizures may be manifested in a great variety of ways. Because the basic mechanism of a seizure still is understood imperfectly, there is some difference of opinion about the implications of the different types.

Generalized Convulsions, Major Convulsions or Grand Mal. The symptoms of a generalized convulsion have been described in the preceding section. Such seizures also are called major convulsions or grand mal attacks. There is always loss of consciousness and postural muscle tone, followed by tonic or clonic movements of the extremities. Older children and adults who have generalized convulsions often describe a constellation of warning symptoms known as an aura. Peculiar feelings, sights, sounds, tastes, smells or involuntary muscle contractions may occur a few seconds before consciousness is lost and may lead the victim to utter a warning cry or noise before he falls. Headache and deep sleep not infrequently follow a generalized convulsion.

Akinetic Seizure. An akinetic seizure is similar to a generalized convulsion except that there is no clonic jerking or tonic contraction of the extremities. The child loses consciousness and postural tone and falls limply.

Lightning Major Convulsion. In young children less than 2 years old, a variant type of seizure called a lightning major convulsion sometimes is seen. It consists of a very rapid forward ducking of the head with simultaneous pulling of the arms and the legs onto the abdomen. The duration is often so brief that the significance of the movement may not be recognized. Such convulsions may occur in bursts, are usually difficult to control and often portend mental retardation.

Focal Convulsions. In focal convulsions consciousness may be retained and postural tone preserved while involuntary convulsive movements of an extremity progress from its tip toward its connection with the body (jacksonian fit). Episodic sensory disturbances may replace the muscle movements in this type of seizure, so that it appears as a temporary disturbance of sight, smell, hearing or taste or as pallor, flushing, hypertension, abdominal pain, changes in heart rate and other manifestations. Differentiation of the last group from other varieties of bodily disorder may be very difficult.

Minor Convulsions or Petit Mal. Minor convulsions or petit mal attacks consist of very brief absences or loss of consciousness without loss of postural tone or abnormal muscle movements. The victim momentarily stops whatever he is doing for a few seconds and then resumes where he left off. He is frequently unaware of the fact that he has had a brief seizure.

Psychomotor Attacks or Epileptic Equivalents. Various abnormalities of behavior of recurrent and often bizarre type are regarded as psychomotor attacks or epileptic equivalents. The child has no memory of his peculiar behavior. Psychomotor attacks usually occur in children who are having other types of seizure in addition.

Recurrent seizures of more than one variety may occur in the same child. For instance, akinetic seizures may precede the appearance of generalized convulsions. A high percentage of children with uncontrolled petit mal attacks eventually will develop generalized convulsions in addition to or instead of the initial form of seizure.

Diagnostic Considerations

Children who have recurrent seizures often require special study either (1) to ascertain that the episodes are really seizures or (2) to attempt to discover an anatomic or physiologic reason for them. When the child suffers from characteristic generalized convulsions there is seldom any doubt about their nature, but recognition of minor attacks and psychomotor attacks may be more difficult. Supporting evidence can be obtained by the use of the electro-encephalograph, a machine which records the cyclic changes in the electric potentials of the brain. The procedure is somewhat analogous to the electrocardiogram applied to the study of heart disease. Most individuals with seizures display abnormal patterns of "brain waves" not only during the seizures but between attacks. In some instances the shape of the waves may be altered by having the child hyperventilate his lungs—a technic which occasionally precipitates an actual seizure. Electro-encephalograms are complex curves which require considerable experience for proper interpretation. Although it is usually true that an individual with seizures has an abnormal pattern, this is not invariably so. Conversely, some persons who never manifest seizures may have abnormal tracings. Electro-encephalograms also may be used to localize areas of abnormal brain discharges in some instances where operative correction is contemplated.

Diagnostic procedures are indicated in many children whose recurrent seizures are suspected of having an anatomic or physiologic basis. In addition to electro-encephalography, which may confirm the presence of seizures and occasionally localize their site of origin, x-ray visualization of the skull is usually desirable. Various abnormalities of shape, proportions and calcification of the cranial bones may give clues to an underlying disorder. A view of the gross structure of the brain itself may be obtained by removing the spinal fluid and replacing it with air (pneumoencephalography). The roentgenograms taken subsequently outline the cavities within the ventricular system and around the surface of the brain and often disclose structural abnormalities.

When there is suspicion of previous infection of the nervous system, various types of specific diagnostic tests may be indicated to exclude virus encephalitis, tuberculosis, syphilis or toxoplasmosis. Abnormalities of carbohydrate metabolism leading to periods of hypoglycemia or of calcium metabolism leading to tetany require special biochemical study. Rickets and lead poisoning produce changes in the x-ray appearance of the ends of the long bones, which may afford etiologic clues.

Treatment

A small number of children with recurrent seizures will be found to have a remediable underlying condition, the correction of which will terminate the seizures. But in most instances the seizures are of unknown causation or are associated with some disturbance which cannot be modified. The main problems in therapy consist of the discovery of a drug regimen that will abolish the seizures or reduce them to a minimum and the guidance of parents and child to an acceptance of a realistic way of life.

Phenobarbital is the most widely used drug for the prevention of recurrent seizures. It is almost devoid of toxic effects and has a large factor of safety which permits liberal dosage even in small children. Its disadvantage is that it is not very effective against petit mal attacks or psychomotor seizures. In large dosage it may cause drowsiness or unsteadiness. For the control of generalized convulsions it may be given in doses of 1 to 3 grains per day, depending upon the size of the child and the frequency of convulsions. The total dose usually is divided into 2 or 3 portions. A level of drug is sought which will prevent attacks without producing drowsiness or unsteadiness. When there is a tendency for the child to have an attack at a certain period of the day, accurate timing of his medicine is necessary to forestall seizures. Attacks that occur during or upon waking from sleep pose a difficult problem that may be solved by administering enteric coated capsules the effect of which is delayed. If a successful regimen can be found, it should be continued until the child has had at least 2 years free from seizures. Slow withdrawal of medication then may be attempted.

When phenobarbital is unsuccessful in controlling generalized convulsions or produces too much drowsiness for the school-age child, other drugs may be used instead of or in combination with it. Dilantin is most commonly used as an adjuvant to or substitute for phenobarbital. The dosage is from 1 to 5 grains per day, depending upon the age of the child. Toxic effects are observed more frequently than when phenobarbital alone is used. These include ataxia, rash and hypertrophy of the gums. A closely related drug is Mesantoin, which has the additional hazard of depressing the blood-forming elements in the bone marrow, a toxic effect which must be sought by periodic leukocyte and differential blood counts in order to terminate the use of the drug at the first sign of difficulty.

Generally, minor convulsions are controlled effectively by Tridione. The dosage ranges from 5 to 20 grains a day. Its ability to terminate petit mal is often dramatic. Disadvantages lie in the side effects which it may produce—rashes, drowsiness, a peculiar sensation of glare and infrequently depression of the blood-forming organs. Paradione is a closely related compound which may be used in its place.

For focal and psychomotor seizures Dilantin is usually the drug of choice.

Phenurone is sometimes useful but is a much more toxic substance.

In children who suffer from both petit mal and major convulsions, a therapeutic problem arises in that Dilantin generally tends to aggravate minor convulsions while suppressing the major attacks, while Tridione may stimulate major seizures while controlling minor attacks.

Bromides and ketogenic diets are mainly of historical interest in the control of seizures. In unusual instances the former may be required for the control of major convulsions. The ketogenic diets will work in the control of petit mal attacks but are very difficult to maintain.

Nursing Care

The nurse has a number of obligations toward the child who is hospitalized for treatment or investigation of recurrent convulsions. She contributes important information by accurate observation of the child and by recording the number and the variety of his seizures. She can help to regulate his daily life in such a manner as to avoid unnecessary anxiety and provide him with as much healthy diversion as his condition will permit. She must be cognizant of the possible toxic effects of the drugs that he is taking and observe him for such adverse symptoms. In addition she may have to help him through diagnostic procedures such as a lumbar puncture or an encephalogram.

Encephalograms are used as a part of the diagnostic regimen in an attempt to find an anatomic cause for the seizures. Cerebrospinal fluid is replaced by air through a spinal puncture needle in order to obtain contrast roentgenograms of the brain. One method for this procedure is to withdraw 10 cc. of fluid and replace it with 5 cc. of air, after which 10 cc. of fluid is replaced with 10 cc. of air, and this process is repeated until no more fluid is obtained. Approximately 100 cc. of air may be injected in this manner. Normally, the air will fill the ventricles and spread over the cortex. A roentgenogram shows the outline of the ventricles and of the cortical convolutions. Distortions and changes from the normal outlines indicate the location and often the nature of the lesion.

Preparing the child psychologically for this procedure is necessary. A preliminary hypodermic of a sedative and an Avertin anesthesia preceded by a cleansing enema usually are ordered. Both procedures should be explained to him, and he should understand the effect that will be produced by the Avertin. In some instances, children are made ill by this procedure. Headaches may be a complaint, and some degree of prostration or shock may appear. Older children react to the aftermath of an encephalogram much better if they have been forewarned of the discomfort that they may experience. Before the anesthesia is given, the blood pressure should be determined. Avertin reduces blood pressure, and the significance of the readings after the procedure is based on the readings prior to anesthesia.

Sterile equipment for an encephalogram consists of spinal-puncture needles, gloves, 20-cc. syringe, medicine glass, spinal manometer and 3-way stopcock, glass graduate, lumbar puncture drape sheet, cotton balls and a gauze dressing to cover the site of puncture.

Two nurses are required for the treatment. The child must be held on the treatment table in a sitting position to allow the injected air to rise and to replace the cerebrospinal fluid. Position can be maintained more easily if a tray covered with a pillow is placed over his lap and his body is bent forward to rest on it. A second nurse assists the doctor, collects samples of spinal fluid, records the amount withdrawn and the amount of air injected and watches for change in the child's pulse and respiration rates.

After the injection of air, the child should be wrapped in a blanket and transported in an upright position to the x-ray department for skull films. A tray containing hypodermic equipment and stimulants should be taken with the child, as emergency stimulants may be indicated by a change in color, pulse and respiration rates and blood-pressure reading. Pulse and respiration rates, temperature and blood pressure should be observed frequently until stabilized. Symptoms of shock and increased intracranial pressure should be watched for.

In many institutions, fluids are given parenterally on return from the x-ray examination to replace fluids lost by withholding nourishment and by perspiration during the procedure. Oral intake of fluid is usually low in the first 24 hours after this diagnostic procedure. Administering oxygen 100 per cent by mask for 2 minutes at hourly intervals for the first 6 to 8 hours aids in the absorption of the injected air, decreases headache and prevents nausea. Helping the child to see the benefits of remaining flat in bed prevents discomfort from headache.

In the presence of brain tumor, a ventriculography is done instead of encephalography. Cerebrospinal fluid is replaced by air through a needle passed into the lateral ventricles through trephine openings in the skull. Ventricular needles, rubber tubing and a 3-way stopcock replace the lumbar puncture needles for this procedure. Maintaining an upright position is not necessary for this procedure.

Postoperative care is the same as for encephalography. However, occasionally it is necessary to remove air from the ventricles that is producing symptoms of increased intracranial pressure. For this reason, a sterile ventricular set should be kept in the child's room for 48 hours after the procedure.

The "whole" child, not merely his seizures, must be studied and treated. The child's personality is influenced by his response to problems and situations created by his symptoms. The convulsion itself does not lead easily or early to personality disintegration. Nor do convulsions always occur in persons with a particular personality type. It is chiefly the significance of the convulsion to the child in his little world that affects his personality development.

Often the child with recurrent seizures is described as being emotionally unstable, egocentric, tempestuous in emotional response, selfish and moody. If these traits exist in the personality make-up of a child, they indicate a need for delving beneath the surface to discover the genesis of his emotional disturbance. Eliminating the pressure points that cause his undesirable behavior will do much toward decreasing the number of attacks and toward helping him to become better adjusted. This does not mean that his attacks are purely psychogenic in origin but it does mean that unwise guidance tends to cause feelings that can precipitate an attack. Such behavior traits as the above are not peculiar to the child with seizures; they are seen as frequently in normal children who come from environments that fail to meet their basic emotional needs.

The nurse interested in the well-being of the child must extend that interest into the home and into his community. Unless convulsions are severe and uncontrolled, school experience with normal children should not be denied him. Teachers who have learned how to handle a child in a convulsion and have understanding of his home background and insight into his needs exert a profound influence on the child's peers and often through them on those in their homes. They help the community to accept him, a point which increases his security and belief in himself and gives him a feeling of "belongingness." Feeling for himself is influenced by the attitudes of his family and the reactions of his group toward him.

At home and in school, relationship experiences that produce anxiety, fear and problems too great for the child to master must be eliminated to give him peace of mind. The more problems there are for which he cannot find satisfying solutions, the less probable is the therapeutic value of any drug.

Assisting the child, his parents and his community in accepting him as he is constitutes one of the greatest responsibilities that society can have. The child must do his own adjusting, but society can assist him in making a comfortable and constructive adjustment to his handicap.

The National Epilepsy League in Chicago does much to help the parents of children with seizures. They provide pamphlet material and direct parents to sources of help in their communities. Personnel in branches of the organization counsel parents and work with nurses and teachers in the schools.

BRAIN TUMOR

Brain tumor is a result of abnormal growth of cells already present in the brain or of malignant cells transported to the brain from their origin elsewhere in the body. Most brain tumors are of the first group.

ETIOLOGY

Brain tumors are approximately one sixth as frequent in children as in adults; nevertheless, they are relatively frequent among the tumors of the body. Most of the brain tumors of children occur in the posterior fossa of the skull cavity, whereas most of the tumors of adults occur above the tentorium. Fully three fourths of the tumors of childhood are composed of glial cells (glioma). These cells are of various types which differ in their invasive ability. The most common type is slow growing and not invasive. The type of glial cell is known as an astrocyte, and the tumor is an astrocytoma. These tumors usually are in the cerebellum.

SYMPTOMS

Most of the symptoms are caused by increase in intracranial pressure. Tumors of the posterior fossa are almost certain to cause hydrocephalus from obstruction of the outflow of cerebrospinal fluid from the basal foramina. Increased intracranial pressure is likely to cause headache and vomiting. Among the nerve changes resulting, one easy to detect is swelling of the head of the optic nerve, as observed by ophthalmoscopic examination ("choked disk"). After a period of persistent swelling, the optic nerve atrophies, causing permanent blindness. In young children, the skull sutures are not united. Therefore, the sutures may separate as a result of the increased pressure and thus delay some of the more severe pressure effects. Increased intracranial pressure is likely to cause slowing of the pulse and may cause increase in blood pressure. Fretfulness, irritability and changes in disposition are common results, followed later by mental dullness and drowsiness. Older children may complain of dizziness.

Symptoms from local destructive effects of the tumor vary greatly and may be lacking. Cerebellar tumors often cause nystagmus and disturbances in gait and ability to stand. Localizing symptoms are produced more often by tumors above the tentorium. Convulsions are common with cerebral and rare with cerebellar tumors.

DIAGNOSIS

Tumors of the brain have an insidious beginning, and often early diagnosis is impossible. The course is progressive and soon or late symptoms suggesting the condition appear. The course of some of the slow-growing tumors at times may be as long as several years before serious symptoms appear. In other instances of tumor, perhaps only a few weeks elapse. The coexistence of headache, vomiting and choked disks is highly suggestive of brain tumor, but these 3 conditions appear together late in the disease. A ventriculogram or an encephalogram is helpful in making the diagnosis and locating the tumor. In some instances, an electro-encephalogram also is helpful. Evidence of increased intracranial pressure may be obtained by direct measurement of the cerebrospinal fluid pressure and in many instances by x-ray examination of the skull. The skull may show separation of the sutures in the younger children and atrophy of bone in the same pattern as the brain convolutions in the older children. Symptoms identical with those of brain tumor may be produced by brain abscess, encephalitis and certain degenerative diseases of the brain. Examination of the cerebrospinal fluid is often helpful in making a differential diagnosis.

TREATMENT

The treatment of brain tumor is surgical removal when this procedure is feasible. An invasive tumor cannot be removed completely, and it is certain to recur after operation. Some of the tumors of children are enucleated easily and removed completely. With such tumors the prognosis is good if the child survives the operative procedure.

NURSING CARE

When a child comes under observation because of possible brain tumor, the nurse should observe symptoms that may be helpful in localizing the lesion. The child of school or adolescent age will talk of his symptoms; the younger child cannot. But if the nurse is observant, she will note behavior that results from partial blindness, visual hallucinations, headache and intracranial pressure. Pulse and respiration rates, temperature and blood pressure should be observed at short intervals, and changes should be reported promptly. Observations as to the following should be made: mental state, drowsiness, sleepiness, irritability, pupillary changes (fixation or dilatation), vomiting with or without nausea, quality of speech, yawning, hiccoughing, sphincter control and details of convulsions.

Wise preparation for the child's operation influences the postoperative course. Frequent nourishing feedings should be given in the days prior to operation. Vomiting usually is unaccompanied by nausea, and in many instances the child is hungry and can be refed. Every effort should be made to understand the child and to gain his confidence so that he may be relieved of emotional strain when physical postoperative discomfort makes co-operation difficult. Suggestions to help the nurse prepare the child for operation are given on page 177. A preoperative enema may be contraindicated because it may increase intracranial pressure. Preoperative drugs may include atropine, but morphine seldom is given because of its depressant action on the central nervous system.

A crib bed should be provided for all children with brain tumor in both the preoperative and the postoperative periods. When the child returns from the operating room he should be placed in bed off the operative site, on his side, with his head level. The nasopharynx must be kept free of secretions and vomitus. The suction catheter should be of firm rubber and should be held closed to prevent injury to the mucous membrane as it is passed through the nose into the throat and then opened to produce suction.

Knowledge of the anesthetic used will guide the nurse in understanding the significance of the recorded temperature, blood pressure and pulse and respiration rates. Observations of these phenomena should be made every 15 minutes until the child's condition justifies longer intervals. If the operative procedure has been extensive, symptoms of surgical shock may be striking. In applying external heat, warm blankets are preferable to hot-water bags, as these children burn easily because of their sensory and motor disturbances. Raising the foot of the bed is considered inadvisable, due to the possibility of increasing intracranial pressure and bleeding. Emergency stimulants, oxygen inhalations, intravenous fluids and small blood transfusions may be indicated, and apparatus to give these supportive measures should be in readiness. Measures to raise blood pressure rapidly to normal levels are not desirable because rapid change predisposes to intracranial bleeding.

When operation has been preceded by a ventriculogram, a sterile ventricular tap setup to remove cerebrospinal fluid which may contain blood and produce both increased pressure and rise in temperature must be included in the equipment always available at the child's bedside. A ventricular tap setup includes ventricular needles, spinal manometer and 3-way stopcock, 20-cc. syringe, rubber catheter (cut off to 3 in. in length, including the wide end), gauze squares, Kelly clamp, lumbar-puncture drape, towels, medicine glass, emesis basin, gloves and materials for a collodion and gauze roll-dressing. Test tubes and a bacterial culture medium should be available to collect samples of cerebrospinal fluid for culture and to determine progress of the bleeding by noting changes in its color from time to time.

If the dressing becomes moistened with blood or cerebrospinal fluid, the doctor may wish to be notified so that the dressing can be changed. Escape of spinal fluid is often advantageous, since it reduces the intracranial pressure. If the child is young or restless, elbow restraints must be applied to prevent him from disturbing his dressing. Before wrist and ankle restraints are applied to children who are dangerously restless, every method possible should be used to allay their anxiety, for it not only makes them uncomfortable but it also may increase intracranial pressure.

Hyperthermia may be due to trauma, to disturbance of the heat-regulating center or to intracranial edema. Control of hyperthermia requires constant vigilance and intensive nursing care. The child's temperature should be taken hourly. When it begins to rise above 101° F. to 102° F., he should be undressed and covered with a sheet. Room temperature should be regulated as changes in temperature occur. When the temperature rises higher after his clothing has been removed, the sheet over the child should be replaced by a cover over the pubic area. The use of a cold water mattress or tepid water sponge baths are often ordered for a rise in temperature to 102° F. In giving a sponge bath the bed should be protected by a bath blanket or bath towels if the child is small. Water at 85° F. should be used initially and then reduced to 75° F. When sponging, only the parts of the body that are warm should be included. The parts that are cold to touch should be covered with a light blanket until warm. Then sponging of these parts may be included. Rectal ice water enemas for a temperature of 103° F. to 104° F. are often ordered. The size of the catheter and the amount of water introduced will be dependent upon the age of the child. The water should run in slowly. Then the tube should be clamped off and after 10 minutes reopened for siphonage and to introduce more water. After this process has been repeated 3 or 4 times, the tube should be removed gently and the temperature taken in 30 minutes. If the temperature continues to rise, warm alcohol sponge baths may be given every half hour. For a markedly elevated temperature (104° F. or over), small retention enemas with aspirin will produce diaphoresis and temperature reduction. In all the above procedure, it is not expected that the temperature will

be reduced to normal; keeping it within a reasonably low range only is desired. Lumbar punctures to remove blood and fluid may be necessary to reduce temperature.

The child's temperature must be taken at half-hour intervals during the period of hyperthermia to prevent it from dropping too rapidly. If it drops as much as 1° below the level of the starting point, the temperature-reducing procedures should be discontinued. If it drops to a subnormal level, the child should be dressed and covered with blankets. However, care must be taken to prevent overheating him to such a degree that his temperature again rises to above 100° F.

Trauma during surgery may produce edema of the face and the eyelids. If the edema is great, circulation of lacrimal secretion over the eye may be impaired, and the eye may become dry and subsequently infected. Drops of sterile sweet oil prevent corneal dryness; gentle warm saline irrigations keep the eyes free of exudate, and elbow restraints keep the child's hands away from his irritated eyes. Swelling of the eyelids can be controlled partially by the application of cold compresses. Care in application should be used to prevent dampening the head dressing.

The extent of the external facial and scalp edema may be indicative of the amount of intracranial edema that exists. When marked external edema develops, with accompanying drowsiness and pupillary change, the nurse should be increasingly watchful for additional signs of intracranial pressure requiring prompt treatment.

When nausea subsides, fluids can be given by mouth. To prevent aspiration, only small sips of water should be given until the swallowing reflex is known to be functioning. A rubber-tipped or a cellophane drinking tube should be used, and when nourishing fluids can be tolerated, amounts should be increased gradually. Too rapid ingestion of fluids is to be guarded against, because vomiting, which increases intracranial pressure, may be induced. Until the child's fluid and food requirements are satisfied orally, infusions are continued.

If the swallowing reflex is absent, gavage feedings may be given. Usually, the catheter is introduced and left in place for a 24-hour period. By withdrawing it an inch or two for saline cleansing of the catheter and the nostril, irritation from the tube can be prevented. When tube feedings are given, distention should be watched for.

As the child's condition improves, solid foods can be introduced. Often encouragement is necessary to help the child eat increasingly larger amounts of foods of high calorie and vitamin content.

Unless meticulous mouth care is given frequently, discomfort results. Use of a tongue depressor to keep the mouth open when cleansing the teeth, the gums and the tongue makes the procedure a safer one.

To prevent pressure sores of the head and the body and hypostatic pneumonia, the child's position should be changed hourly. Pressure sores of the head and the ears develop easily, and cotton "doughnuts" to lie on prevent them from occurring. Until the use of suction is unnecessary, the child should be kept off his back to prevent aspiration. After that period, he can be placed in any position that eliminates pressure over the operative site. His back should be washed and massaged thoroughly every 4 hours. A good preparation for use is a combination of zinc-oxide ointment and castor oil. When changing his position, his head should be supported, and turning should be done

slowly and carefully. Quick movements produce vertigo and increase in blood pressure. In cases in which there is paralysis or spasticity of the extremities, support of the parts with pillows, rolls or other means is necessary. Need for measures to prevent foot drop and pressure sores of the ankles, the heels and the knees often exists.

Intelligent observation resulting in appropriate nursing and a determination to continue supportive nursing, regardless of the seeming outcome, are part of the skill and the spirit which are required to nurse these children. Although to the observer he may appear to be unconscious, conversation that might have a deleterious effect on the child must never occur.

The child's parents need much consideration. If they have been prepared previous to operation, the sight of the child with his bandaged edematous head and the emergency procedures so often required will not be so frightening to them. They must be helped, too, to handle their emotions in the presence of the child.

The child's convalescent care should include guidance that assists him to a greater stage of independence. As function of the body returns, it should be noted, and graduated opportunities to use it should be provided. During the acute stage of his illness he has been waited upon, and his needs have been anticipated constantly; now in convalescence he needs to learn gradually to do things and to play by himself and with others. If in this period the parents observe his increasing abilities, they will continue to foster independence at home. Return visits during the ensuing years are necessary to check progress after removal of brain tumors.

INFECTIONS

MENINGITIS

Inflammations of the meninges are classified according to the bacterial exciting cause. The differential diagnosis is made chiefly by identifying the causative organism in cerebrospinal fluid obtained by lumbar puncture (for technic and equipment, see pp. 528-529).

Tuberculous Meningitis

Etiology. Tuberculous meningitis is caused by the tubercle bacillus (*Mycobacterium tuberculosis*), which gains access to the meninges from a focus elsewhere in the body. The disease may occur in association with a generalized miliary tuberculous infection, in which case the symptoms of miliary tuberculosis elsewhere are likely to be masked by those of meningitis. It often occurs also when symptoms and signs of tuberculosis elsewhere are not manifest and when a careful examination reveals perhaps nothing more than a hilus gland infection. Thus, tuberculous meningitis may appear in a child who previously had had apparently excellent health and nutrition. Tuberculous meningitis may occur at any age, but it is encountered with the greatest frequency under 5 years of age.

Symptoms. The onset is gradual and insidious in most instances and is manifest by some variety of change in behavior. These changes vary with the person and probably are brought about chiefly by increased intracranial pressure caused by an increased amount of cerebrospinal fluid. The child is likely to become cross and irritable. The play habits and reactions to associates change. Drowsiness and mental dullness are common. Because of the increased intracranial pressure, vomiting, anorexia and constipation are frequent, especially in infants, and headache becomes a complaint of older children. The temperature during this period is elevated only slightly. These symptoms of the early stage do not give very definite indication of the cause of the difficulty but after perhaps a week, sometimes longer, the symptoms become more severe and point more definitely to their intracranial origin.

Drowsiness and headache increase. Hyperesthesia appears, and the child prefers to remain undisturbed. Intolerance of noises and bright lights frequently develops. In some cases, the child screams intermittently, the so-called hydrocephalic cry. The reflexes are increased, the pupils are of normal size or small, the neck is stiff, the head is held back, and very often the extremities also are held rigidly. Convulsions sometimes occur. This period of more severe illness has been called the irritative stage. Gradually, the illness goes through a transition into what is known as the paralytic stage. The stupor becomes more marked and continuous and eventually becomes so deep that the child cannot be aroused. Respiration becomes irregular. The pupils are large and fixed. The reflexes diminish until they no longer can be elicited. Various paralyses, often transitory, may be noted. Muscle movements are chiefly automatic and not purposeful. General muscular relaxation increases. Death occurs either quietly in deep coma or in a few instances with terminal convulsions. At the very end, the temperature, which has been relatively low throughout the illness, rises rapidly to a high point.

Prognosis. Before the discovery of streptomycin, tuberculous meningitis was almost invariably fatal. At the present time it is impossible to say how effective streptomycin and the adjuvant drugs used with it will be in the cure of tuberculous meningitis, for widely divergent results are reported from different countries and from different clinics within the United States. Treatment is more likely to be successful with older children than with infants. The best results are reported when treatment can be initiated very early in the course of the disease. Infants under 1 year old and older children who are already in coma at the time of diagnosis recover in less than 25 per cent of the cases. Under the most favorable circumstances, recovery without residual effect may be expected in more than half of the patients treated.

Treatment and Nursing Care. Because of the serious danger to life and to mentality, antituberculous drugs must be used in maximum quantities over long periods of time. Therapeutic regimens differ in detail, but most include daily intramuscular administration of streptomycin or dihydrostreptomycin combined with oral isoniazid or one of its derivatives and a third adjuvant such as Promizole or para-aminosalicylic acid. Long duration of treatment usually means at least 4 to 6 months and sometimes a year or two. Some treatment regimens include intrathecal injections of streptomycin in order to carry the drug in high concentration directly to the lesions in the meninges. Whenever one of the streptomycins is used for such lengths of time the very real risk of damage to the eighth nerve, which controls the functions of hearing and equilibration, must be recognized and accepted as necessary.

Treatment may be handicapped by the formation of meningeal adhesions which prevent the free circulation of spinal fluid and in consequence produce hydrocephalus. Various surgical measures and intraspinal injection of enzyme preparations such as streptodornase, streptokinase, papain and other materials have been used with indifferent success in counteracting this complication. Hydrocortisone is reported to be effective in preventing or dissolving subarachnoid adhesions.

During the prolonged treatment, nursing measures to care for the skin and prevent pressure sores are necessary during the early stages of the disease. Also, nutrition must be maintained by careful feeding, sometimes requiring gavage technic. If the child recovers with residual neurologic difficulties, the same sort of rehabilitative measures as those outlined for the child with motor disabilities must be used. Deafness may be a permanent handicap. Loss of equilibrium is usually a temporary disability for which the child learns to compensate.

Meningococcic Meningitis (Epidemic Meningitis, Cerebrospinal Fever, Spotted Fever)

Etiology. Meningococcic meningitis is caused by the diplococcus, *Neisseria intracellularis* or *meningococcus*. This organism gains entrance to the body by way of the nose and the throat and during the early stage of the disease may be cultured from this locality and from the blood. Therefore, the disease is naturally transmissible. Great variation is shown at times in the ease and the frequency of transmission. Most of

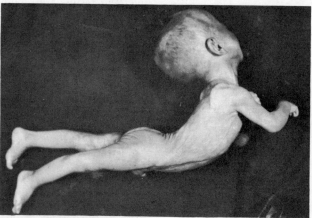

Fig. 96. Opisthotonos position in a baby with meningitis.

the time meningococcic meningitis exists as an occasional sporadic disease but at other times it becomes widely epidemic. In approximately three fourths of all cases, this disease occurs in children under 10 years of age and in nearly half of them, in children under 5.

Symptoms. As with other infectious diseases, this one has its abortive, mild, severe and malignant forms. The symptoms of only the common form will be described.

After a short incubation period, usually less than a week, prodromal symptoms lasting a day or two may appear. More commonly the onset is sudden, with vomiting, prostration, headache, pain in the neck, the back and the legs and frequently convulsions. Although present, fever seldom is high. The head is bent backward, and the neck and the back are held rigidly (Fig. 96). A position of marked opisthotonos may be assumed. The child prefers to be undisturbed, and movement causes much discomfort. Delirium is common. Stupor and coma appear in the more severe illnesses but are not so common in those of ordinary severity. Fretfulness and irritability may alternate with periods of drowsiness or stupor. Herpes may appear about the mouth.

An eruption of purpuric spots varying from pinhead size to large ecchymotic blotches is characteristic of the meningococcus bacteremia that generally accompanies the meningitis. In a few instances the rash is very extensive and is associated with signs of shock which progress rapidly to a fatal termination, presumably due to adrenal failure (Waterhouse-Friderichsen syndrome).

Diagnosis. The diagnosis is made by examination of the cerebrospinal fluid. One or several of the symptoms and the signs enumerated constitute the indication for spinal puncture. This is particularly true of neck rigidity and other signs pointing to irritation of the nervous system. In an infant, the fontanel is full or bulging.

Lumbar puncture reveals increased quantity and pressure of cerebrospinal fluid. At the onset of the illness, the fluid may be fairly clear, although showing a definite increase in cells. However, very quickly the fluid becomes cloudy from the large number of pus cells present. These statements are true also of other varieties of purulent meningitis. The difference between the fluid of meningococci meningitis and that of other purulent forms is solely in the variety of organism present as the cause.

In most cases of purulent meningitis, the causative organism is easily demonstrable in a stained smear prepared from the cerebrospinal fluid. In the few instances in which the organism cannot be found readily, the chances are great that the illness is caused by the meningococcus. The meningococcus is a gramnegative diplococcus and is found chiefly within the pus cells. The causative organism of no other common variety of meningitis has these characteristics. Usually the meningococci can be grown and identified by cultural methods when they are too scarce to be found easily by direct examination. Meningococci can also be found in blood cultures or in smears made from petechial skin lesions.

Prognosis. Before the use of specific serum the mortality rate was approximately 70 per cent. With serum treatment the rate was reduced to 30 per cent or less. With sulfonamide therapy the death rate is usually less than 10 per cent. The mortality rate varies with the age of the child and with the promptness with which therapy is instituted. When appropriate treatment is given on the first or the second day of the disease, the death rate is low. The mortality rate is much higher in the first year than in the second, and higher in the second year than later. With prompt and effective treatment, complications are uncommon. On the other hand, some of the complications are serious. They include mental deterioration, various paralyses and, in infants, hydrocephalus.

Treatment. Until the advent of sulfonamide drugs, the treatment consisted of the use of specific serum developed by immunizing the horse with cultures of the meningococcus. Serum now has been supplanted almost completely by the sulfonamide drugs. Oral administration is satisfactory, although a more prompt effect is obtained by giving a soluble preparation intravenously for the first dose. Sulfadiazine is the preparation usually preferred. It is given in full dosage, which varies in relation to body weight according to the age of the child. Penicillin also is highly effective and may be used in conjunction with sulfadiazine.

Symptomatic treatment consists chiefly of good nursing care. Spinal puncture may be required occasionally in convalescence for the relief of pressure, should pressure symptoms develop.

Influenza Bacillus Meningitis

Except during times when epidemic meningococcus meningitis is present, influenza bacillus meningitis is the most common form of purulent infection of the meninges in children.

Etiology. The disease is caused by the *Hemophilus influenzae,* a gram-negative rod which differs markedly in size and shape under various circumstances of cultivation. The same organism causes respiratory infections among children and in particular is responsible for a severe variety of croup.

Symptoms. The early symptoms are similar to those of meningococcus meningitis except that the purpuric rash is absent. In infants the onset is likely to be more insidious, with unexplained fever, vomiting, lassitude or peculiar cry or behavior as the presenting complaints. In older children the disturbance advances rapidly toward stupor or coma with the usual evidences of meningitis.

Prognosis. Before the discovery of antibiotics, the fatality rate from influenza meningitis was nearly 100 per cent. Prompt diagnosis and treatment now permits survival of 80 to 90 per cent of the victims. Delayed or inadequate treatment carries an increasing hazard of neurologic sequelae, even if the life is spared. Despite optimal treatment, some of the infants afflicted fail to make a complete recovery.

Treatment. Since 1940 a number of substances have been discovered which are capable of curing children with influenza meningitis. Antibacterial rabbit serum, sulfadiazine, streptomycin, chlortetracycline, oxytetracycline, tetracycline and chloramphenicol are included in the list. Because of the propensity of the influenza bacillus to acquire resistance to many of these agents before treatment can be completed, it is now considered prudent to use at least two of the substances simultaneously. Serum is expensive and difficult to obtain. Streptomycin is toxic to the eighth cranial nerve and does not enter the spinal fluid rapidly. Consequently, the preferred method of treatment at the present time is full dosage of sulfadiazine and one of the tetracycline antibiotics or chloramphenicol in addition. At the beginning of treatment these substances usually have to be given by parenteral routes—intramuscularly or intravenously—because of vomiting or coma. Once improvement begins, they may be given orally. Treatment must be continued until repeated spinal fluid cultures have been shown to be free of influenza bacilli.

Other Types of Meningitis

Any one of several varieties of bacteria may cause a purulent type of meningitis similar to meningococci meningitis. The more common varieties of organism are the pneumococcus, the streptococcus, the staphylococcus and the organisms which normally inhabit the intestinal tract. Without specific treatment the outcome is uniformly fatal. The bacteria usually enter the meninges by way of the blood stream, except when there is direct extension from an infected mastoid or cranial sinus cavity. The onset is usually sudden, and the symptoms include vomiting, convulsions and stiffness of the neck with eventual stupor and coma.

Pneumococcic Meningitis. This disorder is seen most frequently in small infants as a complication of pneumonia, otitis media or mastoiditis. Unless it is treated promptly it is rapidly fatal. The symptoms are similar to those of other types of meningitis. Rapid recognition of the disease is usually possible, for the pneumococci are found in large numbers in the spinal fluid and are identified easily by microscopic examination. Treatment consists of heavy dosage with penicillin and sulfadiazine administered by a parenteral route at first and continued until the patient has had sterile spinal fluid for at least a week, since this variety of meningitis is prone to recur if treatment is stopped too soon. The results of treatment depend upon the speed of recognition of the disease. When full treatment is begun within the first few hours of symptoms, recovery may occur in as many as 75 per cent of the children affected.

Streptococcus Meningitis. During hemolytic streptococcus infections the meninges are invaded in rare instances. The symptoms and the management of this variety of meningitis are almost identical with those of pneumococcus meningitis.

Staphylococcus Meningitis. This organism may gain entrance to the spinal fluid from trauma to the skull, from erosion of the sac of a myelomeningocele or in the course of a bloodstream infection with the staphylococcus. The symptoms and the diagnosis of staphylococcus meningitis are similar to those described previously. Treatment is complicated by the fact that the staphylococci present in the environment are not uniformly sensitive to any one antibiotic. It is essential to test each strain, as it is isolated from the patient, for its sensitivity to all the available antibiotics. This procedure takes a day or two to complete in the laboratory. Hence, it is desirable to treat with more than one antibiotic from the start until the best agent can be identified accurately. In general, the newer the antibiotic, the less likely is the staphylococcus to be resistant to it. Penicillin is effective against approximately half of the strains of staphylococcus at the present writing and should be used in conjunction with another substance, such as erythromycin.

Intestinal Organisms. In small infants, in chronically debilitated children and in those who have wound infections following neurosurgical procedures, meningitis may occur due to a wide variety of organisms which ordinarily are found in the intestinal tract—colon bacilli, Proteus, Pseudomonas, Salmonella, *Streptococcus faecalis,* for example. The meningitis so produced tends to be a relatively low-grade chronic process. Treatment depends upon identification of the organism (or organisms, for sometimes mixed infections are found) and laboratory determination of the most appropriate antibiotic, as in the case of staphylococcus meningitis. The difficulty of suspecting and recognizing meningitis in the newborn infant has been discussed in Chapter 10.

Nursing Care of Meningitis

Children with meningitis have all degrees of prostration and illness according to the stage of the disease. In the early stage of purulent meningitis before improvement from therapy has begun, one may have to deal with convulsions, delirium, stupor, cyanosis and urinary retention.

The convulsions of meningitis are

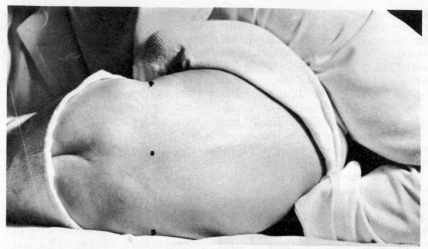

Fig. 97. Illustrating spinal puncture. This shows a method of holding the child and the puncture site.

managed as previously discussed in this chapter. Cyanosis requires administration of oxygen. When stupor is present, special attention is required for management of the food and fluid intake. Depending on the general condition of the child, the food may be given by gavage or, if vomiting is severe, it may be administered parenterally.

Records should be kept suitable for prompt detection of urinary retention, which may require catheterization. Fecal retention also should be watched for, although it does not have the major importance that urinary retention does.

The child with meningitis may be restless or, if disease is fulminating, his movements are limited, and unless he is moved he lies on one side, his back arched in the position of opisthotonos. Good skin care and frequent turning will lessen the incidence of complicating upper respiratory infection and pressure sores about the ears and over the hips. The use of a cold water mattress may be necessary to control high temperature and to make the child more comfortable. If fever is present and orally administered fluids are not tolerated, special mouth care is indicated. If the

meningitis is severe, suction apparatus and stimulants should be on hand for emergency use.

Lumbar punctures are done for diagnostic purposes and to determine the progress of the disease, to give medication intrathecally and to relieve pressure symptoms if they develop. The sterile equipment required consists of lumbar-puncture needles, drape sheet, spinal manometer and 3-way stopcock, hypodermic syringe, needles and procaine, cotton balls, dressing, gloves, medicine glass and medication as desired by the attending physician. Test tubes for spinal-fluid samples should be available.

The technic for spinal puncture in the child differs in no essential way from that in the adult. However, the adult usually can be persuaded to lie quietly, while more often than not this is impossible with children. It is desirable that as much co-operation as possible be obtained from the child, and the situation should be discussed with him to that end if he is old enough to understand and if his consciousness is not clouded by his infection. Even with co-operation, holding usually is desirable to avoid the trauma which might be produced by unexpected and involuntary movement. The manner of holding the child is important; in fact, the success of the puncture depends about as much on the holding as on the skill of the operator. The child usually is in a recumbent position on the right side, the thighs and the legs flexed and the back arched in a curve with the convexity posteriorly. Restraint in a good position is accomplished most effectively when the holder places his right arm about the thighs and his left arm about the neck, bringing the hands together in a locked position at the front of the child (Fig. 97). The struggle can be minimized still further, if necessary, by leaning forward, thus placing some weight on the body of the child. For obtaining cerebrospinal fluid the puncture usually is made between the third and the fourth or between the fourth and the fifth lumbar vertebrae. The appropriate site of puncture may be located by drawing a line across the back at the level of the crests of the ilium. The vertebral space nearest this line is chosen.

At times, as when the spinal canal is blocked, it becomes desirable to make the puncture at the top of the spine. This procedure is designated as "cisternal puncture." The space containing the cerebrospinal fluid (the cistern) is entered by inserting the needle immediately below the edge of the skull, with the needle pointing toward a line between the two ear canals.

Sometimes spinal or perhaps cisternal puncture is done for diagnostic purposes when the child is not sick, as in the case of latent syphilis, for example. If such children are permitted to remain ambulatory, often headache and perhaps vomiting occur. Reactions of this type are avoided by keeping the child recumbent for a period of from 8 to 12 hours.

During convalescence, return of function of the extremities should be ob-served and when it occurs it should be recorded. During this period, too, behavior that might indicate complicating brain abnormality, deafness or symptoms in the infant of developing hydrocephalus should be noted.

ENCEPHALITIS

Encephalitis is a diffuse inflammation of the brain. In some instances the spinal cord is affected also, and the disease is then called encephalomyelitis. There are many inconsistencies in the current use of these terms, for at some times they are applied to diseases that have well-recognized bacterial or viral etiology; at other times they describe conditions in which a known or a presumed toxin is at fault; in still other instances the term is not used in spite of the fact that the disease has all the typical features of encephalitis. From this confusion of terms it is possible to separate out one group of disorders which is due to specific virus infection of the brain and is transmitted in epidemic form by mosquitoes or mites, a second group which represents a complication of some of the contagious diseases and of vaccination procedures, and a third group which results from the influence of known and unknown soluble toxins upon the brain tissue. In a separate listing, the encephalitides which masquerade under some other name will be enumerated.

Virus Encephalitis Transmitted by Insects and Mites

Epidemiology. Since 1930 a number of specific viruses have been shown to cause epidemics of encephalitis in the United States and other parts of the world. Viruses isolated from specific geographic areas can be separated from one another in the laboratory, although the diseases they produce are clinically very similar. Each has acquired the name of the general area and circumstances under which it was first discovered—St. Louis, western (U. S.) equine, eastern (U. S.) equine, Japanese B, Russian spring-summer, Venezuelan. The term "equine" indicates that this form of encephalitis exists primarily in horses rather than in man. Now it is known that each of these forms is transmitted from animal to man by a particular variety of mosquito or mite. In some instances the epidemics are restricted to certain times of the year (usually summer) because of the life cycle of the insect required for the spread of the infection.

Symptoms. The onset of the disease is generally abrupt, with fever, vomiting, stiff neck, convulsions, delirium and coma present in varying degree. In some instances there may be a preceding period of illness that simulates influenza. In many respects the symptoms imitate meningitis, and the distinction must be made from examination of the spinal fluid, which contains relatively few cells, usually lymphocytes instead of polymorphonuclear leukocytes, and is sterile on bacterial culture. The fatality rate and the incidence of enduring neurologic disturbances is higher among infants than in older children or adults. Exact figures depend upon the variety of agent responsible for the encephalitis.

Diagnosis. Usually this is made from the clinical picture and the examination of the spinal fluid. At a later stage in the illness, specific virus antibodies appear in the blood which can be used for laboratory confirmation of the type of illness.

Treatment. No specific treatment is known. General good nursing care, control of convulsions and support of nutrition are indicated until the disease subsides spontaneously.

Encephalitis Following Contagious Disease or Prophylactic Injections

During the course of some of the contagious diseases, symptoms of irritation of the brain may appear at a time when convalescence otherwise might be expected. Such symptoms may be mild —delirium, headache, stiff neck, increase in fever—or more serious events such as convulsions, coma, or paralysis of the eye muscles, the extremities or the bladder. Measles is the contagious disease which is complicated most often by encephalitis. Fortunately, complete recovery takes place in more than 80 per cent of the children thus affected. Occasionally, a similar complication is seen following chickenpox, rubella, smallpox and the process of vaccination against smallpox. During the course of pertussis in infants an unusually severe form of encephalitis may result which leads to prolonged convulsions, stupor or generalized rigidity and usually results in severe mental retardation.

After prophylactic injections against rabies there is a significant incidence of paralysis, usually involving the lower extremities and the bladder. Symptoms commonly begin about 3 weeks after the injections are given and often start with peculiar sensations in the feet, later progressing to paralysis of the legs. Between 10 and 20 per cent of such individuals succumb. The survivors usually make a fairy complete recovery. This unfortunate complication must be recognized in considering whether or not to give rabies prophylaxis to a child who has been bitten by an animal.

In a very few instances severe encephalitis has been described following prophylactic injections against pertussis. The number of such cases is so small that the complication can be disregarded as a significant risk in conducting programs of pertussis vaccination.

Toxic Encephalitis

During the course of acute infectious diseases such as pneumonia, small infants at times may exhibit bizarre and dramatic symptoms of cerebral irritation. These take the form of extreme irritability, diffuse muscular twitching, generalized convulsions or nystagmoid movements of the eyes. The manifestations presumably are due to some toxin produced during the course of the illness. At times recovery is completed as the original infection is brought under control; at other times there may be permanent damage of the brain, with residual mental deficiency. Lead poisoning produces a toxic encephalitis that is characterized by generalized convulsions which are very difficult to control. Treatment is sometimes effective, but too often recovery is followed by persisting neurologic difficulties and mental deficiency.

Tetanus and chorea might be classified as forms of toxic encephalitis.

Other Varieties of Encephalitis

Among the diseases which are really forms of encephalitis but are not so designated are rabies, poliomyelitis and lymphocytic choriomeningitis, a disease which is rare. Mumps often is complicated by encephalitic symptoms; infectious mononucleosis and herpes sometimes are followed by signs of cerebral inflammation.

Encephalitis lethargica (von Economo's encephalitis) is a disorder of considerable historical interest. It appeared in epidemic form during World War I, producing acute symptoms somewhat like those described above for the specific virus encephalitides. In addition, it adopted a chronic form which appeared over a space of years and resulted in a wide variety of peculiar disabilities, of which parkinsonism is one and oculogyric crises is another. In recent years the acute stage of this disease seldom is recognized, but some of the more chronic manifestations are still apparent. No specific virus infection has been demonstrated as a cause, although such an etiology has been suspected for a long time. Many instances of mental retardation and peculiarities of behavior are ascribed to chronic encephalitis. The retrospective diagnosis of this condition is often difficult and tenuous.

Toxoplasmosis is an infection caused by a protozoan parasite which may be transmitted from the mother to her infant during the course of pregnancy or may be acquired by the child later. In the congenital form the infection commonly produces hydrocephalus or microcephaly. In addition cerebral calcification and changes of chorioretinitis are commonly discovered in the eyegrounds. During the acute stage of the disease symptoms of encephalitis may be present, and the parasites are demonstrable in the spinal fluid. After the active disease has subsided, the chorioretinitis and cerebral calcifications may offer a lead to the cause of cerebral damage, a lead which may be confirmed by tests on the blood serum which reveal specific antibody. Treatment of the acute stage of the disease is unsatisfactory, although sulfadiazine may have some effectiveness.

HEREDITARY DEGENERATIVE DISORDERS OF THE NERVOUS AND THE MUSCULAR SYSTEMS

A large number of disorders are recognized among children as hereditarily transmitted processes which, during infancy or childhood, lead to progressive loss of muscular or neurologic function. Fortunately, these disturbances are relatively rare. Unfortunately, their accurate identification is difficult and even may require study by a specialist in child neurology. The nurse cannot be expected to remember the exotic names and complex pathologic processes with which these disorders are endowed, nor can they be treated with any completeness in a brief text. A few representative types of disorder will be described briefly. More detailed information must be sought through the use of standard pediatric or neurology texts. Most of these degenerative disorders lead inex-

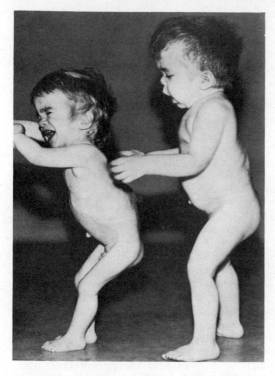

FIG. 98. Two children in the same family, showing the typical features of gargoylism (Hurler's Syndrome). (From Buchanan, D. N., *in* Grulee, C. G., and Eley, R. C.: The Child in Health and Disease, Baltimore, Williams & Wilkins)

orably to death or important permanent handicap. Only a few can be alleviated by any useful form of treatment. Some terminate life during early infancy; others appear during early or even late childhood and produce disability which is carried into a fairly long adult lifetime.

AMAUROTIC FAMILIAL IDIOCY (TAY-SACHS)

This disorder affects infants, frequently of Jewish families, and leads to arrested and then regressing mental development around the age of 6 months. Characteristic changes are visible in the fundus of the eye. The degenerative changes progress so rapidly that life seldom is spared for more than a year after the diagnosis is made. In amaurotic familial idiocy, lipid degeneration is confined mainly to the central nervous system.

Niemann-Pick Disease

This is closely related but attended by additional widespread deposition of lipid substances in organs such as the spleen, the liver, the lungs and the lymph nodes.

Gaucher's Disease

This is an allied but less frequently fatal disease in which the nervous system usually is spared, and a long and fairly normal life is possible.

GARGOYLISM (HURLER'S SYNDROME, LIPOCHONDRODYSTROPHY)

In this hereditary disorder there are widespread changes in the body due to abnormal deposits in the brain, the spleen, the liver, the bone marrow and the cornea of the eyes (Fig. 98). It is recognized easily by the gradual appearance of facial features and body characteristics which are almost identical in all affected children. The appearance is much like that of the Duchess in the popular illustrations of *Alice in Wonderland*. Mental retardation is usually definite but moderate, and the disease often permits the child to survive for a number of years.

OTHER FORMS OF CEREBRAL DEGENERATIVE DISEASE

Schilder's Disease

Among infants a rapidly fatal disturbance known as Schilder's disease is seen occasionally. Generally, it is marked by frequent and severe convulsions, loss of vision or hearing and retardation which progresses within a few months to coma and complete helplessness. No treatment is known.

Wilson's Disease

Among older children the degenerations include Wilson's disease, which combines cirrhosis of the liver with progressively increasing tremor and muscular rigidity.

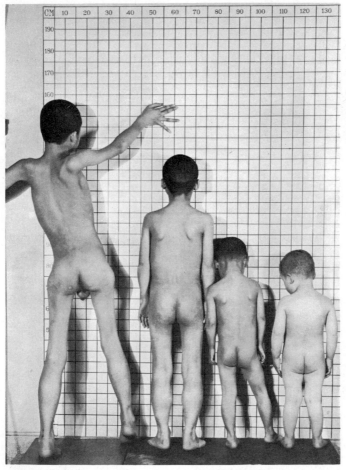

FIG. 99. Pseudohypertrophic muscular dystrophy in four brothers.

Dystonia Musculorum Deformans
(Torsion Spasm)

This peculiar twisting spasm of muscles usually begins in one leg and progresses to the point where the child is bedfast.

Friedreich's Ataxia

In this disease there is unsteadiness of gait and tremor of the extremities, which advances very slowly, and, during childhood at least, may not interfere seriously with activities.

These are only a few of many bizarre and fortunately rare disorders that are encountered.

Pseudohypertrophic Muscular Dystrophy

This is the most common form of muscular dystrophy (Figs. 99 and 100). It affects boys 8 times more frequently than girls. At some time during the preschool years the child begins to show weakness in his legs which generally is

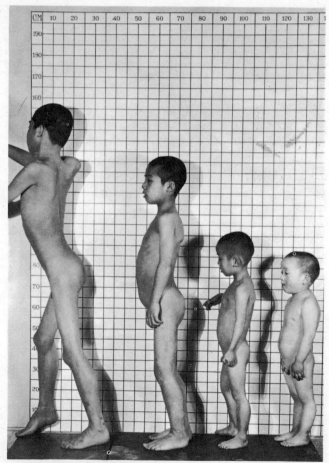

Fig. 100. Pseudohypertrophic muscular dystrophy in four brothers.

accompanied by enlargement of the calf muscles, which feel firm and rubbery. To arise from a sitting posture on the floor such children learn that they must kneel on all fours, then straighten their legs and gain the erect posture by putting hands on knees and "climbing up the legs." This performance is typical and practically diagnostic of the disease. Weakness of the leg muscles and later of the arm and the shoulder muscles progresses gradually, and the victim usually succumbs by early adult life to some intercurrent disease. Periods of bed rest are to be avoided whenever possible, for muscle strength tends to deteriorate more rapidly unless activity is maintained. At present no useful treatment has been discovered.

MYASTHENIA GRAVIS

This peculiar familial disorder is characterized by excessive fatigability of muscle, which usually is most marked in the muscles of the face and the pharynx. Drooping eyelids, a weak smile, difficulty in swallowing and severe fatigue following mild exercise are characteristic. The symptoms are relieved promptly by injection of Neostigmine which constitutes the chief diagnostic test. Unfortunately, there is a tendency toward progression of the symptoms, so that the attacks become more frequent and severe, and the relief obtained from Neostigmine or octamethyl pyrophosphoramide becomes less effective. Death in the severely affected child or adult results from respiratory failure during an unrelieved exacerbation.

MISCELLANEOUS NEUROLOGIC DISTURBANCES

TRAUMA

Concussion

Few children traverse the early years without suffering some variety of head injury. Most of these result only in bruising or laceration of the scalp. In a few there is evidence of temporary disturbance of cerebral functions which is referred to as concussion. In its mild form this may result in temporary dizziness, headache, vomiting or brief loss of consciousness. Sometimes there may be disturbances of vision or of motion of the eyes. Children usually recover rapidly from simple concussion and within a period of a day or two are restored to normal. The important point in management of concussion is to make sure during the early hours after the injury that no intracranial bleeding has resulted from the trauma.

The first 2 to 6 hours after injury is the critical period in which careful observation is required. During this time impending coma must be watched for. The parent or the nurse should test the child's state of consciousness by arousing him periodically. In the hospital, accurate observation of pulse, respirations and blood pressure is desirable. Drastic change in these measurements or inability to arouse the child demand prompt investigation. If signs of bleeding are confirmed, neurosurgical exploration usually is indicated. Even though it be attended by a period of unconsciousness, only a very small fraction of children who suffer head injury will have bleeding, but this small fraction presents a dire emergency.

Skull Fracture

The management of skull fracture is primarily a neurosurgical problem. In many instances there is a linear crack in the skull which causes no displacement of the bones and is not associated with bleeding. Management in such instances is the same as for concussion. More serious disturbances result when the break in the bones occasions tearing of blood vessels or distortion of the brain by compression. Some form of operative relief usually is indicated in such instances. Recognition of depression of a skull fracture depends upon roentgen examination or upon the presence of localizing neurologic findings which indicate abnormal pressure upon specific areas of the brain. With severe injuries the problem of managing shock and intracranial pressure is often of primary importance.

SUBDURAL HEMATOMA

Etiology

The brain is covered by a delicate filmy membrane which encloses the surrounding layer of cerebrospinal fluid. This membrane is known as the pia-arachnoid. Bleeding into the space which it encloses is called subarachnoid hemorrhage, and the blood usually is found circulating freely in the spinal fluid. Between the arachnoid and the tough membrane (dura mater) which lines the inner surface of the skull, there is a potential space (subdural space) which is normally empty because the arachnoid is in close apposition to the dura. Under certain conditions such as trauma or some form of hemorrhagic disorder, bleeding from small vessels may occur into the subdural space. The extent of the bleeding is limited by the pressure required to push away the brain in order to make room for the clot. Once formed, the clot usually liquefies. Its high protein content tends to draw more fluid into the space within the membrane which surrounds the clot. Thus, a slowly enlarging space-occupying mass exists within the rigid confines of the skull and creates an increase in the intracranial pressure. Subdural hematoma in older children is almost always the result of trauma. In infants it often is found in the absence of any obvious trauma other than the more or less normal events of birth and early infancy. It is more likely to be found in poorly nourished infants or those with bleeding tendencies. However, this is not exclusively the case, for it also is seen in otherwise healthy infants.

Symptoms

The bleeding usually takes place rather slowly, so that the symptoms appear insidiously. Abnormal enlargement of the head, slow developmental progress, irritability, convulsions, vomiting and poor weight gain may be present. In many of the infants, hemorrhages are seen in the eyegrounds, and some degree of swelling of the optic nerve head betrays the presence of an increase in intracranial pressure. Occasionally, the bleeding takes place rapidly, and the child passes into a state of shock, coma or uncontrolled convulsions.

Diagnosis

Diagnosis is suspected from the enlargement of the head and from the symptomatology. The finding of hemorrhages in the eyegrounds of an infant is almost certain to mean the presence of a subdural hematoma. Confirmation of the clinical suspicion is obtained by inserting a needle through the dura of the skull and withdrawing yellow, chocolate or bloody fluid from the liquefied clot. In infants with open suture lines, such taps are performed easily between the margins of two separated cranial bones. In older children, exploratory burr holes must be made by the neurosurgeon.

Treatment and Nursing Care

Subdural hematoma is primarily a neurosurgical problem. In older children a craniotomy has to be done, and the clot and its surrounding membrane must be removed. In infants often the same procedure is indicated, but in some instances repeated aspirations through the dura will effect a cure without the need for a craniotomy. Postoperative nursing care is similar to that which is employed after brain-tumor operations. It should be emphasized that early recognition and prompt treatment of the disorder are necessary to permit normal growth of the brain during infancy. Where the diagnosis is overlooked and treatment is delayed too long, permanent damage to the brain and irreversible mental deficiency result.

INFECTIOUS POLYNEURITIS

Infectious polyneuritis is a disorder characterized by generalized, often extensive weakness and pain in various muscle groups. It is ordinarily a self-limited disease which progresses for a period of 2 to 4 weeks and then abates. During this interval there may be considerable atrophy of the involved muscles. The chief importance of this disorder is its confusion with poliomyelitis. Distinction between the two diseases is made from the presence of sensory changes in infectious polyneuritis and from the appearance of the spinal fluid, which usually contains a marked increase in protein but little or no increase in cells. Nursing care of polyneuritis is similar to that for poliomyelitis.

SPASMUS NUTANS (NODDING SPASM)

This queer affliction is confined to infants and runs a self-limited course of a few months. Its cause is unknown, and it is seen with decreasing frequency in recent years. The manifestations consist of a peculiar shaking of the head from side to side or up and down, together with nystagmoid movements of the eyes and a tendency to cock the head on one side when looking at objects. No treatment is known or necessary.

TIC (HABIT SPASM)

A habit spasm or tic is a simple or complex muscular movement which is repeated over and over in the same manner. Tics differ from choreiform movements in that the latter are without order or purpose and never are repeated twice in the same order of progression. Tics most frequently involve the face, but often also the neck, the shoulders or some other part of the body. They may take the form of blinking of the eyes, a facial grimace, shrugging of the shoulders or other movements, or a combination of some of these.

Tics begin as voluntary movements and are repeated until they become habitual and involuntary. Even in the habitual and involuntary stage, the movements can be repeated voluntarily on request. The movements may have had their origin in imitation of another or they may have started as the result of some local irritation or psychic or physical discomfort; they continue long after the exciting cause has disappeared. A tic may leave one part of the body and appear in another. As in chorea, the movements are increased by anxiety and cease during sleep.

Drugs and disciplinary measures are ineffectual in the treatment of tics. The parents should be urged to ignore the symptom as much as possible and to expend their efforts toward relieving stress which may be contributing to the child's feelings of insecurity or unhappiness. If changes in environmental circumstances do not result in cessation of the tic, it probably indicates the need for psychiatric therapy. It is particularly important to differentiate the movements from those of rheumatic chorea, since the treatment of the latter disorder is quite different.

HEADACHE

Among children, headaches occur under a wide variety of circumstances. Severe or persistent complaints require careful exclusion of organic disease of the brain or meninges with accompanying increased intracranial pressure. Among older children headache may be a symptom of strain or refractive error of the eyes, of chronic sinusitis, of fatigue, anemia or toxic or metabolic disorder. Occasionally, it announces the presence of hypertension. Migraine headaches occur in children but with lesser frequency than in adults. They usually are associated with a family predisposition to migraine and occur more frequently in girls. They may have the features of one-sidedness and abrupt onset seen in the older individual. Sensitivity to light and sound, dizziness, spots before the eyes and vomiting are often features of the onset. Treatment with aspirin or phenobarbital or codeine is usually not sufficient to give relief. Ergotamine is sometimes effective. In many instances the headaches appear to be precipitated by emotional tension or unusual fatigue. Detailed examination of the child's environment and way of life may disclose ways in which such pressures can be relieved.

Headaches among younger children often precede the appearance of fever with an infectious illness. For some children they represent the somatic manner in which anxiety is expressed. Headaches are often projected upon small, suggestible children by an anxious mother through questions such as "Are you sick? What's the matter? Does your head ache?" The child in agreeing with the suggestion finds that he receives solicitous attention and may later use the symptom of headache as a method of achieving this secondary gain.

THE VISUALLY HANDICAPPED CHILD

RECOGNITION OF VISUAL DEFECTS

The analysis and the correction of visual defects is a highly technical specialty which can be performed only by those with special training. When there is obvious deformity or abnormal movement of the eyes the child usually is brought quickly under the care of such a specialist. But in many instances the visual defect is a subtle one which is discovered only through the astute observations of parents, nurses, doctors or schoolteachers. In some instances early discovery and proper management are essential to preserve bilateral vision; in other instances it is necessary to prevent problems of social and educational adjustment. Most of the visual defects that are not grossly apparent depend upon errors of refraction in one or both eyes. A few are due to abnormal development or disease of the retina and its vascular or nervous supply.

Visual defects in infants may easily go unnoticed for several weeks or months. Early suspicions may be aroused after the infant has reached the age of 2 months if he fails to observe objects or to follow them with his eyes or to blink when they are brought close to his eyes. During the second half of the first year the child's failure to locate distant objects and his propensity for bringing things very close to his face for inspection may lead to the suspicion that he has severe myopia. In the school-age child, failure to learn, headaches, head-tilting or behavior disorders may be the first indication of a visual handicap.

As indicated above, a child who has a severe refractive error may begin to squint. More importantly, he may begin to favor his better eye and slowly lose the vision in the other eye because of disuse. Unless the poor vision in the defective eye is discovered early and efforts are made to correct it or to encourage the child to use the eye some of the time, its vision may be lost irretrievably.

Unfortunately, it is not always possible to assume that the child's eyes are under proper care merely because he is wearing glasses. In some instances the original fitting may be unskillful. In other circumstances the parents may have assumed that one examination and correction was all that ever would be needed and have failed to return for the periodic examinations requested. In some instances the child's refractive error keeps changing over a period of years, and the initial pair of glasses becomes obsolete.

Fig. 101. This blind child has learned to explore her environment through her other senses. Aided by appropriate stimulation and permission from her mother to try things independently, she is able to attend school and participate in the full program with sighted children. (From Miriam Norris)

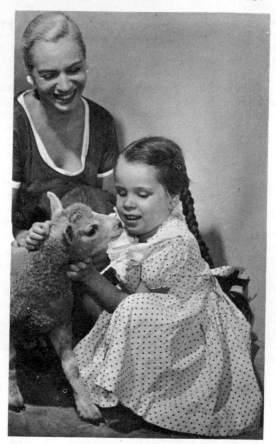

PSYCHOLOGICAL CONSIDERATIONS

Minor or correctable visual defects seldom create important problems of adjustment. Glasses have become so common among young children that the average child soon accepts the fact that he must wear them and makes an easy adjustment.

The parents of infants who are discovered to have serious visual defects or total blindness nearly always require help in adjusting to the handicap suffered by the child, in understanding the normal aspects of his individual development, in recognizing the cues that signal his need for new learning experiences and in seeing the child's urgent need to learn in his own natural way. After a 5-year study of preschool blind children, Norris, Spaulding and Brodie concluded that blind children, including those with retrolental fibroplasia, have the potentialities to grow up into independent, trusting, self-respecting, free functioning individuals who can be compared favorably with healthy sighted children (Fig. 101). Because the nurture of the blind child requires special understanding and skills, the reader is referred to the section which begins on page 164 and to the references which appear at the end of Chapter 8.

SITUATIONS FOR FURTHER STUDY

1. During hospitalization, after a child's mental capacity was established as inferior, if the parents were unable to accept the diagnosis, what problems could you anticipate would result for the child? How would the failure of the parents to accept the fact of his limitations affect the relationship between the child and his siblings?

2. Study a child with seizures. How has he accepted his handicap? How could you help him to adjust to it? Does he seem to be emotionally stable or unstable? What were his adjustment problems in the hospital? Does he say anything that might indicate the attitude of his peers toward him? Does he talk of his convulsions? What does he say? Or does he try to hide the fact that he has them when he is with a group of children? Does he in any way indicate his relationship to his parents, brothers and sisters? What reaction do you have to the parents' attitude toward this child? Are there ways in which you could help them to accept the child's handicap and develop his individual capacities? Visit the child's school and talk to his teacher to determine his progress in school and the teacher's attitude toward him. If the child shows problems of adjustment what community resources are available for his help? How would you interpret the function of the agency to the child? How would you interpret it to his parents to help them understand the need of seeking its aid?

3. Write to the National Epilepsy League, Room 715, 130 N. Wells, Chicago 6, Ill., and obtain literature concerning the needs of the child with seizures. Use it in observing and working with the child you are studying.

4. Write to the National Society for Crippled Children, Inc., 11 S. LaSalle Street, Chicago 3, Ill., for pamphlet material pertaining to the mental hygiene needs of the child with cerebral palsy. Use the literature in studying a nursery or a public school for crippled children.

5. Visit a nursery school for children with cerebral palsy and write a report which answers the following questions: In what ways were the children like normal children? Describe ways in which the teachers helped the children to be more independent, to express themselves creatively and to communicate verbally with them and with other children? How had they adapted equipment to meet the needs of the children? What was the teacher's philosophy in working with the children? What emotional attitudes did the teacher have which helped the children to succeed in gaining increased self-mastery?

6. Study a child of school age with cerebral palsy. What limitations are imposed because of his handicap? What is he capable of doing? Compare his capacities with those of a normal child of the same age. In what ways could you teach him to become more independent? Does the child seem to be normal mentally? If intelligence tests have been given, study the results to increase your insight into his potentialities. What characteristics does he have that would make intelligence testing difficult? What are your observations when the hospital schoolteacher is with him? What help could she give you in understanding him and in gaining insight into ways in which you could be of greater help to him? How has he accepted his handicap? Does his crippling condition affect the parent-child relationship? What is his reaction to other children and what is their reaction to him? How could you help him in increasing association with other children? How could you direct the play activities of the group so that his power could be utilized in group play? What are his interests? Can he express them? What play materials could you present that he could use to express himself in

such a way that some of his basic needs might be satisfied? How does he respond to attention and recognition? How does he seek them? If you were supervising this child's care in the home, what would be your objectives and how would you approach the problem of attaining them? What are the community resources available for his care?

7. What early symptoms might be indicative of the presence of a brain tumor in a preschool child?

BIBLIOGRAPHY

Abel, Marjorie: Feeding the child with cerebral palsy, Am. J. Nursing 50: 558, 1950.

Bridge, E. M.: Epilepsy and Convulsive Disorders in Children, New York, McGraw-Hill, 1949.

Callahan, Margaret: Twenty forgotten children, Am. J. Nursing 55:965, 1955.

Carlson, E. R.: Born That Way, New York, Day, 1941.

Carter, J. D.: Children's expressed attitudes toward their epilepsy, Nerv. Child 6:11, 1947.

Clark, Martha W.: Accepting a child for a lifetime, Nursing Outlook 5:279, 1957.

Coyle, Ione: The public health nurse in the cerebral palsy program, Nursing Outlook 4:95, 1956.

Cruikshank, William M., and Raus, George M.: Parent education and counseling in Cerebral Palsy: Its Individual and Community Problems, Syracuse, N.Y., Syracuse Univ. Press, 1955.

Denhoff, E., et al.: Prognostic studies in children with cerebral palsy, J. A. M. A. 161:781, 1956.

Flory, Mary C.: Administering a program for retarded children, Nursing Outlook 5:466, 1957.

———: Helping parents train a retarded child, Nursing Outlook 5:426, 1957.

Ford, F. R.: Diseases of the Nervous System in Infancy, Childhood and Adolescence, ed. 3, Springfield, Ill., Thomas, 1952.

Glick, Selma, and Donnell, Catherine: Nonmedical problems of the child with cerebral palsy, Nursing Outlook 1:101, 1953.

Gutman, Eleanor B., and Simmons, William D.: Health department leadership in prevention of blindness, Am. J. Pub. Health 46:1525, 1956.

Ingraham, Franc D., and Matson, Donald D.: Neurosurgery of Infancy and Childhood, Springfield, Ill., Thomas, 1954.

Jones, M. H.: The cerebral palsy child, Am. J. Nursing 46:465, 1946.

Kerr, Marion: Nursing responsibilities in cerebral palsy, Am. J. Nursing 46: 469, 1946.

Lewis, R. S., Straus, A. A., and Lehtinen, L. E.: The Other Child, New York, Grune, 1951

MacKenzie, Marguerite, and Baldwin, Maitland: Cerebral seizures, Am. J. Nursing 57:312, 1957.

Michal-Smith, Harold: The Mentally Retarded Patient, Philadelphia, Lippincott, 1956.

Nelson, W. E.: Textbook of Pediatrics, ed. 6, Philadelphia, Saunders, 1954.

Norris, Miriam: What affects blind children's development, Children 3:123, 1956.

———: The blind child in the sighted nursery school, New Outlook for the Blind 50:379, 1956.

Norris, Miriam, Spaulding, Patricia, and Brodie, Fern: Blindness in Children, Chicago, Univ. Chicago Press, 1957.

O'Leary, James L.: Electro-encephalography, Am. J. Nursing 55:1238, 1955.

Perlstein, M. A., and Barnett, H. E.: Nature and recognition of cerebral palsy in infancy, J. A. M. A. 148: 1389, 1952.

Roseman, Ephraim, and Taylor, Anne: Progress in the treatment of epilepsy, Am. J. Nursing 52:437, 1952.

Shechy, Thomas, and Bowden, Mary: Tuberculous meningitis, Am. J. Nursing 55:960, 1955.

Stewart, Mary: The child with cerebral palsy and the nurse, Am. J. Nursing 52:1228, 1952.

Stimson, P. M., and Hodes, H. L.: Common Contagious Diseases, ed. 5, Philadelphia, Lea & Febiger, 1956.

Ward, Moira M.: Toilet seats for disabled children, Am. J. Nursing 57: 483, 1957.

Weaver, H. E.: The nurse and sight conversation, Am. J. Nursing, 51:553, 1951.

The preschool child who is blind, Children's Bureau Folder No. 39, Washington, D.C., Government Printing Office, 1953.

The Backward Child (pamphlet), Ottawa, Canada, Dept. of Nat'l Health and Welfare, 1956.

Attitudes Toward Blindness (pamphlet), obtainable from Am. Foundation for the Blind, New York, N.Y.

The Child Who Is Mentally Retarded (pamphlet), Washington, D.C., Dept. of Health, Education and Welfare, 1956.

CHAPTER TWENTY-THREE

Diseases of the Endocrine Glands

GENERAL DISCUSSION

Knowledge about the endocrine glands, the hormones they produce, their functions, interactions and abnormalities has increased very rapidly within recent years. New concepts are being added daily as biochemical research clarifies the role which these organs play in normal and abnormal growth and in disease. Within a short chapter it is impossible to do more than scratch the surface of the many complicated equilibria which exist. The reader is referred for more detailed explanations and illustrations to the excellent text by Wilkins.

The endocrine glands consist of the thyroid, the parathyroids, the adrenals, the pituitary, the islands of Langerhans of the pancreas, and the gonads (ovaries or testes). The pineal gland is sometimes included in the list, as is the thymus. However, neither has any well-recognized endocrine function.

The endocrine glands secrete hormones which are absorbed into the blood. These hormones are "chemical messengers" which have their effect on other organs of the body. Hormones of several glands may act together and enhance the effects of the others; or they may act antagonistically, maintaining a balance of activity.

The pituitary hormones activate or inhibit secretion in so many other endocrine glands that sometimes the pituitary is spoken of as the master gland. The pituitary gland or the hypophysis has two parts: an anterior and a posterior lobe, each with separate functions. When injected, posterior lobe preparations cause increased blood pressure, increased intestinal tonicity and peristalsis, increased respiratory rate and powerful contraction of the uterus, and they have an antidiuretic effect in diabetes insipidus. The most important hormones of the anterior lobe are those that promote growth and those that increase the function of the generative, the adrenal and the thyroid glands. Many other effects have been recorded.

Several of the hormones of the anterior lobe of the pituitary have been isolated in relatively pure form. Of these, the adrenocorticotropic hormone (ACTH) which stimulates the cortex of the adrenal glands is the most widely used in treatment of children. The gonadotropic hormones, which stimulate the generative organs and the thyrotropic hormone, which increases the activity of the thyroid gland, are also available for therapeutic use. A growth hormone has been isolated, but its effect appears to be confined to experimental animals.

The effect of hormones in some instances depends on the ability of the receptor organ to respond. Abnormally increased secretion of the growth-promoting hormone of the anterior lobe of the pituitary gland results in exaggerated symmetric growth of the body (gigantism) if the epiphyses have not yet fused; as a consequence, the bones have capacity for growth in length. After fusion of the epiphyses, the increased secretion results in acromegaly, a condition of distorted growth in which various parts of the body increase in size without increase in body length.

Carbohydrate metabolism is controlled by the pancreas and the pituitary, the adrenal and the thyroid glands. The internal secretion of the pancreas, insulin, regulates the storage of glucose as glycogen. One of the pituitary hormones is antagonistic to insulin. Hyperpituitarism produces hyperglycemia and glycosuria. Hypopituitarism has the opposite effect. Adrenalin causes increase in blood sugar by calling out the glycogen stores from the liver and has other effects on sugar metabolism. The thyroid hormone causes increased combustion of sugar.

Anterior pituitary hormone stimulates the thyroid gland to increased secretion. Hyperthyroidism may be produced in this manner. Conversely,

through lack of stimulation of the thyroid, decreased pituitary secretion lowers the basal metabolic rate and may produce hypothyroidism.

Growth and maturation of the body are dependent on proper functioning of the pituitary, the thyroid, the adrenal and the gonad or the sex glands. The pituitary is concerned directly with growth and also indirectly through stimulation of the gonads and the thyroid. The general maintenance of growth of body organs, especially of epiphyseal and periosteal bone growth, is the chief function of the growth-promoting hormone of the pituitary. The thyroid also directly affects growth because of its effect on metabolism.

The parathyroid glands control the level of blood calcium, using bone as the reservoir of calcium. Hypoparathyroidism produces tetany from low blood calcium. In addition to producing high blood levels and high rate of excretion of calcium, hyperparathyroidism causes disappearance of bone mineral, with resulting osteoporosis.

The adrenal glands have a medulla and a cortex. The medulla produces adrenalin or epinephrine, a material which increases blood pressure, increases the conversion of glycogen to glucose, stimulates the thyroid and inhibits the internal secretion of the pancreas. The cortex of the adrenal produces hormones essential for the metabolism of sodium, water and carbohydrate. Deficiency causes Addison's disease. An excess causes precocious puberty with masculinizing changes, regardless of sex. In Addison's disease, the major effect of cortical deficiency is on the kidney, which loses its ability to excrete certain materials, such as potassium, and to stop excreting sodium and chloride when these should be retained.

NORMAL SEXUAL DEVELOPMENT

The physical changes characteristic of puberty (see Chap. 2) are dependent

on the presence of gonadal or sex hormones that are formed as a result of stimulation of the gonads by the gonadotropic hormones of the pituitary gland. The amount of secretion of gonadotropic hormones by the pituitary is negligible in early childhood but increases in late childhood to give the impetus to puberty development. These pituitary hormones maintain gonadal activity for many years.

The sex characteristics, particularly the secondary characteristics, are determined by the type of hormone formed in the greatest quantity and by the relative proportions of the two types of sex hormones. The sex hormones, both male and female, are similar chemically. Each person elaborates both types of hormones. The male sex hormones are called androgens; and the female hormones, estrogens. Androgens give the body the male configuration and cause the normal hypertrophy of the male sex organs. Estrogens give the body the female configuration and cause normal hypertrophy of the female sex organs. Both types of gonadal hormones stimulate fusion of the epiphyses through repression of the pituitary growth hormone, bringing growth in length to a stop. The process of epiphyseal fusion is slow, so that growth proceeds for a considerable time after puberty. The gonadal hormones have a powerful influence on psychic attitudes and general health.

The endocrine sex mechanisms in boys are relatively simple in comparison with the complicated cyclic changes which take place with menstruation in girls. The gonadotropic hormones of the pituitary not only stimulate the production of estrogen by the ovary but also stimulate the maturation of ova. As soon as the ovum begins to ripen, the follicle in which it is developing secretes further amounts of estrogen. This increased amount of estrogen causes increased growth of the inner lining of the uterus (endometrium) and increase in its vascularity. After the ovum has matured fully and has been extruded, the follicle site becomes filled with cells

to form what is known as a corpus luteum. This is formed under the stimulus of a luteinizing hormone from the pituitary. The corpus luteum has a hormone of its own. The effect of this hormone on the uterus is to cause still further increase in the thickness, the vascularity and the gland development in the endometrium. The endometrial changes are in preparation for reception of the fertilized ovum. When the ovum is not fertilized it is not implanted in the uterus, and the corpus luteum immediately atrophies, and its hormone progesterone disappears. With the sudden decrease of progesterone, the outer portions of the hypertrophied endometrium slough off, producing menstrual flow.

ACNE

In late childhood or during adolescence a disturbance of the pilosebaceous apparatus of the skin occurs in such a high percentage of children that it (acne) can almost be considered a normal aspect of sexual development.

Under the influence of the sexual hormones of the maturing person an activation of the sebaceous glands occurs which results in an increased production of oily sebum. At the same time there is a tendency for the orifices of the glands to become blocked by dark inspissated material (blackheads or comedones), around which may develop an inflammatory reaction, often with pustule formation. Acne vulgaris is usually prominent about the forehead, the face and the neck. It also may be present on the shoulders and the back and occasionally on the chest. Its extent is quite variable. Some children have little or none during the whole course of their adolescence and early adult lives. Others are affected severely, with permanent scarring of the skin as a consequence of the repeated formation of pustules. Administration of cortisone or ACTH often produces a similar eruption even in young children, but there is seldom any associated infection.

Treatment of mild acne consists of frequent bathing of the skin to remove oil and bacteria and to encourage drying. For the latter purpose various washes that cause mild peeling are useful. Exposure to ultraviolet light is also beneficial, either from the sun or from a lamp. The diet is of some importance in the aggravation of lesions, and the natural tendency of the adolescent to gorge himself with carbohydrate foods must be discouraged if the inflammatory reaction is to be controlled adequately. Expression of the contents of comedones and pustules usually is done by the physician. In severe cases, judicious use of x-ray treatment may be required.

VARIATIONS IN SEXUAL DEVELOPMENT

SEXUAL PRECOCITY

Constitutional or Idiopathic Precocity

Sexual development is regarded as being precocious when secondary sex characteristics appear before the age of 8 in girls (Fig. 102) and before the age of 10 in boys. Such an acceleration is about 4 times as common among girls as it is among boys. In both sexes the most common variety of sexual precocity is called constitutional or idiopathic precocity, signifying that there are no obvious associated abnormalities which might be presumed to set off the maturing effects of the pituitary gland prematurely. In some instances there appears to be a hereditary predisposition within the child's family. The effects of this variety of sexual precocity may be upsetting to the family and to the child because of his abnormally mature appearance. No serious consequences result otherwise, and the child's age-mates eventually catch up to his development. The ultimate height of such boys and girls tends to be below the average, for, although a marked growth spurt usually occurs when sexual development first appears, the process also leads to early epiphyseal closure in the long bones of the skeleton, which in turn limits the duration of growth to an abnormally brief period.

Intracranial Lesions

Intracranial lesions such as a preceding encephalitis or an unrecognized brain tumor may stimulate the precocious appearance of puberty. Usually there are other evidences of neurologic disturbance when this is the exciting cause.

Adrenogenital Syndrome in Boys

Either hypertrophy or tumor of the adrenal cortex may lead to excessive production of androgens which in turn stimulate premature development of male sexual characteristics but without proportional enlargement of the testes. Benign hypertrophy occurs most frequently and is due to perverted activity of the adrenals which are unable to synthesize the normal corticosteroids. Treatment with cortisone results in rapid decrease in the production of androgen, cessation of further virilization and a fall in the level of 17-ketosteroids in the child's urine. If the underlying defect is due to a tumor, this therapeutic result will not be obtained, and other diagnostic procedures are in order.

Tumors of the Gonads

Rarely, tumors of the gonads may be responsible for precocious pubertal development. Interstitial-cell tumors of the testis usually can be recognized by palpation, since they produce enlargement of one testis. Granulosa-cell tumors of the ovary are likewise discoverable by palpation. In such circumstances the tumor must be removed.

FIG. 102. Constitutional sexual precocity in a girl of 7 years.

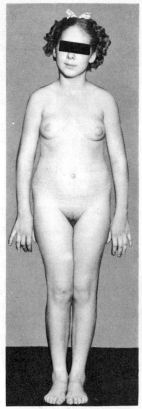

FAILURE OF SEXUAL DEVELOPMENT

Delayed Adolescence

The onset of normal adolescence may be delayed instead of being precocious. For a variety of reasons, delayed puberty in girls is infrequently a cause of parental concern, whereas the failure of a boy to keep up with his age-mates in sexual development is very commonly a topic of unnecessary worry. While the average male begins puberty by 13 or 14 years, some normal boys may wait until the age of 16 or 17 before the first changes occur. A particularly common cause of concern is the high-hipped, mildly or moderately obese boy who matures late. The rare Fröhlich's syndrome referred to below has unfortunately become too popular as a lay and even medical diagnosis which is pinned unjustly upon normal boys of this body build. Treatment of delayed adolescence is usually not justified although occasionally, strong psychological reasons may warrant an attempt to initiate maturation by the use of chorionic gonadotropin.

Hypothalamic Lesions

Disorders of the hypothalamus, the portion of the brain immediately adjacent to the pituitary gland from which it receives nervous stimulation, may be responsible for failure of sexual development. Tumors, congenital defects, and most commonly cysts known as craniopharyngiomas may interfere with the production of gonadotropic hormone by the pituitary. This combination of circumstances due to a tumor prompted the original description of the Fröhlich syndrome which combined sexual infantilism with diabetes insipidus and a feminine type of obesity.

Pituitary Abnormalities

If the pituitary gland itself is ab-normal and unable to produce gonadotropic hormone, sexual maturation fails to occur. It is usually part of a general failure of the pituitary gland (panhypopituitarism) which also leads to dwarfism. Occasionally, it occurs as an isolated defect of the gland in a person of normal stature.

Gonadal Abnormality

If the end-organs (the gonads) which the gonadotropic hormone is destined to stimulate are absent or defective it is obvious that sexual development cannot take place. Defective embryonic development of the gonads is now recognized as leading most commonly to a clinical picture in which female external genitalia are associated with a boyish appearance which does not change at the age of puberty. Other defects are usually present. Short stature is regularly found and webbed neck, hypertension and various skeletal abnormalities are frequent. The latter characteristics may lead to the suspicion of gonadal defect even during infancy. The diagnosis can be confirmed during the prepuberal years when the urinary excretion of gonadotropic hormone (FSH) rises to high levels as the pituitary tries vainly to initiate puberty. A number of variations of the general pattern are recognized. It is interesting to note that a high percentage of these individuals have male sex chromosome patterns in spite of their external appearance.

Hermaphroditism

This term implies the presence of elements of both male and female glands in the same individual. In its true form it is seen with extreme rarity. A variety of combinations of malformations which seem to combine elements of the two sexes are referred to as pseudohermaphroditism. The most frequent and important one is the adrenogenital syndrome in which the cortical adrenal glands produce abnormally large amounts of androgens in an effort to compensate for their inability to fabricate normal corticosteroids. In the developing female infant the influence of such androgens leads to partial masculinization of the developing external genitalia. At birth, a large clitoris and labia majora may be confused with male hypospadias and bifid scrotum. The vagina may be rudimentary or it may communicate with the urethra internally. Recognition of the syndrome is important because treatment with cortisone will suppress the virilizing effects of androgen and at the same time compensate for the congenital deficiency of corticosteroids. Later plastic correction of the external genitalia to agree with the female sex of the child is sometimes necessary.

THYROID DISORDERS

GOITER

The thyroid gland which lies on the anterior surface of the neck has the responsibility of manufacturing thyroid hormone which is an essential regulator of the body metabolism and of growth. Iodine in small amounts is needed in the process. Ordinarily, the gland is seen or felt with difficulty. Under certain conditions it may enlarge and become visible. The resulting tumor is called a goiter. The presence of enlargement does not indicate what the nature of the underlying abnormality is. This must be worked out by additional investigations, particularly of thyroid function.

Simple Goiter

This term implies a physiologic enlargement of the thyroid which occurs particularly in girls at the time of puberty when the gland is called upon to produce an increased amount of hormone. It requires no treatment. It may also occur with pregnancy.

Endemic Goiter

Enlargement of the gland occurs in geographic regions where the soil is lacking in iodine and the local vegetables thus fail to provide adequate amounts for the fabrication of hormone. The enlargement is a response to the attempt to make hormone with insufficient materials. It can be stopped or corrected by administration of iodine. In the United States it has become very rare, since it is prevented automatically by the addition of iodine to most commercial table salt.

Goitrous Cretinism

Cretinism may be due to an inability of the gland to manufacture hormone in spite of an adequate intake of iodine.

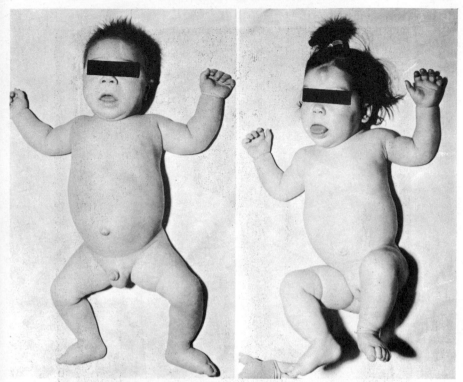

FIG. 103.Two infant cretins, showing characteristic facies, large tongues and trunks which are long in proportion to the extremities.

This variety of hypothyroidism requires the same treatment as that described under the cretinism due to congenital absence of the gland.

Toxic Goiter

This is enlargement of the gland associated with an abnormally large production of hormone. It is discussed below under hyperthyroidism.

Other Varieties

Newborn infants whose mothers have received antithyroid drugs in the treatment of hyperthyroidism during pregnancy may be born with goiters which persist for a few weeks. Tumors and nodules of the thyroid may produce enlargement of the gland. Infection of the thyroid is very rare in children.

HYPOTHYROIDISM

Cretinism

Cretinism is the condition produced by complete absence of thyroid secretion from birth. Cretinism occurs only sporadically in this country but is found endemically in goitrous regions of other countries. Sporadic cretinism is associated with congenital absence of the thyroid gland or with an inability of the gland to make hormone. The mother of the cretin is presumably normal. Cretins develop normally up to the time of birth because of the availability of the mother's thyroid secretion. The effects of lack of thyroid make their appearance gradually. The characteristic physical features do not appear for a period of from 3 to 5 months, although

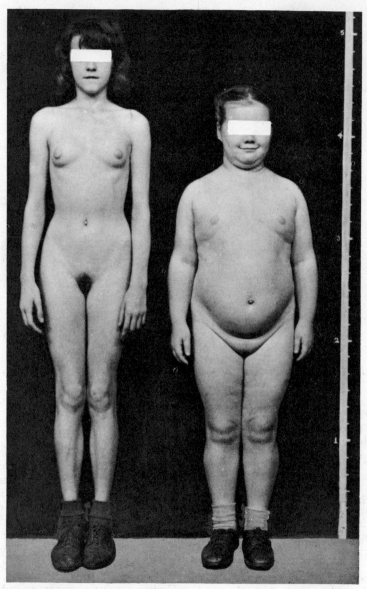

Fig. 104. Normal 12-year-old girl (*left*) contrasted with 13-year-old girl with hypothyroidism.

certain chemical changes in the blood characteristic of hypothyroidism could be detected earlier if examination were made.

Once the condition of cretinism has developed fully it is distinctive and unmistakable, although the inexperienced often confuse it with mongolism. These children are conspicuously backward mentally and have characteristic physical abnormalities. The facial features are heavy and almost pathognomonic, although an adequate word picture of them is scarcely possible (Fig. 103). They lack the slant eyes and the epicanthic folds of the mongol. The tongue protrudes from the mouth; the voice or the cry is hoarse. Two cardinal symptoms of cretinism are absence of sweating and obstinate constipation. The skin is dry, and often the hair is coarse. Generally, growth in length is greatly retarded, the retardation showing itself chiefly in the short extremities. Because of slow bone development, the fontanel remains open far beyond the normal closing time. Roentgen examination of the bones discloses that the ossification centers appropriate for the chronologic age have failed to appear. Tooth eruption is delayed. The poor muscle tone leads to protrusion of the abdomen, and often there is an umbilical hernia.

In addition to the clinical appearance and behavior of the child, various laboratory tests may assist in confirming the suspicion that thyroid function is depressed. Radioactive iodine given by mouth fails to reach a normal concentration in the thyroid gland, as determined by the Geiger counter. Chemical examination of the blood shows an abnormally low level of iodine which is bound to protein (essentially a direct measurement of the quantity of thyroid globulin being manufactured). Blood lipids may be abnormally high. More cumbersome but useful are tests of basal metabolism and creatine excretion in the urine, both of which give low values in hypothyroidism.

The prognosis in cretinism depends on how early and how effectively treatment is given. If an adequate amount of thyroid is given very early, the physical growth will proceed in a normal manner, and the mental development will tend to be relatively normal. It is seldom

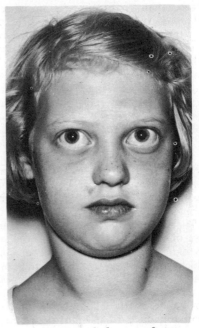

FIG. 105. Exopthalmos and goiter in a girl with hyperthyroidism.

that mental development is fully satisfactory, even when the best methods of treatment are instituted early in infancy.

The treatment consists of the administration of dried thyroid gland by mouth. The amount of thyroid should be the maximum that can be taken without symptoms of overdosage. A cretin infant will require from 0.5 to 1.5 grains daily. The original dose should be smaller, and then the amount should be increased to tolerance. The diet should be complete and should include ample vitamin D. Without vitamin D, rickets is very likely to develop because of the very rapid rate at which the bone will grow when thyroid is first given. The symptoms of overdosage of thyroid are the same as those of hyperthyroidism, notably, vomiting, diarrhea, irritability, fever, rapid pulse and weight loss.

Acquired Hypothyroidism

Occasionally, hypothyroidism of lesser degree than that of cretinism is encountered in childhood. All degrees of hypothyroidism exist, from the obvious to that detected only with special tests. When the condition is of at least moderate degree, both physical and mental growth is slowed (Fig. 104). The basal metabolic rate is decreased. The "bone age" is less than the chronologic age. Puberty is delayed. The child tends to be lethargic, the skin cool and dry and of a poor color. The cholesterol content of the blood is increased, and the phosphatase content is decreased. The creatine output in the urine is below normal.

The treatment of these children consists of giving an appropriate dose of thyroid. The amount should be that which corrects the symptoms and less than that which produces nervousness or other evidence of hyperthyroidism. The child with hypothyroidism has good tolerance to thyroid medication. When thyroid is given in case of an erroneous diagnosis of hypothyroidism, as often happens in obesity, the tolerance is poor, and nervousness develops quickly.

HYPERTHYROIDISM
(TOXIC OR EXOPHTHALMIC GOITER)

Hyperthyroidism as it occurs in childhood is more frequent in girls than in boys and has its onset most often near the time of puberty (Fig. 105). The cause of increased thyroid secretion is not known. Toxic goiter has been observed with pituitary tumor and has been relieved by treatment of the tumor. It is possible, though not proved, that the thyrotropic hormone of the pituitary is responsible in other instances in which no lesion of the pituitary can be demonstrated.

The onset usually is gradual. All the symptoms that develop are attributable to excess thyroid secretion. These include nervousness, increased pulse rate, muscle weakness, easy fatigue, increased metabolic rate and sweating. Fine tremor of the extended fingers and tongue is present. Despite increased appetite and food intake, many have weight loss because of increased metabolic rate. The rate of growth is increased, and the bone age ultimately advances above the chronologic age. The thyroid gland increases in size (goiter), and the eyeballs become prominent (exophthalmos). The urinary excretion is increased, and blood cholesterol is decreased from the normal. In the more severe intoxications, vomiting, diarrhea, cardiac palpitation and dyspnea are likely to be present.

The course of the disease varies, but the illness does not become dangerously severe so often in adolescents as in adults. In some instances it may become progressively and rapidly worse from the onset and cause death if no relief is given. More often, it progresses slowly with remissions. The so-called thyroid crisis is not common in children. A crisis represents a sudden large outpouring of thyroid secretion, resulting in prostration, high fever, vomiting, diarrhea and greatly increased nervous and mental symptoms.

Treatment

Since the introduction of drugs such as propylthiouracil, methylthiouracil and Tapazole which suppress the formation of thyroid hormone, the treatment of hyperthyroidism in children has shifted from a surgical to a medical approach. Initially, a dose of about 300 mg. is given daily which is expected to produce gradual reduction of the metabolic rate and disappearance of the symptoms, including the enlargement of the gland. Prominence of the eyes may not reverse, but it usually does not advance after treatment is started. Addition of thyroid extract to the regimen aids in the decrease in size of the gland.

The antithyroid drugs must be monitored for evidence of toxic reaction in the form of rashes or serious depression of the white blood cell count. In the absence of these complications, hyperthyroidism usually can be brought under sufficient control to allow the child to pursue a normal life. The duration of treatment must be individualized. In many instances the drug has to be continued for several years before the disease burns itself out.

If toxic reactions to the drug cannot be avoided, or if the parents or child fail to co-operate with medical management, surgical removal of part or all of the thyroid must be undertaken. If all of the thyroid is removed, the child will require permanent substitution therapy with thyroid preparations.

CARCINOMA OF THE THYROID

Occasionally, neoplastic change in the thyroid gland is found in girls. Usually there is nodular enlargement of the gland or enlargement of the adjacent cervical lymph nodes to which the tumor has metastasized. The condition is a very slowly progressive one and can often be controlled by removal of the tumor if it is recognized in an early stage. There is strong suspicion that the use of x-ray therapy to the neck and the chest in early infancy may play a role in initiating neoplastic changes in the gland.

PARATHYROID DISORDERS

Primary disorders of the parathyroid glands, which regulate calcium and phosphorus metabolism, are quite rare in children. A familial type of hypoparathyroidism is seen occasionally which gives symptoms of chronic tetany comparable with the acute form observed in rickets. Treatment, consisting of large doses of vitamin D, is difficult to regulate appropriately.

PITUITARY DISORDERS

PITUITARY DWARFISM

Children who remain unusually small but well-proportioned are suspected of suffering from a deficiency of the growth hormone of the pituitary gland. Actually, there are two varieties of symmetric dwarfism which are very difficult to distinguish from one another during childhood. In one type there is actually a lack of pituitary function, but the proof of this fact is not apparent until the child passes through adolescence without maturing sexually. The other type of dwarfism is hereditary or constitutional in type, and the child matures sexually at the expected time.

DIABETES INSIPIDUS

Diabetes insipidus is a condition in which the water excretion by the kidneys is abnormally large, with the result that the intake also must be large in compensation. The kidneys are normal but do not function normally because of lack of the controlling posterior pituitary hormone. This lack causes a lowered threshold for water. Because of the large quantity of water excreted, the urine has a very low specific gravity (1.002).

Diabetes insipidus may be caused by various conditions that disturb pituitary function. Thus, it may occur in cases of brain tumor located in or near the pituitary gland, particularly in the neighboring hypothalamic region. It may occur as a result of encephalitis or other inflammation of the hypothalamic region. In some instances it has resulted from traumatic injury to the brain. In many instances no lesion can be demonstrated, and the disease is on an idiopathic basis.

The symptoms of the idiopathic disease may consist only of drinking and excreting large amounts of water. The nutrition may suffer because the drinking of so much water is likely to interfere with the taking of sufficient food.

The treatment consists of regular daily administration of posterior pituitary hormone and of attention to the underlying brain lesion, when such exists. Such conditions as brain tumor are more dangerous to life than diabetes insipidus. Certain of the brain lesions are not amenable to treatment.

When the disease is idiopathic, administration of posterior pituitary hormone is the only treatment needed. Pitressin tannate in oil is the preparation usually employed. Dosage must be regulated by trial for the individual child, but usually amounts of 1 or 2 cc. per day will bring the volume of urine excretion to normal levels. A pitressin-resistant form of diabetes insipidus is encountered in which the kidney fails to respond to the hormone.

DIABETES MELLITUS

Diabetes mellitus is a condition in which part or all of the ability to utilize sugars has been lost because of deficiency of insulin, an internal secretion of the pancreas.

ETIOLOGY

The disease is less common among children than among adults and apparently more common among children in some parts of the country than in others. The primary cause of the disease remains obscure. Heredity apparently is a predisposing factor in many instances, but this factor is not obvious in many others. Occasionally, diabetes has its onset after an acute infection, but a causal relationship is not certain.

PATHOGENESIS

In diabetic children, digestion and absorption of food are unimpaired. Normally, absorbed sugar is stored as glycogen or converted into fat, and small amounts are being burned constantly to supply energy. In diabetes mellitus the ability to store, convert and burn the absorbed sugar is impaired or lost, and the sugar accumulates in the blood. When the amount in the blood increases above the renal threshold, sugar is excreted in the urine.

SYMPTOMS

The onset of diabetes is usually abrupt, since its preliminary stages may present no symptoms. Sugar may be

discovered in the urine incident to a routine examination. As the disease appears, loss of weight and increased urination, thirst and hunger usually are present. The excess sugar requires water for its excretion, and this accounts for the thirst and the polyuria. Since much of the food is not utilized the child loses weight, and increasing muscular weakness may be noted. When the disease has progressed rapidly from the onset, sometimes these early symptoms are of brief duration and pass unnoticed, the first observed evidence being a state of coma due to the development of severe acidosis.

Acidosis

The capacity of the body to burn fats is limited. When carbohydrate is not available for energy production, fat is mobilized for energy in amounts greater than can be burned completely. Much of the fat is oxidized incompletely, with the resultant accumulation of ketone bodies (acetone, diacetic acid and oxybutyric acid). When neutralized, these substances are only slightly toxic and are excreted readily in the urine. Their chief harmfulness arises because two of these substances are acids and require neutralization. Thus base is removed from the body, giving rise to acidosis, which easily becomes serious and is the usual cause of death of those with diabetes.

COURSE

When untreated or treated inadequately, the diabetic child continues to lose the ability to utilize sugar, and increasing amounts of insulin are required. The rate of downward progress is not constant for various children or even for the same child. Such factors as overexercise, infection, nervous exhaustion and excessive carbohydrate ingestion accelerate it. Soon or late, acidosis and coma supervene, and the child succumbs unless adequate emergency treatment is instituted promptly. Untreated diabetes in the young runs a relatively more rapid and more uniformly fatal course than in older patients. When the management is intelligent and consistent the diabetic child is as healthy as the normal child. Because of the thought and the care given to the diet, most diabetic children who are under good control are in a better physical state than the average nondiabetic child.

DIAGNOSIS

The symptoms that have been enumerated are strongly suggestive of the presence of diabetes but do not prove it beyond question. The finding of sugar in the urine is important but not conclusive evidence, since a few children have a low renal threshold for sugar (renal glycosuria) with entirely normal metabolism and blood sugar. The repeated finding of glycosuria, together with increased sugar in the blood, may be considered as conclusive. In such instances, in the uncommon mild case, the prediabetic phase of the disease or when one wishes to confirm or to exclude the existence of diabetes definitely, a sugar-tolerance test may be made.

Sugar-Tolerance Test

A sugar-tolerance test is useful only for diagnosis and not for the determination of the amount of sugar that may be permitted a diabetic child. The test is made before breakfast after a night of fast. Dextrose is given in solution by mouth in the amount of 1.75 Gm. for each Kg. of body weight, or sometimes a standard dose is given regardless of age. The blood and the urine are examined before and at hourly intervals after the dextrose has been ingested. The normal child will not excrete sugar or have high blood-sugar values in these circumstances, while the diabetic child will. Normally, the blood contains some sugar at all times, the amount varying from 70 to 160 mg. for each 100 cc., depending on the relation to meals. At slightly above this higher level sugar appears in the urine of the normal person. Sometimes a diabetic child has a renal threshold higher than normal.

PHILOSOPHY OF MANAGEMENT

Today there are two distinct ways of approaching the details of the management of a diabetic child. The traditional (strict diet or aglycosuric) method implies that the diabetic child must be controlled closely and meticulously if he is to have the best chance for a long life and freedom from the late complications of his disease. This school uses calculated, weighed diets, permits no departures from them without exact substitution of equivalent food and regulates the insulin dosage so closely that no sugar is excreted in the urine at any time. Advocates of the more recent (free diet, glycosuric) method do not believe that such exact regulation is necessary and that excretion of glucose in the urine is not by itself harmful. They feel that the child should be given freedom to follow a diet of his own choosing, provided that he avoids excesses and that his insulin need be regulated only with a view to keeping him from excreting ketone bodies. This latter school doubts that late complications are any more frequent with this type of management and feels that the child is much better off with the freedom and the lack of regimentation which this system provides. Actually, the general principles of the management of diabetes are the same in each instance, the main difference lying in the exactness with which physiologic correction is sought. Since the two approaches are quite different, each will be described.

STRICT DIET MANAGEMENT

The food requirements of the child are calculated carefully, a diet is prescribed, weighed and measured precisely, and its exact components taken at the same time each day. Insulin doses are arranged so that no sugar will be lost in the urine. Periodic adjustments of diet are made for growth and activity changes, and insulin doses are modified accordingly.

Food Requirements

The food requirements of a diabetic child are the same as those of a nondiabetic child of the same age. These are discussed elsewhere. Since the child has decreased ability to utilize carbohydrate, the concept became established that a large share of the energy requirement should be derived from fat and only a small portion from carbohydrate. However, it now is known that for diets of equal energy value the insulin requirement after stabilization of control remains the same regardless of the relative proportions of fat and carbohydrate. The older concept has been modified almost everywhere, and the general tendency is to have the relative amounts of these food components approximately the same as those found in the diet of the nondiabetic child. These more popular diets allow the child to feel less different from others and thus have a beneficial psychological value.

It is important that the foods selected to fill the specifications of protein, carbohydrate and fat be of such a nature that the mineral and vitamin needs also are supplied. According to one good method of management, the meals should be apportioned so that they are equal, each representing one third of the day's allowance. The food must be weighed carefully and all of it ingested. No other food of any nature is permitted. However, water is allowed.

Use of Insulin

In the case of some diabetic persons, adults more often than children, the nutritional requirements may be satisfied with a closely regulated amount of food which can be handled by the body without the use of insulin. The majority of diabetic children require more food than their unaided tolerance would permit. Insulin should be given in such quantities that sugar is not excreted in the urine, and the blood sugar remains at an approximately normal level. When the child is receiving sufficient food and appropriate amounts of insulin he is in the same metabolic status as a nondiabetic child.

Insulin is prepared from the pancreas of animals. It is supplied in vials in solutions of various strengths designated as U20, U40, U80 and U100. These contain 20, 40, 80 and 100 units, respectively, to each cc. It is valueless by mouth and must be given hypodermically, intramuscularly or intravenously. Syringes graduated in cubic centimeters are entirely satisfactory for insulin administration, but special insulin syringes are available and are commonly used. They are graduated in terms of U20 insulin on one side and U40 on the other or in terms of U40 and U80. It should be remembered that if a certain volume of U40 insulin is required, twice this volume of U20 will be necessary to supply the same number of units, while only half the volume of U80 will be required. The dosage must be measured accurately, and to this end the syringe and the needle should be free from leaks.

Dosage. The dosage of insulin required varies for each child. The less the insulin supplied by the child himself, the more severe the diabetes and the more the insulin required by injection. The dosage is established by intelligently managed, trial-and-error procedure. It is important that the insulin be given as prescribed at the proper interval before a meal. The food allotment for the day is divided equally into 3 meals given the same number of hours apart, but the insulin dosage is not so divided. The child with severe diabetes usually requires 4 doses of insulin daily. A satisfactory distribution of the insulin has been found to be 35 per cent 30 minutes before breakfast, 22 per cent 30 minutes before the noon meal, 28 per cent 30 minutes before supper, and 15 per cent once during the night. When the child has mild diabetes, 3 and sometimes 2 daily doses will be satisfactory.

The initial doses of insulin frequently are based on the amount of excess sugar in the blood, and the subsequent doses on the amount of sugar lost in the urine. For this reason, it is desirable to collect the urine in 4 separate portions: (1) from breakfast to dinner, (2) from dinner to supper, (3) from supper to bedtime or the time of the night dose of insulin and (4) from previous collection until breakfast. By means of this division the adequacy of each dose of insulin is indicated. When diabetes is brought under control in this manner, it is customary to find that the child recovers some of his lost sugar tolerance, and as a consequence the insulin dosage must be lowered. Usually, a stability in the insulin dosage is attained in the course of from 3 to 6 weeks, and the daily dosage becomes relatively constant. Certain uncontrollable factors, such as the amount of exercise and the occurrence of infection, may cause moderate variation from day to day. For this reason, constant checking and alertness are necessary. The insulin requirements will change also with the increased food necessary as the child grows. Blood-sugar determinations should be made at intervals, as it is possible for the blood sugar to be maintained at a level above normal and no sugar to appear in the urine.

Insulin Shock. Occasions will arise when it will be evident that insulin is present in the body in excess of the immediate need. Such a condition may occur because of increased tolerance for food and a lessened need for injected insulin, because of error in calculation and administration of either the insulin or the diet, because some of the prescribed food is not eaten, is vomited or is utilized poorly because of diarrhea, or delay in eating or unusual exertion. In any of these circumstances more sugar is stored than should be, and too little is left for circulation and use. The sugar in the blood falls below normal limits, and insulin shock results. A definite group of symptoms is associated with this event. Any or all of the following may be observed: nervousness, irritability and possibly other personality changes such as silliness; a general drowsiness or lassitude; unusual hunger; either pallor or flushing, accompanied by dilatation of the pupils and sweating; decreased response, perhaps leading to unconsciousness; local jerking or generalized convulsions. In mild insulin shock, only the first 3 or 4 symptoms may appear. The symptoms usually develop within a relatively short time and disappear within a few minutes after the child receives some sugar-containing food. For a mild attack, 1 ounce of orange juice and for a more severe attack, 2 ounces of orange juice should be given. If the attack persists for 15 minutes, the dose of orange juice should be repeated. If the child is unconscious or refuses to co-operate, the orange juice or sugar solution may be dropped into the mouth with a medicine dropper. Dextrose solution may be given intravenously. It is necessary to distinguish between insulin shock with coma and diabetic acidosis with coma. During insulin shock the urine is sugar-free, and the blood sugar is low. In diabetic acidosis, sugar is present in the urine, and the blood sugar is high.

Varieties of Insulin

The type of insulin referred to in the preceding discussion is designated as ordinary or regular insulin. Other varieties have been produced, and some are in common use. Insulin has been prepared in combination with zinc in a crystalline form known as zinc-insulin crystals. It is dispensed in solution in the same unitages as ordinary insulin. A solution of zinc-insulin crystals has the same action as ordinary insulin and presents no advantage over ordinary insulin except that it is less likely to cause reaction at the injection site. Ordinary insulin, like the solution of zinc-insulin crystals, has an effect of relatively brief duration, several injections being necessary every 24 hours to keep diabetes in control. In the endeavor to produce an insulin product which would be absorbed more slowly and so have a more lasting effect, it was found that when insulin was combined with a very simple protein the desired effect was obtained. However, the resultant products are unstable and have poor keeping qualities. When they are combined with zinc, more stable products result.

Protamine Zinc Insulin. This has commercial distribution and is commonly used. The outstanding characteristic of protamine zinc insulin is its slow, continuous absorption. By its use, mild diabetes in some instances can be kept under control by a single injection daily. When the disease is sufficiently severe to require more than 1 dose of insulin daily, it is customary to give only 1 dose of protamine zinc insulin and to supplement this dose with other injections of ordinary insulin. By this means fewer total doses are required.

The advantage of fewer injections through the use of protamine zinc in-sulin may be outweighed by the dangers encountered in its use. Shock resulting from overdosage of ordinary insulin is recognized easily and responds readily to sugar by mouth, whereas shock from protamine zinc insulin tends to develop insidiously, become very severe and respond slowly to treatment, dextrose frequently being required by the intravenous route. The severity of the reaction and the slowness of response to treatment cause great alarm to attendants. When shock has occurred in the home, away from technical and laboratory facilities, it has resulted fatally in some instances.

Globin Zinc Insulin. This form is a more recent commercial product which is absorbed more slowly than regular insulin but more quickly than protamine zinc insulin. By its use it is possible to eliminate 1 or 2 doses of regular insulin. The night dose of regular insulin can be eliminated by giving about 43 per cent of the day's requirement as globin zinc insulin 1 hour before the evening meal and saving half of the milk from this meal to give from 3 to 4 hours later. This change can be made without altering the level of control.

NPH Insulin. This is approximately a combination of two parts of regular insulin and one part protamine zinc insulin. It acts a little more slowly than globin zinc insulin, but its late effects do not persist as long as those of protamine zinc insulin.

FREE DIET MANAGEMENT

With this type of management, excretion of sugar in the urine is permitted, and the precise controls over diet and insulin are relaxed. This does not mean that supervision is abolished. Until the child and his parents learn the general principles of diabetic physiology and the vagaries of the individual child's disease, frequent consultations about diet, insulin adjustment and general hygiene are needed. Regular examination of the urine for the presence of sugar and acetone is required also.

The mother and the child are instructed in the requisites of a good diet. Although an exact intake is not prescribed, regularity and consistency are urged in order that insulin adjustment may be regulated easily. Periodically, the child's food intake is analyzed by the physician or the dietitian in order to be sure that he is meeting his requirements for calories, proteins, minerals and vitamins. If he is lacking in any dietary respect, acceptable modifications of the diet are suggested. Excessive carbohydrate intake and between-meal feedings are discouraged but not forbidden.

Since exact control of glycosuria is not a goal, the administration of insulin usually can be reduced to a single injection of globin or NPH insulin once a day or a combination of protamine and regular insulin given simultaneously in 1 or 2 syringes. The urine is tested 3 or 4 times a day for both sugar and acetone. If there is intermittent glycosuria without acetone in the urine, the regulation is considered as being adequate. If glycosuria is continual but without acetone, periodic quantitative estimation of the amount of sugar being excreted per day is desirable. If more than 30 Gm. is being lost in the average 24-hour period, the glycosuria is considered excessive, and insulin is increased in an attempt to decrease the spillage. When acetone appears in the urine it is regarded as a danger sign which requires consultation with the physician in order to adjust the diet or the insulin or to arrange for an examination to discover an unrecognized infection. If the urine remains consistently free of sugar, usually insulin is reduced in order to avoid the appearance of insulin reactions.

The proponents of the free diet type of management of diabetes recognize the danger that parents and children will become too lax and casual in the regulation of the disease. However, they feel that in the long run most families can achieve a satisfactory regulation while avoiding the social disadvantages and the emotional rebellion which the stricter type of regimen sometimes induces.

MANAGEMENT OF SPECIAL CIRCUMSTANCES

Initial Effect of Treatment

When a diabetic child first comes under adequate care, the insulin requirement is always higher than it becomes subsequently. With the return of blood sugar to normal levels the child's ability to produce insulin increases. The insulin requirement eventually becomes stabilized, the time required depending on the closeness of control and on the state of nutrition. A longer period is required for the undernourished than for the well-nourished child.

Exercise

Exercise has a striking effect in reducing the insulin requirement. Increase in muscular activity requires compensation either by increasing the food intake or by decreasing the dosage of insulin. Failure to make this compensation is the most frequent cause of insulin shock. For spasmodic increase in activity it is better to try to maintain a relatively constant dosage of insulin and give additional food at mealtime. For more prolonged periods of activity it is necessary to decrease the insulin dosage. A boy spending the summer at a camp with its active life requires much less insulin than when he returns to the sedentary life of school in the fall.

Emotional Disturbances

The effect of emotional disturbance may be as severe as that of infection and in the same direction in that the insulin requirement is increased. The insulin dosage is much easier to regulate for the emotionally stable child.

Acute Infections

During acute infections, the ability of the body to use sugar properly is lessened. As soon as the signs of any infection appear it is advantageous to increase the insulin dosage moderately in an attempt to prevent glycosuria. If glycosuria occurs, the insulin should be increased still more, and if symptoms of shock develop, the dose should be decreased. The diet should be made up of easily digested soft or liquid foods. With the more severe infections, fat should be reduced or eliminated. As convalescence takes place, the regular regimen is re-established.

Surgical Operations

Diabetic children withstand operative procedures well if proper care is given them. Details of management vary with the circumstances of operation. Insulin must be given before and during the postoperative period. Crystalline insulin usually is employed because of its short period of activity. If food cannot be tolerated, calories must be supplied by intravenous infusion of glucose. Many children can be restored to their usual regimen on the day after operation.

Acidosis

The mechanism by which acidosis develops already has been described. As long as the ketone bodies are formed in only moderate amounts and the body is able to excrete them without excessive drain on its supplies of base, acidosis does not develop. The condition then is known as ketosis. This is not a desirable or a healthy state of affairs, but the immediate danger is slight. With increased formation of ketone bodies the base of the body is depleted, and acidosis develops. As it becomes severe enough to become clinically manifest, the following symptoms and signs may be noted: the respiration becomes deep, rapid and without pause (air-hunger breathing) and remains thus until the child is in extremis, when it may become slow and shallow; the cheeks are flushed, the skin and the mouth are dry; nausea and vomiting are frequently present; thirst usually is extreme; the pulse is rapid and thready; the temperature is either normal or elevated; the white cells of the blood may be increased markedly; severe abdominal pain may be present.

As the acidosis increases in severity, the child becomes stuporous and then comatose. Death is the usual sequel to untreated diabetic coma. These various signs and symptoms usually do not appear suddenly but increase in severity rather insidiously during several days as a result of some infection or dietary mismanagement. If the urine is tested daily, as it should be, sugar and increasing amounts of diacetic acid will be found, giving warning and making it possible to prevent or to relieve the acidosis promptly.

If the urine contains much diacetic acid and sugar but symptoms of acidosis have not developed, the child should be confined to bed, kept comfortably warm and given abundant fluids. The diet should consist of liquids; most of the fat-containing foods should be excluded. The dextrose equivalence of the previously prescribed diet or of a diet slightly lower in energy value should be maintained. The insulin dosage should be increased sufficiently to make the urine sugar-free. Usually this also will cause the disappearance of diacetic acid. The amount of insulin needed cannot be foretold. When the sugar excretion has lessened demonstrably, the extra insulin administration should be discontinued and the child put on the regimen described under treatment of diabetes.

If symptoms of acidosis are present, the treatment is similar to that just described but it must be more vigorous. The sugar content of the fluids ingested should be recorded, and every 2 to 4 hours the child should receive one unit of insulin for each gram of sugar ingested in the preceding period. If the child is vomiting excessively, it may be necessary to give intravenously 5 per cent dextrose in normal salt solution, to which insulin has been added, one unit for each gram of sugar; 250 cc. an hour can be given with benefit. In addition, extra insulin will be needed to consume the excess of sugar already present in the body. The amount needed will depend on the amount of sugar in the blood and the severity and the duration of the symptoms.

When acidosis is extreme, it is often useful to supplement the treatment as outlined with the intravenous administration of alkali or potential alkali. During the period of recovery from severe acidosis it is desirable to administer solutions containing potassium, which is lost in large amounts during the acute stage of metabolic disturbance. Parenteral potassium is administered cautiously and only after renal flow has been established. When the child is able to take oral fluids, liquids such as tea, fruit juice and milk will provide significant amounts of potassium. After the acidosis has disappeared, as evidenced by the disappearance of diacetic acid from the urine, the subsequent treatment is directed toward the re-establishment of the child on a regimen of suitable diet and insulin dosage, as already described. It is desirable to use a liquid diet for a day or two after recovery from acidosis, the fat content being kept lower than would be necessary later. Usually it is safe to give the child his calculated diet requirement within 2 or 3 days.

NURSING CARE

Because the symptoms that accompany the onset of diabetes, acidosis or insulin reaction are threatening to the child and his parents, the nurse needs to be as sensitive to their psychological needs as she is to the child's need for immediate medical therapy. The child with symptoms of diabetes, acidosis or of an insulin reaction cannot help feeling less stable physically. He responds with changes in behavior and signs that indicate that he is also threatened psychologically. His parents and the hospital personnel are concerned about his symptoms. Their anxiety is often communicated to the child, which heightens his feelings of apprehension. The child needs to know the purpose of each test to which he is being subjected. If he is too young or too ill to understand, he must be supported adequately, because his response to initial physical care will color his feelings about all subsequent care that he will require. If the child is supported initially, the possibilities of developing wholesome attitudes toward his disease and its treatment will be greater.

Observation of the child's personality characteristics is essential in detecting signs that indicate a change in his physical status. The nurse must be able to distinguish between emotional upset and temporary personality change caused by low blood-sugar. If insulin shock is suspected, the child should be put to bed. If no sign of improvement is detected in 10 minutes, the doctor should be notified. He may order dextrose water, orange juice or part of the milk from the next meal. Close observation should continue until the child's behavior becomes normal again.

Alleviating the child's anxiety is another facet of nursing care with which the nurse must be concerned. Carbohydrate metabolism can be altered by emotional disturbances. Therefore, it is imperative that the child have the help he needs to adjust to his disease and to its associated treatment. Most children with diabetes have concerns about their physical status, their prognosis and the reasons why they have to have insulin and a dietary regimen that is different from that of other children. Some children feel guilty about their hostility and view their illness as punishment for misbehavior or evil thoughts and wishes. Discovering the child's concept of his disease, its treatment and the meaning that it has for him personally should precede teaching. Unless unrealistic notions are corrected, the child will derive little therapeutic value from the instruction.

When insulin is administered, the same care as when giving any hypodermic medication should be taken but with the following additions: the syringe should be dry before measuring the insulin; there must be no bubbles in the syringe; a cotton pledget should be held firmly over the site of injection for a few seconds to prevent leakage of insulin; and the site of injection should be selected with care. Injections may be given in the upper or outer part of the arms and the thighs. Repeated injections in one area cause "insulin pads." To prevent them from developing, the legs and the arms should be used in rotation, and the injections should be given in rows.

Teaching the young child to cleanse the area and to choose one of the various sites of injection of insulin will stimulate his co-operation. As he indicates his capacity and interest to learn to give himself insulin, he should be encouraged to do so. If the child can be helped to gain feelings of success, he will become increasingly interested in his treatment. His interest and the use of his own power in giving the insulin will help him to master his fear of the procedure. Some 5-year-old children are capable of injecting the prepared insulin. With supervision, the average child between the eighth and the tenth years can be taught to measure the required dose in the syringe. Because insulin will be a daily requirement, it is imperative that the child learn to accept his need for it. Initially, he will undoubtedly rebel and misinterpret the reasons why it is being given. Encouraging verbal expression of his feelings concerning it gives the nurse understanding of the meaning it has

for him and helps him work his problem through to the point where he can accept himself and the insulin that he requires.

When there are several children with diabetes in the ward, it is desirable to group them together for meals and for insulin administration. Instead of having insulin at their bedside, they can have it in the treatment room. Insulin should be given first to those children who already are well adjusted to their medical regimen. This gives the child with recently diagnosed diabetes an opportunity to observe children who have adapted themselves to insulin administration.

The collection of specimens of urine must be done methodically. When fractional specimens are desired, sufficient bottles plainly labeled with the date and the times at which collection began and ended (e.g., 7 to 11 A.M.) should be at hand. Gradually, the child can learn to prepare and take the specimen to the laboratory, test it and report the results to the doctor or to his parent if he is being cared for in his home.

Because the occurrence of glycosuria is such an important factor in the plan of treatment, collection of specimens may become an irksome routine for the older child and for the adult who must assume the responsibility for the preschool child. If diabetes has developed after bladder control has been attained, the collection of the specimen will pose few difficulties if the preschool boy's need for privacy in urinating is maintained. If the child has not attained bladder control, care must be taken to prevent the problems that result from coercive toilet training. The nurse must attempt to handle her anxiety if she has concern in relation to her ability to collect a specimen. If she is fearful of her capacity for success, the child will feel it and be without the support he needs to gain control of his body functions. Accomplishments should be rewarded with the nurse's responsiveness;

accidents should be accepted with patience and understanding. Gradually, the child should be helped to assume the responsibility for collecting his specimens for examination. When problems arise in collecting specimens from a male child, the help of the father should be elicited. During preschool years and during adolescence, feelings toward the mother may create anxiety in the male child and prevent him from co-operating fully.

Infections and injuries should be prevented in such a way that the child does not come to feel that he is being overprotected because of his disease. Early symptoms of infection should be noted so that change in treatment may be begun before sugar tolerance has become greatly affected.

Although the diet is prescribed by the doctor and prepared by the dietitian, it is the nurse who helps the child accept his food happily. The child who is placed on a restricted dietary regimen must be helped to face the fact that his food in some ways differs from that served to other children or adults. Segregating him from the group because of food differences protects him from temptations that he eventually must learn to meet. It also will tend to make him feel different, which is an unwholesome attitude for him to acquire. If he is served at the table with other children, opportunities for teaching will present themselves. Little by little, the nurse can give him understanding of his particular dietary needs.

When planning menus for the child, his food likes and dislikes should be respected. Forcing and urging a child to eat large quantities of disliked foods creates personality problems which are more difficult to treat than the diabetes. As the child matures, he should be given opportunities to assist in the planning and in the preparation of his food.

When a child's appetite is unsatisfied the temptation to eat forbidden foods is increased, and he easily falls victim to it. The power of resistance to temptation is a matter of slow growth. A child with diabetes often is faced with a temptation that he has not learned to resist. The temptation may be greater at some times. When the blood sugar is low, the child becomes extremely hungry and is driven to satisfy his needs.

When a child gives in to temptation in the hospital or at home, he needs understanding help. Many children give into temptation because they have not lived long enough to develop controls from within. Scolding, labeling them as thieves or un-co-operative beings and punishing them provoke feelings of hostility, rebellion and resistance. Instead, they need help in building up their tolerance for frustration. Facing the desire for forbidden foods with the child is a helpful means of supporting him in his fight to resist temptations. When his problem is faced with him by an understanding adult he gets the strength that he needs for growth. The adult's faith in the child must be maintained consistently. When it is, the child will acquire a sense of responsibility for his own care.

Preparation for the child's home-going is imperative. In the hospital the parents' attitudes toward the child and his problems should be observed as a basis for guidance. The parents' attitudes toward the child, his disease and its treatment will become reflected in the child's feelings about himself. They will determine the kind of adjustment that he will make to his disease and the requirements of his care. Oversolicitude and overprotection often arise from guilt and anxiety. Overprotection increases the child's anxiety and places undue emphasis upon his disease. The feelings underlying overprotection also limit the parents' opportunity for emotional comfort and prevent them from handling their problems constructively.

Before discharge the parents should be studied so that environmental problems which might complicate the child's treatment or influence his adjustment to it may be eliminated. The child's parents often need repeated reassurance that the prognosis is favorable when adequate care is given. Many times the nurse will need to help the parents gain confidence in their capacity to care for the child. Until parental anxiety is relieved they will not be able to cope with their problems. Nor will they be able to accept the child as he is and provide him with support that makes it possible for him to make a healthy adjustment to the reality that he must face.

Confidence can be developed through learning experiences that produce confidence. The parents can be taught to calculate diets and to prepare and administer insulin. They also can be taught to recognize the early symptoms of acidosis and insulin shock and to carry out the emergency treatments for them should they occur. Parents cannot know too much about their child's disease, for it is through knowledge and wholesome attitudes that self-assurance is gained. The child also needs to know about his disease and the values of treatment in supplying his body with what he needs for health. Self-responsibility is the outgrowth of self-acceptance and knowledge. Self-understanding is the child's birthright. Denying him this privilege robs him of his right to self-mastery!

For many parents the administration of insulin will be the most difficult feature of the child's care. Understanding supervision of the mother is essential. Her feelings need acceptance. Permitting her to voice her feelings will give the nurse clues concerning the meaning of the procedure to the mother. She may see the treatment as punishment. If she does, she may be inhibited in learning. If she has ambivalent feelings toward the child, insertion of the needle may be too great a threat for her. If she feels that it is an act of punishment,

she will need help to see its therapeutic value—that it is in reality an act of giving what is necessary to keep her child in a state of health.

The adolescent with diabetes manifests problems which are different from those seen in the younger child. Adolescence is a period of reappraisal of the self. The struggles to find himself, identify his role and attain feelings of self-acceptance and self-competence is existent in every adolescent. The child with diabetes will need additional support to surmount the developmental tasks of the period. Frequently, feelings of despondency and of inferiority are discovered in adolescents with diabetes. They need help in acquiring a mental attitude that will enable them to face life in a reasonably contented way. There is no cure for diabetes. The adolescent must face, accept and handle this fact. Everyone has a handicap of one kind or another. The wholesome solution is to face it with the feeling that it is a surmountable problem that need not hinder the individual's capacity for self-realization and productivity.

It has been estimated that approximately 50 per cent of cases of coma occur between the ages of 10 and 15. Prepubescent physical growth accounts for some, but psychological change seems to have a greater bearing on the occurrence of complications. During preadolescence and early adolescence, self-discipline becomes more difficult. There is a strong urge for recognition, to be like others and for self-expression and independence. Parental devaluation and doubt of parental control increases, and the adolescent tends to rely on his own judgment, which too often has not become strengthened through sufficient experience. All routine to the adolescent is irksome, and the routine that diabetes requires adds duties which are viewed as "boring," "bothersome" and sometimes even "useless." He exceeds his dietary regimen, not always because of physical needs but because of psychological needs produced by growth. The adolescent is driven to express his independence, to be like others and to rebel against authority. One excess in diet produces no immediate catastrophe, but a cumulative effect may occur without his realization.

To survive, the child with diabetes must learn self-control and achieve the capacity to take responsibility for himself. This growth can come only with experience that provides opportunities to develop his inner resources. The preadolescent and the adolescent need guidance that is different from that which is appropriate during the school-age period. They have grown. They want a new status and freedom within bounds to develop the inner resources they need to feel competent for independent activity. The teen-ager with diabetes has the same needs as the normal youngster and has equally as much capacity for acquiring self-direction. Democratic guidance gives him the support that he requires to achieve responsibility for his own behavior.

Many of the problems of adolescence could be prevented if opportunities for self-direction were given gradually as the child matured. Not all parents are able to do this without help. Some mothers *need* their adolescent dependent upon them to meet their own emotional needs. Sometimes a mother uses her child's handicap to justify keeping him tied to her. When this happens the child's problems are compounded. His conflict between dependence and independence becomes intensified, which becomes manifested in any number of ways. The example* which follows serves to illustrate the way one boy manifested his conflict, resentment and anxiety. It also serves to illustrate the way a social worker can help a mother

* Material pertaining to the case of Gus was prepared by Mrs. Betty Butler, Director of Social Service in the Pediatric Department of the University of Chicago Clinics.

to gain insight into her use of her child's handicap to solve her own problems. The importance of the father's participation in implementing a plan of home care is also demonstrated.

Gus was a 12-year-old undersized boy who had been under medical care for diabetes for 3 years. His general adjustment had been satisfactory until his 12th year. Then his behavior began to change. His parents became alarmed when the school authorities notified them that their son was failing. Gus's doctor requested the social worker's help in evaluating the situation in order to determine the source of the difficulty. In the early interviews with Gus's mother, the social worker discovered that the parents had many marital problems and that Gus had become increasingly rebellious about following his diabetic regimen. He refused to eat breakfast; he refused to permit his mother to test his urine; and he had "skipped school" and refused to reveal his whereabouts. In spite of the mother's concern and her plea for "any solution," she was reluctant to arrange for her husband to be interviewed by the social worker. It was not until Gus was admitted to the hospital for insulin regulation that he and his father were seen by the social worker. Once Gus's father began talking over his role in the family it became clear that the marital difficulty was the major problem of the family. Gus's mother had sought to keep him "her little boy." She used his small stature and his disease as a means of exercising control. Gus vacillated between wanting to be at home and to prove that he was as adequate as other boys. He refused to talk with either of his parents for several days at a time and remained aloof from all ward activities. At the same time, the nurses reported that Gus was not eager for discharge. Gus had complained that his mother had looked at his urine "just like you'd check on a baby."

In evaluating the family relationships, the social worker concluded that Gus's father had the capacity to change his role within the family. Gus's mother complained that her husband left all decisions up to her. At the same time, however, she was able to admit that she had "hidden problems" from him, including the fact that Gus had been out of diabetic control for several days prior to admission to the hospital.

Before Gus's discharge from the hospital, the doctor, the social worker, the head nurse and the dietitian discussed the total situation together and made specific plans for helping the family. Gus was given the responsibility of testing his urine with his father supervising the activity. Gus's mother felt this meant that the staff did not "trust" her. She needed further help from the social worker to see that this was a step which she could take in a more positive direction. With help the mother was able to regard the change in the routine in the light of Gus's developmental needs. Gradually, she became more aware that she had used Gus as a threat against her husband. Eventually, both parents were able to see their need to discuss their marital problems with an appropriate family agency, and a referral was made.

SITUATIONS FOR FURTHER STUDY

1. If diabetes were discovered while a 5-year-old child was hospitalized for treatment of appendicitis and you had the responsibility of giving his first injection of insulin, how would you proceed?

2. If a child 4 years old with diabetes were eating at the table with a group of normal children, what would you do if he reached for a cookie from the nondiabetic children's supply? If a diabetic child 8 years old were seen taking cake from the food truck, what should be done?

3. Study a teen-ager with diabetes. At what age did the diabetes develop? What is his attitude toward the disease? Is he well-informed about his needs as a diabetic? Does he accept insulin in a matter-of-fact way? Can he prepare and give it to himself independently? How well-developed socially is he? Does he enjoy being with a group or does he prefer solitude? Does he show feelings of inferiority? Is he irritable or emotionally unstable? What type of situations produce excitability? Does he accept his diet pleasantly or does he make suggestions that should be used in planning his diet? What characteristics of adolescence does he manifest? How does his developmental status influence his attitude toward his diabetic regimen? What is his relationship with his parents? Have they encouraged independence and self-reliance or have they tended to overprotect or neglect his need for growth? How have their attitudes toward him and his disease influenced his behavior? How could their insight into the developmental needs of a teenager be increased?

BIBLIOGRAPHY

Blake, F. G.: Development and care during the preadolescent period 10 to 12 years, p. 360, and development and guidance during adolescence, p. 381, *in* The Child, His Parents and the Nurse, Philadelphia, Lippincott, 1954.

Brown, G. D.: The development of diabetic children with special reference to mental and personality comparisons, Child Develop. 9:175, 1938.

Bruch, H., and Hewelett, E.: Psychologic aspects of the medical management of diabetes in childhood, Psychosom. Med. 9:205, 1947.

Fischer, A. E.: The emotional factors in the treatment of diabetic children, Proc. Am. Diabetes Assn. 7:217, 1947.

——: Factors responsible for emotional disturbances in diabetic children, Nerv. Child 7:78, 1948.

Fischer, A. E., and Horstmann, D. L.: Handbook for Diabetic Children,

New York, Intercontinental Medical Book Corp., 1954.

Joos, T. H., and Johnston, J. A.: A long term evaluation of the juvenile diabetic, J. Pediat. **50**:133, 1957.

Robinson, P.: A child with diabetes, Am. J. Nursing **51**:690, 1951.

Root, H. F., Roehrig, C. B., and Pond, M. R.: Diabetic coma, Am. J. Nursing **55**:1196, 1955.

Wilkins, L. W.: Endocrine Disorders in Childhood and Adolescence, ed. 2, Springfield, Ill., Thomas, 1957.

Wilkinson, M.: Diabetes mellitus in adolescence, Am. J. Nursing **50**:126, 1950.

CHAPTER TWENTY-FOUR

Viral and Rickettsial Infections

General Discussion

The various infectious diseases differ greatly in the ease with which they may be transferred from one person to another. Certain of them cannot be transmitted by contact. To this group belong those diseases which are transmitted by biting insects. The group includes yellow fever, plague, dengue, malaria, relapsing fever, typhus and Rocky Mountain spotted fever.

Those infectious diseases which have their portal of entry by way of the alimentary tract are not easily communicable by contact. The causative agent must be ingested. This group includes cholera, dysentery, typhoid, Salmonella infections and probably poliomyelitis.

More easily, but not highly, communicable by contact are some of the infections of the skin and the mucous membranes. The group includes erysipelas, impetigo, tularemia, syphilis and gonococcus infections.

Some infectious diseases are highly communicable and require only casual contact for transmission. These infections have one feature in common, namely, the causative agent has easy access to the body and easy exit from it. For most of the highly communicable infections the respiratory tract constitutes the portal of entry as well as the channel of exit for the causative agent. The responsible organisms are expelled easily from the infected person by coughing, sneezing or even talking and, as a part of the particles thus propelled into the air, they are inhaled easily by persons in the immediate vicinity. Of course, these same diseases may be

568

transmitted by crude infection instead of by droplets: saliva and discharges may be transmitted grossly.

Thus, the most common means of transmission of the more highly communicable infections is by contact of a susceptible person with one who has the disease or with one who is a carrier of the causative agent.

Certain of the communicable diseases may be transmitted by a third or intermediate person or by means of articles such as books and toys. Diseases that are transmitted more easily in this manner are those whose causative organisms are relatively long-lived, for example, scarlet fever and diphtheria. In the case of such diseases as measles and chickenpox, the virus dies quickly after leaving the body, and transmission by indirect contact is difficult. However, in institutions or in circumstances in which the interval between contacts is brief, indirect contact assumes importance for all communicable infections.

Although communicable diseases sometimes seem to appear out of nowhere when there has been no known direct or indirect contact with an afflicted person, it is not appropriate to consider these diseases as air-borne. They can be air-borne in only a limited sense. When droplets containing the causative agent are expelled from the mouth, they may be carried several feet by favorable air currents. The water of the droplets may evaporate, leaving an infectious nucleus floating. Such material may be carried somewhat farther than droplets. Contaminated dust may be a similar menace with improper sweeping and dusting. However, these events would not affect neighboring houses and are not within the usual meaning of air-borne infection. When a communicable disease appears without apparent relationship to the same disease in another person, the source is usually an unsuspected carrier or a person having the disease in an exceedingly mild and unrecognized form.

The diseases that are highly communicable by direct or indirect contact have been designated as *contagious diseases*. Since different diseases present all gradations of infectivity by contact, no sharp dividing line exists between the highly contagious diseases and those of low communicability. For practical purposes, it is customary to make such a division in hospital practice by putting persons with certain diseases in quarters separate from the general wards and keeping those with other diseases in the general wards with certain precautions.

The diseases for which isolation is customary are diphtheria, measles, smallpox, streptococcus infections, whooping cough, chickenpox, mumps, poliomyelitis, meningococcus meningitis, gonococcus infections, influenza, erysipelas, open tuberculosis and typhoid fever.

No isolation is required for any variety of meningitis other than meningococcic, for closed tuberculosis or syphilis, for malaria or rheumatic fever or for a large group of local infections such as appendicitis and pyelitis.

ISOLATION

A child who is suspected of having a contagious disease should be separated from others until a diagnosis can be made. One who has the disease should be isolated until the danger of transmitting it to others no longer exists. The period appropriate for isolation depends on the duration of communicability of the disease. For some diseases, this period is determined easily by the presence or the absence of the causative agent; in others, the causative agent is identified with difficulty. In this latter group, an arbitrary isolation period is determined on a statistical basis. Statistical studies show that after a certain time has elapsed the child no longer transmits the disease to susceptible persons. By means of such observations, suitable isolation periods have been established for each disease.

The practice of quarantine in which

the families of children with contagious diseases were confined to their homes until the household was deemed no longer infectious has been given up except for smallpox and diphtheria. Local boards of health and school systems have also liberalized their regulations in respect to the exclusion of nonimmune contacts of contagious disease from school.

Need for Immunization

Although there can be no question as to the value of isolation in limiting the spread of communicable diseases, they never can be exterminated by this means alone for they will continue to be spread by (1) carriers, (2) persons with mild illness and (3) persons in the prodromal stage of the disease.

A carrier is a person who harbors the causative agent without showing evidence of the disease. He may or may not have had the disease in the past but in order to be a carrier without showing evidence of the disease he must be immune. The carrier state is recognized in diphtheria, meningococcic meningitis, poliomyelitis, typhoid fever and several other infections and without doubt exists in many more.

Communicable diseases manifest themselves with all degrees of severity. Sometimes the mildness of the disease is due to resistance of the host and sometimes to the low virulence of the causative agent. In either case, the person may not be ill enough to call a physician, or the physician may not be able to recognize the disease in its mildness. A disease acquired from one who is mildly ill is not necessarily mild—often quite the reverse.

Most of the communicable diseases which have a prodromal stage are highly infectious during this stage. The disease is not recognized in this early stage, and isolation is not instituted.

Since it is impossible to prevent exposure of all susceptible persons to communicable diseases, it is desirable to immunize against as many of them as constitute a menace. Methods of immunization are discussed under those diseases for which means of protection are known. Completely satisfactory methods of active immunization exist for smallpox and diphtheria; partially satisfactory methods exist for whooping cough and poliomyelitis. Passive immunization is useful for temporary prevention when exposure is known to have occurred. Means for passive immunization exist for diphtheria, measles and whooping cough. A very high proportion of deaths from measles and whooping cough occur under 3 years of age. Obviously, it is desirable to protect children, at least until they are past this age period, against those diseases that affect the young so seriously.

Aseptic Technic

It is possible for persons with different communicable diseases to be cared for in adjacent rooms by the same attendants without the transmission of the disease of one patient to another (cross-infection) and without the attendants themselves becoming infected. For such accomplishment a special technic is necessary. The technic employed is known as medical asepsis or aseptic technic. In many respects, this technic is the reverse of surgical technic. When ready for a surgical operation, the patient as prepared is "clean," as are also the instruments and the instrument tables: anyone entering the room unprepared is "dirty" or contaminated as far as the technic is concerned. In the care of persons with communicable disease, anyone entering the room is presumably clean until contaminated by touching the patient or anything which the patient has contaminated.

One may enter a contaminated room and, if nothing is touched, not become contaminated. Minor offices often may be done for the patient with contamination of only the hands, which when washed are again clean.

For prolonged or intimate nursing care, protection of the clothing by a gown becomes necessary. In some institutions, a gown is worn only once. After giving care to a child, the gown is removed and discarded in a special hamper, the hands are washed, and the nurse is again clean. In other institutions, gowns are reused and are kept clean inside by a special technic described below.

When the nurse must care for patients with contagious disease for long periods, it is preferable that she not only wear a gown while with the patient but that she also exchange her street clothing or usual uniform for a special uniform before entering the sickroom or the isolation ward.

General Rules and Considerations of Aseptic Technic

All floors are considered to be contaminated. Nothing dropped on the floor should be used again without cleaning. The infant's toys should be tied to his bed. A toy bag should be attached to the head of the older child's crib or bed, and its use demonstrated as soon as the child is well enough to play. The bed, the bedside table and the wall near the patient are contaminated. If gowns are hung to be reused, the place where they are hung is contaminated. The inside of the sink bowl is contaminated, but otherwise the sink is considered to be clean. All other areas are kept clean.

Gown and Mask Technic

A mask is worn over both nose and mouth to prevent the spreading of disease and the inhaling of infectious material. The gown should be long enough to cover the skirt and the apron. The gown should have its opening in the back and should overlap sufficiently to prevent separation. An additional tie at the waistline aids in holding the gown in place when the nurse bends over the bed. When the gown is used only once, the ties are untied, the gown is removed

and discarded, and the hands are cleansed thoroughly.

If the gown is used for a 24-hour period, special technic in putting it on, taking it off and hanging it up is required. The gown is folded and hung in the unit with the contaminated side out. For removal of the gown, the waist ties are loosened before cleansing the hands. Cleansing before the gown is removed is necessary to keep the inside clean. After cleansing the hands, the clean neckband ties are loosened, the fingers of the right hand are inserted under the cuff of the left sleeve, and the left sleeve is pulled over the left hand. The cuff of the right sleeve is grasped on the outside, and the sleeve is removed by the left hand still covered by the left sleeve. Next, the clean hands are used to bring the ties of the neckband together. Then the hands become contaminated as they are used to bring the shoulders of the gown together and to hang it over a hook in the child's unit. The gown is hung in such a way that the inside remains clean and so that the attendant's clothing is protected from contamination. Handling the outside of the gown to hang it in the unit contaminates the hands, and another cleansing is necessary to make the attendant clean.

Hand-Washing Technic

Facilities in institutions differ, but the equipment always consists of soap, running water, brush and towels. The brush is commonly kept in a disinfectant solution on or near the sink. The hand-operated faucet is kept clean by using the brush to turn it. In the cleansing of the hands, plain but thorough soap-and-water washing (lathering and rinsing at least 3 times) is all that is necessary unless the hands are grossly contaminated with bodily secretions. In instances where there is gross contamination, cleansing the hands and the nail beds with a brush is required. The use of antiseptic solutions in addition is not necessary and certainly should not replace disinfection by washing. The towels, usually of paper, may be kept on a clean shelf above the sink. Keeping the hands free of cuts and abrasions and preventing chapping with the use of hand lotion is important for the nurse not only to protect her own health but also because chapped hands are a deterrent to thorough disinfection.

CONCURRENT DISINFECTION

This term is used to designate the disinfection which must be carried out more or less continuously while the patient remains isolated. It includes the disinfection of contaminated materials such as dishes, eating utensils, instruments used for examination or treatment and bedding which are to be used again for other patients. It also includes the disposal of excreta and sputum.

Upon admission to the isolated unit each patient is provided with his own personal equipment, including a face basin, a soap dish, a toothbrush, thermometer and other equipment as indicated. These articles remain within the room and are considered unclean until subjected to the procedures for terminal disinfection when the isolation is concluded. Housekeeping measures such as sweeping and dusting should be carried out with a damp technic so as to limit the dispersion of infected materials into the air of the room. Treatment of blankets, drapes, furniture coverings, dust clothes and mops with an oily preparation has been shown to be of great help in limiting the contamination of the air about the patient.

Articles which enter the room and are contaminated by contact with the patient must be disinfected before re-use. Bedding, laundry, gowns and eating utensils are usually sterilized by heat, either by autoclaving or boiling. Instruments, thermometers and other glass or metal objects should be cleansed with soap and hot water or with 70 per cent alcohol. Objects such as blood pressure cuffs, clothing, mechanical equipment and personal articles must be exposed to air and either sunlight or an ultraviolet lamp for an arbitrary period which is considered sufficient to kill residual infectious particles.

To feed the patient, certain preparations must be made in advance. The trays are prepared in the kitchen by a dietitian or by a nurse who remains clean. The trays of those who must be fed are served last. After the meal, the trays are collected carefully, with contamination of only the hands. No hand washing is necessary in the course of the collection. The contaminated trays are carried to the kitchen and placed on a paper-covered table, the paper preventing contamination of the table. Food remnants are scraped into a garbage can. Paper tray-covers and napkins are placed in a can provided for the purpose. The trays and all dishes and utensils are disinfected by boiling for 20 minutes and then are washed. The disposal of garbage and waste depends on local facilities. With adequate city sewage disposal, no special handling is required. Otherwise, either chemical disinfection or burning in an incinerator is necessary.

Discharges from the body, such as sputum, stools, urine, vomitus or surgical drainages, must be disposed of in similar fashion. Depending again upon the local sewerage arrangements, it may be possible to empty them directly into toilets or hoppers and dispose of the containers by burning or by autoclaving or boiling. When sewage arrangements do not permit the use of toilets and hoppers directly, the discharges must first be treated by immersion in 5 per cent cresol solution or some other appropriate disinfectant.

TERMINAL DISINFECTION

Discharging a patient from isolation is simple, provided that there are convenient bathing facilities. All contaminated clothing is left in the sickroom, and the patient takes or is given a thor-

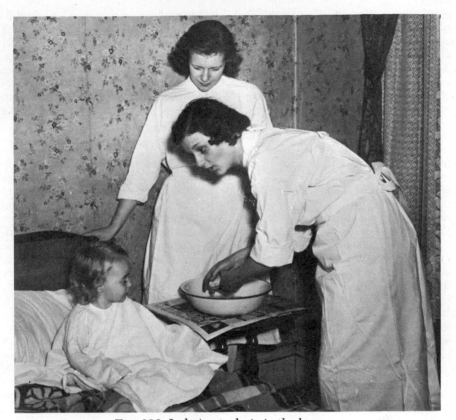

Fig. 106. Isolation technic in the home.

ough cleansing bath, washing of the hair included. Then in a clean room he dresses with clean clothing. The use of antiseptic solutions in addition to the bath is unnecessary.

The terminal disinfection of a room is aided greatly by having very simple furnishings. Rugs, carpets and hangings serve to collect contaminated dust and to make the cleaning of the room more difficult. However, if they have been used, they should be either autoclaved or exposed to light and air for a long period. After disinfection by house-cleaning, the room should be aired thoroughly for at least 24 hours before being used again. This period may be shortened to a few hours by the use of an ultra-violet portable lamp.

Isolation in a Home

Such isolation may offer more difficulties than in a hospital equipped for the purpose. Often running water is lacking in the sickroom, and there are many other similar minor difficulties. Two rooms *en suite* serve better than one. The anteroom should be kept uncontaminated and may serve many purposes. The nurse may use it as a place in which to have her meals and exchange her contaminated clothing for her street clothing. It also may be used for boiling or soaking linen. The family should be kept out of the sickroom as much as possible. Any member of the family who enters the room should observe the same technic as is prescribed for the nurse.

Even though the nurse is unaccustomed to doing the work of a housemaid, it is advisable for her to take the responsibility of keeping the room wiped up daily with a moistened dust cloth. The nurse also should supervise the boiling of the dishes and other disinfection procedures.

In some instances, it is necessary to teach the mother the details of isolation technic (Fig. 106). Some improvising often is necessary. Contaminated material to be carried from the sickroom should be so wrapped or prepared as to permit its being transported without contamination of the person carrying it. Papers can be spread outside the door as a place on which to deposit contaminated linen. Then the linen can be wrapped without contamination of the outside of the paper and can be carried to the place of boiling. The food can be brought on a tray or in a pan and removed to the table for eating, the pan being kept clean for use in carrying away the dishes for boiling after the meal.

It is customary to require other children of the household to remain home from school and not to play with the children of the neighborhood. Such children should remain at home for the entire period of the illness of the patient or should be removed to another home for the incubation period of the disease. Removal of a sick child to a hospital will shorten the stay of the well children at home to the incubation period of the disease.

HOSPITAL ADMITTING WARD

Institutions for the care of sick children should be provided with facilities suitable for the separate isolation of those newly admitted children who have a communicable disease. For this purpose, some hospitals have cubicled admitting wards in which isolation technic is carried out. All newly admitted children pass through this ward, even though no indication of communicable disease exists. The need for special admitting wards to accommodate all newly admitted children is much less than formerly, in a large measure because of the greatly decreased number of diphtheria carriers. Usually at present isolation is practiced only for those children suspected of having a communicable infection.

Viral Infections

Viruses, which cause a number of our common infectious diseases, are minute submicroscopic particles with certain common properties. In some measure these properties explain the characteristics of virus infections. The general remarks about viruses which follow are not strictly applicable to each of the virus infections subsequently described but they may give the reader a theoretic framework which will aid in the understanding of the symptomatology, the prevention and the treatment.

Unlike the bacteria, viruses cannot survive for long unless they are in intimate relation with living cells. Some viruses are quite precise in their requirements and must parasitize not only a certain type of tissue cell but even require also a certain species of animal. Virus particles are regarded as incomplete forms of life which must borrow enzyme systems from living cells in order to carry out their metabolic processes and to reproduce themselves. Once furnished with an appropriate environment, many of them will increase at an extraordinarily rapid rate and overwhelm the tissues which they infect. Recent laboratory technics have made it possible to support virus life outside the animal body by supplying the proper living cells in tissue culture media.

In general, viruses enter the body and

PLATE 4

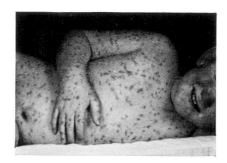

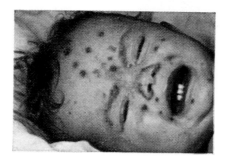

(Top) The rash of measles.
(Bottom) The rash of chickenpox.

PLATE 5

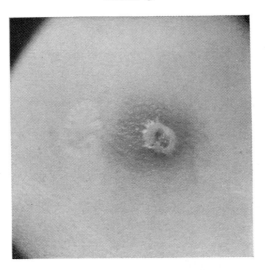

A taking vaccination with scar of previous vaccination next to it, demonstrating that immunity is not necessarily permanent. (From Franklin H. Top, M.D., *Communicable Diseases*, St. Louis, Mosby, 1955, and *Therapeutic Notes*, Parke, Davis and Company)

PLATE 6

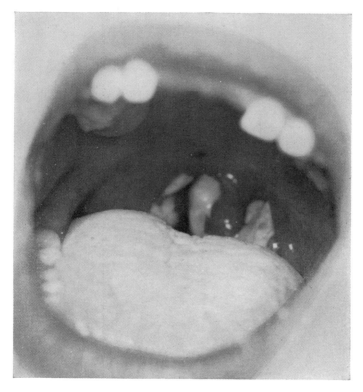

Diphtheritic throat showing membrane on the tonsils.
(From Franklin H. Top, M.D., *Communicable Diseases*,
St. Louis, Mosby, 1955, and *Therapeutic Notes*, Parke,
Davis and Company)

then remain clinically dormant through an incubation period which is at least a week in length and sometimes much longer. During this period they presumably are migrating toward the cells which they wish to infect. Symptoms of disease do not appear until virus multiplication is well advanced and the favored cells are being attacked. Thus, by the time a clinical diagnosis can be made, the virus already has gained a foothold in the tissues which it seeks to invade.

Treatment of most virus infections is relatively ineffectual in controlling the growth of virus particles which already have entered cells. In this sheltered location it is impossible for specific antibody or antibiotics to affect them. (There are a few exceptions to this statement.) Under natural circumstances the disease is brought to a conclusion when the body begins to produce specific antibody against the infecting virus. This antibody probably does not enter the cells but it limits infection to those cells which already have been attacked and disposes of virus which is circulating among or being released from them. In some instances artificially given antibody or antibiotic may speed this process but in general they have little advantage over natural controlling mechanisms. Clinical recovery is frequently abrupt and probably corresponds to the point at which antibody has gained the upper hand over the infecting virus. For most of the diseases which will be discussed subsequently, the quantity of antibody production is sufficiently great to result in a long period of protection from reinfection—often the protection lasts for the rest of the person's life.

Prevention of virus diseases may be achieved in two ways: (1) by artificially stimulating the body to produce antibody through the administration of a vaccine and (2) by administration of antibodies which have been formed previously by another person who has had the infection. The first method (active immunization) is used before the person encounters the disease in question and is the best method of providing a long-standing protection. Unfortunately, it is not available for many virus diseases. The second method of passive immunization may be used during the incubation period when known exposure has occurred but before the virus has been able to get an irreversible foothold in the tissues.

MEASLES (RUBEOLA, MORBILLI)

Measles is a disease having symptoms of respiratory infection and a characteristic enanthem and exanthem (Plate 4).

ETIOLOGY

Measles is caused by a virus which, during the active stage of the disease, is present in the nose, the mouth, the throat and the eyes and in the discharges from them. Measles is one of the most highly communicable diseases. It is communicable from the beginning of the respiratory symptoms and before the appearance of the rash. The period of greatest communicability is at the height of the respiratory symptoms, and it diminishes as these symptoms subside.

Measles occurs chiefly in the late winter and the early spring. Infants under 6 months of age usually do not acquire measles even though thoroughly exposed to it, because their mothers transmit protective antibody to them via the placenta. After this age, the susceptibility at all ages is great. One attack usually protects permanently against a second attack. Second attacks occur occasionally, but in most instances of reported recurrence one of the two illnesses probably was due to some disease other than measles. Relatively few adults acquire measles because of the protection afforded the majority by a previous attack in childhood.

Symptoms

The symptoms of measles begin to appear after an incubation period of from 10 to 11 days. Approximately 14 days elapse between exposure and development of the rash. The invasion is gradual, with fever and coryza. During this early stage, it is difficult to distinguish measles from an ordinary cold. The enanthem appears on the second or the third day, and the exanthem on the third, the fourth or the fifth day. The original respiratory symptoms continue and extend. Lacrimation and photophobia are associated with the conjunctivitis. The discharge from the eyes becomes purulent. Sneezing is frequent at the onset, and complaint is made of soreness of the throat. The infection may extend to the ears and cause otitis media. It always extends to the larynx, the trachea and the bronchi, and frequent cough, sometimes modified to a "brassy" sound by the laryngitis, is a distressing symptom. By secondary invasion of other organisms—usually streptococci—bronchopneumonia becomes a relatively common complication. The white count is normal or low throughout the course of measles except when pyogenic complications occur.

The fever reaches its height within a few days of the onset and remains high until the rash is fully developed over the body. In a few instances, a transitory decrease in fever occurs just before the appearance of the eruption. In the absence of complications, the fever either ceases by crisis or decreases rapidly by lysis with full development of the rash. The constitutional symptoms usually correspond in severity and duration to the course of the temperature. Irritability, malaise, drowsiness and often chilly sensations are present. Headache is common, and delirium may occur. As with other infections, the child may be affected mildly, moderately or severely. The illness may be so severe that the child dies before the rash appears, or the rash may be hemorrhagic. Such severe varieties of measles are uncommon, and death seldom occurs as a direct result of measles but only as a result of complications.

Enanthem

The most characteristic feature of the enanthem is bluish-white spots, pinpoint size, surrounded by a red areola on the mucous membrane of the mouth. These spots are known as Koplik's spots and are important in the early diagnosis of measles before the rash appears on the skin. Koplik's spots disappear quickly, sometimes by the time the rash has appeared.

Exanthem

The exanthem or rash appears first somewhere on the head and spreads gradually over the body. From 3 to 4 days are required for it to reach its greatest extent and then it persists for from 1 to 6 days longer. The rash consists of small dark-red papules which increase in size and coalesce into groups. Between these groups of papules the skin appears to be normal. The contrast between the blotchy, raised areas of redness and the normal skin surrounding them produces the appearance characteristic of the rash of measles. The character of the rash is thus very different from that of scarlet fever, in which the appearance from a distance is that of diffuse redness with no normal skin in the same area as the rash. Unlike scarlet fever, the rash of measles always involves the face in the same manner as other parts of the body. After the rash has faded, there remains in the same blotchy areas a pigmentation of the skin which persists for several days.

The superficial layer of skin begins to desquamate during the second week in very fine flakes, the desquamated skin never being of the size or the thickness found after scarlet fever. This process lasts from 5 to 10 days. In rare instances when the illness and the rash are unusually severe, petechial hemorrhages occur in the areas of eruption, causing what has been termed "black measles."

COMPLICATIONS

Bronchopneumonia is the most important of the common complications of measles. Otitis media, though frequent, is not so serious. The stomatitis which is a part of measles in the early stage usually causes no difficulty and requires no special attention but it prepares the way for the more serious ulcerative variety which sometimes occurs as a complication. Nephritis is infrequent. Encephalitis, although not common, occurs approximately once in a thousand cases. It is a cause of death in a few instances. Complete recovery may be expected in more than half the cases, residual defects of varying severity persisting in the remainder. Measles is reputed to be an activator of pre-existing tuberculous infection. In severe measles, as in any other severe infection, the intoxication may be great enough to affect the myocardium and cause dilatation of the heart and a rapid feeble pulse. If the circulation fails for this reason during the eruptive stage, the rash fades or even disappears. The popular fear of the "rash going in" has no foundation except as this event may be dependent on circulatory failure. Keeping the rash well out by the use of heavy clothing or a hot room is more of a disadvantage than otherwise.

ISOLATION PERIOD

The isolation period of measles should be for the duration of the catarrhal symptoms. This period is from 1 to 2 weeks after the beginning of symptoms and from 2 to 3 days after the temperature becomes normal. In most instances, 5 days after the appearance of the rash is a sufficient isolation period.

PROGNOSIS

The prognosis in measles is dependent in part on the age and also on the previous condition of the child. The younger the child and the poorer the physical condition, the more likely is the disease to result seriously. In the general population, the mortality rate is seldom more than 1 per cent and it is usually less. In a hospital where children already are ill, especially in a ward for infants, the mortality rate may be expected to be several times that in the general population.

PREVENTION

Active immunization against measles is at present in the experimental stage and is not yet available. Temporary passive immunity may be conferred by means of convalescent serum, by means of "immune globulin" prepared from human placenta or by means of gamma globulin extracted from pooled blood plasma. If immune serum or globulin is given parenterally within a few days of exposure to measles, development of the disease will be prevented. If 5 or 6 days are allowed to pass before serum is given, measles will develop, but in a mild and modified form. After symptoms of measles have appeared, serum has no effect on the course of the disease. In the case of young or ill children or children in an institution, complete prevention is desirable, and the serum should be given as soon as possible after exposure. In the case of older and healthy children in their own homes, it is often desirable to give the serum late in order to permit the development of the disease in a controlled mild form, and perhaps confer lasting active immunity. Serum given late tends to prolong the incubation period.

DIAGNOSIS

Typical measles offers little difficulty in making a diagnosis. The rash of measles may be simulated by that of German measles, in which condition respiratory symptoms are mild or lacking, and Koplik's spots never are present. Some drug eruptions may resemble measles for a short time. These rashes may be distinguished from measles by the history of drug ingestion and by the absence of respiratory symptoms.

TREATMENT AND NURSING CARE

The child should be kept in bed as long as fever persists and as much longer as cough and physical signs of lung infection are present. No special diet is indicated, except that in any acute febrile illness the diet during the acute stage should be light and easily digestible, consisting chiefly of liquids. Because of photophobia, the eyes should be protected from light until it is no longer unpleasant. For this purpose, some means other than darkening the room is preferable. The child's bed may be placed in such a position that he does not have to look directly into the light of a window. Wearing dark glasses or placing a screen behind the bed will shield the child's eyes from bright light. Unusually high fever is controlled by hydrotherapy. Cough is controlled by sedatives when severe enough to disturb sleep and rest. Often moist air is used in the management of laryngitis or bronchitis. Any itching associated with the eruption may be controlled as suggested for scarlet fever.

All of the complications of measles except encephalomyelitis are the result of bacterial invasion of mucous membrane surfaces which have been debilitated by the infection with measles virus. Antibiotic therapy controls these complications. In some instances antibiotics are given during the febrile period of measles in order to forestall bacterial invasion.

RUBELLA (GERMAN MEASLES)

Rubella is a contagious disease characterized chiefly by a skin eruption and mildness of constitutional and associated symptoms. It is a relatively unimportant disease because of the slight and fleeting incapacity produced. Its chief importance is from the standpoint of diagnosis because of its resemblance to measles or scarlet fever.

ETIOLOGY

Rubella is caused by a virus which is present during the early stage in the upper respiratory tract. The incubation period varies from 7 to 22 days. The disease does not commonly occur in the first 6 months of life. The immunity produced by the disease is permanent, and recurrences are rare.

SYMPTOMS

Symptoms of invasion are often absent. When present, they consist of slight fever and malaise and mild catarrh. The fever rarely lasts more than 2 days, usually less. The catarrhal symptoms consist of coughing and sneezing. Congestion of the mucous membranes of the nose and the eyes is present. Even though no complaint may be made of sore throat, there is to be seen almost constantly a diffuse redness of the pharynx and often slight swelling of the tonsils. In many cases, there is an enanthem on the soft palate, consisting of red spots pinhead in size. Koplik's spots never are found. Slight general glandular enlargement occurs. Enlargement of the posterior cervical and occipital glands is of some diagnostic importance. The white blood count is normal or low.

Rash

Soon after the onset of the symptoms of invasion or in their absence, the eruption appears on the face and in the course of from a few hours to a day spreads over the body. The first thing calling attention to the disease may be the finding of a rash covering the body. Sometimes the rash has faded from the face and the neck by the time the extremities are involved. The total duration of the rash is not more than from 2 to 4 days, often less. The eruption consists of erythematous spots, slightly papular, which vary in size from that of a pinpoint to several millimeters, and they are usually discrete. In some areas these spots may become confluent and assume somewhat the blotchy appearance of measles. The eruption is subject to considerable variation, even in different cases in the same epidemic. It may be of such a character as to resemble closely the rash of measles in one case and that of scarlet fever in another. A faint desquamation similar to that found in measles sometimes follows the eruption.

COMPLICATIONS

On rare occasions encephalitis occurs as a complication of rubella. The only other complications of importance are certain congenital malformations of the fetus when the mother develops the disease. If rubella affects the mother during the first 3 months of pregnancy, the fetus may develop congenital cataract or malformation of the heart or both. Later in the pregnancy rubella has no effect upon the fetus.

ISOLATION

Isolation is not considered necessary except in institutions if the diagnosis is certain. By the time the diagnosis is made the remaining infective period is brief. The child probably is not a source of infection after the rash has faded.

PROGNOSIS

The prognosis in rubella is good except in those few instances in which encephalitis occurs as a complication. In many instances, recovery from encephalitis is complete.

PREVENTION, DIAGNOSIS AND TREATMENT

Sometimes prevention is attempted when a susceptible woman is exposed during the first trimester of pregnancy. Gamma globulin is used, but its efficacy is not well established.

Diagnosis is relatively easy in an epidemic but difficult in sporadic cases. The disease can be simulated by various toxic and drug eruptions and by very mild scarlet fever. It lacks Koplik's spots and the more severe catarrhal symptoms of measles.

Treatment other than brief isolation is not required.

EXANTHEM SUBITUM (ROSEOLA INFANTUM)

Exanthem subitum is a benign, presumably infectious, disease of infancy and early childhood characterized by fever of from 3 to 5 days in duration which terminates by crisis and by a morbilliform eruption which appears as the temperature declines.

ETIOLOGY

The causative agent has not been identified but probably is a virus. Although direct communicability is not evident and no epidemics have been reported, sporadic cases tend to occur in a community at approximately the same time. The disease occurs predominantly in infancy and nearly always under 3 years of age, though a few cases in older persons have been reported.

SYMPTOMS AND COMPLICATIONS

The onset is abrupt, with fever which rises to between 102° and 105° F. in a few hours. Accompanying the fever may be a moderate amount of restlessness, fretfulness, irritability and food refusal, but these are not constant. Despite the high fever, the child does not appear to be toxic and even may be playful and apparently comfortable. On examination, no abnormality other than fever may be noted. One constant characteristic of the disease is leukopenia, with relative increase in lymphocytes. In different cases the white count varies from 2,500 to 7,000, and the proportion of lymphocytes is between 75 and 85 per cent.

A few children present slight redness of the throat. In some groups of cases reported, moderate enlargement of the superficial glands of the neck has been present; in other groups, this has been absent. The glandular enlargement, if present, appears on the second or the third day. The fever continues for approximately 4 days, with some tendency to slight morning remissions. The fever ends usually by crisis, and at the same time the characteristic eruption appears. With the cessation of fever and the appearance of the eruption, any previous indisposition disappears, and the child seems to be as well as ever.

Eruption

The eruption is macular or at times slightly maculopapular. The early individual lesions are pink or pale red and about 3 mm. in diameter. They tend to increase in size and to coalesce, in this respect resembling measles. The color disappears on pressure. As the lesion becomes older, it tends to fade at the center and irregularly acquires a slightly bluish color, similar to some lesions of erythema multiforme. No unanimity exists in published reports as to the site of first appearance of the eruption, and one is led to the conclusion that no uniformity exists. Regardless of where it begins, it spreads rapidly to its maximum extent and when fully out is most extensive and prominent on the trunk or perhaps the trunk and the neck, and the lesions are relatively sparse on the face and the extremities. Usually the eruption reaches its height in 24 hours or less and disappears in another 24 hours or more. Either no desquamation, or at most a very faint branny desquamation, follows.

No complications or fatalities ever have been reported.

ISOLATION

No isolation is required. Any transmissibility that the disease may have probably is terminated by the time the rash appears and the diagnosis is made.

DIAGNOSIS AND TREATMENT

The diagnosis cannot be made with certainty before the eruption appears. After it appears, the diagnosis presents no difficulty. The two diseases with which it might be confused are measles and rubella. It does not have the catarrhal symptoms or the Koplik's spots of measles. High prodromal fever is absent in rubella.

No treatment is needed.

SMALLPOX (VARIOLA)

Smallpox is a highly communicable disease with severe constitutional symptoms and a generalized pustular eruption which tends to leave permanent pitted scars.

ETIOLOGY

Smallpox is caused by a virus which, in the course of the disease, is present in the skin and the mucous-membrane lesions, the nose and the throat, the blood, the alimentary tract, the feces and the urine. The disease is contagious from the beginning of the earliest symptoms and until all lesions are healed. It is transmitted easily by a third person and by air pollution.

Smallpox occurs in any exposed person, regardless of age, who is not immune by reason of a previous attack or of vaccination. Were it not for vaccination, smallpox would be chiefly a disease of childhood. Smallpox may occur as a mild illness because of partial but waning immunity from vaccination many years previously. It may occur as a mild illness also because of low virulence of the virus strain. A few epidemics are caused by a strain of fixed and relatively low virulence.

SYMPTOMS

After an incubation period, which averages from 11 to 12 days, the symptoms of invasion appear. The onset is abrupt, with headache, backache and fever, and with the temperature rising to between 103° and 104° F. The sudden rise in temperature often causes a chill or a convulsion. With high fever, delirium is likely to be present. Prostration is severe. Vomiting and constipation are common. After from 1 to 2 days of illness, there appears a prodromal rash which may resemble that of scarlet fever or of measles. It is of brief duration.

Eruption

Approximately 3 days after the onset of symptoms, the characteristic eruption begins. It tends to appear first on the forehead and the wrists. In the next 1 to 3 days it spreads over the remainder of the body, with a greater concentration of lesions on the head, the arms and the legs than on the trunk. Thus the distribution is centrifugal.

The earliest lesion is a small round macule. Rapidly and within a few hours, the macule becomes a papule, which enlarges. In approximately 3 days, the papule becomes vesicular with a depressed center (umbilicated). The lesion becomes definitely pustular during the next few days. The course of the lesion is similar to that of vaccinia. The lesion of smallpox is deep-seated in the skin. In the papule stage it feels shotty. The early vesicle is pearl-colored and it never has the clear, watery appearance of an early varicella vesicle. After the pustule has developed fully, it begins to dry, and a firmly adherent crust forms. The crust gradually loosens and falls off in from 4 to 6 weeks after the onset of the disease.

The pustules often become confluent on the face and sometimes on the extremities. Discrete pustules have a red areola. The severe inflammation of the pustule causes edema. Where the lesions are grouped closely, as on the face, the edema may be severe. Usually many pustules become ruptured, and some become infected secondarily with pyogenic bacteria. The odor of the free pus is unpleasant. When smallpox is very severe, blood may extravasate into the skin lesions and thus change their appearance markedly.

Enanthem

The lesions of smallpox may occur on any mucous surface. They are easily visible in the mouth and the throat. When they occur on a surface constantly moist, they lose their covering quickly and appear as ulcers. At times these lesions interfere seriously with the ingestion of food. When they occur on the cornea, careful treatment is required to preserve vision. If they occur in the larynx, tracheotomy may be necessary.

COMPLICATIONS

The most common complications are those caused by pyogenic bacteria which have invaded the pustules. Furunculosis, erysipelas or septicemia may result. Because of the virus nature of the infection, myelitis or encephalitis may occur. As in any severe toxic disease, bronchopneumonia may be a complication.

PROGNOSIS

Except in those instances in which the virus is of low virulence, the mortality from smallpox among the unvaccinated is in the range of from 25 to 35 per cent. It is higher among infants and young children than among those older. Most of the deaths occur within the first 2 weeks of the disease.

PREVENTION

Vaccination with cowpox virus is a fully adequate and satisfactory means of prevention. Not more than a dozen cases occur in the United States in any given year. Vaccinia is discussed separately.

DIAGNOSIS

Diagnosis before the eruptive stage is difficult and may be impossible with certainty. If an epidemic is present, the diagnosis may be strongly suspected from the symptoms of invasion. During the eruptive stage, varicella is the chief disease to be considered in differential diagnosis. The lesions of smallpox are more deep-seated in the skin. At no stage do they have the clear, watery appearance of the varicella lesion in its early stage. The lesions of smallpox are more abundant on the extremities than on the trunk. In chickenpox the reverse is true. Varicella lesions appear in crops, and in any one area several stages in the evolution of the eruption are to be found. In smallpox, all lesions of any one area are in the same stage of development. Usually, varicella is a mild disease, and variola is severe. Difficulties in diagnosis arise when smallpox occurs as a mild disease.

TREATMENT AND NURSING CARE

An important phase of the management is isolation. The isolation technic must be far more rigid than for any other communicable disease. A completely separate unit is preferable for the hospital care of those with smallpox. Closed technic is desirable. With such technic, no contaminated article and preferably no contaminated person should leave the smallpox unit before disinfection. Vaccination of everyone in the vicinity is desirable. Isolation should be continued until all crusts are off and should be terminated with a thorough bath.

Discomfort is great during the invasion period and again later during the height of the pustular stage. Sedatives usually are indicated for these periods. An icebag is useful for the headache and a hot-water bottle for the lumbar backache of the invasion period. Soreness of the mouth during the pustular stage may require local treatment. If eating is prevented, fluids must be given parenterally.

The skin lesions usually require no treatment until pustule formation is well advanced. At this stage, many pustules are likely to be ruptured, and many more are likely to become infected with pyogenic bacteria. Boric-acid compresses are useful in keeping the skin clean and in minimizing inflammation. They also help to allay itching and subsequently to hasten detachment of the crusts. Infected pustules should be treated by local application of some antiseptic such as 3-per-cent gentian violet. Antibiotic therapy also is useful during the period when infected pustules are present. During the pustular stage, it is desirable to keep the bedcovers away from the skin by means of a cradle. The use of an air mattress also helps to protect the pustules.

VACCINIA

Vaccinia is a local skin lesion produced by the inoculation of cowpox virus for the purpose of protecting against smallpox. Cowpox is a pustular disease affecting cattle and is communicable to man. It is a less virulent and less serious disease for both cattle and man than is smallpox for man. A man who has had cowpox is thereafter immune to smallpox. This view was current among the country folk of England during the life of Edward Jenner (18th century). Jenner was the first to take advantage of this knowledge by making the experiment of inoculating a human being with cowpox (1796). Since then, cowpox vaccination has become customary in many countries and compulsory in some.

Cowpox acquired naturally is a generalized disease, as is smallpox. Inoculation into the skin produces only a local lesion but it gives immunity to both cowpox and smallpox. The virus of cowpox is contained in the pustules of this disease. Early in the history of vaccination, inoculations were made from the pustule of one human to the skin of another. Complications were not uncommon. Sometimes pyogenic and other bacteria were carried along with the virus. Inoculation is no longer made from the human. In commercial production the virus is obtained from the calf under most carefully controlled conditions. The safeguards are such that complications of the variety mentioned are all but impossible. Some of the available vaccine is produced by growing the virus in the chorio-allantoic membrane of the chick embryo with still further elimination of the hazard of bacterial contamination.

VACCINATION

Vaccination or the inoculation of cowpox virus may be carried out as follows: The skin of the site chosen for inoculation is washed first with soap and water and then with ether or acetone. After drying, the skin is scratched or punctured through a drop of the prepared vaccine. The object is to infect the skin with the virus and with the virus alone. If the scratch procedure is used, 2 or 3 short parallel scratches are made with a needle, not deep enough to draw blood. If the multiple puncture method is used, the skin is punctured lightly several times with the needle. Usually the needle is held almost parallel with the skin surface in order to control the depth of puncture. After the inoculation, the vaccine remaining is wiped off. No dressing is applied.

Inoculation Site

The inoculation site usually chosen is the left arm at the insertion of the deltoid muscle. In the case of girls and women, the lateral surface of the calf of the leg is sometimes chosen, or the inoculation may be made on the thigh. (In these areas the risk of secondary infection is greater.)

Course of the Lesion

After the lapse of 2 or 3 days, the inoculation site should appear normal except for slight evidence of the original trauma. On the fourth or the fifth day, a papule appears (Plate 5). This increases rapidly in size and becomes vesicular. The vesicle is pearly gray and surrounded by an area of redness. The vesicle is a pustule or quickly becomes pustular. It increases in size and reaches its maximum extent by the ninth or the tenth day. At this time, there may be some swelling of the axillary glands and constitutional symptoms consisting of fever, malaise and irritability. After the tenth day, the pustule begins to dry and the neighboring inflammation to disappear. The constitutional symptoms subside rapidly. The crust which forms as a result of the drying of the pustule gradually loosens and falls off, usually late in the third week, leaving a scar which later becomes white and depressed and is characteristically pitted.

Management of the Lesion

Many prefer no dressing at any stage of the lesion. Some suggest that gauze be pinned inside the sleeve over the pustule. A very good procedure is to place a plain gauze dressing over the pustule and hold it in place by adhesive tape in such a manner that constriction of the swollen arm by the tape is not possible. The object of the dressing is to prevent secondary infection in case the pustule should be broken accidentally. If the pustule should rupture, the dressing will adhere to it. Then if it is desired to change the dressing, the outlying portions of the gauze are cut away, leaving the small circle of gauze stuck to the lesion. Then a new dressing is applied over the old one. A "vaccination shield" should not be used.

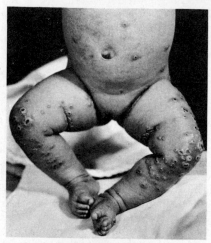

FIG. 107. Generalized vaccinia.

COMPLICATIONS

Complications in vaccinia are uncommon. The most common are those arising from secondary infection of the pustule, such as erysipelas and sepsis. Sometimes a child will rub the freshly vaccinated spot with a finger, then with the same finger rub the skin elsewhere and produce a second lesion. Generalized vaccinia or cowpox is a rare complication but potentially serious (Fig. 107). Infants with exuding eczema are particularly susceptible. They should be neither vaccinated nor exposed to others who have been vaccinated recently. Also rare is encephalitis, a serious complication when it does occur. For the 60 to 70 per cent who survive, recovery is complete. Encephalitis is more rare in infancy than later.

TREATMENT OF SYMPTOMS

Usually the constitutional symptoms are not severe enough to require treatment. For severe symptoms, remaining in bed is sufficient. The treatment of any pyogenic complication is that which is applicable irrespective of vaccinia. The treatment of encephalitis and of generalized vaccinia is symptomatic.

VACCINATION FAILURE

Vaccination may fail to "take" because of faulty performance of the procedure. When properly done, two reasons exist for failure. It will be unsuccessful if the person is immune because of previous vaccination or smallpox. In these circumstances, an immune reaction will appear. This reaction consists of the development of a small area of induration and redness within a day or two of vaccination. More often, vaccination is unsuccessful because the virus used is no longer living. The virus as dispensed commercially will remain living for many months if kept cold and away from sunlight. Continued exposure in a warm room will soon make it useless.

REVACCINATION

Although a single vaccination may protect for life, immunity for so long a period cannot be relied on. Vaccination in infancy and revaccinations from 12 to 14 years and at from 25 to 30 years are to be recommended. When the first vaccination is performed in early infancy, the reaction is much less severe than at later periods of life. After successful vaccination all subsequent vaccinations tend to have milder reactions.

CHICKENPOX (VARICELLA)

Chickenpox is a highly communicable virus disease in which the chief feature is a generalized vesicular eruption (Plate 4).

ETIOLOGY

The virus of chickenpox is present in the nose and the throat, in the vesicles of the eruption and probably in the crusts resulting from the drying of the vesicles. The disease is rare in the first 3 months of life but occurs at the first exposure after this age. It is one of the most highly communicable diseases.

SYMPTOMS

The incubation period is from 14 to 16 days. Prodromal symptoms usually are absent or are limited to a slight fever of which no complaint is made. Rarely, high fever may be present and even convulsions. Commonly, the first thing noted is the rash, which appears first on the face or the trunk and a little later on the extremities. New lesions continue to appear over the entire body for a period of from 3 to 4 days. The individual lesion appears first as a macule, which quickly develops into a vesicle, or first a papule and then a vesicle. The vesicle rapidly increases in size to 3 or 4 mm. in diameter within 24 hours of the first appearance of the macule. The characteristic mature chickenpox lesion is a vesicle with a red areola and filled with clear fluid. The vesicle then dries gradually, first becoming depressed at the center, and later becomes a flat crust. The crust falls off in from 1 to 3 weeks.

After the eruption has been present for a day or two, all stages of it may be seen on the skin in the same area. In the same general area may be seen macules, papules, immature and mature vesicles and crusts of dried lesions. The presence of many stages of eruption at the same time is due in part to the development of the lesions in successive crops and in part to beginning retrogression of a large number of lesions before maturity, perhaps because of developing immunity.

The lesions of chickenpox also appear on the mucous membrane of the mouth and the vagina. In these areas no vesicles are seen, but the appearance is as if a vesicle had been present and the top rubbed off, that is, a gray-white spot surrounded by a ring of redness.

COMPLICATIONS

Complications are infrequent. Scratched or traumatized lesions offer a portal of entry for pyogenic bacteria, with resultant local suppuration and sometimes the development of erysipelas. The virus of the disease sometimes causes encephalitis, but complete recovery is the rule. Unlike measles, the small infant obtains little temporary immunity from his mother. At this age the disease tends to be more severe.

ISOLATION PERIOD

An isolation period of from 10 to 14 days is generally considered sufficient, but in institutions that care for children it is preferable that isolation be continued until all crusts are off.

PREVENTION

When chickenpox occurs among children in their own homes, preventive measures other than isolation are not carried out because of the mildness of constitutional symptoms and the rarity of serious complications. On the other hand, the disease becomes important when it occurs in a children's hospital, where it may cause postponement of the treatment for which the child was admitted, for example, of a surgical operation. Other obvious reasons exist as to why an epidemic cannot be allowed to continue in a hospital.

Convalescent serum and gamma globulin are not effective as sources of passive immunity.

DIAGNOSIS AND TREATMENT

The disease most likely to be confused with chickenpox is smallpox. Usually, smallpox is a serious disease with great prostration but it may be mild and resemble chickenpox. Smallpox has only one crop of lesions in any one skin area, and all are in the same stage of maturity at any one time. Smallpox affects more prominently the exposed parts, the extremities and the face, while chickenpox affects chiefly the trunk, with scattered lesions on the face and the extremities. The vesicular lesions of chickenpox are superficial in the skin, and the early lesions contain obviously clear fluid. Smallpox lesions are more deeply seated in the skin, and the early vesicular lesions have a pearly appearance, never that of containing obviously clear fluid.

Usually, no treatment is required. Scratching and picking at the lesions should be prevented by applying petrolatum, by using elbow restraints and by keeping the fingernails cut short. Itching may be relieved by the application of ointments or lotions containing calamine and antihistaminics.

HERPES ZOSTER (SHINGLES)

This disorder, commonly known as shingles, consists of a group of itching or painful blisters that are confined to the distribution of one of the sensory nerves emanating from the posterior root ganglia of the spinal cord. It is recognized by its sharp limitation to one side of the body within a skin area corresponding to a dermatome. It is now thought that herpes zoster is caused by the same virus as chickenpox. Today it is also thought that herpes zoster often represents a second attack of chickenpox in a person who had his first attack years ago. The disease is not very common in children.

MUMPS (EPIDEMIC PAROTITIS)

Mumps is an acute contagious disease affecting chiefly the salivary glands, especially the parotid glands. It causes swelling of these glands, local discomfort and usually moderate constitutional symptoms.

ETIOLOGY

Mumps is a virus disease. It occurs infrequently under 2 years of age and is not common in adults. The period of greatest incidence is between 4 and 15 years. Closer contact is required for the transmission of mumps than for most of the contagious diseases, and only a small proportion of those exposed acquire the disease. One attack usually protects from subsequent attacks. The incubation period varies. It is usually between 2 and 3 weeks, with an average of 18 days.

SYMPTOMS

In most instances there are no prodromal symptoms. When present, they consist of slight fever, malaise, headache and anorexia. These are of short duration before the swelling of the parotid gland begins, associated with local, dull, aching pain. Sometimes both parotids are involved simultaneously; sometimes the disease remains limited to one; but more often one parotid gland is involved first, and after an interval of several days the disease in the other parotid becomes manifest.

The parotid becomes greatly swollen, tender and painful. Much individual variation exists in the amount of local and general symptoms. In the majority, the disease is mild, and most of the discomfort is local. It is difficult to confine such children to bed. Some children have high fever and are prostrated. Opening the mouth may be impossible because of swelling and pain. The swelling begins to subside within 2 or 3 days, and at the same time the constitutional symptoms subside rapidly. By the eighth to the tenth day the swelling and all signs of the disease usually have disappeared.

Frequently, the submaxillary and the sublingual salivary glands are involved coincidentally with the parotid glands. Occasionally, the submaxillary or the sublingual glands alone are affected.

COMPLICATIONS

Although complications occur frequently in some epidemics among adults, they are uncommon in childhood. The most common complication among males past puberty is orchitis. This occurs usually 1 week (sometimes up to 2 weeks) after the onset of mumps, and the local and the general symptoms are severe. The testis becomes greatly swollen and subsequent atrophy occurs in about half the cases. A similar inflammation may occur in the ovaries, the uterus, and breasts or the external genitalia of the female. Pancreatitis is occasionally suspected when mumps is accompanied by abdominal pain.

Meningo-encephalitis of mild degree is the most common complication in the younger child. Increase in the pressure and the cellular content of the spinal fluid may be suspected when headache, vomiting or delirium is marked. Relief of symptoms often follows a lumbar puncture. Recovery is complete in all instances.

Deafness also rarely occurs as a complication, but when it does it is usually unilateral and permanent.

ISOLATION

Isolation of those with mumps should be continued for 2 or 3 days after the swelling has disappeared. Thus, most children can be released by the end of 2 weeks. Any complication prolongs the course of the disease approximately 1 week.

PREVENTION

No proved means for active immunization exists. Convalescent serum given parenterally within a few days of exposure prevents the development of the disease. An appropriate amount of serum is 10 cc.

DIAGNOSIS

A common error in diagnosis is confusion of cervical lymphadenitis with mumps. The lobe of the ear is at the center of parotid swelling, while the swelling of lymphadenitis is slightly lower in the neck. An aid in diagnosis is redness and swelling of the outlet of the parotid duct in the mouth. The blood leukocytes are normal in number or decreased in uncomplicated mumps and increased in acute lymphadenitis.

Laboratory assistance in confirming the suspicion of mumps is now available by looking for the appearance of specific antibodies in the blood. A skin test with inactivated virus is useful in distinguishing between persons who are susceptible and those who are immune. An inflammatory response at the site of injection of the killed virus indicates immunity.

TREATMENT AND NURSING CARE

Treatment and nursing care are symptomatic. Often no treatment is required. For local pain, the application of heat usually gives relief. It may be necessary to restrict the diet to articles of food which do not require chewing. Acid foods tend to increase the pain. Many children are not sick enough to wish to remain in bed. It is common belief that rest in bed helps to prevent complications. Observation of soldiers in World War I showed that this was not the case, particularly as regards orchitis. Complications usually require treatment in bed.

POLIOMYELITIS (INFANTILE PARALYSIS)

ETIOLOGY

Poliomyelitis is caused by a small virus which, when it gains access to the central nervous system, produces dysfunction or death of nerve cells, particularly those in the anterior horn of the spinal cord and the corresponding regions of the brain, i.e., the cells that supply motor nerves. Three general types of poliomyelitis virus have been separated by immunologic methods. These are designated Type I (Brunhilde), Type II (Lansing) and Type III (Leon). In nature, the viruses infect man alone; experimentally, the disease can be produced readily in monkeys and under special circumstances in a few other animals. The work of Enders,

Weller and Robbins, which won a Nobel prize, has accelerated the study of poliomyelitis by providing a simple means of cultivating these and other viruses in tissue culture media and of rapidly testing for antibody against them.

METHOD OF INVASION

The manner in which the virus enters the body and gains access to the cells of the spinal cord or the brain has been under study for a great many years but is not understood thoroughly. Entrance into the body is probably through the mouth, the pharynx and the intestinal tract, perhaps occasionally through the nose. For a brief time early in the disease the virus can be recovered from throat swabs, but a more consistent source is the stools. From some time before the onset of symptoms and often until a month after recovery, virus can be recovered from the contents of the lower intestinal tract. This, together with other experimental evidence, suggests that the chief site of virus multiplication is in the intestine. Recently, its presence in the blood has been determined during a brief period of the illness. In experimental infection of monkeys and in examination of tissues of children who have died, the virus is recovered from various parts of the nervous system. The exact pathway from the intestinal tract to the central nervous system is not settled. Originally, it was believed that the spread occurred along the nerve trunks from their branches in the intestinal wall backward to the cord or the brain. Recently, the mediation of the blood stream as an avenue has been demonstrated.

There is reason to believe that asymptomatic infection with the poliomyelitis virus is a common, almost a universal, event among children. During epidemic periods virus is found in the stools of children living in association with poliomyelitis victims, children who themselves show mild or no evidence of disease. It is judged that fewer than 1 out of 10 children who excrete virus in the stools will have evidence of clinical disease. Furthermore, examination of the blood of adults shows that a high percentage have antibodies against poliomyelitis, even though they never have had the disease. The belief is growing that most children acquire virus infection early in life but that only a few permit the virus to migrate from their intestinal tracts to their nervous systems. The reasons why some fail to keep it localized have yet to be discovered. Vaccination against poliomyelitis presumably will provide the child with a better defense against the transmission of virus from intestine to nervous system.

EPIDEMIOLOGY

There are some peculiarities about the spread of poliomyelitis which require an explanation before any theory of its epidemiology can be accepted. The disease is of little importance in tropical regions but appears with regularity in both north and south temperate zones during the period of the year when hot weather is prevalent. In small geographic areas it fluctuates in importance from year to year, but some areas have more poliomyelitis than others. In large cities it may run in cycles. It seldom attacks small infants. Formerly, it attacked children from 1 to 5 almost exclusively, but in recent years the incidence among older children, adolescents and adults has been rising steadily. The disease tends to be more severe in older children and adults. It is surprisingly uncommon to have more than one person in a family affected, in spite of the fact that others in the family or in the immediate environment can be shown to harbor virus in their intestines.

An intriguing theory which explains many of these facts but is not yet fully substantiated is the following: tropical regions with their steady warm climate and relatively poor sanitation provide favorable circumstances for maintenance and dissemination of poliomyelitis virus present in the stools. Small infants acquire temporary protection from their mothers by passage of antibodies through the placenta before birth. While still having some protection from this source and during a relatively favorable age period they become exposed to virus and acquire an active immunity of their own without suffering from the paralytic disease. Thus much of the populace in tropical areas grows up immune to poliomyelitis. By contrast, the children in temperate zones are reared in a region where virus is present in the community only during a portion of the year and then is removed carefully by modern sanitary facilities. Such children are more likely to grow up without having any contact with the virus until they reach an older age, at which time they are more susceptible to the paralytic form of the disease.

TYPES OF DISEASE

Infection with the virus of poliomyelitis can result in a great variety of clinical manifestations. For convenience these are usually grouped into the carrier state, abortive infection, nonparalytic and paralytic poliomyelitis. The last category is subdivided into spinal and bulbar forms of the paralytic disease. Since the management of each type is somewhat different, they will be considered separately.

The Carrier State

This merely signifies that the child has poliomyelitis virus in his stools but has no evidence of the disease. The condition goes unrecognized except when special epidemiologic studies are in progress. No treatment is required.

Abortive Poliomyelitis

During epidemic periods a large number of children are observed with illnesses which are suspected of being the initial symptoms of poliomyelitis. In some instances this is a correct presumption which can be confirmed by isolation of virus from stools. In other instances it is impossible to be sure what the nature of the illness really is. The symptoms may include brief fever, headache, sore throat, mild diarrhea, abdominal pain, nausea and vomiting. Signs of involvement of the nervous system are lacking, and the spinal fluid is normal. Since the symptoms subside rapidly, no treatment is necessary except limitation of activity and a brief period of observation to be certain that further manifestations are not going to appear.

Nonparalytic Poliomyelitis

This is similar to the foregoing, except that symptoms may be prolonged over several days' time, and in addition there is clinical evidence of meningeal irritation. The latter is manifest by pain in the neck or the back with limitation of flexion of the spine. There may be increased sensitivity of skin or muscles and peculiar sensations such as tingling or transient weakness of muscles. The spinal fluid shows an increase in the number of lymphocytes and a slight increase in protein content. Treatment consists of bed rest and observation until the fever and the other symptoms disappear and it is clear that no paralysis will occur.

Spinal Form of Paralytic Poliomyelitis

Symptoms. In what might be called the average or typical case, the onset is sudden, with fever, headache and prostration, sometimes vomiting, and rarely convulsions. The fever, the headache and the prostration continue. Irritability, general or local hyperesthesia and neck and back rigidity develop. The child may be mentally clear or drowsy. In severe infections, coma may occur. These symptoms constitute the essential features of the preparalytic stage. In most instances, constipation is present, though diarrhea has been a feature of some epidemics. Frequently, the child sweats profusely. Acute upper respiratory infection has been associated with early symptoms in some epidemics.

In many instances, the symptoms enumerated are preceded by a short period of fever with varying minor symptoms, none of which is indicative of the nature of the infection. An afebrile period of from 2 to 3 days intervenes between this vague illness and the more characteristic illness already described. When the disease produces these two "humps" of fever, sometimes it is spoken of as the "dromedary" type (although it is the camel that has two humps).

After the symptoms described have persisted for a variable period, often from 2 to 3 days, paralysis and other phenomena appear. Such true paralysis as occurs is flaccid in type, and the muscle fibers affected cannot function and therefore cannot exhibit spasm. Either the maximum amount of paralysis appears at once or it increases in degree and extent for a period of 3 or 4 days. In the order of their frequency, paralysis occurs in the following parts of the body: one or both legs, one or both arms, combined arms and legs, legs and trunk. The legs are involved in the majority of cases; other parts, to a much less extent.

True paralysis is dependent on the effect of the inflammation on the anterior horn cells and their motor neurons. This effect may be destructive by action of the virus directly on the anterior horn cells, or the effect may be through functional impairment, such as in edema. The indirect effects of the inflammation may be temporary, and in some instances perhaps the direct effects may fall short of destruction and be temporary. Usually, not all of the nerve supply of any muscle is destroyed, although for some muscles all the nerve supply may be thrown out of function temporarily. During the period of temporary dysfunction of the nerve supply, the intact muscle fibers are subject to the harmful effects of spasm. The muscle spasm of this condition is reflex. It is painful and usually tonic, but visible twitching and tremors may be noted. The spasm of an affected muscle causes dysfunction of its antagonist. The muscle spasm is aggravated by manipulation of the affected parts as well as by splinting in a fixed position.

The constitutional symptoms characteristic of the early stages of poliomyelitis seldom last more than 6 or 7 days. Sometimes the hyperesthesia and the irritability last longer. After the paralysis has developed fully, it remains stationary from 1 to several weeks. Although no change occurs in the paralysis during this time, those muscles or portions of muscles which already are paralyzed undergo more or less atrophy. After this short stationary period, improvement in power of the paralyzed parts takes place. Some show complete recovery in a few weeks; others will be completely well in 3 months. The most rapid improvement occurs in the first 6 months. After this time, recovery is slow but may continue for as long as 2 years. After 2 years, nearly half of the children will have recovered completely, while the remainder will show permanent paralysis of varying extent. If the permanent paralysis extensively involves a limb, its further growth, in both size and length, is stunted, the skin is cold and mottled from poor blood supply, and unless proper care is given, contractures occur and result in deformity.

Treatment and Nursing Care. In the absence of useful specific therapy, the treatment is symptomatic and supportive. Seldom in childhood is the fever high enough to require relief. When caused by increased intracranial pressure and if severe enough, headache may be relieved justifiably by spinal puncture. Care of the bladder and the bowel is an important part of the early treatment in many cases. Parasympathetic stimulants such as Furmethide may stimulate bladder contraction. Often the bladder overfills, and catheterization becomes necessary. Some advocate irrigation of the bladder several times daily with 1:1,000 solution of Merthiolate to prevent infection from repeated catheterization. Often spasm of the lower back and the abdomen cause difficulty in emptying the bowel. If constipation is present, appropriate measures should be taken for relief. Prostigmin is sometimes effective. Since the stools contain virus, they should be considered as infectious and treated in the same way as the stools of those with typhoid fever or dysentery.

Maintaining a good bodily alignment is necessary to prevent deformities. The child should be placed on a firm, flat mattress. In those instances in which the legs are affected, the mattress may be pulled away enough from the foot of the bed to allow the heels or the toes to extend over the end. A board should be attached to the foot of the bed to maintain the feet at right angles when the feet are resting against it. The position of the child should be changed frequently.

The diet should be that suitable for the severity of the illness. Usually a soft diet is appropriate except when bulbar involvement causes difficulty in swallowing. Although the fluid intake should be maintained, fluids should not be forced.

The older treatment included immobilization of the paralyzed parts in splints or casts and the relief of pain with sedatives. Neither of these measures is now common practice. Immobilization causes normal muscle units to atrophy and delays recovery of paralyzed muscles. Freedom of motion maintains the normal individual muscle units in good condition, and with appropriate treatment these units of a single muscle may hypertrophy to compensate for damaged portions of that muscle, with no loss of total function.

The pain of poliomyelitis is chiefly from muscle spasm, and the spasm is relieved within a short time by hot applications (Kenny treatment). For the first few days, in most instances the application of hot compresses or packs is the chief treatment used. When spasm and pain have been relieved, passive motion is carried out by moving the part gently throughout the normal range of motion 4 or 5 times daily. The passive motion serves to maintain muscle nutrition and joint sense. Active motion is permitted and encouraged when such activity does not increase spasm and tenderness. When conditions permit and if desired, active motion may be carried out under water within a few days. All manipulation, passive or active, must be limited to that which does not cause pain, spasm or fatigue. The services of a trained physiotherapist are desirable.

The majority of children over 6 years of age suffer from acute anxiety. They have heard about "polio" over the radio and from their peers and parents. They react to their parents' anxiety and they fear that they will be crippled as others have been. Discovering the child's fears is of vital importance in his care. After his fears have been verbalized, he needs to be kept informed about his progress and given help in facing the possible outcome of the disease.

The next step in the treatment is muscle training and re-education. This procedure begins with the use of active motion. Throughout the early treatment period and for as long as any spasm or tenderness remains, the hot packs are applied regularly every day. For a long subsequent period, overactivity may cause return of muscle spasm and dysfunction.

The kind of treatment described can be carried out best in a hospital and by personnel specially trained in the necessary procedures. With this type of treatment, contracture from muscle shortening is prevented, and, as compared with the older methods, the proportion who recover is higher, and the residual disability is less. If possible, hospital treatment should continue for as long as evidence exists of return of muscle function. In those instances in which the legs are paralyzed and a stage has been reached at which the physician desires the child to attempt walking, braces or splints may be prescribed for support.

The final steps in treatment may require operative procedures to improve the efficiency of permanently paralyzed extremities.

Bulbar Poliomyelitis

Symptoms. When the inflammatory reaction of poliomyelitis attacks the higher portions of the central nervous system, especially the bulb, or medulla oblongata, nervous control of vital functions becomes threatened, and the prognosis for survival is reduced. In favorable instances the muscles of the eye, the face, the jaws or the palate alone may be affected. Recovery is complete in most cases, and no serious effects are suffered from the temporary disability. But when the lower cranial nerves and the upper portions of the spinal cord are involved there may be serious disturbance of swallowing, of respiration or of the central control of circulation. Paralysis of swallowing prevents not only the intake of food but also interferes with the disposition of the normal accumulations of mucus and saliva in the pharynx. Aspiration into the trachea may result in pneumonia or atelectasis. When certain areas of the brain stem are involved there may be serious disturbance of the general circulation with progressive cyanosis and weak, feeble pulse. Disturbances of respiration may be due either to involvement of the respiratory center which governs the automatic effort to breath or to paralysis of the muscles of respiration such as the diaphragm, the intercostal muscles and the pectoral muscles. Most of the fatalities in poliomyelitis are caused by disturbances of the circulation or the respiration.

Bulbar poliomyelitis has had a variable incidence in different epidemics, from 5 to 20 per cent of paralytic cases. It is more common in adults and is particularly prone to affect pregnant women. An increased risk of the bulbar form of the disease is observed in children who have had recent tonsillectomies.

Treatment and Nursing Care. The management of bulbar poliomyelitis is frequently difficult and demands the best medical judgment and skillful attentive nursing. If the child's difficulties are limited to an inability to swallow, repeated gentle suction of the pharynx and postural drainage may be sufficient to protect his airway until his ability to swallow returns. Feeding is accomplished by gavage or by a nasal tube left in place. Parenteral fluids may be required if a satisfactory intake cannot be achieved in this way. When the child has respiratory difficulties in addition, it may be impossible to keep his airway clear without performing a tracheotomy.

Patients who require care in a respirator because of failing respiratory muscles present a complicated problem which is handled best by a staff of doctors and nurses who are specially trained for this purpose. Some of the difficulties which must be met are those of maintaining an airway, preventing aspiration, providing mechanical aids in exchanging air, maintaining nutrition and morale, physiotherapy, prevention of intercurrent respiratory and urinary tract infections and eventually rehabilitation of a patient who sometimes is paralyzed extensively and fearful of being weaned from the respirator.

DIAGNOSIS

The diagnosis of poliomyelitis after paralysis has occurred presents no difficulty. Diagnosis in the preparalytic stage with any degree of certainty is obviously not so easy. The preparalytic symptoms which have been enumerated, together with the results of an examination of the cerebrospinal fluid, will give strong presumptive evidence of a correct diagnosis. The cerebrospinal fluid in poliomyelitis, whether preparalytic or abortive, always shows moderate but definite abnormality. The cells are increased, often up to 100, seldom to 500 for each cubic millimeter, and rarely sufficiently to cause the fluid to be definitely cloudy. The proteins of the fluid are increased, and the colloidal tests (Lange, etc.) are positive.

Poliomyelitis may be confused with other infections of the central nervous system such as Coxsackie virus disease, mumps encephalitis, infectious polyneuritis or the virus encephalitides. Spinal fluid examination usually permits a ready distinction between poliomyelitis and acute meningitis.

ISOLATION PRECAUTIONS

To limit the spread of virus from a hospitalized child with known infection, the same sort of precautions as those taken with typhoid fever are required, namely, careful disposal of stools and aseptic technic. The period during which this must be continued is determined arbitrarily and usually is set at about 2 weeks after the onset of symptoms. The child who is cared for at home already has contaminated his environment with virus by the time his disease is discovered, so that enforcement of such isolation measures is probably futile.

PREVENTION

Active immunization with a satisfactory and safe vaccine would be the desirable method of preventing poliomyelitis. The extensive trials and use of the Salk vaccine in the United States in recent years offer hope that significant control can be achieved. Preliminary results indicate that proper immunization will lower the incidence of paralytic poliomyelitis by 75 to 80 per cent. Passive protection of exposed children by administration of transfusions, convalescent serum and pooled gamma globulin preparations has been tried in the past, but to date there is no scientific evidence to indicate that these procedures influence the course of an epidemic. Quarantine measures, closing of schools during an epidemic and isolation of children from one another likewise have failed to have any observable influence. Generally it is considered wise to keep susceptible children from entering households which are known to be contaminated and to prevent chilling and overexertion during the polio season.

COXSACKIE VIRUS DISEASE

This peculiar name (pronounced cook-sock-ee) is applied to a recently discovered family of virus agents which often travel with poliomyelitis viruses and may be isolated simultaneously from the same patient at times. Clinical symptoms of infection include meningeal irritation, pain in the muscles of the chest and ulcerative lesions in the mouth. Fever is usually present for a few days. The infections are self-limited. Complications never occur, and the infections are not known to cause death. The chief importance of these infections lies in the confusion with poliomyelitis which they may occasion.

RABIES

Rabies is a uniformly fatal disease resulting from a specific virus infection of the nervous system usually acquired through the bite of an animal afflicted with the disease. Presumably, all warmblooded animals are susceptible, although in settled communities the dog is the animal most commonly affected. Rabies occurs at any season. The season of "dog days" has no connection either with dogs or rabies, but some increase of the amount of rabies in dogs takes place in warm weather, beginning in April.

The virus of rabies is present in the saliva of rabid dogs and is introduced into the body by means of a bite. The virus travels along nerves, eventually reaching the central nervous system by this route. The time of travel represents all or most of the incubation period, which is widely variable, depending on the quantity of virus introduced, the virulence of the virus, the nerve supply and the distance of the point bitten from the central nervous system. Rabies from bites about the head has a short incubation period. The incubation period is rarely shorter than 2 weeks and may be as long as 6 or 7 months. The average time is from 1 to 2 months. If the virus is introduced in small quantity in an area poorly supplied by nerves, the disease may never develop. Bites through thick clothing are not very dangerous because of the small quantity of virus inoculated. Only from 15 to 20 per cent of those bitten by rabid animals develop the disease.

Symptoms

Regardless of the length of the incubation period the symptoms are equally severe when they occur. The onset and the course are rapid. An outstanding feature is hypersensitiveness and increased reaction to external stimuli. The hyperirritability may be local at first but it rapidly involves the entire body. One of the early symptoms is convulsive contracture of the muscles of swallowing when ingestion is attempted. Soon the convulsive seizures are general and they may occur at the slightest stimulus. There are periods of excitement in which the child may rage about, become destructive and perhaps

attempt to escape. The convulsive and the excitement periods sometimes are interspersed with times of apparently complete normality. Usually the mind is clear throughout this stage of the disease, except during the brief periods of excitement. During convulsions, the child experiences acute agony. Death may occur during the convulsive stage 2 or 3 days after onset of the disease. If the child survives longer, the hyperirritability is replaced by increasing weakness and finally by complete paralysis; death occurs from respiratory paralysis or cardiac failure 3 or 4 days after the onset.

In some instances, the convulsive stage is largely lacking, and in its place a general trembling precedes the paralytic stage. This is spoken of as the paralytic, or in animals the "dumb," type of rabies in contrast with the "furious" type already described. Children with paralytic rabies usually live 1 or 2 days longer than those with the convulsive type.

Treatment and Prevention

Treatment is entirely symptomatic and completely futile.

The only hope in the management of rabies lies in its prevention. The first step in prevention is proper treatment of the wound, and the second is active immunization. Bleeding from the wound should be encouraged. The wound should be cleansed promptly and thoroughly and then either cauterized with fuming nitric acid or irrigated thoroughly with a 20-per-cent solution of soft soap. Tincture of green soap is as effective as nitric acid and is not tissue-scarring. Such treatment of the wound gets rid of much of the virus and thus tends to prolong the incubation period. It may even prevent the disease. Immunization is delayed pending the diagnosis of the condition of the dog, unless the dog has escaped and is not available.

If the dog shows undoubted symptoms of rabies, it should be killed and examined. If the dog is apparently normal, it should be confined for 2 weeks. If the dog remains well for 2 weeks, it did not infect the child with rabies. A dog with manifest rabies does not live longer than 4 or 5 days. The dog's saliva is infective for 3 to 4 days before the symptoms appear. The symptoms of rabies in dogs are not very different from those already described for man. First, there occurs a change in disposition, either to one of sullenness and irritability or to one of unusual affection and desire to be petted. The dog becomes restless and is startled easily. Then occurs either the furious or the dumb type of rabies. In the furious type, the dog runs away and wanders aimlessly, biting whatever animals or humans get in the way. Soon the difficulty in swallowing and convulsions appear, with death in from 3 to 5 days after the onset of the symptoms. In the paralytic type, the dog usually remains at home and is not so much of a public menace. The incubation period in dogs is usually 14 days or less.

The dog should not be killed for examination until the symptoms of rabies are established very definitely, for the reason that satisfactory examination cannot always be made in the early stages. For examination, the dog's head and part of the neck are sent to a suitable laboratory. If the weather is warm, and the distance great, the head should be packed in ice for preservation. Rabies is diagnosed by the findings of inclusion bodies, known as Negri bodies, within the cells in smears or sections of material from certain parts of the brain and the spinal cord. If rabies is diagnosed in the dog, immunization of the bitten child should be begun at once.

In the procedure advocated by Pasteur immunization is carried out by daily injections of active, living but attenuated virus contained in the spinal cords of rabbits in which it has been propagated. The attenuation of the virus is brought about by drying the cords for periods of from 2 to 8 days. The cords are pulverized and suspended in water for injection. The more attenuated virus is injected first, and virus of increasing virulence subsequently. By this procedure, 3 weeks are required to give all the necessary injections. Another satisfactory procedure is to inject gradually increasing quantities of rabbit-cord virus of known and constant virulence. By this method, the necessary injections may be given in 2-weeks' time. A more recent procedure is to use killed virus for immunization. For all methods, the same doses are employed for children as for adults. From 4 to 5 weeks are required for the development of full immunity, 2 or 3 weeks of this time being occupied by the injections. Death from rabies of persons immunized in the manner described is limited largely to those instances in which the incubation period was short or the immunization delayed. Even with these handicaps, the death rate is less than 0.5 per cent of those bitten by rabid animals in contrast with from 15 to 20 per cent among the unimmunized.

The immunization injections are given subcutaneously in the abdominal wall and are spaced as widely as possible. Usually some local reaction occurs, particularly in the second week, with redness, soreness and itching. Occasionally, a slight constitutional reaction is experienced, including urticaria. The immunization is relatively safe, accumulated statistics ascribing to the injected material approximately 1 death in 10,000 immunizations. The deaths are chiefly among adults and never in young children. The cause of the deaths has not been explained.

Recently a hyperimmune serum has been produced to offer passive immunity while awaiting definitive diagnosis of rabies.

INFLUENZA

Influenza is a specific respiratory virus infection caused by a group of closely related virus agents. The symptomatology is well-known—chills, fever, muscular aches, headache and sore throat. A similar train of symptoms may be observed with other acute respiratory infections which are not due to the specific virus of influenza, and differentiation is possible only by special laboratory examination or by suspicion during the course of an epidemic. In general, children are not so seriously affected as adults, and for this reason, prophylactic immunization with influenza vaccine has found little favor. Treatment consists of bed rest, aspirin for relief of symptoms and protection against superimposed bacterial infections.

CAT-SCRATCH FEVER

Cat-scratch fever is a benign disease presumably caused by a virus closely related to that which produces lymphogranuloma venereum in the adult. The agent is carried by cats and may be inoculated into the skin by a scratch or into an open cut. A small local lesion results which heals slowly and may flare up at a later date when the child shows evidence of fever, malaise and enlargement of the lymph nodes which drain the infected area of skin. The symptoms persist for a few days, but the lymph node enlargement may last longer. The disorder may be confused with tularemia, tuberculous adenitis or pyogenic adenitis. Diagnosis is achieved by discovery of a positive skin reaction to a preparation from infected lymph nodes. No treatment is required, since the lesions heal spontaneously, albeit slowly.

VIRUS CONJUNCTIVITIS

Viruses are the cause of inclusion blennorrhea, trachoma and the primary conjunctivitis of measles.

Inclusion Blennorrhea

This disease is more common in the newborn period than at other times. In the newborn the infection is acquired from the vagina of the mother. The disease becomes manifest in from 7 to 12 days after birth. The acute stage has a duration of from 2 to 3 weeks and is followed by a chronic stage lasting from 6 weeks to 6 months. It is a harmless disease in that no serious complications or sequelae develop. The diagnosis is made by finding inclusion bodies in epithelial cells scraped from the conjunctiva and stained. Local antiseptics have no effect. Sulfonamide in standard dosage for 10 days is effective in control.

Trachoma

Trachoma is a result of a virus infection which is endemic in some parts of this country. The inflammation of the conjunctiva and the cornea is low-grade and chronic, often lasting over many years. Inclusion bodies are found in conjunctival scrapings. In the early stages of the disease the conjunctivitis is catarrhal or only moderately purulent. As the inflammation becomes chronic, follicles of hypertrophied conjunctival epithelium appear, and blood vessels invade the cornea. In the course of time, these lesions are associated with scarring in the conjunctiva and clouding of the cornea; such damage is permanent. Formerly, no treatment used was wholly satisfactory. At present, sulfonamide seems to be curative in that the virus is destroyed and the disease process is arrested. Existing scarring is likely to remain. Approximately half the standard dosage of sulfonamide is given for about 3 weeks.

Rickettsial Infections

The infectious agents called rickettsia are larger than viruses and barely visible by the ordinary microscope. They are agents which primarily infect ticks, mites, fleas and lice but may be transmitted to man in some instances. Like the viruses they are incapable of surviving unless in close association with living cells. The rickettsial diseases of man are not transmissible from man to man but require the mediation of one of the small parasites mentioned above. The diseases that rickettsia produce have some common characteristics—fever, headache, skin eruption, leukopenia, self-limited course and favorable response to chlortetracycline (Aureomycin), oxytetracycline (Terramycin) and chloramphenicol. Detailed description will not be given because these infections are uncommon in the United States, and each of them has a rather limited geographic area of prevalence.

ROCKY MOUNTAIN SPOTTED FEVER
(TICK TYPHUS)

This is the most severe rickettsial infection seen in the United States. As the names suggest, it is found in the Rocky Mountain area and is transmitted to man by infected ticks. The onset is abrupt with high fever and severe headache followed by a measles-like rash which generally is more marked on the extremities than on the trunk. The prognosis of the untreated disease is rather serious, but rapid response to chlortetracycline or its related antibiotics is to be anticipated. A vaccine is available for active immunization.

MURINE TYPHUS

Murine Typhus is transmitted to man by fleas and mites which live on rats. It is seen in the southern part of the United States. The symptomatology is similar to tick fever but less severe. It responds to the same treatment.

RICKETTSIALPOX

This is a new disease which thus far has been observed only in New York City. A mouse mite is responsible for its transmission to children. A local lesion develops at the site of the infecting bite and before the appearance of the rash which is distributed over the entire body except palms and soles. The disease is self-limited and improves under chlortetracycline treatment.

Q FEVER

This is a rickettsial infection which simulates protracted influenza. It is derived from infected cattle; the mechanism of transmission is imperfectly understood. It too responds to chlortetracycline.

SITUATIONS FOR FURTHER STUDY

1. How do symptoms of German measles differ from those of rubeola? Do infants under 6 months of age acquire measles? What is the period of greatest communicability in measles? In what age period is the mortality rate of measles the highest?

2. Compare the lesions of chickenpox and smallpox. How do they differ? What is the difference in the distribution of the lesions?

3. What specific protective measures against communicable disease can be given during the period of infancy?

4. When caring for a child in the acute stage of poliomyelitis, how could you assist in preventing deformities?

5. What is entailed in the convalescent care of a child with poliomyelitis? What problems would he need help in facing during the convalescent period?

6. A child has been bitten by a neighborhood dog. The mother asks you for advice. What suggestions would you make?

7. What should parents teach their children about dogs?

BIBLIOGRAPHY

Chant, H. L.: Rabies, Am. J. Nursing 47:391, 1947.

Lowman, C. L., Siedenfeld, M. A., and Newton, Kathleen: Poliomyelitis: I. The management of poliomyelitis: II. Psychological considerations in poliomyelitis care: III. The nurse in poliomyelitis, Am. J. Nursing 47:367, 1947.

McKhann, C. F., and Wilson, J. L.: Acute anterior poliomyelitis *in* Brenneman's System of Pediatrics, vol. 2, Hagerstown, Md., Prior, 1948.

Parise, C. Di P.: The patient in a respirator, Am. J. Nursing 51:360, 1951.

Rivers, T. M.: Viral and Rickettsial Infections of Man, ed. 2, Philadelphia, Lippincott, 1952.

Stevenson, J. L.: Nursing for the polio-myelitis patient, Am. J. Nursing 48:290, 1948.

Stimson, P. M., and Hodes, H. L.: A Manual of the Common Contagious Diseases, ed. 5, Philadelphia, Lea & Febiger, 1956.

Webster, L. T.: Rabies, New York, Macmillan, 1942.

Wright, J.: The respir-aid rocking bed in poliomyelitis, Am. J. Nursing 47:454, 1947.

Nursing for the Poliomyelitis Patient (pamphlet), Joint Orthopedic Nursing Advisory Service of the National Organization for Public Health Nursing, New York, 1948.

Psycho-Social and Educational Adjustment of the Child with Poliomyelitis, Nerv. Child (entire issue), vol. 11, no. 2, January, 1956.

CHAPTER TWENTY-FIVE

Bacterial, Fungous, Spirochetal and Protozoal Infections

Bacterial Infections

A large number of bacteria are known to produce infection in man. In this text only a few of the more important pediatric conditions will be considered. Some of them are discussed in other chapters—gonorrheal ophthalmia in Chapter 10, bacterial meningitis in Chapter 22 and dysentery in Chapter 13. In contrast with the viral infections, the incubation period tends to be short, and the course of the untreated disease is prolonged. The degree of immunity which is achieved is variable but in most instances does not result in life-long protection. For most of these diseases some form of antitoxic or antibiotic treatment is available; hence, their prompt and accurate recognition becomes important in order to provide optimum therapy. Isolation of the infecting organism is possible in all of them except tetanus.

DIPHTHERIA

Diphtheria is characterized by the growth of the specific bacillus of this disease on an epithelial or mucous-membrane surface with the production of an exudative membrane and with the production and the absorption of toxin which has severe and destructive effects locally and in distant tissues and organs.

ETIOLOGY

The disease is caused by the diphtheria bacillus, *Corynebacterium diph-*

599

theriae. Diphtheria is endemic in all large communities that have not yet suppressed it with programs of mass immunization of infants. It occurs to some extent in all seasons. With the coming of winter the incidence increases, sometimes to the extent of an epidemic, and it declines in late spring. Diphtheria occurs at all ages, but with the greatest frequency between 2 and 6 years. Older children and adults are more common victims in countries which have comprehensive immunization programs for infants. Because antitoxin is used in treatment and because toxin does not produce immunity in the presence of an excess of antitoxin, one attack protects against subsequent attacks in only about one third of the cases.

Symptoms

The characteristic lesion of diphtheria is destruction of superficial epithelium at the site of the infection, with exudation of fibrin and pus cells to produce a pseudomembrane by coagulation of the fibrin in a thick layer. The most frequent location of the infection is in the throat, particularly on the tonsils. It occurs also in the nose and in the larynx and the trachea, and sometimes on the skin. It may be limited to any one of these sites or it may affect several of them simultaneously.

Faucial Diphtheria

Diphtheria of the tonsils and the tonsillar region is known as faucial diphtheria and is the variety most frequently observed. It has an incubation period of from 1 to 4 days. In the average or typical case the symptoms consist chiefly of fever, sore throat, malaise, headache and often general aches and pains. An early throat redness is followed quickly by an exudate which coalesces, becomes thicker and resembles a membrane. The membrane at first is grayish white but later it becomes a dirty gray. The breath has an unpleasant and rather characteristic odor. When the membrane is removed forcibly, a bleeding surface remains. When no treatment is given, the membrane spreads in all directions. It may involve the posterior pharynx, the uvula and the soft palate. The cervical lymph glands are moderately to greatly enlarged, with proportionate visible swelling of the neck. Prostration increases as the disease progresses. Death results in a high proportion of those who are untreated.

Diphtheria may occur with degrees of severity other than that described. It may be of a rapidly fatal fulminating type or it may never become more than a mild catarrhal inflammation manifest by redness and slight soreness. Other organisms, particularly streptococci, are capable of producing a membrane indistinguishable in appearance from that of diphtheria. On the other hand, the lesion produced on the tonsils by diphtheria bacilli, especially in the early stages, may have an appearance identical with that of follicular tonsilitis produced by other organisms. The points of follicular exudate, when caused by diphtheria bacilli, usually continue to increase in size until they meet each other and coalesce to form a membrane (Plate 6).

Nasal Diphtheria

When the lesions of diphtheria are limited to the nose, little and often no constitutional disturbance results. Internal examination of the nose reveals areas of membrane. Nasal discharge is present, sometimes thickly purulent, but more often thin and tinged with blood. The discharge excoriates the upper lip. The disease may extend to the pharynx and the fauces. Nasal diphtheria tends to remain chronic over a period of weeks. Because of the relative infrequency of paralyses and other usual complications of diphtheria, it may be concluded that a lesser amount of toxin absorption occurs in nasal diphtheria.

LARYNGEAL DIPHTHERIA

Diphtheria may occur primarily in the larynx and remain limited to it. More commonly, laryngeal diphtheria occurs in association with and probably as an extension from faucial diphtheria. When the process is limited to the larynx, usually little constitutional disturbance, except that produced by obstruction to the passage of air, is present. The absorption of toxin from this area is relatively poor. Obstruction is caused by inflammatory edema and by membrane and sometimes by an additional factor of spasm of laryngeal muscles excited by the infection. A croupy cough is present, and the voice is lost because of involvement of the vocal cords. Otherwise, the symptoms are chiefly those of respiratory difficulty. The breathing is noisy or stridulous on both inspiration and expiration. The accessory muscles of respiration are brought into use by voluntary effort. Retraction of the tissues of the neck above the clavicle, of the intercostal spaces and often of the abdomen at the chest margin occurs during inspiration. Cyanosis is present, the degree depending on the amount of obstruction. Death from asphyxia is frequent.

The membrane of laryngeal diphtheria frequently extends down the trachea and into the larger bronchi. Symptoms of such extension usually are absent or overlooked because obstruction to respiration is limited to the larynx. The trachea is relatively large, and the laryngeal space between the vocal cords is small. Sometimes laryngeal diphtheria is spoken of as membranous croup, in contrast with catarrhal or spasmodic croup, which has symptoms similar in some respects.

EFFECTS OF DIPHTHERIA TOXIN

The only important damage produced by the diphtheria bacillus is that caused by its toxin. The toxin causes degeneration and death of tissue. At the site of the diphtheria membrane the toxin has killed the superficial tissues. From this site the toxin is absorbed and carried over the body by the blood stream. The effects on the various tissues of the body are proportionate to the amount of toxin absorbed. Certain of the body tissues show the effect more strikingly than others.

Degeneration of the heart muscle (myocarditis) is one of the most serious effects of diphtheria toxin. If myocarditis becomes manifest, it usually becomes evident in the third week of the disease, after all local signs of diphtheria have disappeared. The heart often becomes dilated, the pulse rate changes markedly from the normal, and death from cardiac failure is a frequent outcome, particularly in patients who receive antitoxin late in the course of their infection. Myocarditis which appears before the end of the second week has a very grave prognosis.

Diphtheria toxin also causes degeneration of nerves. In cases of faucial diphtheria, the first nerves to show this effect are those of the soft palate. Paralysis of the soft palate occurs in the second week of the disease. It causes a "nasal voice" and difficulty in swallowing, with frequent expulsion of fluid through the nose because of this difficulty.

It is in the third week or later that other paralyses appear. Paralysis may be general or it may be more conspicuous in one part than in another. The most serious paralysis is that of the muscles of respiration. Complete recovery from all these paralyses always occurs, provided that interference with vital functions (respiration) is not great enough to cause death. Even with respiratory paralysis, recovery occurs if the child can be kept breathing by means of a respirator.

COMPLICATIONS

The direct effects of diphtheria toxin are parts of the disease rather than complications. Otitis media is not uncommon as a complication. Pneumonia occurs occasionally when the illness has been severe.

ISOLATION

Isolation is maintained until several consecutive cultures of the nose and the throat fail to grow the diphtheria bacillus.

PROGNOSIS

In general, the mortality rate is between 5 and 10 per cent. It is higher with laryngeal diphtheria and lower when the infection is limited to the nose. For those who live, complete recovery is to be expected.

PREVENTION

In the event of known exposure of a nonimmune child, temporary protection can be given by antitoxin, which usually is injected intramuscularly for this purpose. A satisfactory prophylactic dose is 2,000 units. A previously immunized child should be given a booster dose of toxoid.

Active immunization produces longlasting immunity. It is used extensively and is to be recommended strongly. The procedure is carried out by means of injections of diphtheria toxin which has been modified in such a manner as to make it harmless. Three varieties of preparation are available, namely, a toxin-antitoxin mixture, a toxoid and an alum-precipitated toxoid. Alum-precipitated toxoid is the one in most common use and usually is combined with tetanus toxoid and pertussis vaccine. Although a single injection of this material may give satisfactory immunity, it is preferable to give 3 injections a month apart. The time required to produce satisfactory immunity varies from 2 weeks to 6 months. The majority are immune within 2 months. It is desirable to verify the existence of immunity subsequently by means of the Schick test. If the test is positive, the child should

have more immunizing injections. Some physicians give booster injections every 3 years arbitrarily without Schick testing.

Schick Test

The Schick test consists of injecting into the skin 1/50 of the minimum lethal dose of toxin for the guinea pig. This amount of toxin is contained in a volume of 0.1 cc. A positive or nonimmune reaction consists of redness, swelling and later pigmentation. In the performance of the test on adults and older children, it is desirable to make a control injection, using material identical with that used for the Schick test except that it has been heated to 100° C. for 5 minutes. Heat destroys diphtheria toxin. Any reaction which occurs with the control solution is due to other proteins which it contains and not to toxin. By comparing the test with the control, the amount of reaction due to the toxin can be determined. The reaction from protein reaches its height usually within 24 hours, while that from toxin does not attain a maximum for several days, at which time the protein reaction usually has disappeared.

DIAGNOSIS

The diagnosis of diphtheria is made by means of the clinical features which have been described and by the finding of the diphtheria bacillus in material from the site of the local lesion. These organisms are found with the greatest reliability when inoculations are made from the diseased area onto a special culture medium (Löffler's blood serum) and the culture is incubated for from 8 to 12 hours or longer. The cultural growth is placed on a glass slide, stained and examined microscopically. Certain throat infections may resemble diphtheria closely. These are distinguished from diphtheria by identification of the causative organism by culture. Not all diphtheria organisms produce disease; only those capable of excreting toxin are pathogenic. Laboratory tests of the capacity to produce toxin take several days to complete. Though valuable in clinching the diagnosis of diphtheria, treatment must be initiated before results of a virulence test can be known.

TREATMENT

The administration of diphtheria antitoxin is of primary importance. It alone can neutralize the effects of free toxin which has not yet become attached to cells. It probably has no effect on toxin which already is combined with cells. A single dosage with antitoxin is to be preferred to repeated small doses, and the common practice is to give 40,000 units intramuscularly. In children who exhibit symptoms of severe toxicity, an additional 40,000 units may be given intravenously. In either circumstance it is imperative to test the child first for sensitivity to horse serum. Unlike toxoid, antitoxin is prepared in horses and is capable of producing a severe or even fatal reaction in a child who is sensitive to it. Testing is done by conjunctival or intracutaneous inoculation of a small amount of the diluted material. An immediate inflammatory reaction appears if the individual is sensitive.

Several of the antibiotics are effective against diphtheria bacilli. The neutralization of the antitoxin should be followed by full dosage with penicillin or one of the broad-spectrum antibiotics such as oxytetracycline, chlortetracycline or tetracycline.

In addition to administration of antitoxin and antibiotics, certain other treatment measures are important. The child should be kept in bed until afebrile in all cases—for at least 2 weeks in cases of moderate severity and for at least 3 weeks in cases of greater severity.

Cleansing gargles or similar appropriate measures add to the comfort of the child. The diet should be modified according to the amount of soreness of the throat and the degree of prostration. If myocarditis should develop, absolute rest in bed is the chief therapeutic measure of importance. Confinement to bed should be maintained until the child has recovered entirely and for several weeks thereafter. The necessary inactivity should be aided by full doses of morphine or other sedative at short intervals. Digitalization is usually employed to augment the activity of the cardiac muscle.

Laryngeal Stenosis

If laryngeal stenosis is present, the breathing of warm moist air (croup tent or steam room) and the administration of such drugs as antipyrine and ipecac will relieve whatever part of the stenosis is caused by spasm of the larynx but will have no effect on stenosis due to edema and membrane. The several possible ways of relieving stenosis due to edema and membrane require special equipment and a certain amount of skill. Cotton swabs passed into the larynx may dislodge and remove membrane sufficiently to allow adequate passage of air. Similarly, aspiration by means of a suction tube may accomplish the same purpose.

A tube shaped to fit the larynx may be inserted into the larynx by way of the mouth (intubation) and left in place until the inflammation has subsided sufficiently to permit satisfactory breathing without it. A tube may be placed in the trachea through an incised opening in the neck (tracheotomy).

The choice between intubation and tracheotomy depends chiefly on the availability of expert medical care. With the decline in the incidence of diphtheria the medical profession has lost the art of intubation for want of practice. Almost without exception hospitals now resort to tracheotomy when relief of laryngeal obstruction is indicated. The nursing care has been discussed in Chapter 17 under laryngo-tracheobronchitis. Tracheotomy tubes are left in place until the membrane formation has been controlled by specific treatment—usually only a matter of a few days.

DIPHTHERIA CARRIERS

Individuals who are found to harbor diphtheria bacilli in their throats with-out being ill themselves are known as carriers. They are a potential menace to the community and should be isolated until freed of their organisms. Penicillin in full dosage for from 1 to 2 weeks is usually effective. If it fails, one of the broad-spectrum antibiotics should be used. If this too fails, removal of tonsils and adenoids or thorough drainage of infected sinuses may be required.

TETANUS

Tetanus (lockjaw) is a disease characterized by tonic muscular spasm, either local or generalized, the spasm being a manifestation of toxic effects on the nervous system produced by the exotoxin of the tetanus bacillus. Unlike diphtheria, it is not contagious or transmissible by contact. It resembles diphtheria in that symptoms are due to a soluble exotoxin which disseminates from the infecting bacilli.

The tetanus bacillus (*Clostridium tetani*) commonly is found in the soil and in the fecal discharges of man and animals. It is a spore-forming organism and in its spore stage can live for an indefinite period of time in dust and under other unfavorable conditions. It is harmless in the alimentary tract. When introduced into the body by way of a wound, it frequently finds conditions favorable to its growth. The organism is anaerobic. An anaerobic environment often prevails in injured tissue. Puncture wounds, crushing injuries and burns are particularly apt to provide favorable soil for the tetanus bacillus. Its growth produces no identifiable local tissue damage and therefore no characteristic lesion. Its growth is accompanied by the production of an exotoxin. The toxin has a special affinity for nervous tissue and finds its way to the central nervous system along the various motor nerves.

Motor nerves of the region of the wound may carry the earliest and largest supply of toxin in some cases, thus accounting for the occasional occurrence of local tetanus. However, usually the toxin reaches the blood by way of the lymph channels and is carried to all the motor nerves of the body, entering them presumably by way of the motor end plates. The interval between the time of infection and the development of symptoms depends on the rate of toxin production, which in turn depends on whether conditions in the wound are favorable for growth of the organism, on the number of organisms introduced and on their virulence or ability to produce toxin. Thus it is that the shorter the incubation, the more severe the disease and the more likely it is to prove fatal. Incubation periods vary from 3 days to 1 month or more, falling between 7 and 14 days in a high proportion of cases. It has been stated as a rule, not strictly true, that the prognosis is bad when the incubation period is less than 9 days and relatively good when the incubation period is longer.

SYMPTOMS

Sometimes the earliest symptom is twitching of the muscles in the neighborhood of the wound. More often—in fact, usually—the first symptoms are in association with the shortest motor nerves of the body, namely, those of the head. Thus a stiffness of the muscles controlling the jaw, a condition known as trismus, is the outstanding first or early symptom. The jaw is held tightly closed and it cannot be opened. Involvement of the muscles of the throat and the tongue causes difficulties in swallowing and in speech. Soon the muscles in the distribution of the spinal nerves are affected, first those supplied by the shorter nerves (the trunk) and then those supplied by the longer nerves (the extremities).

All the voluntary musculature of the body becomes affected and is in a tonic state. Superimposed on this state of continued tonicity are to be observed paroxysms of increased muscular spasm. These paroxysms are termed convulsions, though they differ considerably from the cerebral type of convulsion. Consciousness is not lost or impaired, unless through asphyxia from spastic fixation of the thorax. The convulsions are precipitated by relatively small external stimuli, such as noises, bright lights or jarring of the bed. When all the muscles of the body are in strong contraction, the position of the body is determined by the strongest muscle groups. The characteristic position is one of opisthotonos, often extreme, with the head drawn back and the back arched (Fig. 108). Such strong muscular contractions are very painful, and pain is felt particularly in the back and the head. During the severe paroxysms, the thorax is held immovable, so that the respiratory movements are feeble or absent. This results in cyanosis and anoxia and in many instances in death by asphyxia.

The disease in its most characteristic form increases in severity and then, in those who recover, it gradually decreases in severity. During the stage of increasing severity, the convulsions usually are preceded by twitchings which become more frequent and more severe and gradually merge into the convulsive stage. The convulsions increase in frequency and violence, and the continued tonicity between convulsions becomes greater. The interval after the onset of symptoms required for the full development of the convulsive stage varies from a few hours to 2 days, with an average of about 24 hours.

In the children who survive, the symptoms remain unchanged for a period of from 5 to 10 days or more, after which time they gradually subside, their complete disappearance requiring from 2 to 3 weeks or longer. The temperature may be normal throughout the course of the disease or it may rise to 104° or more. In those who die, terminal pyrexia is common. Death may occur from exhaustion or from aspiration pneumonia. The most common cause of death is asphyxia from fixation of the respiratory

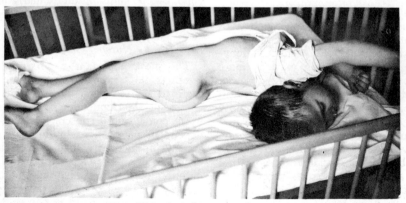

FIG. 108. Opisthotonos of tetanus.

muscles. Bad prognostic signs are a short incubation period, early complete trismus, rapid general development of spasms and high fever. Without treatment by antitoxin the average mortality from tetanus was as high as 80 to 90 per cent. With antitoxin and modern methods it has been reduced to 20 to 50 per cent.

PREVENTION

Passive Immunization

Tetanus may be prevented by parenteral administration of antitoxin soon after the injury which permitted the introduction of the tetanus bacilli. The antitoxin is similar to that used in diphtheria and is prepared in the same manner in horses. Testing for sensitivity to horse serum is essential before it is used. The usual prophylactic dose is 1,500 units. If the wound is large or grossly contaminated, it is sometimes desirable to repeat the dose within a week or 10 days. Decision as to which wounds require antitoxin administration and which do not is sometimes difficult. In cases of doubt the antitoxin should be given. Burns, compound fractures, wounds from explosives (e.g., Fourth-of-July accidents) and any wound in which soil contamination is likely require tetanus prophylaxis.

Active Immunization

Immunity produced by injection of tetanus toxoid (alone or in combination with diphtheria toxoid) produces a long-lasting immunity which may be more or less permanent. At least 2 doses of toxoid are required, spaced from 1 to 3 months apart. The basic immunity thus established may be reactivated within 4 to 6 days if a booster injection is given. Thus in children known to have basic immunity, fluid toxoid rather than antitoxin is given as prophylaxis. No test for horse serum sensitivity is necessary when toxoid is used.

ISOLATION

Isolation is not necessary, since the infecting organisms are harmless unless inserted into a deep wound.

TREATMENT

The treatment of tetanus, once the symptoms have appeared, may be considered as having 3 phases: (1) the performance of any necessary surgery; (2) antitoxin treatment; and (3) symptomatic treatment.

Surgical Treatment

The indications for surgical treatment of the causative wound are the same as for a similar wound in the absence of tetanus. Any foreign body should be removed, any cellulitis or inflammation treated appropriately. The existence of tetanus does not call for radical or emergency operative measures, for the reason that antitoxin will neutralize any toxin that is present or that will be formed in the wound. In most instances, the wound will be healed and require no attention by the time tetanus develops.

Antitoxin Treatment

Enough antitoxin to neutralize all the free toxin within the body and any which is being newly formed in the wound should be given at once. Tests for serum sensitivity are imperative before the dose is administered. For a child, 50,000 units intramuscularly and an equal amount intravenously suffices.

Symptomatic Treatment and Nursing Care

The most important factors in the symptomatic treatment of tetanus are those measures which are effective in decreasing the frequency and the severity of convulsions. The convulsions are dependent on changes in the nervous system produced by toxin which has been "fixed" in the cells. Antitoxin has no effect on the fixed toxin and, consequently, no effect on convulsions. Further fixation of toxin in the cells is prevented by the antitoxin administered. The effect of fixed toxin on the nervous system will continue unaltered for a period of from 5 to 10 days or more, during which time the convulsions will continue to recur unless brought under control by medication. It is important that convulsions be controlled as completely as possible. It is because of the convulsions that many of these children die, and the importance of their control has not been stressed sufficiently. The duty of first importance is to carry out the measures necessary for control of convulsions. This procedure takes precedence over antitoxin administration and all other nursing and medical procedures.

For the control of convulsions it is necessary to employ sedatives in large dosage and in addition to have the child in such a location that he will not be disturbed by noises, bright lights or anything else that is irritating to him. The sedative used will depend on the preference of the physician in charge but could be chloral hydrate, Amytal, Avertin, one of the barbituric acid derivatives or some other drug. With such a drug as Avertin it is possible not only to prevent convulsions but also to maintain a state of relaxation which in the milder illnesses will permit the ingestion of food with relative ease and comfort. Relaxation usually can be obtained well within the toxic limits of the drug and in some cases without disturbing appreciably the consciousness of the child. Some of the drugs mentioned have only a small margin of safety between the therapeutic and the toxic dose. If the child is conscious, an anesthetic should be used for any painful procedure.

The ideal sedative management includes the giving of a dosage which maintains the child continuously in a relaxed state but is no larger than is required for this purpose. Rectal Avertin lends itself well to this kind of management. When this drug is used, the rectal tube should be kept constantly in place, ready for injection at any time. The Avertin fluid is kept in a constant-temperature water bath at body temperature ready for immediate use. After the initial large dose and after relaxation has been attained, subsequent doses of Avertin should be small and given frequently, if necessary, rather than large doses given infrequently. An even level of sedation is desirable. Various criteria may be used as indications for further sedation, but the recurrence of rigidity of the abdominal muscles serves well.

The life of the child depends in large measure on meticulous nursing and medical attention. A nurse should be with the child constantly, and the presence of both a nurse and a doctor is desirable. Without constant watching, suddenly the child may develop a convulsion and die. When the tetanus is severe, the amount of sedative required is sufficient to make the child unconscious, and in some instances the state of unconsciousness must be maintained for a week, or even 2 weeks, continuously. An unconscious child requires many things not needed by one whose reflexes are intact. Food must be given by gavage, and the fluid intake requires special attention. Parenteral fluid administration is often necessary. Bowel and bladder functioning must be watched. Accumulated mucus must be kept aspirated from the throat. The pneumonia that occurs in these circumstances is extremely severe and is very likely to cause death. Frequent respiratory stimulation with a breathing mixture of carbon dioxide and oxygen is desirable. The only use for a respirator would be when an overdose of sedative had been given inadvertently; it has no place in the treatment of asphyxia from muscle spasm.

Frequently, the management of pharyngeal and laryngeal spasm and of mucus accumulations is made easier if a tracheotomy is performed early in the disease.

PERTUSSIS (WHOOPING COUGH)

Whooping cough is characterized by paroxysms of coughing and a crowing sound with each quick intake of air during the course of the paroxysm.

ETIOLOGY

Whooping cough is caused by a bacillus, *Hemophilus pertussis,* described originally by Bordet and Gengou. The disease commonly occurs under 6 years of age and rarely after 10. Very young infants are susceptible, for immunity is not conducted across the placenta as in measles. It occurs in epidemics and endemically. One attack may be expected to confer lifelong immunity, though it does not do so in all instances. Second attacks of the disease occasionally occur.

SYMPTOMS

The incubation period varies. It is between 7 and 14 days. The disease begins as an ordinary bronchitis with only slight fever and little or no prostration. The cough becomes increasingly severe and finally assumes the peculiar paroxysmal nature characteristic of pertussis. The early stage is known as the catarrhal stage. Its duration is about a week but it may vary from 2 days to 2 weeks. The stage of severe cough is known as the paroxysmal or spasmodic stage. The duration of this stage also is variable but is usually from 2 to 3 weeks.

The typical paroxysm of pertussis consists of a series of explosive coughs rapidly repeated on a single expiration with no time for a breath between them. When the breath is expired to such an extent that no more coughing is possible, there is a rapid intake of air, and the coughing continues. This procedure may be repeated 3 or 4 or even more times.

Each inspiration during the paroxysm is accompanied by a peculiar crowing sound or whoop. The sound is produced by a spasm of the glottis. A severe paroxysm is a serious and terrifying ordeal for the child. Due to inability to breathe over such a long period, there is a feeling of impending suffocation. At first the face becomes red because of the coughing effort. As the attack progresses, the face becomes darker in color, the eyes and the veins of the neck become prominent, the tongue protrudes with each cough, and tears, saliva and perspiration flow freely.

The paroxysm continues until the mucus which was the immediate exciting cause is dislodged. Toward the end of the paroxysm this mass of ropy mucus may be expelled a considerable distance from the mouth. Vomiting is frequent immediately after a paroxysm, often making the nutrition of the child a serious problem. The paroxysms vary in number, from only a few up to 50 or 60 in 24 hours. They are more frequent at night. In small infants the typical paroxysm consists of a smothering spell rather than a whoop.

Unless the child suffers from loss of sleep because of frequent cough and from loss of food by vomiting, he passes through the paroxysmal stage with unimpaired nutrition and in apparent good health. In the absence of complications there is no fever. As in other infectious diseases, pertussis occurs with varying degrees of severity. Sometimes the paroxysms are infrequent and mild, and no doubt there are many instances of pertussis infection in which the symptoms are so mild that the conditon is not diagnosed.

After the paroxysmal stage comes the stage of decline, lasting from 2 to 3 weeks. The attacks decrease gradually in severity and frequency. The development of simple bronchitis may prolong the paroxysmal cough indefinitely. Sometimes bronchitis acquired several weeks after complete recovery from whooping cough will cause paroxysmal cough and even whooping. The second attack is not pertussis; the peculiar cough is the result of habit or neurosis. The total duration of pertussis is from 6 weeks to several months.

COMPLICATIONS

The most frequent serious complication of pertussis is bronchopneumonia. Moderate bronchitis, which is a part of pertussis, produces increased susceptibility of the lower respiratory tract to secondary infection. Infants especially are likely to develop pneumonia, and as a consequence the mortality of pertussis in infancy is high. When pneumonia is present, the cough loses its paroxysmal character.

Hemorrhage is common in whooping cough but usually it is not serious. Hemorrhage from the nose is frequent. Hemorrhage beneath the conjunctiva occurs occasionally. Brain hemorrhage is infrequent. Hemorrhages are caused by the intense congestion incident to severe paroxysms of cough.

Convulsions, paralyses, coma and other cerebral symptoms sometimes occur. Occasionally, these are caused by gross brain hemorrage, but more often they are not. The exact cause is not always easy to determine. These symptoms may be due to edema of the brain from passive congestion or vascular changes. Sometimes petechial hemorrhages are present as a cause, and occasionally inflammation of the meninges.

When paroxysms of cough are severe, the increased abdominal pressure may cause hernia. In some instances it may cause rectal prolapse. The dragging of the tongue over the lower incisor teeth during the cough may cause traumatic ulcer of the frenum of the tongue.

ISOLATION

Usually isolation is continued until whooping has ceased, which is from 2 to 3 weeks after the beginning of the paroxysmal stage.

PREVENTION

Active immunity is produced by injections of vaccine, which are given in a series of 3 injections at weekly or longer intervals and in a total dose of at least 80 billion bacilli. The immunity thus produced may be of relatively short duration, modified whooping cough sometimes developing after exposure a year after the injections. Even though immunization is not as satisfactory as that for diphtheria and smallpox, it is to be recommended for the infant and the young child because of the seriousness of the disease at this age. Frequently, pertussis vaccine is combined with diphtheria and tetanus toxoid and given as a "triple vaccine."

Passive immunity produced by injection of convalescent serum or by hyperimmune human or rabbit serum is effective in prevention if given soon after exposure to the disease. This procedure is useful in controlling epidemics in institutions and in deferring the disease in the infant and the young child.

DIAGNOSIS

Diagnosis is usually easy after the cough has become typically paroxysmal and difficult before this period. By the time the cough has become paroxysmal, the white cells of the blood are increased definitely and often markedly, with relatively large predominance of lymphocytes. When the child is caused to cough onto a culture plate containing an appropriate medium, the organisms of the disease will grow and can be identified.

TREATMENT AND NURSING CARE

No specific means of treatment now available seems to be entirely satisfactory, although good results are claimed from the use of large doses of hyperimmune serum and antibiotics. Hyperimmune serum is produced by giving a series of injections of vaccine to adult humans who have had whooping cough. A similar serum may be prepared in rabbits. Reliance must be placed largely on symptomatic management. No treatment is required when the disease is mild. Confinement to bed is unnecessary except as required by complications. Living or playing out of doors diminishes the frequency and the severity of paroxysms and is to be recommended when weather permits.

Sulfadiazine, oxytetracycline, chlortetracycline and chloramphenicol all have been useful in lessening the severity of pertussis, although they do not always stop the symptoms completely.

Much dependence is placed on sedative drugs for the control of paroxysms. Ether dissolved in oil and given by rectum is preferred by many for severe whooping cough. The barbiturates are useful, as also is codeine. Careful nursing is of the greatest importance in the management of a child with severe whooping cough, especially if the patient is an infant or a young child. Expert attention is needed during a severe paroxysm. During a paroxysm, an infant should be turned on his side to prevent aspiration of vomitus or mucus. Keeping the child's nose free of secretion is of value, especially in preparation for the night. Such management tends to lessen the paroxysms. The throat should be kept free of mucus. Sodium bicarbonate mouthwashes cleanse and dissolve the mucus that may initiate coughing.

The vomiting associated with coughing paroxysms is not associated with nausea. After an infant or a child has vomited, he should be refed because he is likely then to have an interval of freedom from cough. The child's diet should be an easily digested, bland type. Supplying the necessary fluids between meals rather than with meals tends to lessen vomiting. Because pressure on the diaphragm stimulates coughing, distention should be prevented.

After a paroxysm, care must be taken to prevent chilling. Rest periods prior to meals and during the day prevent overstimulation and emotional reactions which increase the frequency and the severity of the paroxysms. The nurse should be careful not to give the child an exaggerated amount of sympathy during the paroxysms. A child whose affectional needs are not satisfied may learn quickly that coughing brings him the attention he craves. To prevent undue attention becoming associated with the paroxysms in such instances, the nurse must support wisely during them and give him the attention he craves during the periods he is free from coughing episodes.

STREPTOCOCCAL INFECTIONS

General Considerations

Streptococci

The streptococci are a large and ubiquitous family of bacteria which have in common the properties of round shape, positive staining by Gram's method and a tendency to form chains during the process of reproduction. They are of great importance in human disease, particularly in pediatric infections. Unlike the typhoid bacillus, there is not one single variety of streptococcus but rather a large family, the members of which have widely differing abilities to create disease. Some are natural inhabitants of the body; others are harbingers of important disease. A general understanding of the classification is desirable in order to interpret bacteriologic reports.

To differentiate among the streptococci it is first necessary to discover what type of hemolysis the growing colony produces on a blood agar plate. Streptococci that are productive of *alpha* or *gamma* type of hemolysis are common inhabitants of the upper respiratory and the gastro-intestinal tracts, and their presence does not indicate disease in these locations. On the other hand, if found in blood cultures or in urine cultures, they assume pathogenic importance. The streptococci that are of major importance in pediatric disease produce a type of hemolysis that is known as *beta* hemolysis. The more nearly exact term "beta-hemolytic streptococcus" often is shortened to "hemolytic streptococcus" in everyday usage. Actually, there are about a dozen groups of beta-hemolytic streptococci which can be identified by immunologic methods. Only those in Group A are important in human disease. However, few laboratories actually test the grouping of the streptococci but assume that a beta-hemolytic streptococcus isolated from a person with an illness is probably a member of Group A. Occasionally, this assumption is wrong, and the streptococcus that is isolated turns out to be a harmless member of one of the other groups (B to N).

Group A beta-hemolytic streptococci can be subdivided further into some 40-odd types by a different immunologic procedure. Determination of these types has utility in the investigation of certain aspects of epidemiology but is not practiced commonly in clinical medicine. Group A streptococci produce a number of substances which exude from the bacterial cells and have a bearing upon the type of disease which results. Among these substances are erythrogenic toxin (or Dick toxin), streptolysin O and streptolysin S, streptokinase (or fibrinolysin) and hyaluronidase. As a result of streptococcal infection the body may produce antibodies against these substances which are known respectively as streptococcal antitoxin, antistreptolysin, antistreptokinase and antihyaluronidase. Fuller discussion of these substances can be sought from the bibliography.

Types of Streptococcal Disease

The most common site of infection with Group A beta-hemolytic streptococci is the upper respiratory tract. Many of the infections discussed in Chapter 17 (pharyngitis, tonsillitis, cervical adenitis, otitis media) are initiated by these organisms. The same sort of infection by a strain that produces a large amount of erythrogenic toxin and happens to affect a person who has no antitoxin immunity will result in scarlet fever. These upper respiratory infections constitute the common form of beta-hemolytic streptococcus infection in childhood.

In another group of disorders, the hemolytic streptococcus infection is not a primary one but is favored by previous illness such as measles, pertussis or diphtheria. Secondary streptococcus infection of this sort is particularly troublesome after the virus infections.

The skin may be invaded by hemolytic streptococci in 3 characteristic ways: erysipelas, impetigo and cellulitis. Erysipelas will be described below. Impetigo has been discussed in Chapter 15. Cellulitis usually results from the invasion of a break in the skin by beta-hemolytic streptococci. It is a diffuse erythema and edema of the skin which surrounds the local wound. It may be accompanied by lymphangitis and local adenitis.

The Group A beta-hemolytic streptococci have an additional role in human disease. Glomerular nephritis, rheumatic fever and perhaps some other systemic diseases are preceded regularly by hemolytic streptococcus infections. The resultant disease is not due to direct streptococcal invasion of the organs affected but is rather a secondary phenomenon associated with the development of antibodies during the recovery from the local streptococcal disease.

Hemolytic streptococci also may be responsible for pneumonia, septicemia, osteomyelitis, pyogenic arthritis or meningitis. Fortunately, these are rare varieties of infection.

Epidemiology

Streptococcal disease is endemic in

most areas of the United States. It tends to become more prevalent during the winter and the early spring, probably due to the collection of children indoors during the school year and during inclement weather. It is most prevalent in those who are in the first or the second year of schooling and presumably in the process of having their first contact with such organisms. In families where there are several children the school-age children may be responsible for introducing the infection into the family and transmitting it to preschool siblings or even infants. In the latter the disease is likely to be more severe and persistent. Younger children who suffer from repeated infections over many months sometimes are said to have "streptococcosis" analogous to the first infection with tubercle bacilli.

In addition to infected school contacts, children may acquire the infection from carrier adults who are well or suffer only minor symptoms in spite of the fact that they harbor virulent streptococci in their noses and throats. Search for and treatment of such carriers is often essential before the recurring infections of the child can be terminated.

The density of streptococcal infection varies in a given community from one winter to the next. Usually, the incidence of scarlet fever, nephritis and rheumatic fever parallels the amount of general streptococcal infection in any given year.

Scarlet Fever (Scarlatina)

Etiology

Scarlet fever is an upper respiratory infection with Group A beta-hemolytic streptococci accompanied by a generalized erythematous skin eruption and toxic manifestations due to the effects of erythrogenic toxin upon a susceptible person. In occasional circumstances the initial streptococcal infection is in a wound or a burn rather than in the upper respiratory tract.

The disease occurs rarely in the first year. The incidence is at its height between 5 and 8 years, after which time it decreases. The disease occurs chiefly in the fall and the winter months, only rarely in summer.

The incubation period varies from 1 to 7 days; most frequently it is from 2 to 4 days. The period of greatest communicability is during the height of the febrile period, the first 3 to 5 days. The causative streptococcus is abundant in the throat and in all discharges from this site. Streptococci gradually decrease in number and may be expected to have disappeared within 5 weeks of the onset.

Symptoms

The onset of scarlet fever is sudden, with sore throat, vomiting, prostration and fever. The onset is so sudden that the mother often can state an exact time. The appearance of the throat is that of acute tonsillitis. Within from 24 to 36 hours both an enanthem and an exanthem appear, and the fever reaches its height. This period is marked by restlessness, great thirst and often delirium. Also, the pulse rate is high and out of proportion to the temperature. After reaching the maximum, the temperature remains elevated continuously for several days, then gradually declines, reaching normal in from 10 to 14 days after the onset in the untreated child.

Enanthem. The enanthem consists of closely packed, minute, dark-red macules on the palate and the fauces, which later spread to the cheeks and the gums. The macules may fuse to a diffuse redness. The tongue in the beginning is coated, then first the edge and finally the entire tongue becomes clean. As the tongue clears, a swelling of its papillae is apparent. Very early in the disease, usually after the third or the fourth day, the tongue assumes the appearance known as "strawberry tongue," due to the general redness and the swollen papillae extending above the surface. Although strawberry tongue occurs in most cases of scarlet fever, it occurs also in other diseases and is not characteristic of any disease. The changes in the tongue are a part of the enanthem.

Exanthem. The exanthem, or rash, starts about the neck and the upper trunk, spreads over the body and attains its maximum in from 12 to 24 hours. It lasts from 3 to 7 days and gradually disappears. It is followed by desquamation, which begins about the 8th day or later and lasts 4 or 5 weeks. The rash from a distance looks like a diffuse red blush but on closer inspection is seen to consist of small points of redness, closely grouped. The appearance on the face is that of a diffuse blush, with the exception of a narrow area about the mouth, which by contrast appears to be white. When the rash is fully developed, the entire surface of the body is red except for the small area of pallor about the mouth. When the disease is mild, the skin, especially of the extremities, may be involved incompletely by the eruption.

The extent of skin desquamation is dependent on the severity of the eruption preceding it. When the eruption is mild, there is little desquamation. The desquamation on the body is usually in fine flakes ("branny") and involves the skin only superficially. On the hands and the feet it is more extensive and involves thicker layers of skin. In no case is the entire thickness of the skin involved in the desquamation, there being left an intact and adequate skin covering. These scales are not infectious, except as they have been contaminated by discharges from the throat. The duration of the desquamation is not a criterion of termination of isolation.

Variations of Severity

The preceding description of scarlet fever corresponds to a case of average severity. Great variations in the severity of scarlet fever are to be observed. In one instance, the disease may be so mild that it is difficult to recognize, and in another so severe that the child succumbs within a few days, sometimes before a rash has appeared.

Complications

The most common complications are otitis media, cervical adenitis and nephritis. Less common are arthritis, carditis and pneumonia. The otitis and the adenitis are extensions of the process in the throat. Although nephritis may appear earlier or later, it starts most commonly in the third week. Carditis and pneumonia may be expected to occur only when the illness is severe.

Isolation

The isolation period should be based on the persistence of streptococci in the throat. With the occurrence of complications with suppuration, such as otitis media, mastoiditis or empyema, the child remains a source of infection for a longer period than with the uncomplicated disease. Often the child is a source of infection for as long as discharges from these lesions continue.

Prognosis

In general, scarlet fever as it occurs at the present time is less severe than that of former years, and few deaths result directly from the toxic effects of the disease. Children nearly always recover from the nephritis of scarlet fever. The infectious complications tend to be more serious than the toxic effects.

Phases of Scarlet Fever

Scarlet fever may be divided into two distinct parts. One part consists of an infection with specific hemolytic streptococci; the other is a reaction to erythrogenic toxin produced by the streptococci. Perhaps some immunity to streptococcic infection exists, but the chief immunity to scarlet fever consists of immunity to the toxin of the bacterium. Thus, one may have a streptococcic infection of the throat or elsewhere without having the rash of scarlet fever. If a person susceptible to scarlet fever is given an injection of the toxin, he develops a rash without having an infection. The conditions due directly to the infection are the sore throat and the accompanying malaise, fever and leukocytosis. Such complications as otitis, mastoiditis and cervical adenitis are dependent also on the infection. The phenomena caused by the toxin include fever, the initial vomiting, slight general glandular enlargement, the enanthem and the exanthem.

Dick Test

The Dick test consists of the injection into the skin of a small amount of the toxin obtained by filtration of a broth culture of scarlet fever streptococci. If a local reaction occurs, the result is positive, and the person is susceptible to scarlet fever. The amount used for injection is that which will produce a moderate local reaction in a person known to react to this material. This amount is known as a skin-test dose. A positive reaction to the Dick test begins to be evident in from 4 to 6 hours after injection and proceeds rapidly to its maximum. It should be read in 24 hours. The Dick test gives information as to susceptibility to the rash and associated phenomena of scarlet fever, but none as to susceptibility to streptococcic infection.

Diagnosis

Eruptions similar to the rash of scarlet fever may be produced by certain drugs. In such instances, sore throat and other characteristic symptoms are likely to be absent. Sometimes erythematous eruptions from other causes are distinguished from the rash of mild scarlet fever with some difficulty. In such instances, the Schultz-Charlton test is of value.

Schultz-Charlton Reaction. The injection of immune serum into the skin in an area of scarlet-fever eruption, if made early in the course of the eruption, will cause a blanching of the rash in the area surrounding the site of injection. No other rash responds in this manner.

Prevention

Active immunization against scarlet fever has been accomplished in the past by repeated injections of toxin. It has not been accepted generally because the resulting immunity is only against the toxin and does not prevent hemolytic streptococcal infection and because the reactions to the injections are frequently quite uncomfortable. Children known to be exposed to scarlet fever or other hemolytic streptococcus infections can be protected in many instances by prophylactic administration of a small dose of sulfadiazine, penicillin or other antibiotic given early during the incubation period.

Treatment and Nursing Care

In most instances the treatment is the same as that for any hemolytic streptococcus respiratory infection. Penicillin is the antibiotic of choice unless the child is sensitive to it. Sulfadiazine, oxytetracycline, chlortetracycline and tetracycline are also effective. Occasionally, a child with severe symptoms of toxicity may benefit from convalescent serum or antitoxin administered intramuscularly. During the second and the third weeks of the disease urinalysis is generally desirable to discover the child who occasionally develops nephritis as a sequel.

ERYSIPELAS (ST. ANTHONY'S FIRE)

Etiology

The causative hemolytic streptococci gain entrance to the skin through a wound or other skin lesion. It affects people of all ages. In childhood, it is more common in infancy than later.

Symptoms

The lesion of erysipelas is red and tender. The edge is demarcated sharply and raised above the level of the neighboring normal skin because of swelling. The inflammation spreads by way of the skin lymphatics. Streptococci are present in the skin in large numbers at the edge of the advancing lesion. The speed and the extent of spread of the lesion vary. In a few instances it may migrate over a considerable portion of the body, clearing up behind as it advances. The affected areas subsequently desquamate.

The constitutional symptoms include fever, which tends to be high and irregular. Very young or weak babies may have no fever. Varying degrees of intoxication are present. Appetite is lost, at least some drowsiness is present, and loss of strength occurs. Leukocytosis is nearly always present. The disease is self-limited and with the older methods of treatment lasts from 6 to 9 days.

Prognosis

Erysipelas used to be feared as a serious disease, particularly in debilitated infants. It seldom is seen in recent times and is controlled readily by antibiotic therapy.

Treatment

As with any other hemolytic streptococcus infection, prompt response to penicillin or another suitable antibiotic can be anticipated. No local treatment is required.

STAPHYLOCOCCAL INFECTIONS

The group of organisms known as staphylococci are very common saprophytic (presumably harmless) bacteria which are found on the skin and in the dust of homes, schools and hospitals. Under usual circumstances these agents are not important incitors of disease, for the bodily defenses prevent them from invading. When resistance is low, they may initiate infection of the skin (furunculosis or impetigo) or may extend beneath the skin to form abscesses, or may even gain access to the blood stream and produce a bacteremia with distant foci of infection such as osteomyelitis, meningitis, or pneumonia. The circumstances which permit their invasion by reason of lowered bodily resistance are those of chronic debility from other disease or certain age factors notably prematurity and the newborn period and to a lesser extent adolescence. Occasional sporadic generalized staphylococcal infections are encountered in individuals who do not have any obvious reason for such reduced resistance. Treatment is based upon isolation of the organisms, determination of antibiotic sensitivity, and heavy dosage with the appropriate antibiotic. Pneumonia, osteomyelitis and meningitis may require special mechanical procedures to aid in the drainage of localized collections of pus.

During the past few years it has become apparent that the staphylococci capable of invading the body have a great facility for acquiring resistance to the antibiotics which are in general use. Thus, although penicillin was originally a potent weapon against most staphylococci, today only one quarter or less of the organisms isolated are found to be susceptible to it. The more recently discovered broad-spectrum antibiotics are effective against a wider range of staphylococci. In some institutions serious epidemics of resistant staphylococcus infections have erupted among surgical patients and in newborn nurseries. Transmission of such infections is usually through the medium of the hospital personnel who act as carriers of the organisms which reside in their noses. Control of such epidemics is often a difficult matter. The nursing problems in the care of these infants and in the protection of other infants in the unit are of great magnitude.

TYPHOID FEVER

Typhoid fever is an acute infectious disease most typically characterized by fever, prostration, stupor, enlarged spleen and inflammation of the intestine.

ETIOLOGY

The causative bacterium is the bacillus typhosus, *Salmonella typhosa*. The portal of entry is the alimentary tract. In areas where water supplies are supervised and sewage disposal is adequate, typhoid fever is uncommon. In such areas, the infection is acquired chiefly from persons who have the disease or are carriers of the typhoid bacillus. Typhoid fever has its greatest incidence in late childhood and early adulthood (15 to 25 years). It is uncommon, though not rare, in infancy and early childhood.

SYMPTOMS

The incubation period is variable and because of the insidious onset it is difficult to determine. In general, it may be stated as being from 1 to 2 weeks.

The symptoms vary greatly with the age of the child. The younger the child, the less severe the disease. As children approach the age of puberty, the disease occurs with a severity approaching that observed in the adult.

The prodromal symptoms may be malaise, anorexia, headache and thirst. In a few cases in childhood, the disease develops abruptly without prodromal symptoms. In the more severe case, the fever is high and usually remittent. It reaches its peak within the first week. Prostration is severe. The mental state is affected sometimes by delirium, sometimes by stupor. It is the stupor that gives rise to the term "typhoid state."

The infection is implanted first in the intestinal tract, and the greatest anatomic damage occurs at this site, but the organisms also reach the mesenteric lymph glands and the blood stream and are distributed throughout the body. The organisms are found in the blood during the first week of the disease but usually not subsequently. It is the lymphoid tissue (Peyer's patches) of the intestine that is affected most severely. The patches of lymphoid tissue become swollen and then ulcerated. The ulcerations may cause hemorrhage within the intestine, or an ulcer may extend entirely through the bowel wall into the peritoneal cavity and cause peritonitis. The inflammation of the intestinal mucosa, other than in the lymphoid tissue, is only moderate but it is sufficient in most instances to cause diarrhea. In a few cases, constipation is present. Abdominal distention is the rule, often requiring special treatment measures. The pulse rate is low, out of proportion to the fever. The white cells of the blood are not increased and frequently are decreased. The spleen becomes palpable during the first week of the disease and remains enlarged throughout the illness. Late in the first week an eruption (rose spots) appears on the abdomen in a large proportion of cases. The rash disappears within a few days. When the disease is severe, degenerative changes may occur in the liver, the heart and the kidneys. Albuminuria may be present.

In the young child, the disease is less severe. The onset is often indefinite and ill-defined, and the disease is of shorter duration, often only from 2 to 3 weeks. The nervous symptoms may be more marked than the gastro-intestinal but they are less severe than in the adult. A few children have meningismus. Severe typhoid states are seldom seen, although apathy and sometimes slight nocturnal delirium may be present. Many children show no prostration, remain comfortable and scarcely have the appearance of being ill. Others are fussy and irritable. Gastro-intestinal symptoms often are negligible. Either constipation or diarrhea may be present. Even with diarrhea, the stools are not passed involuntarily, as they frequently are in adults. Usually only moderate abdominal distention is present. Vomiting, especially at the onset, is sometimes a feature of typhoid fever in children, while it occurs seldom in adults. In infants, typhoid fever may manifest itself chiefly by vomiting and diarrhea and resemble in every way, except duration and response to dietary therapy, a gastro-intestinal disturbance due to improper food or to parenteral infection.

Anatomically also the disease is milder in the infant and the young child. The younger the child, the less the ulceration in the intestine, the process often being limited to simple hyperplasia of Peyer's patches. Intestinal hemorrhage occurs almost exclusively after the age of 10 years. Intestinal perforation also is unusual and is limited chiefly to late childhood. The symptoms of perforation in childhood are more indefinite, and the diagnosis is more difficult than in adults. The temperature curve is similar to that of adults, except that in children the fever is of shorter duration and is less likely to be markedly remittent. Occasionally, it ends by crisis. Bronchitis is frequent. Relapse, although infrequent, occurs about as often as in adults.

COMPLICATIONS

Intestinal hemorrhage and perforation are the usual complications and are the cause of most of the deaths in childhood.

ISOLATION

Isolation should be continued until several successive stool cultures fail to grow the typhoid bacillus.

PROGNOSIS

The mortality in children is less than half that in adults because of the relative mildness of the disease and the infrequency of complications.

PREVENTION

Typhoid vaccine is as useful for children as for adults. It is to be recommended especially if the family is sojourning in places where the food and the water supply may be subject to poor sanitation. The vaccine is used in the same manner as for adults in ½ the adult dose for a child; ¼ for an infant. Children have less reaction to the vaccine than do adults. Seldom does it cause inconvenience. Protective immunity may be expected to last for from 2 to 3 years.

DIAGNOSIS

Diagnosis in the young child may be difficult because of the lack of characteristic symptoms. At any age a diagnosis can be made if the organisms are found by culture in the blood, the urine or the stool. An agglutination test (Widal) is useful. A positive result may be expected by the end of the first week, with subsequent increase in titer. Both agglutination tests and cultures are useful in diagnosing Salmonella infections and undulant fever, diseases that may simulate typhoid fever. Dysentery also may be excluded by stool culture.

TREATMENT AND NURSING CARE

To the symptomatic treatment of typhoid fever there has been added recently an effective antibiotic—chloramphenicol. The child should be kept in bed regardless of the mildness of the illness or how well he feels. The diet should be complete with high energy value but with little rough residue. Foods should be finely divided and of a character which will not aggravate existing diarrhea. Milk, eggs and puréed fruits and vegetables should be prominent in the diet. Sugar may be used to increase energy value. Hydrotherapy for nervous symptoms and fever is not indicated as often as in adults. When children are found to react poorly to hydrotherapy it should be discontinued.

When diarrhea is present, specific nursing care is indicated (see Diarrhea). Dehydration is especially likely to occur in infants. Moderate anemia is common with severe typhoid fever. Sometimes transfusions are desirable to promote quick recovery. When a child is confined to bed for a long period, especially if he is in a state of stupor, special nursing care is required to keep the skin free from pressure areas and to keep the mouth clean. Nursing measures to prevent distention are required.

When the disease is severe, the nurse

should be alert for symptoms that indicate intestinal hemorrhage or perforation. Restlessness, rise in rate and change in quality of the pulse, abdominal pain and distention are symptoms of perforation that require immediate attention.

Chloramphenicol is highly effective in shortening the course of typhoid fever. Administration in high dosage (50 to 100 mg./Kg. of body weight per day) usually will produce reduction of fever and sterilization of the blood stream in from 24 to 48 hours. Treatment is continued for at least 3 weeks in order to assure the eradication of organisms from all recesses of the intestinal tract.

In instituting aseptic technic the nurse must bear in mind that the alimentary tract is the portal of entry and the chief exit of the typhoid bacillus. The stools contain an abundance of the organisms. For a short period early in the disease, the organisms are present also in the urine in many instances.

SALMONELLA INFECTIONS

The Salmonella group of organisms is a very large family that has characteristics similar to the typhoid bacillus. Unlike the latter, infection generally is spread to man from contact with the products of infected animals. The resultant disease is in some instances quite similar to, although usually milder than, typhoid fever, requiring the same sort of diagnostic measures, isolation precautions and treatment. Occasionally, these organisms produce acute food-poisoning. In small infants there may be insidious infection with unexplained fever and mild diarrhea. As long as the infection remains confined to the intestinal tract it tends to be mild, albeit often protracted. If a heavy infection of the blood stream occurs, there may be more serious consequences, such as osteomyelitis or meningitis, which are more difficult to eradicate.

BRUCELLOSIS
(UNDULANT FEVER, MALTA FEVER)

Brucellosis is a generalized infection by organisms of the genus *Brucella*. The disease is characterized chiefly by intermittent fever without definitely pathognomonic symptoms.

Three different strains of the causative organism are recognized, namely, the bovine (cow) strain *Brucella abortus*, the porcine (swine) strain *Brucella suis* and the caprine (goat) strain *Brucella melitensis*. The caprine strain is the cause of Malta fever. It is the most highly infective strain for man but it is not common in this country. Both the bovine and the porcine strains have wide distribution, and their prevalence in this country is extensive. *Brucella abortus* is the cause of infectious abortion in cattle. For man it is the least infectious of the 3 varieties when ingestion is the means of transmission. Cattle may become infected also with *Brucella suis*. The Brucella organisms are present in the milk of infected cows, and humans may be infected with either strain through the medium of cow's milk. Apparently, large numbers of organisms must be ingested by man in order to produce an infection. The infection is transmitted much more easily through an abrasion and by contact. Consequently, brucellosis in this country is commonly an occupational disease of handlers of meat and milk. Brucellosis is relatively uncommon in childhood, partly for reasons just stated and perhaps also because of an assumed relative immunity in the young. Nevertheless, the disease does occur in the young, and unless the possibility of its presence is considered in relation to fevers of obscure causation, a correct diagnosis cannot be made.

SYMPTOMS

The incubation period varies from 1 to 3 weeks and occasionally it is longer. The onset of the disease is insidious and indefinite. As the illness gradually becomes definite, the symptoms most likely to be present are irregular fever, with chills or chilliness, malaise, general weakness and loss of appetite. There also may be general aches and pains, often migratory. In some cases sweating is profuse during sleep. The symptoms usually are sufficiently severe to cause the child to be confined to bed, although the illness may be mild and the child ambulatory. Examination of the child reveals little of significance. Ofter evidence of weight loss is apparent. The spleen may be enlarged. Blood examination shows slight anemia and usually moderate leukopenia. A red macular eruption is found at times on a few children, but this may be merely miliaria or "sweat rash." Fever is the only constant symptom and this has its remissions. The temperature may be nearly normal in the morning and high in the afternoon. The disease runs a variable course, from a few weeks to many months. An average duration is approximately 2 months for the older person and somewhat shorter for the younger. Eventually, the disease subsides, usually without serious complications or sequelae.

DIAGNOSIS

The diagnostic aid of first importance is the obtaining of the causative organism in blood culture. A special medium is used, and a period of from 10 days to 3 weeks or more is required for the organism to grow sufficiently for recognition. A positive blood culture makes the diagnosis certain but does not appear early in the course of the disease. Agglutination and skin tests are available to aid in diagnosis but must be interpreted cautiously. Conclusive proof of brucella infection is often difficult to obtain.

TREATMENT

The prognosis for life in cases of brucellosis always has been good, but chronic forms of the disease were attended by prolonged or recurring periods of fatigability and vague symptoms. Chlortetracycline now appears to be able to terminate these symptoms if given in full dosage for a period of from 2 to 3 weeks. The efficacy of the newer "mycin" drugs has not yet been established, but presumably oxytetracycline, chloramphenicol and tetracycline also will be effective. Symptomatic nursing care should include rest in bed until the fever has been brought under control.

TULAREMIA (RABBIT FEVER)

This disease is acquired from contact with infected animals, usually wild animals such as rabbits, squirrels, skunks, deer and woodchucks. The bacterium responsible (*Pasteurella tularensis*) is able to penetrate skin and mucous membrane surfaces rather easily, so that mere handling of infected animals may be sufficient to produce human infection. Symptoms develop in from 2 to 5 days' time after exposure and depend upon the site at which the organisms enter the body. In one form a local skin ulcer appears, associated with enlarged and painful lymph nodes (ulceroglandular type); in another form (oculoglandular) the portal of entry is through the conjunctiva, so that conjunctivitis and enlargement of lymph nodes about the eye are the presenting symptoms; in another type entry occurs through the tonsil and the cervical lymph nodes; in some instances the site of entry is obsure, and the symptoms may simulate typhoid fever. The diagnosis can be confirmed by isolation of the specific organism from the blood or by detection of agglutinins which appear in the blood in the second week of the disease. Thus far, streptomycin, chlortetracycline and chloramphenicol have been demonstrated to be effective in treatment.

Complications are unusual, and fatalities are rare even in the absence of treatment. Since spread from man to man is unknown, strict isolation of the patient is unnecessary unless open discharging lesions are present.

TUBERCULOSIS

Tuberculosis is the result of infection by the tubercle bacillus (*Mycobacterium tuberculosis*). The most frequent source of this infection is human, and for the child this source is most often the home. Infection may occur also from more casual human contacts or from tuberculous animals. The common animal source is the cow, and the infection is conveyed by means of contaminated milk. With present-day precautions in inspecting dairy herds and in the handling and the treatment of milk, relatively few infections occur from this source in this country. The infection is communicable at all ages. At no age is susceptibility to the primary infection greater than at any other age. Often it has seemed that young infants are more susceptible, but this impression may be due largely to the fact that when an infant is exposed at all, he is likely to be exposed constantly and to massive doses of the organisms. It may be also that susceptibility to primary infection is greater than that to reinfection because of moderate immunity conferred by the first infection.

INCIDENCE

The general frequency of tuberculous infection varies widely between different communities and different countries. The skin tuberculin test, when positive, means that the person has a tuberculous infection, although not necessarily tuberculous disease. Surveys by means of this test have shown that in some communities 10 per cent or less of the children have been infected by the time they have reached adolescence. In other places, the incidence of positive tests at this age has been 50 per cent, and in still others, 90 per cent. Regardless of how low the incidence may be in a community, it is high in a tuberculous family. Tuberculosis is a family disease, and when one member develops the disease in an infectious form and remains in contact with the family, the other members will be infected in the course of time in a high proportion of instances.

PRIMARY INFECTION

Tubercle bacilli gain entrance to the body by way of either the respiratory or the alimentary tract. Because the common source is human, the most frequent portal of entry is the respiratory tract, and the primary lesion is most frequently in some part of the lung. The initial lesion often is small and relatively insignificant, especially if the dose of tubercle bacilli was not large. In these circumstances, it usually causes no symptoms and presents no physical signs. On the other hand, especially if the exposure has been intimate and prolonged, the primary focus may be more extensive and sometimes, when in the lung, it may involve the whole lobe in an exudative process. Organisms from the primary infection site travel along the lymphatics to the lymph glands that drain the region. Here the tissue reaction and changes are often more marked than at the primary focus. Part or all of the gland undergoes necrosis, and the necrotic areas have the consistency of cheese (caseation).

If the number of organisms is not large and the body defenses are reasonably good, the disease progresses no further and ultimately undergoes healing.

In the process of healing, often calcium is deposited in the necrosed areas, and the primary infection site and the regional glands become the seat of dense calcium deposits. Roentgenograms of the chest frequently show a solitary calcified tubercle (Ghon tubercle) in the parenchyma of the lung and calcium deposits in the regional glands. With more massive infection, the essential lesions are the same, although they involve a larger area and the organisms are not so easily confined to the site of infection. If they filter past the lymph glands, the organisms pass on through the lymph channels into the blood stream and are distributed to other organs or, depending on the numbers, to the entire body, thus giving rise to miliary tuberculosis or to tuberculous meningitis or to various lesions of bones and joints.

An attempt is made to distinguish between clinical tuberculosis and tuberculous infection without clinical disease. Tuberculous disease is present when the evidences of activity are revealed on examination. When those evidences are not apparent and the presence of tuberculosis is shown only by a positive result of a tuberculin test or a calcified pulmonary or gland tubercle, the condition is referred to as tuberculous infection. The dividing line between disease and infection is entirely artificial and is based on the limitations of diagnostic ability. Frequently, there are found at necropsy foci of active infection which were entirely unsuspected and in such locations that they could not be demonstrated during life.

ROLE OF ALLERGY

The majority of infected persons survive the primary infection, but accompanying this initial infection there develops a state of specific allergy which affects the future of these persons. The allergy is produced in response to the proteins of the tubercle bacillus. The skin tuberculin test gives evidence of this allergy and is a means of testing for it.

A positive tuberculin reaction may be obtained 4 weeks or more after the primary infection. Because of the existence of allergy, the body behaves differently to later infections than it does to the primary infection. Sensitized cells tend to fix the tubercle bacilli and not to let them pass on to the regional glands. The tissue reaction at the site of the primary infection tends to be nonspecific, that is, the tissue reacts as it might to a number of different irritants, while the reaction at the site of a later infection is specific. By then the cells have become sensitized to this particular irritant and react in a more violent inflammatory manner. Long ago Koch observed that if tubercle bacilli are inoculated subcutaneously in an animal previously infected, the inoculated area rapidly sloughs out and subsequently undergoes healing. Thus, along with the violent and destructive allergic response is associated a certain degree of immunity.

FIRST AND LATER INFECTIONS

From the preceding discussion it is apparent that tuberculosis associated with the first infection differs much from that resulting from later infection. Both the first and the later infections are predominantly pulmonary in initial location. The resultant pulmonary disease differs strikingly in the two instances. In the later infections, the disease tends to be confined to the lungs, while with the first infection the regional glands always are involved, and occasionally from these sites organisms are carried to other parts of the body. Thus, glandular tuberculosis, miliary tuberculosis, bone and joint tuberculosis and tuberculosis of other locations are associated almost entirely with primary infections and only rarely with later infections. The confinement of the disease chiefly to one location in the late infection is perhaps indicative of increased resistance.

Pulmonary infection as it results from infection subsequent to the primary infection is observed chiefly in late adolescence and adult life. It will not be discussed here except in comparison with the first infection or "childhood type." The childhood type has a strong tendency to heal without much loss of tissue, while the reinfection or "adult type" tends to slough out, leaving cavities. Healing in the childhood type is by resorption of exudate and calcification of the necrosed areas, while in the adult type healing is largely by means of scar tissue (fibrosis). In the adult type, the regional glands are not as heavily involved. The pulmonary lesion in the adult type is nearly always in the apex, while the primary lesion may be located in any part of the lung.

SYMPTOMS

Pulmonary tuberculosis as it results from the primary infection has been described to some extent in the preceding discussion. The area of inflammation about the original focus may be so small that it is missed easily by the most careful and complete examination or it may extend throughout an entire lobe. The extension beyond the original focus is in the nature of a consolidation brought about by exudate. Necrosis usually occurs only at the original focus, and not always even there. Upon healing, the exudate resorbs, leaving no trace of its former existence. Only the caseous area of the primary focus becomes calcified. With moderate involvement of the lung no symptoms are associated, and often a frank and progressive lesion gives rise to no symptoms whatsoever. In the more extensive infections, one may encounter cough, fever and loss of weight or the symptoms of mild pneumonia. In the average case, physical examination is of little help, although an extensive consolidation may present the signs of pneumonia. Besides the skin tuberculin test, a roentgenogram of the chest gives the most important and conclusive diagnostic evidence. In primary tuberculosis, usually little or no exudative material is free to be coughed up, yet frequently tubercle bacilli are carried up to the pharynx and swallowed. Thus tubercle bacilli may be found in material washed from the stomach after a brief fast.

TUBERCULOSIS OF THE LYMPH GLANDS

This is the predominant type of tuberculous disease during childhood. The tracheobronchial and the hilum glands of the lung are the ones most frequently affected. The development and the course of hilum-gland tuberculosis have been discussed already. The symptoms are vague or entirely lacking, though in infants the enlargement of the tracheobronchial glands may give rise to an expiratory stridor. Frequently, the glands are not discernible in a roentgenogram. Their presence may be diagnosed by this means only when they show some calcification or when they form a mass large enough to encroach on the lung field. Thus, tuberculosis in the hilum glands may be active and progressive without giving conclusive evidence of its presence and location.

Tuberculosis of the Mesenteric Glands

This is not so frequent as that of hilum glands in this country. It is to be found particularly when the portal of entry has been the alimentary tract.

Tuberculosis of the Cervical Glands

This infection occurs when the portal of entry is the upper respiratory tract or the tonsils. The clinical course of the disease in the glands of the neck is observed more easily than that of the disease in glands elsewhere. In the neck, the swollen glands are palpable, and the swelling is visible externally. The chronicity of the disease, as well as the great variability of the course, is apparent. In cases of more severe involvement, the process extends beyond the glands and involves the skin; the skin becomes red, and an area of softness is felt in the center of the indurated mass. Finally, the necrosis may extend to the surface, and a discharging sinus may result from it. Tuberculous sinuses tend to remain open with drainage for long periods. In other cases, after a time the process recedes before it has become extensive and finally heals with calcification.

MILIARY TUBERCULOSIS

This is a condition in which tubercle bacilli have been disseminated in large numbers by way of the blood stream, usually from the breakdown of infected glands. Thus many foci are set up, and the disease runs a rapid course, so rapid that by the time of the death of the child the tuberculous lesions are still very small. The distribution may be in both the pulmonary and the general circulations or it may be limited to one of them. The diagnosis of miliary tuberculosis often is difficult because of the lack of characteristic symptoms. Fever, weight loss and increasing prostration may be the only manifestations. In the systemic form, the spleen enlarges. When the distribution is pulmonary, lung signs are few or lacking, though a roentgenogram is definitely diagnostic. When meningitis (Chap. 22) occurs as a part of the general distribution, the symptoms of this localization usually are sufficiently prominent to overshadow those produced by tuberculosis elsewhere.

TUBERCULOUS PLEURISY

Tuberculous pleurisy of the fibrinous adhesive type occurs regularly with the adult type of tuberculosis, particularly near the site of the apical disease. The kind of pleurisy that occurs with the childhood type of tuberculosis is exudative. It seldom occurs before 5 years of age and is not frequent in childhood. This type of pleurisy usually represents a state of marked allergy. The onset is with pain, which stops quickly as the pleural surfaces are separated by exudate. The exudate is a clear serous fluid that usually is resorbed within a short time, especially if the child is kept at rest. Although one might expect the pleurisy to have its origin in a lesion of the adjacent lung parenchyma, such a lesion is not always found by available methods of examination.

TUBERCULOUS PERITONITIS

Tuberculous peritonitis may be of the same exudative type as that described for pleurisy and it may have the same favorable prognosis. In other instances, the exudate is fibrinous, and the peritoneal surfaces tend to become adherent. In this latter type, the prognosis is not so favorable, but a large proportion of the children recover when well cared for.

TUBERCULOSIS OF BONES AND JOINTS

Tubercle bacilli transported by the blood stream may lodge in bones and there set up tuberculous disease. In the long bones, the site of the lesion may be in the shaft but most frequently it is near an epiphysis, in which case the line of least resistance for extension is toward the neighboring joint. It is in this manner that tuberculosis of the joints most frequently originates. The weight-bearing joints are affected most frequently, possibly because resistance is lowered by trauma. Joint tuberculosis is characterized clinically chiefly by pain, muscle spasm, limitation of motion and early muscle and bone atrophy. The prognosis as to life is good, especially in childhood. The outlook for function depends somewhat on the adequacy and the promptness of treatment. In some instances good function results, but in most a stiff joint may be expected.

The spine is a common site for bone tuberculosis, and the thoracic spine is the part most frequently affected. The disease always arises in the anterior portion of the vertebra and erodes the vertebral body. The erosion soon permits a kyphos, which is the characteristic deformity. Muscle spasm and referred pain are constant when the spine is not at rest in a good position.

TUBERCULOUS ABSCESSES

Tuberculous abscesses are common in bone and joint tuberculosis. These usually progress slowly and may burrow for considerable distances before coming to the surface. Often they are referred to as "cold abscesses" because of the lack of heat characteristic of the usual pyogenic·abscess. With good treatment of the bone and joint tuberculosis, the abscesses often are resorbed without having been drained. The treatment for bone and joint tuberculosis consists of the general care suitable for a child with any type of tuberculosis and, in addition, mechanical or surgical measures which immobilize the parts in proper positions.

TUBERCULIN TEST

This is a test for allergy to the proteins of the tubercle bacillus. With a few exceptions, a negative reaction to a test properly performed indicates that the person does not have a tuberculous infection. Infection in a young child cannot be very old and therefore is either still active or latent. However, in the adult the infection may have been in the distant past and may be well healed, the allergy alone remaining. Thus one encounters the belief that in the adult and the older child a tuberculin test gives little information of value. On the other hand, it is possible that the allergic state gradually disappears as the original infection becomes completely cured, in which case a positive reaction would mean that some focus is still more or less active. If this is true, a positive tuberculin reaction is of real significance at any age. Whatever the merits of these concepts, a highly allergic state at any time is considered as a menace if the person should be exposed to tuberculosis, despite some degree of immunity that accompanies this state.

Several methods are available for performing the tuberculin skin test. In the patch test, tuberculin-impregnated material is attached to the skin by adhesive tape. This method has a high degree of reliability but it is not as dependable as the Mantoux test. The Mantoux, or intradermal, test consists of the injection into the skin of a measured amount of tuberculin. The dose most commonly employed for intradermal injection is 0.1 mg. of tuberculin contained in 0.1 cc. diluent. For greater certainty in excluding the presence of tuberculosis, a negative intradermal test should be followed by the injection of a larger dose of tuberculin, e.g., 1 mg. The tuberculin referred to is called old tuberculin (O.T.). A somewhat purer preparation known as purified protein derivative (P.P.D.) is now available. It is prepared in two strengths, the first of which can be used to detect sensitivity of a high degree. A negative response to the second strength offers conclusive proof that allergy is lacking.

DIAGNOSIS

The diagnosis of tuberculosis is based on the factors already discussed, namely, positive skin tuberculin reaction, roentgen-ray examination in suitable cases and finding tubercle bacilli. The history of exposure and the previous course of the illness often are helpful, but the symptoms in some varieties of tuberculosis are useless for diagnosis in that they do not differentiate between tuberculosis and other infections.

PROGNOSIS

The prognosis in tuberculosis has been described to some extent under the various forms of tuberculosis which have been discussed. The ability of the body to overcome the primary infection is usually good at all ages. When exposure to extraneous infection has been discontinued, the majority of persons with a first infection will recover from their disease. The mortality during infancy and adolescence is much higher than during the preschool and school years. Case fatality rates as high as 50 per cent have been reported in infants before antibiotic therapy was available. When exposed, the infant usually suffers repeated and heavy dosage from close contact with the infectious person. In the adolescent and the young adult the reinfection type of tuberculosis in the rapidly growing person carries a high mortality rate unless specific treatment is instituted.

PREVENTION

General Measures

In the prevention of tuberculosis it is clear that the factor of greatest importance is the avoidance of exposure. Much already has been accomplished in this direction. Accomplishment has been noteworthy in elimination of tubercle bacilli from the milk supply. Dairy herds are tuberculin-tested, and the reactors are eliminated. A high proportion of the milk supply is pasteurized. It is chiefly because of these measures that abdominal tuberculosis has almost disappeared in this country.

Another fruitful field of activity is the attempt to prevent tuberculous disease when tuberculous infection is present. This objective is to be accomplished by special care and observation of those who have been infected. In many communities, special schools and facilities have been established for this purpose. In these schools, extra food and hours of rest, as well as medical supervision, are provided. It is to be remembered that tuberculosis, especially of the glands, may remain latent for many years or even a lifetime, despite the fact that some calcification may have taken place. Infected persons should be kept under observation and their nutrition and general health maintained as well as possible. A latent focus may have its activity renewed by some illness, such as measles, pertussis or influenza, or by any factor that greatly lowers resistance. Another predisposing factor is overcrowded living quarters with insufficient light and fresh air.

In the public-health field, "case-finding" measures have been useful. These measures include tuberculin testing in the schools and x-ray examination of the reactors. They include also the examination of members of a household in which a tuberculous person has been found. So that these measures may be effective, appropriate care must be given to those found to have infection or disease.

Immunization

By propagating bovine tubercle bacilli through successive transplants on artificial media for many years, Calmette produced a strain (*Bacillus Calmette-Guérin* or BCG) of low virulence with which he claimed to be able to produce immunity of perhaps several years' duration. He advocated its use especially for infants of tuberculous parentage. The vaccine was given in 3 doses by mouth on alternate days in the first 10 days after birth. Currently in the United States this vaccine is administered by multiple puncture, scarification of the skin or intracutaneously. The infants are isolated from the tuberculous parents for at least 4 weeks. If a positive skin tuberculin reaction does not develop or if the skin reaction later becomes negative, vaccination is repeated. The procedure is used extensively in Scandinavian countries and elsewhere, not only for infants but also for older persons who have negative tuberculin tests. It has had only limited and experimental use in this country, where there has been a steadily declining tuberculosis rate despite the absence of an immunization program. Although the vaccine is believed to be relatively safe, its value as an immunizing agent remains controversial. It should not be regarded as a substitute for approved hygienic measures or public-health practices. If it is to be used, use should be restricted to selected groups of nonreactors most likely to be exposed to tuberculosis.

TREATMENT AND NURSING CARE

General Measures

Removal of the child from continued contact with his source of tuberculous infection is the first requisite of adequate care. When this cannot be accomplished, an attempt to control the amount of exposure by the use of appropriate isolation precautions should be made. The diet ought to provide a liberal intake of calories and of protein of high biologic value. The tuberculous child should be shielded from intercurrent infections (measles in particular) which may have an adverse effect upon his disease. The use of cortisone and ACTH generally is contraindicated, since these hormones lower the resistance to infection.

Rest in bed is often desirable over long periods of time, whether specific drug therapy is being used or not. If hospitalization is necessary, continuity in his relationships is imperative to provide the experiences that the child needs for psychological growth.

Drug Therapy

A number of drugs are now available which are able to impede the multiplication of tubercle bacilli. Unfortunately, no one of these substances is capable of serving as an ideal therapeutic weapon. Each of them creates toxic reactions in the patient under treatment; each must be used over a long period of time, and some of them lose their effectiveness because of the emergence of strains of tubercle bacilli that are resistant. In spite of these disadvantages the treatment of major tuberculosis has been improved to the point where even a large fraction of children suffering from meningitis can be saved (see Chap. 22), and most of those with miliary tuberculosis survive. In combination with newer surgical technics, many of those with cavitational tuberculosis also can be salvaged, although the effectiveness of drugs is impaired somewhat by mechanical factors in this type of disease.

Ordinarily, drug therapy is reserved for the more severe types of tuberculosis and is not used in primary infection of the usual severity. The logic of this attitude is still under debate, for in many ways it would seem better to attack the organisms during the earliest possible form of the disease.

Streptomycin and dihydrostreptomycin given intramuscularly are effective agents. They have the disadvantage that they produce toxic damage to the eighth cranial nerve when used over long periods of time in heavy dosage. Deafness or loss of equilibrium may result. In addition, the strain of tubercle bacillus under treatment gradually may become resistant to their antibiotic effects. For these reasons, streptomycin usually is used in conjunction with another tuberculostatic drug. Promizole (or other sulfone compounds) or para-aminosalicyclic acid is used for this purpose. A third group of substances which is effective against the tubercle bacillus is the isonicotinic acid compounds, of which isoniazid appears to be the most useful. The sulfones and the isonicotinic acid derivatives are given orally.

The drug treatment of tuberculosis is still in the experimental stage, and many regimens are being tested to discover the most effective one. Generally speaking, at least 2 and sometimes 3 of the effective agents are employed in order to reduce the likelihood of toxic reactions and to prevent the development of drug resistance. Prolonged treatment for 6 months to a year is considered necessary for any of the extensive manifestations of disease.

Some of the toxic reactions to which the nurse should be alert can be listed as follows:

Streptomycin and dihydrostreptomycin—deafness, dizziness, ataxia, exfoliative dermatitis, fever, peculiar sensations.

Promizole and other sulfones—anemia, red pigmentation of the urine, goiter, enlargement of the breasts. Isonicotinic acid derivatives—excitement, convulsions, dizziness, difficulty in starting the urinary stream, increased sensitivity to drugs such as adrenalin and ephedrine.

Fungous Infections

The common varieties of fungous infection in man are superficial invasions of the skin (epidermophytosis) or of the oral cavity (monilia). A few varieties of fungus are capable of producing systemic disease. Both coccidioidomycosis and histoplasmosis are similar to tuberculosis in their clinical manifestations.

COCCIDIOIDOMYCOSIS
(SAN JOAQUIN VALLEY FEVER)

This disease is confined to the southwestern portion of the United States where the climate is hot and arid. The fungous spores are disseminated with the dust and gain entrance into the body either through the respiratory tract or through cuts and abrasions of the skin. The initial invasion may be accompanied by an influenzalike illness or it may be unrecognized. Roentgen examination of the chest reveals enlargement of hilar lymph nodes, soft patches of infiltration in the lung fields and occasionally cavities. Allergy to the fungus may be demonstrated by a skin test similar to the tuberculin test. Erythema nodosum is present in some instances during the onset of allergy. Widespread dissemination of the fungus takes place in a small fraction of infected persons. Manifestations similar to those of disseminated tuberculosis, including meningitis, may occur. No specific therapy is available. Ordinarily, the disease is self-limited, but the uncommon generalized form carries a significant mortality.

Differentiation from tuberculosis may be difficult on clinical grounds but usually can be achieved through skin test reactions and immunologic procedures.

HISTOPLASMOSIS

Histoplasmosis is the result of infection with a fungus that occurs widely in the Mississippi Valley and to a lesser extent in areas along the eastern seaboard of the United States. It, too, is confused frequently with tuberculosis but generally is discovered accidentally through roentgen examination of the chest. The early lesions simulate primary tuberculous infection, and the healed lesions calcify. Differentiation is made through the use of skin tests which demonstrate allergy to the protein of the fungus.

In most instances the disease is asymptomatic and presents purely academic interest. In a few children the infection may be heavy and produce severe pulmonary disease with cavitation or a generalized blood stream involvement which is progressive and usually fatal. In regard to this latter type of disease no known treatment has proved to be effective.

TINEA (RINGWORM)

Superficial fungous infections of the skin commonly are called ringworm and technically are known as tinea. The varieties of tinea are designated by the part of the body or the shape of the resulting lesion. Thus, ringworm of the scalp is *tinea tonsurans* or *capitis;* of the body, *tinea circinata;* of the nails, *tinea unguium* or *onychomycosis;* of the inguinal region, *tinea cruris;* of the feet, *tinea pedis* or *dermatophytosis* or *athlete's foot.* A number of fungi, some of which are obtained from young domestic animals, may be involved. Accurate identification of the fungus requires special laboratory facilities but is sometimes essential to direct adequate treatment.

RINGWORM OF THE SCALP

This infection may have its start at the site of a single hair, but the lesion increases in extent up to an inch or two in diameter. The patches are roughly circular. The base of the hair is invaded by the spores of the fungus. The hair becomes brittle and breaks off close to the skin, leaving the area apparently bald. The skin of the area is scaly and shows no other evidence of inflammation except that secondary infection may occur with the formation of pustules in the hair follicles. Mycelia of the fungus are found in the scales.

The treatment is unsatisfactory in that response to it is slow. The lesions should be washed thoroughly every day, and local application should be made. The application may be tincture of iodine, a sulfur ointment or some other fungicide, according to preference. Complete removal of the hair of the area hastens recovery. The hair may be removed with forceps or by x-ray irradiation. The latter must be used with caution in order to avoid permanent baldness. In pustular ringworm, the hairs pull easily, and removal by forceps is a satisfactory method of treatment.

If the ringworm has been acquired from animal pets or farm animals, as is common in rural areas, the lesion is more likely to be inflammatory and pustular. In such cases there is an elevated, intensely red, pus-exuding inflammation with much crusting. The application of strong fungicides, iodine or sulfur preparations to this variety of scalp ringworm is contraindicated. Application of bland wet dressings, such as potassium permanganate or boric acid, is preferable. Unlike the less inflammatory form of the disease, this type tends to be self-limited. Too vigorous treatment is more likely to result in sensitivity reactions, scarring and permanent baldness.

RINGWORM OF THE BODY

This differs unimportantly from ringworm of the scalp, except that hair is not affected so obviously. The lesion occurs also on the face. In any location the lesion extends by enlargement at the edges: the newer part is pinkish and slightly elevated; the older part at the center is paler or pigmented and moderately scaly. Thus the lesion may be suggestive of a ring. Itching may be present, but little inflammation is apparent except where the origin was animal, and then there may be much inflammation. The responsible fungus is found in the scales. A customary treatment consists of the application of Whitfield's Ointment, which relieves the itching promptly. However, the cure of the lesion requires a long period of applications of some fungicidal substance, such as tincture of iodine or an ointment containing undecylinic acid (Desenex).

RINGWORM OF THE FEET

This infection is located most often between the toes. The moisture of these regions prevents the usual scale formation; instead, the macerated superficial epithelium tends to desquamate, leaving a raw surface with fissures and often with vesicles. The itching is likely to be intense. Like all ringworm, the disease is contagious. It is acquired in gymnasiums, at swimming pools and other similar places where people go barefooted. For the purpose of avoiding this infection, it is desirable to wear foot covering when walking where others walk barefooted. Also, it is important to keep infected persons away from places where people are likely to walk barefooted.

Treatment for the ordinary type, such as occurs between the toes or on the soles of the feet, consists of application of an ointment such as Desenex. Other and often more vigorous methods of treatment are advocated by various physicians. The more vigorous methods are much more likely to cause treatment dermatitis. In addition to treatment of the skin, the foot coverings previously worn should be sterilized or discarded. Thin, ventilated shoes help to avoid the sweating that aggravates the condition.

OTHER FUNGOUS INFECTIONS

In rare instances children may be infected with other types of fungus such as actinomycosis, blastomycosis and sporotrichosis. The characteristics of these infections are not distinctive in children, and their rarity makes them unsuitable for discussion in a brief text. For specific information reference should be made to the standard treatises on internal medicine.

Spirochetal Infections

SYPHILIS

Syphilis is a chronic infection with a motile spirillum, *Treponema pallidum,* which may persist over many years. It has acute, subacute and latent phases.

ETIOLOGY

Although syphilis is looked upon as a venereal disease, and its victims are thereby stigmatized, it must be recognized that by most children it is acquired innocently. The organism gains entrance to the body before birth by way of the placenta, and after birth by way of a lesion of the skin or orificial mucous membrane. From a superficial lesion containing spirochetes the infection is easily communicable to the skin or the mucous membrane of another person. The infection is not conveyed easily through a dry, healthy, intact skin. A baby with active syphilis of the skin can be handled without danger of infection if the hands are washed immediately afterward and if it is certain that no breaks in the continuity of the skin are present. Because it is impossible to be sure of this latter condition, it is safer to wear gloves. The *Treponema pallidum* dies quickly on exposure and lives for only a brief period on such surfaces as doorknobs and toilet seats. On contaminated linen it is killed quickly by drying or by ordinary washing.

Syphilis in children acquired after birth is relatively rare, and the initial lesion in most instances is extragenital, often on the lips. Acquired syphilis in children runs essentially the same course as it does in adults.

PRENATAL TRANSMISSION

The evidence that all mothers of congenitally syphilitic children are syphilitic seems to be entirely satisfactory. It is based on serum reactions and the finding of spirochetes in certain groups of mothers who were subjected to special study. The infection of the fetus is accomplished by the implantation of spirochetes at the placental site and their growth into the placenta. From this location they are distributed to all parts of the fetus by way of the blood stream.

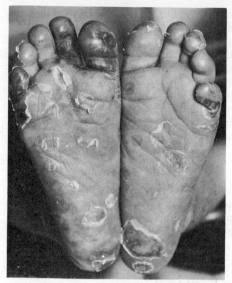

FIG. 109. Congenital syphilis showing shiny erythema and desquamation of feet before treatment.

SYMPTOMS

Fetus

The effects of syphilis on the fetus are variable. Both miscarriages and premature births are 2 to 3 times as fre-quent in syphilitic as in nonsyphilitic women. Infection of the fetus apparently does not occur before the fifth month of fetal life. Perhaps in the majority of instances the infection of the fetus takes place late in the pregnancy. A severe infection is likely to lead to the death of the fetus before birth. Thus, syphilis is a rather common cause of stillbirth. In other instances the baby, though infected, is born alive, and a living syphilitic child is the result.

Infant After Birth—Early Lesions

On rare occasions an infant will show evidences of syphilitic infection at birth, but more commonly it is between the 3rd and the 8th weeks that such evidences appear. As a rule, the earlier they appear the more severe the infection. Syphilis is capable of producing many different lesions but never do all of them occur in one infant. Therefore, the average or typical case cannot be described.

Rhinitis. Of the various lesions, rhinitis ("snuffles") is the most frequent. The inflammation in the nose, together with the discharge, interferes with breathing. The condition often resists treatment rather obstinately. If it is

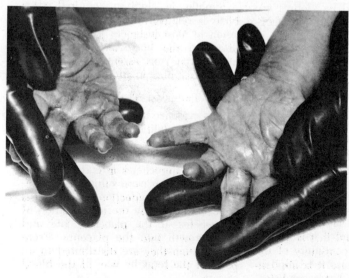

FIG. 110. Congenital syphilis showing shiny erythema and desquamation of hands after treatment.

severe and continues over a long period, growth of the nasal bones is disturbed and results in the deformity known as "saddle nose."

Rash. Skin eruptions are frequent. Often these are of the copper-colored macular variety seen in the secondary stage of acquired syphilis. In a high proportion of cases, the palms and the soles become reddened and thickened, with later desquamation (Figs. 109 and 110). This same type of inflammation may occur in the skin about the mouth. When it does, it is accompanied by fissures that radiate in all directions from the mouth (Fig. 111). Untreated, these fissures tend to remain for a long period and finally to heal with permanent scarring. The radiating scars are known as rhagades and are considered as pathognomonic of a former syphilitic infection.

Bones. Syphilitic inflammation at the ends of the long bones is a common occurrence. Often it becomes severe enough to cause pain to the extent that the part is not moved voluntarily. This pseudoparalysis of syphilis occurs almost exclusively in the first 6 months of life. The lesion is commonly designated epiphysitis, but the term osteochondritis is more nearly accurate.

Neurosyphilis. Syphilitic infection of the central nervous system occurs in approximately one third of all syphilitic infants, but it is manifest in less than 10 per cent. In those without external evidence, the diagnosis is made by examination of the cerebrospinal fluid. These babies are candidates for later development of manifest neurosyphilis.

Other Conditions. Syphilis of the eye is relatively uncommon in infancy, although in the older child it is the most common of all lesions. A high proportion of babies with syphilis have enlargement of the spleen, and approximately one third have fever in some degree during the acute stages, but this usually is not high.

Severity. The severity of syphilis in infants varies markedly. In some the infection is so mild that the baby appears to be in excellent health, and the examination reveals no abnormality except a positive Wassermann reaction. In others, especially with severe visceral involvement, prostration is obvious, weight loss is rapid, and the baby dies in the course of a few weeks. Between these two extremes all degrees of severity are encountered.

Comparison With Acquired Syphilis. The symptoms that have been enumerated as occurring in the infant correspond to those that occur in the secondary stage of acquired syphilis. Since the infant with inherited syphilis has had no primary lesion, these secondary symptoms are referred to as constituting "early" or "infantile" hereditary or congenital syphilis. Except for the primary

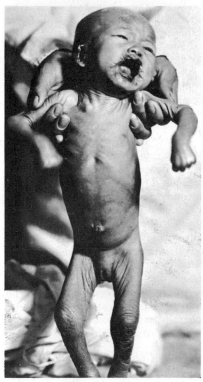

Fig. 111. Illustrating some of the skin manifestations of syphilis.

stage, the inherited and the acquired diseases go through precisely the same stages, but with certain differences in severity and in the type of manifestations. In the early or secondary stage the high infant mortality has no counterpart in the acquired syphilis of adults. Certain developmental defects (e.g., Hutchinson's teeth) occur as a result of infantile syphilis. These could not occur in a person fully developed. Skin inflammation in infantile syphilis is often much more severe than that ever seen in the adult. The presence of rhagades about the mouth is evidence of this fact. In infantile syphilis the metaphyses of the long bones are commonly affected, whereas in syphilis of the adult this does not happen. Most of the differences between inherited and acquired syphilis are in the early or secondary stage. Only two other later events are outstandingly different. These are the frequent occurrence of interstitial keratitis and the relative absence of cardiovascular syphilis as a result of the inherited infection, in contrast with the opposite state of affairs as the result of acquired syphilis.

Infant and Young Child—Late Secondary Lesions

After the subsidence of the secondary or early symptoms, a group of lesions sometimes develop. To this group belong condylomata, mucous patches and skin syphilides. These are most frequent in the 2nd or the 3rd year of life but they may occur earlier or later. Condylomata are wartlike growths which appear about the mucocutaneous junctions, most often at the anus. Mucous patches are seen chiefly in the mouth. Both these lesions contain large numbers of spirochetes and are potential sources of contagion.

The Child—Late Lesions

After the secondary stage, the infection becomes quiescent. The period of latency before the development of some late lesion varies widely with different children. During this latent period, except for possible scars of preceding activity, the only evidence of the presence of syphilis is a positive Wassermann reaction.

At about 6 or 7 years, sometimes sooner, often much later, there begin to appear lesions which are of a type usually very different from those characteristic of the infection in infancy. In the inherited infection, this group of symptoms constitutes the "late" stage of the disease, which corresponds to the tertiary stage of the acquired infection.

Eyes. The most frequent lesion of late congenital syphilis is interstitial or parenchymatous keratitis. This condition develops soon or late in fully half of all syphilitic children. Clinically, it is seen as a clouding of the cornea with prominence of the blood vessels immediately around the cornea. Vision is impaired greatly and remains so as long as the cornea is clouded. Photophobia is present in the acute stage. Keratitis responds slowly to treatment, but with early and vigorous treatment vision eventually is unimpaired. In cases of neglect, more or less permanent clouding of the cornea may cause even complete blindness.

Other affections of the eyes occur but with far less frequency than keratitis. Choroiditis causes impairment of vision in proportion to the extent of the lesion. Loss of all useful vision is not rare. Choroiditis does not respond to treatment, chiefly for the reason that by the time the child is brought to the physician with complaint of impaired vision, the damage that has been done to this specialized tissue is irreparable. Loss of vision through atrophy of the optic nerve is considered in this text with lesions of the nervous system.

Neurosyphilis. As stated previously, approximately one third of all syphilitic infants have changes in their cerebrospinal fluid which show that the central nervous system has been infected. The infection of the nervous system of most infants is latent, but it is these babies who are candidates for later development of manifest neurosyphilis. Examination of the cerebrospinal fluid of older syphilitic children reveals evidence of infection in approximately one fifth of them. The difference in incidence among infants and older children may be due to the infant mortality in this group. As those who survive become older, an increasing proportion develop manifest signs of neurosyphilis. Neurosyphilis is second in frequency among the syphilitic manifestations of older children. Any one or several of a number of conditions may develop. Some of the more common occurrences are altered pupillary reflexs, optic atrophy, various paralyses and dementia. Tabes and general paresis, if they occur, are more likely to be found in late childhood or early adulthood. Most of the conditions mentioned are the result of inflammation of the meninges and their blood vessels, which in turn affects the underlying structures. Destruction of nervous tissues causes permanent damage; repair is impossible. Little can be expected from treatment after neurosyphilis becomes clinically evident, except the arrest of its progress. Thorough treatment before these conditions develop usually will prevent their occurrence.

Bones. Third in frequency among the syphilitic lesions of older children are those of the bones. Although any bone may be involved, the tibia is the one most frequently affected. Usually the lesion is bilateral. The lesion most commonly encountered is periostitis. The periosteal thickening is detected easily by a roentgenogram, and often the swelling is visible and palpable externally. The chief symptom is pain, and this symptom causes the seeking of medical attention. Pain is relieved quickly by treatment, and the bone eventually becomes normal. Sometimes the inflammation extends much deeper into the bone than the periosteum. The bone gumma thus produced may be extensive enough to cause pathologic fracture or it may break down to the surface and give rise to a draining sinus. Bone gumma also responds to treatment, although sometimes surgical measures are necessary in addition.

Joints. Of the various joints that may be affected by syphilis, those at the knees are involved most often. The common lesion is synovitis, which produces chronic swelling of the joints from excess of fluid within them, with little or no pain and with only moderate loss of function. Less commonly, the joint lesion causes acute pain, with consequent complete loss of function. The painful variety responds to treatment rapidly, while arthritis of the other type usually persists for many weeks after treatment is started.

Gummas of the skin and the mucous membranes occur in the same manner as in the acquired infection of adults, but less frequently. These may give rise to perforations of the nasal septum or the palate, or to chronic ulcerations of the skin. They heal rapidly with treatment.

DIAGNOSIS

Some of the lesions of syphilis are so characteristic that the diagnosis can be made with reasonable certainty when they are present. Other lesions require corroborative evidence for diagnosis. When the infection is latent, the diagnosis can be made only by serologic reactions, but the diagnosis may be suspected when such stigmata as Hutchinson's teeth, rhagades and corneal or retinal scars are present. Any early lesion contains large numbers of spirochetes, and the diagnosis may be made definitely by the finding of spirochetes in material from an accessible lesion. However, this method of diagnosis is applicable in only a small proportion of cases. Examination of the serum by means of the Wassermann test or one of the flocculation tests is the diagnostic measure most universally to be depended on.

The Wassermann reaction (or other serologic test for syphilis) is not positive in all newborn syphilitic babies but it becomes so in the course of 2 months. In a few instances, a syphilitic mother transmits to her infant the positive Wassermann reaction without transmitting the infection. In all such instances, the reaction quickly becomes negative in the baby. Thus, without interpretation the Wassermann reaction is not wholly reliable in the first 2 months of life. However, after this time all syphilitic babies have a strongly positive reaction, and all uninfected babies have a negative reaction. The reliability of the Wassermann reaction continues throughout childhood. Only in later childhood, and then but rarely, will be found a child with an active lesion of syphilis and a negative Wassermann reaction. Syphilis should be diagnosed in a child with a negative Wassermann reaction only when the evidence for this infection is otherwise indisputable and proved.

During the course of several diseases the serologic tests for syphilis may give "biologic false positive results." Thus a positive serology cannot be taken as conclusive evidence of syphilis in the older child.

The presence or the absence of syphilis in an infant or a child cannot be determined by examination of the parents. While it may be expected that syphilitic parents will transmit the infection to their children, they do not always do so. On the other hand, a child may be syphilitic by heredity when the parents have negative serologic reactions. In fact, in more than 40 per cent of the fathers of syphilitic children the infection has become latent to the extent of a negative Wassermann reaction by the time the disease is recognized in the child.

PROGNOSIS

With the exception of neglected cases and those discovered after the occurrence of neurosyphilis, the general statement may be made that with adequate treatment the prognosis for the syphilitic child is good. In some instances, treatment must be continued for several years, but ultimately cure is effected, although the child may bear scars of the former presence of the disease. Even in cases of manifest neurosyphilis, the child often may be cured of the infection, but because of dementia or convulsions there can be little pride in the accomplishment. Certain children are spoken of as being "Wassermann fast," because long-continued intensive treatment has not affected the strongly positive Wassermann reaction. Children with neurosyphilis contribute the greatest proportion to the Wassermann-fast group, and it is in the latent neurosyphilis group especially that treatment should be persistent in order that manifest neurosyphilis may be prevented, even though treatment over many years is required.

PREVENTION

It is easy to prevent transmission of syphilis to the child if the infection is discovered in the mother. Even though treatment of the mother is given in the course of her pregnancy, it is highly effective in protecting the infant. Many states now have laws which require serologic testing of pregnant women in order to discover infection of the mother before the birth of the child. Where such programs are enforced properly, the occurrence of congenital syphilis can be virtually eliminated.

TREATMENT

The older methods of treatment with heavy metal injections have been superseded completely by penicillin given in a dose of 100,000 to 1,000,000 units per kilogram of body weight over a period of 3 to 5 days. With the possible exception of spirochetes which have long been entrenched in the central nervous system, this treatment can be expected to kill all the organisms present in the body. Of course, it cannot be counted on to undo the scars of previous damage. Although the need for additional therapy is remote, generally it is agreed that children should be kept under surveillance for 1 to 2 years after treatment. Reversal of the blood serology from positive to negative occurs in all but a small fraction of the cases. The broad-spectrum antibiotics are generally effective against the spirochete of syphilis when penicillin sensitivity makes its use inadvisable.

OTHER SPIROCHETAL INFECTIONS

In the United States there are few other infections in which spirochetes play a part. In one form of ulcerostomatitis (Vincent's infection) a spirillum is found which is thought to be at least partially responsible for the symptoms. It responds readily to penicillin therapy. Rat-bite fever is an uncommon infection with a specific spirochete which, as the the name implies, is transmitted to the child by the bite of an infected rat. It too is terminated by penicillin treatment. Leptospirosis is a spirochetal disease also acquired from rats but usually transmitted by way of well or sewage water which has been contaminated by the urine of infected rats. In addition to general symptoms of infection there may be jaundice or meningitis. Penicillin is of doubtful therapeutic value.

Protozoal Infections

A few of the ailments of children are due to infection with protozoa. Amebiasis is considered in Chapter 20. Malaria is still present in some of the southern portions of the United States. Toxoplasmosis is a form of granulomatous encephalitis which is discussed in Chapter 22.

Parasitic Infestations

PEDICULOSIS

Three varieties of lice are found inhabiting the hair or the clothing of children.

The most common form is *pediculosis capitis*, in which the lice dwell in the hair of the scalp and lay their eggs or nits on the shafts of the hairs. The lice themselves are often difficult to see, but the nits are small, fixed, ovoid, white bodies which can be seen with the naked eye. Scalp lice cause itching which eventually may lead to infection of the scalp by pyogenic bacteria at sites of trauma from constant scratching.

Body lice (*pediculosis corporis*) actually live in the clothes but irritate by their excursions onto the skin surfaces for the purpose of biting and feeding.

Pubic or crab lice (*pediculosis pubis*) dwell in the pubic hair of older people but may invade the eyelashes or the eyebrows of younger children. The nits are seen easily; the lice themselves are found less commonly.

Modern treatment of louse infestation is relatively simple and quite effective. Clothes can be laundered or dusted with 5 per cent DDT in talc, which kills both lice and nits. Various preparations for use in the hair are available. Topocide contains DDT and benzylbenzoate as its main constituents; Kwell and Eurax contain other types of synthetic pesticide. Usually, 2 applications about 12 hours apart are sufficient to eradicate the lice and the nits.

SCABIES

Scabies is a contagious skin disease caused by *Acarus scabiei* (*Sarcoptes scabiei*) or itch mite. The human disease is caused exclusively by the female acarus, which burrows into the skin for the purpose of depositing eggs. The parts of the body involved are chiefly those in which the skin is thin and moist. In the older person, one may expect to find the lesions most abundant between the fingers, on the underside of the wrists, in the axillae and about the genitalia. In the infant, they may be almost anywhere. The most characteristic lesion in infants is the infected burrow on the palm, present as a small pustule with the black wavy line of the burrow on the surface. The primary lesions are the burrows produced by the travels of the acarus. These usually are less than ½ inch in length. With a hand lens they are seen as dark or black lines, the color being produced by fecal deposits of the parasite. Typical burrows may be difficult to find because of secondary inflammation. Scabies causes severe itching. The reaction of the parasite, together with infection produced by scratching, causes inflammatory changes which may take the form of papules, vesicles or pustules.

The treatment of scabies is similar to that for pediculosis as noted above. Occasionally, the modern agents are not available, and the old-fashioned sulfur ointment (5%) may be used. It is important to discover all of the infested members in a family so that they may be treated simultaneously in order to kill all the mites within the household and prevent return of the disturbance.

TICKS

Ticks (and mites) are small arthropods which have biting and sucking parts and attach themselves to man or animals for the purpose of sucking the blood. After satiating themselves they let go and drop off. In the process of feeding they may transmit virus or rickettsial infection to a child or may cause paralysis or fever by the injection of toxic substances. These latter events depend upon the presence of poisons or infections within the particular tick which is biting. In the United States, most ticks are harmless, and the bite is inconsequential except for the local discomfort. Some of the diseases which may be transmitted by ticks or mites are Rocky Mountain spotted fever, St. Louis encephalitis, typhus fever and rickettsialpox. The uncommon circumstance of tick paralysis clears up when the tick is discovered and removed.

SITUATIONS FOR FURTHER STUDY

1. If respiratory difficulty were observed in a child with diphtheria, what emergency equipment would you assemble? What care would a child with a tracheotomy require?

2. How can tetanus be prevented? If you were notified that a 3-year-old child with tetanus was coming into the children's ward, what preparation for his care would you make? What equipment

should be in readiness for his medical and nursing care?

3. Study the mortality rate of whooping cough. At what age is the mortality rate the highest? Why? How could the rate be reduced? What help would a mother require to give adequate care to her 3-year-old child with whooping cough?

4. What are the common complications of scarlet fever? How can they be prevented?

5. How do the symptoms of typhoid fever differ in infancy and in childhood? How does nursing care differ in infancy and in childhood?

6. To confirm a diagnosis of tuberculosis, sputum examination often is desired. How would a sputum specimen be obtained from a 2-year-old child? What equipment would be necessary? How would you help a child meet the experience?

7. What supervision would a child with tuberculosis require? How can tuberculosis be prevented?

8. What care would an infant born of a tuberculous woman require?

9. What care would an infant with syphilis require?

10. Is the Wassermann reaction wholly reliable during the first 2 months of life?

11. How can congenital syphilis be prevented?

BIBLIOGRAPHY

Brennan, Florence: Brucellosis, Am. J. Nursing **50**:358, 1950.

Dubos, René: Bacterial and Mycotic Infections of Man, ed. 2, Philadelphia, Lippincott, 1952.

Harris, Isabel, and Shapiro, S. K.: Tetanus, a challenge to nursing, Am. J. Nursing **50**:362, 1950.

Jeans, Philip, and Cooke, J. V.: Prepubescent Syphilis, New York, Appleton, 1930.

Kohn, Jerome, and Olson, Elsie: Whooping cough, Am. J. Nursing **50**:1723, 1950.

Shapiro, Charlotte: Typhoid fever, Trained Nurse & Hosp. Rev. **120-121**:118, 1948.

Steigman, Alex J., and Epting, Mary H.: Diphtheria in children, Am. J. Nursing **57**:467, 1957.

Stimson, P. M., and Hodes, H. L.: A Manual of the Common Contagious Diseases, ed. 5, Philadelphia, Lea & Febiger, 1956.

Tebrock, H. E., Fisher, M. M., and Mamlok, E. R.: The new drug—isoniazid, Am. J. Nursing **52**:1342, 1952.

Thirlaway, Jean: The new look in typhoid fever, Canadian Nurse **46**:729, 1950.

CHAPTER TWENTY-SIX

Other General Diseases

ALLERGY

The term "allergy" is used to designate an altered or abnormal degree of sensitivity to various materials which act as antigens—substances having the power to cause the production of counteracting substances or antibodies. The altered susceptibility is caused by the presence of antibody to the antigen. In practically all instances the antibody is present because of response to previous introduction of antigen. Thus, antigen causes production of antibody to the antigen, and thereafter, whenever antigen is present, a symptom-producing reaction takes place between the antigen and its antibody. The responsible antigen most frequently is a protein, but it may be a nonprotein chemical substance which combines in the body with protein to form an antigen.

If a material such as horse serum is given parenterally, antibody to the foreign protein* may develop. If a large amount of serum has been given, antibody may develop in quantity before all the foreign protein has been excreted or destroyed. In such an instance, the period required to develop antibody in quantity is from 8 to 13 days. Thus, an allergic reaction may develop as a result

* "Foreign protein" emphasizes its origin from a different animal species. Horse serum and rabbit serum are foreign proteins for man, but human plasma, convalescent human serum and gamma globulin are not.

638

of a single injection. The reaction thus produced is called a *delayed reaction.* Subsequent injections of serum are likely to produce an immediate or early reaction because of the presence of antibody at the time of injection. Smaller initial injections may produce no symptoms, but subsequent injections may cause a reaction because of the antibody produced by the first injection. This type of reaction is not limited to serum; serum is used as an example. When the allergic state develops as a result of a previous introduction of antigen in a person whose capacity to become susceptible is not a hereditary constitutional trait, the allergic response to further introduction of antigen is known as *anaphylaxis.* Often the term "atopy" is used synonymously with allergy, but it is more nearly correct to restrict its use to certain allergies present in those with a hereditary constitutional capacity to develop allergy. In the restricted atopic group belong hay fever, asthma, some urticarias (hives) and certain of the eczemas.

Another type of allergy is that associated with certain infections. For example, in tuberculosis the body becomes sensitive to tuberculoprotein in approximately 30 days after the initial infection. Thereafter a positive skin reaction is obtained with tuberculin, the reaction being an allergic one. Positive skin reactions are obtainable in a similar manner in other infectious diseases, including undulant fever, histoplasmosis and streptococcal infection. The allergy is not only manifest by a skin reaction, but in these and other infections the subsequent course of the chronic infections and the course of the acute illness of recurring infections are also altered importantly because of the allergy. The adult type of tuberculosis differs from the childhood type (primary infection) because of the allergic response of the body. The tertiary lesions of syphilis differ from the earlier lesions because of allergy.

Allergic phenomena occurring spontaneously are usually caused by sensitivity to either foods or materials inhaled or in some instances to both. Hay fever (allergic rhinitis) and allergic asthma commonly are caused by inhalants. The general principles which should underlie the management of allergy to inhalants are discussed under asthma. The general principles of the management of allergy to foods are discussed under eczema. Certain of the allergies in these two groups lend themselves to complete or partial desensitization; others do not. In any case, the desensitization is a slow and tedious process, and in many instances, especially in the case of foods, it is easier to avoid the offending material. Desensitization in the case of inhalants is carried out by hypodermic injections of extracts of the material in gradually increasing doses, with less than the amount which produces symptoms always being given. Food desensitization is accomplished by giving the material by mouth in gradually increasing amounts but in amounts which do not cause reactions.

SERUM DISEASE

An allergic illness which does not occur spontaneously as the result of fortuitous ingestion or inhalation of offending materials, and the one most frequently encountered, is that caused by the prophylactic or therapeutic injection of various sera. All manufacturers of commercial therapeutic sera refine their products in such a manner that the final product contains only the pseudoglobulin portion. Such sera are much less allergenic than the original raw sera. In addition, some therapeutic sera are partially digested in the final stages of the preparation and by this process have lost much more of their allergenic property.

It already has been pointed out that allergic illness from serum may occur with the first injection as a delayed reaction or with subsequent injection as an immediate or early reaction. These reactions are anaphylactic. In certain constitutionally atopic persons, immediate illness may result from the first injection. It is most important to recognize constitutional atopy, since it is probably only persons with this condition who are likely to die as a result of serum injection.

Serum sickness occurs with various degrees of severity. In the most common variety the illness is mild. One may expect moderate fever, local redness and itching or pain at the site of injection and a generalized skin eruption which most commonly is urticarial but may be morbilliform or scarlatiniform. The child is uncomfortable but not particularly ill. A more severe and less common variety includes also several or more of the following symptoms: malaise, albuminuria, joint pains, swelling of the mucous membranes with hoarseness and cough, vertigo, nausea and vomiting. A rare and still more severe variety produces extreme weakness approaching collapse; the temperature may be subnormal and the pulse weak; catarrhal or hemorrhagic enteritis may be present. The most rare type of reaction is that which produces immediate shock, usually fatal. Usually the duration of the common varieties of serum sickness is 3 or 4 days. The more serious effects of serum sickness may be controlled to a large extent by the administration of epinephrine or ephedrine, which must be repeated from time to time as indicated by the recurrence of the symptoms. Urticaria also responds to epinephrine and to cortisone, but usually the skin lesions may be managed adequately by the application of antipruritic lotions.

Serum is used frequently in the prevention and the treatment of various diseases. Therefore, it becomes important to know the proper approach to its administration. It is customary and appropriate to make sensitivity tests as a preliminary procedure, but it is well to remember that these may be misleading. The chances of death from serum administration are extremely small. It has been estimated that not more than 1 in 70,000 injections has caused death. Practically all the deaths have occurred in association with the first injection of serum, when no previous sensitizing dose had been given. From this point of view, the fact that the child has had a previous injection of serum gives good assurance that death will not occur from a second or subsequent injection, regardless of the result of sensitivity tests. In fact, a few deaths have occurred among those with negative sensitivity reactions. Because of the possibility of sudden death, foreign serum should not be given or should be given with the greatest caution to those with hay fever and allergic eczema and particularly to those with allergic asthma.

If the child has no history of atopic disease, a suitable skin-test procedure is to give intracutaneously 0.1 cc. of the serum to be used. If no wheal results or if the wheal is no larger than ¾ in. within 20 minutes, the full dose of serum may be given. If a greater degree of hypersensitiveness exists, as shown by a larger wheal, the first dose of serum should be from ¼ to ½ cc. If no systemic reaction has occurred within 20 minutes, the full dose may be given. Small amounts of serum, such as would be used for a customary dose of diphtheria antitoxin, are safe for nonatopic children, even though the skin test is positive. Serum sickness may develop, but the reaction will not be fatal.

If the child has a history of atopic disease, the sensitivity test should be made with greater caution. A suitable procedure is to give 0.05 cc. of a 1:100 dilution intradermally or to place one drop of this same dilution into the conjunctival sac. If a reaction occurs, further serum is contraindicated. In some instances, as in the case of diphtheria, the decision to give no serum is difficult to make. Desensitization sufficiently rapid to permit the administration of serum in the treatment of acute illness probably is impossible. One may decide to risk giving the serum in minute doses serially, starting with 0.1 cc. In such cases, epinephrine should be in a syringe ready for use. It is probable that most of the severe reactions could be managed by prompt and appropriate use of epinephrine.

DRUG SENSITIVITY

The symptoms of serum disease, particularly urticaria, may occur when a child acquires sensitivity to any of several drugs. Penicillin is much the most frequent and important offender and in these circumstances the symptoms are often delayed until 10 days or even 3 weeks after the penicillin therapy is begun. Any of the features of serum disease may be mimicked. Immediate severe reactions to penicillin are almost unknown in the child but can occur in the adult.

ASTHMA

Asthma is really a complicated pulmonary symptom rather than a specific disease. The mechanical changes in the bronchial tree that lead to the characteristic obstruction, dyspnea and wheezing are the same in all patients, but the factors that produce the mechanical disturbances are varied and often complex.

Etiology

Children who have asthma are generally considered to be allergic subjects. This implies a constitutional predisposition toward abnormal sensitization and in many instances the trait is clearly inherited. Among infants and young children the appearance of asthma is usually restricted to periods when there is obvious acute infection of the respiratory tract and the symptom abates when the infection is treated adequately. Infection may play a role in

older children too, but the relation between it and asthma is usually less obvious. Frequently, the obstructing mechanism is set off by specific sensitivity to an inhalant such as ragweed, house dust or an animal dander. More often, specific sensitivities are suspected but cannot be identified clearly. In some children emotional disturbances alone appear to be capable of setting off an attack of asthma; in the majority of cases emotional factors play an important role in determining the length and the severity of symptoms. Thus, one can recognize constitution, infection, specific sensitivity and emotional factors as playing a part in the production of asthma. The degree to which each participates is a matter that must be determined by study of the individual child.

Symptoms and Diagnosis

The lungs are afflicted by the same sort of disturbance as that described in Chapter 17 for obstructive bronchitis of infancy. There is widespread narrowing of the small branches of the bronchial tree due to a combination of spasm of the circular muscles surrounding them, of edema of the mucous membrane which lines them, and of thick mucus contained within their lumens. The obstruction to air flow is more marked during expiration than during inspiration. Air tends to be trapped in the alveoli, producing overdistention of the lung and requiring the child to make a forcible effort during expiration in order to push air through the narrowed bronchioles. The result is an overdistended (emphysematous) chest with rapid, shallow inspirations and prolonged wheezing expirations.

A typical asthmatic attack usually occurs in a school-age child abruptly at night and without antecedent illness. There is no fever. The child develops a hacking cough and has difficulty sleeping because of the necessity for making a conscious effort to breathe. He finds that he must push during expiration and that he is more comfortable if he is propped up in bed. Characteristically, he is quiet, less upset than his parents are about the symptoms and tends to resist efforts to assist him. He seems to prefer to be left alone to cope as well as he can with the necessary task of breathing. Mild cyanosis may be present. Asphyxiating asthma is rare in children, except in those who have repeated attacks over a long period of time. After the symptom has persisted for a day or two the child may produce thick tenacious secretions during coughing spells. The symptoms tend to become worse at night and to clear somewhat in the daytime. Sleep and the ingestion of food may be seriously curtailed during prolonged attacks. Single attacks may be as brief as an hour or may last for several days to be followed by an additional period of bronchitis.

The diagnosis is made by observation or from the accurate description of an attack by the parent. It is confirmed by physical examination and analysis of the character of the respirations. Prompt relief following the injection of adrenalin helps to substantiate the diagnosis. Determination of the precipitating factors for the individual child is usually a difficult and protracted process which may involve allergic technics or the services of a child psychiatrist, or both.

Treatment of the Acute Attack

Adrenalin administered by injection or by inhalation usually gives relief for a brief period of time. Ephedrine and aminophylline operate more slowly but have a longer-lasting effect. Treatment is usually more effective if used early after the appearance of symptoms. Sedation with barbiturates is helpful in reducing the child's anxiety and encouraging sleep. If the attack is prolonged or severe, removal to a hospital is usually desirable. For reasons which probably are grounded in the relief of emotional tension, treatment of asthma in a hospital setting is rapidly effective in nearly all instances, even though the same measures have been tried previously at home without very much improvement. Unusually severe attacks of asthma may require oxygen administration or the use of ACTH or cortisone.

Prevention of Future Attacks

To forestall future attacks of asthma it is necessary to understand the importance of the various factors that precipitate attacks in the individual child. Sometimes the task is relatively simple. If attacks occur only at certain seasons in the year, pollen sensitivity is likely to be responsible, and the offending agent can be discovered by allergic skin testing. Treatment then depends upon the individual's avoiding the pollen in question, or if this is not feasible, in receiving desensitizing injections over a period of several weeks. When asthmatic attacks are clearly related to the onset of respiratory infections, the attention must be directed toward clearing up sources of chronic infection in the nose and the throat if such can be identified. When the child is losing an excessive amount of sleep or is unable to attend school because of recurring respiratory infections with asthma, sometimes it is desirable to keep him on small doses of sulfonamides or oral penicillin throughout the winter months as prophylaxis against reinfection—a technic which is commonly used for the child with rheumatic fever.

When the factors which precipitate asthma are not so obvious, prolonged allergic or psychiatric study may be required to bring the symptoms under control. Since both of these technics are likely to be long, arduous and upsetting to both the child and the parents, generally they are reserved for children whose asthma is frequent, disabling or so severe that permanent damage to the structure of the lung is threatened if they continue. Severe prolonged asthma almost always stems from an emotional conflict between the child and some member of his immediate family. The most careful and extensive program of desensitization, drug management or change of climate may be unavailing if no consideration is given to the psychological implications of the disorder.

CHRONIC NEURODERMATITIS

A few infants who suffer from eczema (Chap. 15) will have a persistence of lesions beyond the third year of life. Older children occasionally develop a similar eruption without having had the infantile form of the disease. The etiology is variable but constitutional, allergic and emotional factors influence the course. The eruption in its mildest form is a dry transverse cracking about the flexor surfaces of joints, particularly the wrist, the elbow and the knee. From these areas erythema and weeping may extend to involve adjacent areas of skin. In severe cases most of the skin of the extremities, the face and the neck may be affected, but the trunk is usually spared. The eruption tends to improve in summer and with exposure to ultra-violet light. It is aggravated by emotional disturbances which also increase the degree of scratching. Specific food and contact sensitivities are often demonstrated in an individual child, and an important part of the treatment is to shield the child from such allergens in so far as feasible. Constitutionally, these individuals are usually energetic, ambitious and sensitive. It seems as though their frustrations, annoyances and anxieties are converted into itching and eruption of the skin. Sedation with phenobarbital is commonly used but has little effect unless pushed to a degree which makes them drowsy. Partial relief of itching is obtainable through the use of ointments and protective dressings to the skin. Steroid therapy is almost always beneficial but presents a problem, since long-term use may not be without hazard. Improvement can be expected with maturation, since many of these children learn their limitations and organize their lives within bounds which keep their skin troubles minimal. Psychiatric help can aid in this adjustment.

AGAMMAGLOBULINEMIA

A rare but interesting disorder in which the child is unable to manufacture gammaglobulin, the portion of the plasma which contains antibodies, has been observed in recent years. Usually male children are affected, and the disease is a sex-linked recessive inherited characteristic. Early in infancy the child suffers a series of severe major infections, such as pneumonia, meningitis, pyoderma, or bacteremia. He is unable to acquire resistance to infectious agents or allergy to injected antigens. Tuberculin, Dick and Schick tests are invariably negative, and the child does not have the normal blood-group agglutinogens. Life may be sustained by repeated injections of gammaglobulin and by prompt antibiotic treatment of infections.

THE COLLAGEN DISEASES

The term "collagen disease" is applied to a group of disorders which have as their common feature destruction and degeneration of the supporting connective tissue of the body. The name "collagen" refers to the fibers that can be seen under the microscope. There is evidence too that the ground substance between and among fibrils also is disturbed. The etiology of each of these disorders is obscure or at least under debate at the present time. They all improve under the influence of adrenal cortical steroid therapy. In general their symptomatology is sufficiently distinctive to permit sharp grouping into diagnostic entities, but in a few cases it may be difficult to decide which diagnosis to apply to an individual child. In pediatric medicine, rheumatic fever is much the most common representative of the group; rheumatoid arthritis and disseminated lupus erythematosus are uncommon; dermatomyositis, scleroderma and periarteritis nodosa are distinctly rare.

RHEUMATIC FEVER

Rheumatic fever is a systemic disease that causes characteristic involvement of many organs and tissues, most important of which is its effect upon the heart. The common manifestations are migratory joint pains, various skin eruptions, subcutaneous nodules, chorea and carditis. The acute and the chronic effects of rheumatic fever upon the heart have been considered in Chapter 18.

Etiology

The causative mechanism in rheumatic fever is the subject of controversy. The facts seem to be sufficient to warrant certain tentative conclusions. The primary underlying factor is infection in the throat with Group A beta-hemolytic streptococcus. As a result of chronic infection or repeated acute infections, the body becomes sensitized to the organism. Continued infection or repeated infection after sensitization leads to allergic response, the response varying in nature and degree according to the degree of sensitization. Before sensitization, the throat infection has apparent effects only locally. After sensitization, the systemic phenomena consist of certain proliferative and exudative changes with their accompanying symptoms (carditis, arthritis, skin eruptions, rheumatic nodules).

Incidence

The stated cause of rheumatic fever explains its age incidence. Rheumatic fever is rare in the first years of life, not because infections are uncommon, but because the development of allergy requires time. The curve of incidence of onset gradually rises. It has reached a fair height by 5 years of age and is at its peak between 7 and 10. After this time it declines. Rheumatic fever is most prevalent in those parts of the world (temperate zones) and in those seasons of the year in which respiratory infections are most frequent. Rheumatic fever has a relatively high family incidence. A hereditary predisposition to the disease is recognized. The environment and the living conditions are often such that respiratory infections are induced easily, and the causative organism is transferred easily. It is well recognized that rheumatic fever is more frequent in the low-income than in the high-income levels. No doubt this difference is explained in part by living conditions, but nutritional status also is known to be important.

Symptoms

The symptomatology of rheumatic fever is extremely variable in its type and severity. Some children are affected so mildly that the symptoms are vague, and even the most careful and extensive study by laboratory methods leaves some doubt about the validity of the diagnosis. Other children are assailed by a severe, fulminating disorder that rapidly threatens life.

Unlike many of the infectious diseases, the medical problem in rheumatic fever involves more than the management of a single episode of disease, for the child who has experienced one attack is vulnerable to recurrences. Each return of rheumatic activity carries with it the threat of additional cardiac damage. Consequently, it is very important to know which children have suffered from rheumatic fever in order to shield them from additional attacks, even though the first one may have been mild. Conversely, it is undesirable to classify a child as rheumatic unless good evidence is available, for in some instances this leads to unnecessary anxiety and restriction of activity, which hamper normal physical and emotional development.

The symptoms of rheumatic fever may be grouped into major manifestations and minor manifestations. If present in characteristic form, any one of the major manifestations is presumptive evidence of rheumatic fever. The minor manifestations may or may not be due to rheumatic fever, but when several of them are present alone or in conjunction with a major manifestation they add to the suspicion. The major manifestations are polyarthritis, carditis, chorea and subcutaneous nodules. In the young child carditis is apt to be the presenting manifestation, with polyarthritis present in mild degree. In the older child polyarthritis and chorea are more common as presenting complaints.

Polyarthritis. The arthritis of rheumatic fever tends to involve the larger joints such as the knee, the elbow, the ankle, the wrist and the shoulder. However, it may be present in any joint, including the spinal articulations and the mandibular joint. Pain, tenderness and restriction of motion are present. In the young child these symptoms tend to be mild and to endure for only a few days but they may return in a different joint. More severe joint manifestations usually are seen in older children, in whom the part may be swollen, visibly inflamed and exquisitely tender to touch or manipulation. Spontaneous subsidence within a few days even without treatment is characteristic, but migration to other joints may persist over a period of weeks.

The arthritis of rheumatic fever has two distinctive characteristics—it is relieved rapidly by salicylates and it never results in permanent deformity of the joint. The pathologic changes are those of exudation of fluid into the joint and inflammation of the surrounding structures.

The problem of differentiating rheumatic pains from "growing pains" is often a difficult one. Usually the latter are limited to the night hours after the child has fallen asleep. They seldom interfere with his daytime play or provide visible evidence of pain or restricted motion. They tend to recur nightly for long periods of time and are not associated with other manifestations of the rheumatic state.

Carditis. Acute rheumatic carditis is discussed in detail in Chapter 18. The pathologic changes consist of exudation and proliferation. In the pericardium the early changes are those of acute inflammation with exudation of fibrin between the two layers. When healing takes place the exudate may be converted into pericardial adhesions. In the myocardium there is swelling and degeneration of muscle fibers and the appearance of minute granulomas called Aschoff bodies. During healing these areas are converted into microscopic scars. Some of the cardiac muscle fibers are lost in the process. In the endocardium there is at first an acute inflammatory reaction which later becomes an organizing fibrinous exudate. On the valve leaflets this may result in warty growths called vegetations. During healing the scar tissue which forms tends to contract and deform the valve orifices and the adjacent structures. Such scarring may leave the valves unable to close completely, so that blood regurgitates back past them, or the orifices may be narrowed abnormally, so that blood cannot pass through them at the accustomed speed. The maximum effects of the contracting scar tissue are not apparent until several years after the original acute inflammation. These late complications are responsible for the manifestations of chronic valvular heart disease which are discussed in Chapter 18.

Chorea (Sydenham's Chorea). Chorea

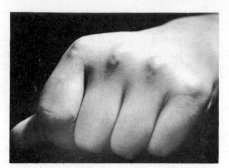

FIG. 112. Subcutaneous nodules of rheumatic fever.

is characterized by involuntary, purposeless, irregular movements commonly involving all the voluntary musculature but occasionally affecting one side of the body more than the other.

The greatest incidence of chorea is between the ages of 6 and 15 years. It is much more frequent in girls than in boys and more frequent in the spring than at other seasons. It has been suggested that a nervous tendency is necessary in addition to an infectious cause. Chorea is said to be more frequent in neurotic families, and it has been assumed that heredity plays a role.

The most prominent symptom in chorea consists of peculiar body movements. These are jerking, spasmodic, in-co-ordinate and without regularity. They cannot be suppressed by volition; in fact, they are made worse by attempts to inhibit them, as well as by the mental stress of excitement or embarrassment. In severe chorea, these movements may be so extreme that the child will be bruised and injured by tossing and jerking against the sides of the bed unless the bed is padded. Such children cannot walk, talk, sit or feed themselves and are incontinent. Fortunately, in most instances the disease is not so severe. To be seen are all grades of severity from that described to such mildness that recognition of the condition requires close observation. Frequently, one half of the body is affected so much more than the other half that the condition is spoken of as hemichorea.

All attacks begin gradually, with signs of increased nervousness. Difficulty in the finer movements such as writing or buttoning clothing is evident early. The child stumbles easily and often drops articles being handled. Food is spilled, and soon, because of the jerky movements, self-feeding becomes impossible. The involvement of the muscles of the face causes grimaces. In-co-ordinate movements affecting the mouth and the tongue make speech difficult or impossible. When one part of the body is involved more than the remainder, as in hemichorea, the chief complaint often is stated as "paralysis." The paralysis is apparent and not real and is due to inability to use the parts purposefully. Choreic movements are absent during sleep.

Children with chorea often are very emotional. Little or nothing obvious is required to produce a fit of giggling or of weeping, and the mood may shift rapidly from one extreme to the other. These children are irritable and fretful. The appetite usually is poor, the sleep disturbed, headaches are common, and the child is easily fatigued. Fever is a feature only in the more severe disease.

Spontaneous recovery is to be expected in from 1 to 2 months. Relapses and second attacks are frequent. Relapses may prolong the illness to 4 months or longer. Complete recovery is the rule, and attacks never recur after puberty except during the course of a later pregnancy. When the disease is extremely severe, death may result from exhaustion. However, death is rare unless due to associated cardiac disease.

Subcutaneous Nodules. Nodules are not a very common manifestation of rheumatic fever but when they do occur they are almost certain confirmation of the diagnosis. They consist of accumulations of fibrous tissue proliferation which are located beneath the skin near the larger joints or along the spine or in the scalp. Small ones are difficult to find and are easily missed unless careful palpation is carried out. The larger ones are often visible through the skin (Fig. 112). They are painless and persist for weeks or months before they disappear gradually.

Minor Manifestations. Rheumatic fever is accompanied by a number of other symptoms which by themselves are not necessarily rheumatic. Lassitude, pallor, fatigability and loss of appetite are seen frequently.

FEVER is usually present, but its degree may be very variable. In severe rheumatic fever it is regularly present and may be high. Sometimes it is present only during the period when arthritis is evident. At other times it may appear as a low-grade protracted elevation which extends over many weeks during the activity of the rheumatic process. However, absence of fever cannot be regarded as equivalent to absence of rheumatic activity, for the two features are not always parallel.

MUSCLE PAINS which are transient or mild may or may not have a rheumatic basis.

NOSEBLEED is a traditional but actually not very frequent symptom that may be present during rheumatic activity. The amount of bleeding is usually mild and creates no significant problem in management.

ABDOMINAL PAIN is an important symptom because it may be severe enough to lead to the diagnosis of appendicitis and an exploratory operation. The exact mechanism of such pain is poorly understood but is attributed ordinarily to peritoneal inflammation or mesenteric lymph node enlargement.

ERYTHEMA MARGINATUM is a faint, changing skin eruption which consists of small red circles, wavy lines or portions of circles which appear and disappear rather rapidly on the trunk and the abdomen. The characteristic eruption seldom is seen except during the progress of rheumatic fever and is regarded by many people as being a clear evidence of rheumatic activity. It creates no symptoms and is not necessarily associated with fever.

Laboratory Aids to Diagnosis

Very often the clinical task of deciding whether an individual child does or does not have rheumatic fever is a difficult one. It would be highly desirable to have a specific laboratory test which indicated the presence of the disease and the degree of its activity. Unfortunately, no specific test is yet available, although several give useful nonspecific information. Each such test requires interpretation in the light of the patient's entire clinical picture.

An increase in the sedimentation rate of the red blood cells indicates the presence of an inflammatory reaction or a disturbance of the plasma proteins. It is a relatively simple procedure which is widely used as a means of following the course of rheumatic activity after the diagnosis has been established by other means. Of course, it can be influenced by inflammatory processes that have nothing to do with rheumatic fever.

Determination of the C-reactive protein of the blood is a similar indicator of the presence of an inflammatory reaction.

Leukocytosis also indicates inflammation but is a less sensitive index than the other tests named.

Since it now is believed that rheumatic fever almost invariably follows beta-hemolytic streptococcus infection, the detection of evidence of such an infection adds weight to the suspicion that symptoms are being produced by rheumatic fever. Usually the streptococcal infection is sufficiently distant or has been treated adequately, so that the organisms are not present in the throat culture at the time that rheumatic symptoms appear. However, certain antibodies may have been formed against the streptococcus products; by laboratory means it is possible to detect *antistreptolysin, antifibrinolysin or antihyaluronidase.* Of course, their presence merely proves that the person has suffered a streptococcal infection and does not indicate the presence of rheumatic fever specifically.

The electrocardiogram provides valuable evidence of the presence of carditis. The most frequent alteration is a prolongation of the P-R interval.

Course and Prognosis

The prognosis for children with rheumatic fever depends entirely upon the effect that the disease has upon the heart. Except for the carditis, none of the other manifestations is likely to be lethal or to leave any permanent aftereffects. The common form of first attack (monocyclic) consists of a period of activity which lasts from 1 to 4 months and during which about half of the children will have evidence of cardiac involvement. More serious is the polycyclic form of the disease in which continuing waves of activity keep the disease process going for many months or even a year or two. It appears as though treatment is able to suppress the activity temporarily but not to shorten the course of the disease.

Once the child has passed through an initial attack he is a candidate for a recurrence if he suffers another beta-hemolytic streptococcal infection. Studies indicate that the risk of recurrence is greatest during the first 5 years after an initial attack and that it declines rapidly thereafter. Each attack or period of prolonged rheumatic activity carries with it the threat of additional heart damage from carditis.

Prophylaxis

Once the child has been identified as a rheumatic subject it becomes very important to prevent future episodes of infection. Since recurrence will depend upon reinfection with beta-hemolytic streptococci, this objective can be attained if he is protected adequately against these organisms. It now is recognized that children with rheumatic fever may be so protected by administering a small daily dose of sulfadiazine or penicillin by mouth or by monthly injections of long-acting penicillin preparations. The administration must be continuous so that the child has a constant low level of the drug present in his tissues to protect him from the very first minimal exposure to streptococci. Many clinicians feel that such prophylactic drugs should be taken during the 5 years following the first attack.

Treatment and Nursing Care

General Considerations. In the main, the treatment of rheumatic fever is the treatment of acute rheumatic carditis, which is discussed fully in Chapter 18. Even when the child has little or no evidence of cardiac involvement during a first attack, usually he is given suppressive treatment with salicylates or hormones in the hope of warding off any important cardiac damage, and at the same time he is kept relatively inactive until it can be demonstrated that his stage of rheumatic activity has passed.

Treatment and Nursing Care of Chorea. The treatment of chorea is largely palliative and symptomatic. Neither the salicylates nor the hormones have any effect upon this aspect of rheumatic fever. As soon as the disease is recognized, the child should be confined to bed, all excitement avoided and the nutrition guarded carefully. In the milder attacks, no specific care is required. When the disease is more severe, sedative drugs are required. Prolonged warm baths often are useful as a sedative measure.

In the later stages of chorea, especially if the attack has been prolonged and if at the time the manifestations are only moderate and if all laboratory evidence of infection has disappeared, often children will do better if they are allowed out of bed and have a fair amount of liberty.

Children with chorea have uncontrolled body movements, often to the point of helplessness, but they do not feel ill. Until they can do things for themselves, everything must be done for them. Not only must all their needs be supplied by others, but also in many instances their needs must be anticipated because they have lost their ability to talk. They must be fed, and the process must be a slow and safe one because of the in-co-ordinate movements of the head, the mouth and the muscles of swallowing. If movements are severe, a fork never should be used in feeding the child with chorea.

Children with chorea need physical and emotional rest. Usually they rest best if they are in a room by themselves where protection from stimuli can be avoided. However, occasionally an isolated child will show increased restlessness and a need for the companionship of another child. Reaction to his environment should be noted and his needs supplied as the physical condition warrants.

The child's reaction to, and behavior after, parental visiting should be noted. The onset of chorea is gradual, and often the acute symptoms are preceded by symptoms of nervous instability. In this period, when the child's family is unaware of his disease, behavior changes may initiate unfortunate forms of discipline. In the period preceding the onset of choreiform movements, the child may show increasing instability by frequent quarreling with siblings, less attention to schoolwork, recurrence of tantrums and fears, or by fretfulness and willfulness which try the patience of those with whom he lives and plays. If a poor parent-child relationship develops during this period, visiting periods may have to be shortened until a good relationship has been re-established.

Special attention must be given to the skin of the elbows, the knees and other points of contact which are constantly being rubbed and chafed because of his uncontrollable movements. Massaging the skin over the joints with zinc oxide ointment and keeping the extremities covered with flannel pajamas will protect these areas from irritation. When chorea is severe, continuous nursing is desirable in order to prevent self-injury and to perform the many duties required by a helpless but mentally active child. He should be cared for in a crib bed with padded sides, and those toys which might prove injurious should be eliminated.

These children often are malnourished. Their constant movements use energy, and though their appetites are usually good, they are underweight and anemic. Frequent feedings of foods which are high in protein, calories, vitamins and iron should be provided.

Understanding the instability of the child with chorea will help the nurse to use patience, consideration and insight in all her relations with him. When chorea develops in an intelligent, sensitive child, personality changes often manifest themselves. At the onset of the disease, the child does not understand his inability to concentrate and to control the expression of his emotions. Often, too, he does not feel that his parents have responded fairly to his uncontrolled behavior. Tendencies toward introversion and introspection develop, and often it is with these personality characteristics that the nurse first sees the child.

A nurse who is poised, unhurried, thoughtful of the child's needs and sensitive to the origin of the personality traits can do much toward building up the child's confidence that perhaps was shattered when he did things that were so annoying to himself and to those in his immediate environment. Listening intently to his defective speech, reading his favorite stories, playing records that soothe and delight him, placing appropriate pictures and pots of growing

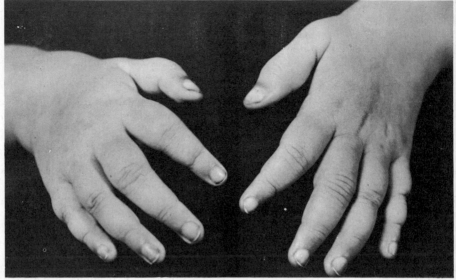

FIG. 113. Spindle-shaped swelling of finger joints characteristic of rheumatoid arthritis.

plants where he can see them, talking calmly of things that interest him—all help him to sense a genuine interest in his well-being. It is the nurse who gradually can increase the child's understanding of his parents' previous reactions to his uncontrolled behavior. She can help, too, in eliminating the parents' feeling of guilt when they realize the situation and reflect on their attitudes and behavior in the prodromal stage of the child's illness. In this way, wholesome relationships can be re-established and compensating overprotection lessened.

During convalescence, when movements are controllable, play materials appropriate to the child's needs should be provided. At first, materials that require use of the larger muscles should be provided. Then, as improvement manifests itself, materials that require fine co-ordination, such as drawing, clay modeling, sewing or airplane construction, can be presented. In this period, the child needs materials to work in order to regain skills lost during his acute illness. Feelings of self-esteem can be restored through well-directed activity programs.

RHEUMATOID ARTHRITIS

Rheumatoid arthritis is a chronic systemic disease which has as it distinguishing feature protracted and deforming inflammation of the joints. It is not very common among children but may be seen at almost any age. The onset may be with joint swelling or may be in a nonspecific fashion. Fairly high fever with splenic and generalized lymph node enlargement is common in the acute stage. The small joints of the body (Fig. 113) are attacked most regularly, but the larger joints and the spine also may be involved. In contrast with rheumatic fever, the disease has no apparent relation to streptococcal sensitization; the arthritis is not readily relieved with aspirin; the symptoms remain in the joints originally involved; the inflammation runs a protracted course and may result in permanent disability of the joint. Although the course of the disease is utlimately self-limited, the spontaneous subsidence of symptoms usually does not take place until the person has been sick for several years. During this period, joint deformity and muscle atrophy may progress to a point where complete restoration to normal cannot be expected. Occasionally, the heart is involved during the course of rheumatoid arthritis, but this is the uncommon exception rather than the expected complication that it is in rheumatic fever.

Before the steroid hormones were available for treatment, a great many measures were used in an attempt to relieve symptoms and terminate the disease. None of these measures was regularly successful. Cortisone, ACTH and compound F will suppress the manifestations of the disease, as in rheumatic fever, by controlling fever and reducing the inflammatory reaction in the joints. (Sometimes compound F is injected into the joint cavity to relieve acute inflammation.) The administration of these substances must be continued for very long periods of time, and the appearance of toxic reactions to them limits their effectiveness. However, they are tremendously superior to the older methods of treatment.

The symptomatic nursing care of rheumatoid arthritis includes shielding of joints from unexpected motion during the time they are acutely inflamed. This is achieved by the use of splints or bivalved lightweight casts which are applied at night while the child sleeps. During the acute stage of the disease the child may need to be fed, dressed and bathed by the nurse because of the restricted usefulness of his hands. For those with the severer forms of the disease there may be long periods of hospitalization during which the nurse and the occupational therapist can do much to keep the child constructively occupied, growing socially and emotionally and to maintain his morale. The importance of emotional stress as a factor in rheumatoid arthritis is recognized, and not infrequently exacerbations of the disease are related to psychic disturbance. Whether such emotional stress is the primary cause or merely a secondary product of the protracted illness is a debated question.

DISSEMINATED LUPUS ERYTHEMATOSUS

Disseminated lupus is an uncommon disorder seen mainly in adolescent and young adult females. It is a slowly progressive and usually fatal disorder, and the multitudinous symptoms depend upon a widespread abnormality of the vascular tree. Prolonged fever, recurring arthritis, pleurisy, erythematous skin eruptions upon portions of the body exposed to the sun, chronic nephritis, endocarditis and hypersplenism are some of the features that may be present clinically. Diagnosis usually is suspected from the combination of some or all of these findings in a girl. The skin eruption and a persistent leukopenia are the features which most often direct attention to the correct diagnosis. Confirmation is obtained by finding characteristic polymorphonuclear leukocytes that contain large masses of amorphous substance (L. E. cells). These cells may be found in bone-marrow preparations or in leukocytes which have been incubated with the patient's serum. The underlying disturbance is thought to be an abnormality of protein metabolism which affects nucleic acid in particular. Accumulation of the same sort of material as that seen in the typical L. E. cell takes place beneath the endocardium to create a verrucous endocarditis and beneath the endothelium of small vessels anywhere in the body, resulting in occlusion of such vessels.

Treatment with steroid hormones is temporarily effective in obtaining remission of symptoms. Unfortunately, these persons tend to become easily sensitized by sulfonamides and other substances, including the hormones.

Eventually, therapy becomes less effective or progression of the renal disease takes place, and the child succumbs to it. Nursing care is that of any protracted and ultimately fatal illness.

OTHER COLLAGEN DISEASES

Other collagen diseases which are seen very infrequently among children are dermatomyositis, scleroderma and periarteritis nodosa. The reader is referred to the bibliography for full description and discussion of these disorders which, like lupus, involve widespread changes in many tissues with a progressive and usually fatal course.

RETICULOENDOTHELIOSIS

Disease of the reticuloendothelial system may result in widespread involvement of bones, skin, lymph nodes, spleen and liver or may be confined to one or a few localized lesions in such tissues. The name *Letterer-Siwe disease* is applied to a rapidly advancing diffuse form of reticuloendotheliosis which is seen occasionally in infants and small children. A diffuse skin rash and seborrhea of the scalp often initiate the symptoms and are followed by enlargement of liver, spleen and lymph nodes with progressive wasting. Recently, some dramatic relief has been obtained through the use of ACTH and corti-

sone. Eosinophilic granuloma is a localized lesion of bone which is usually discovered incidentally in roentgenograms taken for some other purpose. Roentgen-ray irradiation therapy or surgical excision may be curative. Between these two extremes lies the Hand-Christian-Schüller syndrome. This disorder is characterized by multiple lesions of the skull and the long bones which, in its classic form, produces diabetes insipidus and protrusion of the eye. Therapy is not entirely predictable, but some improvement usually results from the use of ACTH or roentgen-ray irradiation therapy.

NEOPLASMS

Children and even infants may suffer from neoplasms of practically any of the types seen in the adult. The incidence of malignancy is very low except for leukemia, brain tumors, Wilms's tumor and neuroblastoma of the adrenal. Other varieties are rarely observed. All of the above have been discussed in previous chapters except for neuroblastoma of the adrenal.

NEUROBLASTOMA OF THE ADRENAL

This tumor affects infants or young children. It arises from sympathetic nervous system tissue, usually of the adrenal gland but sometimes from ganglia elsewhere in the body. It tends to spread quickly and widely so that recognition of its presence is often achieved

by discovery of the metastases rather than the original tumor. In addition to a local tumor in the adrenal region, enlargement of the liver or multiple metastases in the bones may be the presenting symptoms. In the latter form it can be confused with leukemia or with rheumatic fever because of the diffuse pains in the extremities. Diagnosis is accomplished by finding microscopic metastases in the bone marrow or by examination of tumor material removed at operation. Treatment consists of removal of the major tumor and treatment of the metastases by irradiation or with nitrogen mustard, ACTH or one of the antimetabolites used in leukemia. The prognosis is poor but not invariably so.

LEAD POISONING

In the adult, lead poisoning usually results in a chronic illness marked by abdominal colic and weakness due to peripheral neuritis and anemia. The infant or the young child who suffers from lead intoxication is more likely to present a medical emergency because of the rapid appearance of cerebral edema with vomiting, headache, stupor, convulsions or coma. Early recognition of the disorder is highly important, for the longer the symptoms of encephalopathy persist the more certain it is that the child will suffer irreparable damage to the brain.

ETIOLOGY

The infant or the small child may ingest or inhale lead in a variety of ways. In the past, small infants have been poisoned by lead derived from lead nipple shields or from ointments containing lead which were used on the mothers' breasts. Teething powders, drinking water which passed through lead pipes and food contaminated by paint are other sources. One of the most common mechanisms of lead poisoning is that of pica, or perverted appetite, which leads the small child to chew on any and all objects, including painted toys, furniture, household fixtures and plaster. In the course of time he consumes a significant amount of lead if these objects are coated with lead-containing paint. In the United States all children's toys and furniture must now be painted with lead-free paint by the manufacturers. However, this does not control the type of paint used by the amateur in his home. Lead also may be derived from inhaled gases such as burned storage battery casings or from the fumes of gasoline containing tetra-ethyl lead.

Lead that is taken into the body is deposited and stored in many tissues. In the bones it accumulates at the rapidly growing epiphyseal lines, where it is visible on roentgen examination. Its deposition in the brain leads to edema and signs of increased intracranial pressure. It is released slowly from the tissues when the blood level begins to fall and is excreted in the urine.

SYMPTOMS

The symptoms of lead poisoning vary with the degree of cerebral irritation that is produced. Sometimes there will be warning signs of loss of appetite, periodic unexplained vomiting, irritability, changed disposition or ataxic gait. More frequently the encephalopathy appears abruptly with persistent major convulsions which are very difficult to control and may be followed by stupor or coma. A small fraction of children suffer from a more chronic form of the disease with anemia, weakness, colic and peripheral neuritis as the chief symptoms.

DIAGNOSIS

The diagnosis is suspected from the history of lead exposure in combination with the appearance of symptoms as above. Several laboratory tests aid in its confirmation. An anemia is usually present which is associated with basophilic stippling of the red blood cells seen on the smear. There may be a mild degree of glycosuria. The spinal fluid ordinarily has an increased quantity of protein without much or any increase in the number of cells. It is under high pressure when encephalopathy is present. X-ray examination of the bones will demonstrate a band of increased density at the epiphyseal line. The width of this band gives some indication of the length of time that the lead ingestion has been in progress. Conclusive diagnosis can be reached by measuring the level of lead in the blood or the amount that is being excreted in the urine. Precautions are necessary in obtaining specimens in receptacles which are scrupulously freed of lead, for the amounts to be determined are minute, and contamination may result in a wrong interpretation.

TREATMENT AND NURSING CARE

The main problem in treatment is to get the lead out of the tissues, particularly out of the brain, and have it transported through the blood for excretion by the kidneys. To be effective this must be engineered in such a way that additional lead is not taken up by the brain during the process. In the past it was customary to give large doses of vitamin D and sodium phosphate in the hope of removing lead from the blood stream and depositing it in the growing bones. The more recent approach is to give some substance that will tie up the lead in a chemically inactive form in the blood stream while it is being transported to the kidneys for excretion. Sodium citrate has been used in this manner, and more recently BAL. A new type of chemical known as a chelating agent is now under study. This substance is called Versene or Ca E.D.T.A. (calcium ethylenediaminetetra-acetate).

In addition to such attempts to immobilize lead in the blood stream, measures must be taken to terminate or prevent the convulsions that accompany encephalopathy. The usual sedatives such as phenobarbital are less effective than under ordinary circumstances and must be used in large dosage. Magnesium sulfate given intramuscularly in the same fashion as for hypertensive encephalopathy may aid in the control of cerebral edema. Surgical measures of decompression have been tried but are usually ineffective. Once the acute phase has passed, it is desirable to shield the child from acute infections that may reactivate his disease. Months are required to complete the process of deleading the tissues and thus removing the threat of recurrence.

The specific nursing care is that of a child with convulsions from any cause. Avoidance of unnecessary handling is desirable in order to give a minimum amount of stimulation to the central nervous system. In protracted coma it may be necessary to resort to gavage feedings and the skin care that is accorded to any unconscious patient.

PROGNOSIS

In general the prognosis following lead poisoning is not very good. The mortality from acute encephalopathy even with early treatment is significantly high—around 25 per cent—and of those who survive, a high percentage will show evidence of neurologic disturbances, including mental retardation. How many of these victims were retarded children before the acute onset of encephalopathy is always hard to judge. The retarded child is more likely to be one who develops a perverted appetite for lead-coated objects, but pica certainly is not confined to the retarded group. Children who do not have acute encephalopathy, whose lead intoxication can be terminated early in its course, have a much more favorable prognosis for full recovery.

PROPHYLAXIS

Because of the generally unsatisfactory results of treatment it is most important to try to prevent lead poisoning. The approach has been made through the passage of laws which forbid the use of lead paint on articles designed for use by children and through public education calling attention to the dangers of lead intoxication and indicating the common sources from which the child obtains lead. The nurse visiting a home can do much to discover and point out to the parents such potential dangers.

BURNS

GENERAL CONSIDERATIONS

Burns are relatively frequent in childhood and when of more than slight extent are serious. The effects are general and not limited to the burned area. Between 65 and 75 per cent of the deaths occur within the first 48 hours, and in general the prognosis depends upon the extent and the depth of the burn. If as much as 20 per cent of the body surface is burned, shock is almost certain to ensue unless immediate measures are taken to prevent it. When from one third to one half of the skin surface is involved, the chances for recovery are slim.*

SYMPTOMS

Shock

The first serious effect is that of shock, the symptoms of which appear soon after the accident. These include rapid pulse rate, subnormal temperature, pallor, prostration and low blood pressure. If the child survives the shock, the symptoms disappear to a large extent within 12 hours.

Toxic State

The second serious effect is a toxic state which develops within from 1 to 2 days. It is characterized clinically by prostration, fever and a rapid pulse rate. Cyanosis, vomiting and edema may occur. The urine decreases in volume, sometimes to complete suppression. These symptoms may become pro-

* A rough means of estimating the percentage of surface involvement in the adult is to allow 9 per cent for the head, and for each of the four extremities; and 18 per cent for the anterior trunk and the remaining 18 per cent for the back. In the infant this scheme must be modified to allow about twice as much for the head and proportionately less for each of the extremities.

gressively worse and lead to coma and death. In other cases, they may continue for days or weeks. No general agreement exists as to the cause of the toxic symptoms. They may be due in part to delayed effects of the initial shock, which disturb the function of such vital organs as the kidney and the liver, in part to severe electrolyte imbalance or in part to the absorption of toxic substances from the destroyed tissue or from bacteria invading the burned area.

Problems of Convalescence

Children who are burned extensively and yet survive the early dangers of shock and toxicity face a long period of convalescence and complicated care. Attempts must be made to prevent secondary infection of the wound, to provide protection for the delicate epithelium which grows in to replace dead tissue and to prevent the formation of contracting scars and keloids during the healing stage. When the tissue destruction is deep and the gap too wide to be bridged by natural healing, skin grafts must be made to cover the defect. Many of these procedures require prolonged and arduous immobilization. Both the effects of the original burning and those of protracted convalescence interfere with nutrition by hampering the regeneration of serum proteins and red blood cells. Prolonged inactivity and discomfort are likely to interfere with the child's appetite and make it difficult for him to take in the necessary nutriments to speed his recovery. In addition to physical rehabilitation there is much to be done in maintaining his morale and helping him to accept whatever residual handicap and disfigurement he may have to bear. At all stages the management of severe burns is a complicated and difficult procedure.

TREATMENT AND NURSING CARE

Management of Shock and Toxicity

In severe burns the first consideration must be given to the prevention of shock (or the treatment, if shock has appeared already) and of the toxic state that may ensue. In some instances, local treatment of the burn will be deferred until these dangers are over. Where it is necessary to carry out a débridement early, adequate anesthesia or sedation is essential not only for humanitarian reasons but also to minimize pain which may otherwise aggravate shock.

In shock the blood volume becomes reduced, due to the passage of its fluid element, the plasma, through the walls of the blood vessels and into the tissues. The circulating blood then becomes reduced in amount, and as a consequence the circulation becomes sluggish. The normal function of vital organs may be impaired by anoxia and by slow interchange of nutrients and waste products with the blood stream. The loss of plasma in the blood results in an increased concentration of the red blood cells. This affords a simple means of measuring the severity of the shock and the effectiveness of its treatment. Either the red blood-cell count or the hematocrit of the blood may be used as a rough guide. The main element of treatment is to attempt to restore blood volume by the intravenous injection of plasma in amounts large enough to counteract the losses through the capillary walls. In addition, the patient may require oxygen to combat anoxia and sedation to relieve pain. Adequate but not excessive external heat should be applied to maintain body temperature without causing dilatation of peripheral vessels.

Once the blood volume has been supported adequately, it may be necessary to provide additional parenteral fluids such as salt solution, glucose or sodium lactate in order to maintain an adequate fluid intake, promote urine formation and counteract acidosis.

During the early care of a burned patient the nurse's activities must be concentrated upon close observation of his vital signs and the state of the peripheral circulation, in order that she may inform the doctor of changes in the child's condition. In addition, she must do what she can to make her patient comfortable and to give him encouragement and support.

Physical Hygiene

First-degree burns produce only simple erythema and require nothing more than local application of an ointment or an oily dressing to relieve pain. Unless they are extensive there is often no need for hospitalization or elaborate treatment. Burns of greater intensity and extent require careful attention.

Difference of opinion exists concerning cleansing and preparation of the burned area for the first dressing. Some advocate thorough surgical cleansing, while others maintain that no need for washing exists, and that washing should be restricted to the unburned areas. Some advocate the opening of blisters and débridement (removal of contaminated, macerated or lacerated tissue); others maintain that débridement is unnecessary and that the blebs protect the underlying tissue. Simplicity in treatment is advantageous and should be practiced to the extent compatible with the welfare of the child.

The methods of further management are multiple; the one chosen will depend on the preferences of the physician in charge. The goal in any case is the avoidance of infection and the promotion of healing. Some prefer ointment dressing exclusively (antibiotic ointment or gentian violet jelly), regardless of the location of the burn. It is generally agreed that this type of dressing is greatly to be preferred for burns of the face, the hands, the joints, the genitalia and the perineum. When used for other parts of the body, it is

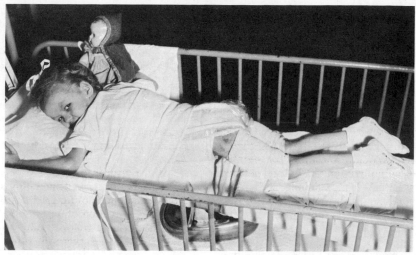

Fig. 114. Illustrating the care of a burned child on a Bradford frame. Waterproof material is used to protect from contamination the burned areas on the thighs. To collect urine specimens from an incontinent child, waterproof material should be used to construct the trough leading into the bed pan.

common custom to retain the ointment in place by a snug-fitting bandage and leave the dressing undisturbed for a period of from 5 to 10 days before changing, except that the bandage is retightened to snugness from time to time.

Other methods of managing burns include wet dressings, exposure to air and the formation of eschars by early spraying of the burned area with gentian violet, tannic acid, silver nitrate or other substances which coagulate the proteins and form a protective crust. Since skin grafting will not be successful unless a clean, uninfected granulating base can be obtained, it is desirable to try to prevent infection of the burn whenever possible. If this fails, careful bacteriologic study of the invading bacteria and their sensitivities to various antibiotic agents is indicated so that the appropriate local or general treatment can be given. Similar scrupulous care is necessary after the grafts have been placed.

Selection of the exact method of treatment must be varied to suit individual needs. Nursing care also must vary. The plan of nursing care will be influenced by the type of treatment instituted, by the location and the extent of the burned areas and by the age and the needs of the particular child. The use of a Bradford frame in extensive trunk-and-extremity burns is highly desirable (Fig. 114). Contractures can be prevented by maintaining good posture; urine specimens can be collected when the child is incontinent; and wound contamination from feces and urine can be lessened or prevented. If the head of the Bradford frame is hung higher than the foot, gravity will produce a downward flow of urine. By using 2 pieces of waterproof material, each 6 x 18 in., to form a trough leading into a bedpan placed beneath the opening of the frame, urine can be collected more easily. One piece of the material should be placed under the buttocks and over the edge of the frame, while the other should be secured over the pubes and brought down over the perineum and into the bedpan. To determine kidney function, accurate measurement of urine must be recorded.

Pressure areas can be prevented by turning these childern at 3-hour intervals and giving them skin care. When 2 beds with Bradford frames are available for a burned child, discomfort from moving can be reduced. Instead of lifting him on to a stretcher while his frame is being recovered, he can be turned and lifted directly onto a clean frame. Skin around the burned area can be kept free from irritating exudate and in good condition by frequent cleansing, massaging and application of petrolatum. When the lower extremities are burned, pressure on the heels can be prevented by supporting the thighs on small pillows to elevate the heels from the frame or the bed.

Measures to prevent foot drop are required. When the child is lying on his abdomen, a pillow placed beneath his thighs will keep his feet in good position.

Every precaution must be taken to prevent infection, which retards healing and growth of the grafts. Gown-and-mask technic should be used to prevent cross-infection, and the hands should be washed thoroughly before any care is given. Sterilized linen placed over the Bradford frame or the bed and over the dressings is an added preventive measure. When the child is young, and the burned area is irritating, arm restraints may be required to keep him from infecting the area with his hands. However, many times, snug coverings which keep the wound inaccessible can be applied. If the child is not too ill, suitable play materials will interest him and divert his attention from the skin irritation. When dressings are changed without anesthesia, a face mask should be put on the child to prevent self-contamination.

When the buttocks and the genitalia are burned, care to lessen dressing contamination and to promote healing is indicated. If enemas are necessary, waterproof materials must be used to prevent dressing contamination. After bowel evacuation, the perineum should be cleansed with cotton balls and oil, and in some instances careful irrigation of the area with warm normal saline solution will help to cleanse the fecal material completely from the burned area. When the penis and the scrotum are burned, frequent cleansing and application of dressings saturated with 1 per cent Mercurochrome reduce the incidence of infection. When the child is on his abdomen, a diaper sling under the frame opening will support the edematous organs and maintain the position of the dressing.

Maintaining a desired position is necessary to prevent contractures and to keep a grafted area at rest. When the neck is burned anteriorly, a roll under the shoulders will hyperextend it and prevent disfiguring contractures. Sandbags or specially applied restraints may be indicated for immobilization. Constant supervision is essential to readjust appliances which prevent crippling complications that require traction or plastic surgery to correct.

Nutrition

Frequent feeding of foods high in calories, protein and iron is imperative to lessen the degree of hypoproteinemia and anemia. During the early stages of the illness, loss of nitrogen is great. It is lost when it passes from the surrounding areas into the burned tissue, when it is excreted from the body by way of the urinary tract, and when exudate is formed. Frequently, poor appetite is encountered, and when protein intake is insufficient hypoproteinemia develops rapidly. In some instances amigen, a casein digest, is given orally. Through use of this material larger amounts of protein may be given than when unhydrolyzed protein alone is used. Often, vitamins B and C are given to accelerate healing and to stimulate appetite. Iron therapy is used when anemia begins to develop. Grafts do not grow well when the red blood-cell count and the hemoglobin are low.

Encouraging ingestion of fluids aids the body in eliminating toxins, maintains body-fluid requirements and prevents kidney damage when sulfonamide therapy is used to prevent or control infection. During the first few days, thirst from dehydration may be increased, and care must be taken not to give fluids too rapidly, for nausea and vomiting are produced easily. After this period, encouragement is usually necessary to keep the intake at desired levels. Accurate intake records must be kept. When intake is compared with output, the onset of kidney impairment may be detected.

Emotional Support

Long periods of immobilization, isolation from family and playmates and painful and frightening experiences involve mental attitudes that must be understood if the burned child is to receive the help he needs. The accident itself is a harrowing experience for the child. If it resulted from doing things that his parents had cautioned him not to do, or if it resulted because he did not have his mother's protection when he needed it, the trauma to his psyche may be nearly as great as the trauma to his body. The child needs reassurance and understanding to build up his tolerance for all the forthcoming experiences. A burned child requires frequent trips to the operating room for dressing changes and for grafting; the type of preparation that he receives may influence the course of his illness. If he anticipates the trips with horror and apprehension, the anxiety produced will affect his personality, his appetite and his total well-being. Evidences of regressive behavior and problems of nursing will become increasingly more evident. The nurse should discover the child's fears and give him comfort. She must help him to face his fears and to use whatever resources he has to handle them.

The child needs help in handling dreaded experiences. Children react differently to painful experiences. Some seem outwardly to accept them, yet on closer observation one sees signs of anxiety. To react to pain with shrieks is more trying to the nurse in attendance, yet it may be that child's way of reacting to pain, and it may give him far greater release than if he were to remain silent. If a nurse whom the child enjoys accompanies him to the operating room and remains to support him in ways she has found successful, trips there can be tolerated. When operating-room nurses and attendants greet the child in a friendly fashion and let him talk of the things which are of concern to him, anticipation at seeing friends there may supplant his former dread. When the ordeal is over, showing recognition of growth in the way he met the situation increases his courage and helps him to continue handling his disagreeable experiences constructively.

Unless arms and hands are burned, equipment for independent play should be provided. A folded sheet brought under the Bradford frame and pinned to the sides of the crib will form a hammock that will provide support for the child's arms and space for his toys. The use of the hammock will prevent position changes which result when a child retrieves his fallen playthings from beneath the frame.

The child will enjoy being read to and played with, and his need for companionship should be met. Placing his bed so that he may look out of the door or the window or into a ward of convalescent children will stimulate his individual activities and increase his desire to get well enough to join the group. In the convalescent period he will need the companionship of children and an environment that gives him increasingly more opportunities to prepare him for life at home.

Through conversation or observation of the parent-child relationship, feelings of guilt often will be detected in the parents. If the accident resulted from lack of protection during play or because the parents failed to teach the child or failed to remove dangerous objects from his environment, parental remorse undoubtedly will be felt. Parental feelings of guilt may be expressed verbally but more often they are expressed unconsciously as they attempt to compensate by oversolicitude. If the feelings of guilt are strong and if they adversely influence their attitudes toward the child or toward themselves the help of a social worker is indicated.

Assisting in a program of burn prevention is the responsibility of the hospital and the public-health nurse. The mortality rate due to preventable accidents that produce burns is tremendously high. Little children are social beings. They enjoy the kitchen because they are with their mothers and because there is much there to interest them. For this reason kitchens must be made safe. Preschool children should be taught caution in the use of matches and in observing bonfires. Fires are fascinating to children, and admonition will not stifle their interest in them. Instead, positive direction should be given to teach children *how* to light a match and *when* they may do it and to teach them *how* to watch a fire safely. Adults must be taught to keep inflammable materials out of children's reach and to supervise all bonfires in their neighborhood. If these measures could be instituted, the incidence of burns would be reduced markedly.

OBESITY

Obesity is the result of the ingestion and the absorption of food in excess of the body's energy needs. The need may be relatively small, and the amount of food average; or the need may be average, and the food excessive. In either case the result is the same. This generalization applies in all instances of obesity.

The amount of food energy needed by the body is determined by the amount of energy necessary for basal metabolism, growth and activity. The one component of this group subject to great variation in childhood is activity. An amount of food satisfactory for an active child would cause obesity in an inactive child of the same age. Striking illustrations are found in children confined to bed for long periods by conditions which do not impair appetite. A child who becomes obese from any cause frequently exercises decreasingly as the obesity progresses, thus increasing the disproportion between the amount of food required and that ingested.

A familial or individually inherent tendency to obesity has been assumed to exist; obesity occurs with the ingestion of average amounts of food. In such persons, the obesity is said to be from endogenous causes; that is, causes within the body such as superior utilization of food in contrast with the exogenous cause of excessive intake. Evidence for the existence of endogenous obesity is meager, and it seems likely that inactivity is the chief cause of obesity when the food intake is not excessive. The occurrence of obesity in families and in several generations may be due more to familial dietary habits of generous food intake than to inheritance of endogenous factors.

ENDOCRINE DYSFUNCTION

Despite a widespread belief to the contrary, obesity is caused by endocrine dysfunction in few, if any, instances.

The thyroid and the pituitary glands are the ones commonly held responsible for endocrine obesity. In hypofunction of either of these glands, retarded growth is a characteristic feature, whereas accelerated growth almost constantly is associated with obesity in childhood. Obese children are taller than the average for their age, and their skeletal development (bone age) is in advance of that normally expected.

Fröhlich's syndrome is frequently stated as the diagnosis in cases of obesity in childhood, especially in boys. True, Fröhlich's syndrome is a result of pituitary disease and includes retarded growth with small stature, girdle distribution of fat and retardation in sexual development. The basal metabolic rate usually is normal, although it is thought to be low for reasons discussed subsequently. The obesity is caused by inactivity or increased food intake or both. Fröhlich's syndrome is rare. The sexual infantilism of ordinary obesity is only apparent, not real. The genitalia are buried in fat; they are seen to be of normal size for the age when the fat is pushed aside. The apparent infantilism disappears at puberty.

Basal Metabolic Rate

Estimations of basal metabolic rate made in the customary manner give low values for the obese child, whereas the actual rate is *greater* than average. The weight of the child enters into the customary calculation. In the obese child a large proportion of the weight is from fat. Actually, the basal rate is in proportion to the amount of active or heat-producing tissue and is wholly unrelated to the fat of the body. The heat-producing tissues are increased above the average in the obese child, but the relative increase is not so great as that of the fat. The obese child may have from 30 to 40 per cent less heat-producing tissue than the average child in proportion to the body weight. Such a child might have a true basal rate of plus 20 per cent or more, yet have a minus value by customary calculations. Customary methods of estimation serve satisfactorily only when the body is of average proportion.

From the preceding discussion it is evident that obese children show evidence of abundant nutrition by accelerated growth; they have an increased metabolic rate; they mature earlier than average. Such findings are not compatible with concepts of endocrine causation of obesity.

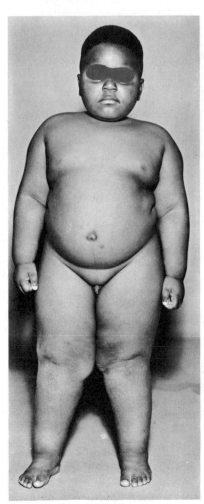

Fig. 115. Obesity.

SYMPTOMS

The symptoms associated with obesity are few. The tendency to decreased activity has been mentioned. Sometimes the posture becomes faulty in the endeavor to carry with greater ease the extra load of fat (Fig. 115). In occasional instances, ingestion of water is increased abnormally. Medical advice is most commonly sought because of the social and psychological problems that result from the child's being markedly different from his associates.

DIAGNOSIS

When an obese child comes under care, the possibility of endocrine dysfunction should be excluded. If the stature and the bone age are in excess of the average, endocrine diseases commonly held responsible for obesity are not present. The basal metabolic rate may be determined but must be interpreted with caution. In any case, the food energy intake is in excess of the need. Sometimes this excess is not obvious and is denied by the parent and the child. However, it usually is revealed by detailed observation of the child's diet. A diet may be relatively low in bulk and yet high in energy value, particularly if fruits and vegetables are present in minimum quantity. Some children obtain an excess of food between meals.

TREATMENT

In the usual case of obesity, the indications are to decrease the food intake and to increase the energy output. Energy output is increased by exercise. The type and the intensity of the exercise must be fitted to the child. For the markedly obese, attempts at violent exercise may be actually harmful, although activity may be made increasingly strenuous as the child becomes thoroughly accustomed to it. Decrease in the amount of food is much more rapidly effective in reducing weight than is increased exercise.

For the child who is young and only moderately obese, it may be satisfactory to reduce the diet only enough to maintain the weight at a fairly constant level over a prolonged period. During this period the child is growing and eventually will be of suitable weight for the height and the age. For the markedly obese, this procedure is not satisfactory because many of these children weigh more than they should were they fully grown. In such circumstances it is desirable to remove at least some of the excess fat. This objective is accomplished only by supplying food in such reduced quantity that the body fat must be burned to supply the necessary energy. When the regimen is managed carefully, a loss of from 2 to 3 pounds of body fat a week may be brought about with safety and at the same time permit increasing activity.

Even though the diet is greatly reduced in energy value, it must be "complete" at all times. Reliance is placed on the stores of body fat for some of the energy, but all other nutritional essentials must be supplied. The full requirement of protein, minerals and vitamins must be furnished, and sufficient carbohydrate must be present in order that fat may not be called on for fuel in excess of the ability of the body to burn it completely. In the beginning of a reduction regimen, it is advisable to start with a diet that is only slightly below the calculated average requirement in energy and then to make the decrease gradually until the desired rate of loss in weight is reached. Weight loss that is too rapid is undesirable and presumably harmful.

The sample diets presented are suitable for children of the ages stated. Such diets always must be adjusted to the individual child and increased or decreased according to rate of weight loss. The older child could have a glass of skimmed milk at bedtime, if he is hungry.

LOW-CALORIE DIETS FOR OBESITY

CHILD OF 6 OR 7 YEARS 1,000 CALORIES	CHILD OF 10 OR 12 YEARS 1,200 CALORIES
Breakfast	*Breakfast*
½ orange	Whole orange
1 egg	1 egg
8 ounces skimmed milk	8 ounces skimmed milk
	½ slice bread or small potato
Noon	*Noon*
2 ounces lean beef	3 ounces lean meat
½ cup vegetable	⅔ cup vegetable
Leaf of lettuce	Lettuce
Ripe peach	Ripe peach
8 ounces skimmed milk	8 ounces skimmed milk
	½ slice toast
Supper	*Supper*
Egg or meat	Egg or meat
⅓ cup vegetable	Celery
½ slice bread	⅔ cup vegetable
Fresh fruit	Fresh fruit
8 ounces skimmed milk	½ slice bread
	8 ounces skimmed milk
Evening	*Evening*
8 ounces skimmed milk	8 ounces skimmed milk
Vitamin concentrate	Vitamin concentrate

PSYCHOLOGICAL ASPECTS

Certain psychological aspects of obesity often are important for successful management. In many instances, the excessive eating that has produced the obesity is part of an emotional and compensatory mechanism in a child poorly adjusted to his environment. In such instances, relief of the maladjustment is necessary in order to obtain permanent results from treatment. Bruch's studies of obese children and their families emphasize the frequency with which the mothers are anxiously overprotective and ply the child from earliest infancy with food in place of more wholesome satisfactions. Many of the more severely obese children were found to be helplessly dependent upon their mothers and unable to make satisfactory social adjustments. In the management of obesity the attitudes of the mother are thus very important and not always clearly apparent upon superficial study.

SITUATIONS FOR FURTHER STUDY

1. How can a child become desensitized to foods that produce an allergic reaction?

2. Study a school-age child with asthma while you give him care. What is his health problem? How does he respond to it? Describe his behavior during an attack. Describe your response to his symptoms and behavior. Describe his relationship with his mother and father and with you. If he is having psychiatric therapy, what help did you get from his therapist which increased your understanding of his needs? What problems did you have in implementing his suggestions for his

care? What changes in behavior did you notice when you were able to follow the therapist's suggestions?

3. Study a preschool child with neurodermatitis in the above way.

4. What early symptoms are indicative of rheumatic fever? What are the common manifestations of rheumatic fever? How can recurrences of rheumatic fever be minimized? What does convalescent care of the child with rheumatic fever include? How is it determined?

5. What are some of the problems that you have encountered in nursing a child with rheumatic arthritis? What problems does he have? What problems did you have in giving him care?

6. Study mortality rates of burns. At what age period is the rate highest? What are some of the causes of burns in the periods of infancy, childhood and adolescence? When making home visits, how could you help a mother learn to keep her infant's environment safe? What would you teach that would prevent accidents from burns?

7. Study a child who is hospitalized with burns in a manner similar to the outline suggested at the end of Chapter 8. How did you discover he felt about his burned skin and the fact that he had not been sufficiently protected by his mother? How did the child's parents respond to him during the period of hospitalization? What changes did you note during the period you cared for the child?

BIBLIOGRAPHY

Afremow, M. L., and Odenal, Josephine: Lupus erythematosus, Am. J. Nursing 51:383, 1951.

Armistead, N. B.: Preventing deformities following severe burns, Am. J. Nursing 50:162, 1950.

Bland, E. F., and Jones, T. D.: Rheumatic fever and rheumatic heart disease; a twenty year report on 1,000 patients followed since childhood, Circulation 4:836, 1951.

Bruch, H.: Obesity in childhood, physiologic and psychologic aspects of the food intake of obese children, Am. J. Dis. Child. 59:739, 1940.

Clise, Marjorie H.: Disturbed children are disturbing children, Nursing Outlook 5:638, 1957.

Coolidge, John C.: Asthma in mother and child as a special type of intercommunication, Am. J. Orthopsychiat. 26:165, 1956.

Ennis, J. M., and Harrison, H. E.: Treatment of lead encephalopathy with BAL, J. Pediat. 5:853, 1950.

Evans, E. L., Purnell, O. J., Robinett, P. W., Batchelor, A., and Martin, M.: Fluid and electrolyte requirements in severe burns, Ann. Surg. 135:804, 1952.

Goldring, David, Behrer, M. R., and

McQuarter, Florence: Rheumatoid arthritis in children, Am. J. Nursing 56:1437, 1956.

Hench, P. S., Slocumb, C. H., Polley, H. F., and Kendall, E. C.: Effect of cortisone and pituitary adrenocorticotropic hormone (ACTH) on rheumatic diseases, J. A. M. A. 144:1327, 1950.

Herschfield, J. W.: The treatment of thermal burns, Am. J. Nursing 46: 156, 1946.

McLaughlin, J. T., Zabarenko, R. N., Diana, P. H., and Quinn, P.: Emotional reactions of rheumatoid arthritis to ACTH, Psychosomat. Med. 15: 187, 1953.

Mohr, George, Gerard, Margaret, and Ross, Helen: Summary of psychoanalytic study of asthmatic children, Psychosom. Med. Monographs 1:81, 1939-1941.

Overall, James C.: The symptomatic treatment of asthma, A. M. A. J. Dis. Child. 93:246, 1957.

Rantz, L. A.: The Prevention of Rheumatic Fever, Springfield, Ill., Thomas, 1952.

Tuft, Harold S.: The development and management of intractable asthma of

childhood, A. M. A. J. Dis. Child.
93:251, 1957.

Wallinger, Elsie: Burns and their nursing care, Am. J. Nursing **42**:1000, 1942.

Wittkower, Eric, and Russell, Brian: Emotional Factors in Skin Diseases, New York, Hoeber, 1953.

Woodhead, Barbara: The psychological aspects of allergic skin reactions in childhood, Arch. Dis. Childhood **21**: 98, 1948.

Index

Hormone(s)—(*Continued*)
  effects in newborn, 227
  estrogen. *See* Estrogen
  gonadal, influence on psychic attitudes
    and general health, 545
  gonadotropic, action in therapy, 544
    chorionic therapy, cryptorchidism,
      500-501
    influence on normal sex development,
      544-545
  growth, experimental use on animals, 544
    pituitary, repression of bone growth,
      545
  luteinizing, role of, in formation of
    corpus luteum, 545
  pituitary, 543-544
    anterior, action, 544
    posterior, deficiency, in diabetes in-
      sipidus, 553, 554
  sex, influence on bone development, 25
  therapy, side effects, 417-418
  thyrotropic, action in therapy, 544
Hospital, admitting ward, viral and rickett-
    sial infections, 574
  first built for care of women and chil-
    dren, 2
  pediatric. *See* Pediatric department or
    hospital
Hospitalization, of child, preventive mental
    health work for, 121
Hostility, in hospitalization period, play as
    therapy, 177
Humerus, fracture, during birth, 232
Hunger, 33
  in diabetes mellitus, 554, 557, 563
  infant, 55-56
Hurler's syndrome, 532-533
Hutchinson's teeth in syphilis, 632, 633
Hyaluronidase, 611
Hydroceles, in newborn, 227
Hydrocephalus, 358-363
  communicating, 359-360
  congenital, vomiting with, 286
  cry, in meningitis, tuberculous, 523
  diagnosis, 360
  etiology, 359-360
  in meningitis, tuberculous, 524
  noncommunicating, 359
  nursing care, 360-363
  separation of sutures of skull with, 25
  symptoms, 360
  from toxoplasmosis, congenital, 531
  treatment, 360
  from tumor of brain, 519
  ventriculo-ureteral shunts for lessening
    intracranial pressure, 361
Hydrocortisone, 214
  therapy, adhesions, subarachnoid, 524

Hydrocortisone, therapy—(*Continued*)
  eczema, 329
  leukemia, 447
Hydrogen peroxide, prevention of caking
    of exudate in otitis media, 383
  therapy, Vincent's infection, 457
Hydronephrosis, 287, 352
Hydrops fetalis, 229
Hydrotherapy, fever, in measles, 578
  in pneumonia, bacterial, primary, in in-
    fants, 396
  typhoid fever, 617
Hygiene, physical, in burns, 656-658
Hykinone therapy, hemorrhagic disease,
    316
Hymen, imperforate, 354
Hymenolepsis nana, 474
Hyperesthesia, in meningitis, tuberculous,
    523
Hyperglycemia, from hyperpituitarism, 544
Hyperparathyroidism, 544, 553
Hyperpituitarism, 544
Hyperpyrexia, in pneumonia, kerosene, 399
Hypersplenism, in disseminated lupus
    erythematosus, 651
Hypertension, alkalosis from, 512
  in carditis, rheumatic, acute, 417
  headache from, 537
  in nephritis, chronic, 489
  from prolonged or high-dosage adminis-
    tration of ACTH or cortisone,
    213
  in tumor of brain, 519
Hyperthermia. *See* Fever
Hyperthyroidism, 544, 552-553
Hypodermoclysis, 201-202
Hypoglycemia, in vomiting, recurrent, 462
Hypoparathyroidism, 544
Hypopituitarism, obesity from, 661
Hypoplasia, in anemia, types of, 439-441
Hypoproteinemia, in burns, 658
  in colitis, ulcerative, chronic, 469
Hypospadias, 353-354
Hypothalamus, disorders, 547, 553
Hypothermia, in serum disease, 640
Hypothyroidism, 544, 549-552, 661

Icterus index, 476
Icthyol ointment therapy, eczema, 329
Id of personality, 51
Idiocy, amaurotic familial, 532
  microcephalic, 364, 365
  Mongolian, 362-365
Ileostomy, for colitis, ulcerative, chronic,
    469
Imbecility, Mongolian, 362-365
Imitation of parents by children, socializa-
    tion period, 81, 82